PeriAnesthesia Nursing Care

A Bedside Guide for Safe Recovery

Edited by

Daphne Stannard, PhD, RN, CCRN, CCNS, FCCM
Associate Chief Nurse Researcher and
PeriAnesthesia Clinical Nurse Specialist
University of California San Francisco Medical Center
San Francisco, California

Dina A. Krenzischek, PhD, RN, MAS, CPAN, FAAN
Nurse Manager
Johns Hopkins Hospital
Baltimore, Maryland

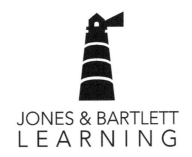

JONES & BARTLETT
LEARNING

World Headquarters
Jones & Bartlett Learning
40 Tall Pine Drive
Sudbury, MA 01776
978-443-5000
info@jblearning.com
www.jblearning.com

Jones & Bartlett Learning books and products are available through most bookstores and online booksellers. To contact Jones & Bartlett Learning directly, call 800-832-0034, fax 978-443-8000, or visit our website, www.jblearning.com.

The authors, editors, and publisher have made every effort to provide accurate information. However, they are not responsible for errors, omissions, or for any outcomes related to the use of the contents of this book and take no responsibility for the use of the products and procedures described. Treatments and side effects described in this book may not be applicable to all people; likewise, some people may require a dose or experience a side effect that is not described herein. Drugs and medical devices are discussed that may have limited availability controlled by the Food and Drug Administration (FDA) for use only in a research study or clinical trial. Research, clinical practice, and government regulations often change the accepted standard in this field. When consideration is being given to use of any drug in the clinical setting, the health care provider or reader is responsible for determining FDA status of the drug, reading the package insert, and reviewing prescribing information for the most up-to-date recommendations on dose, precautions, and contraindications, and determining the appropriate usage for the product. This is especially important in the case of drugs that are new or seldom used.

Production Credits
Publisher: Kevin Sullivan
Editorial Assistant: Rachel Shuster
Production Assistant: Sara Fowles
Marketing Manager: Meagan Norland
V.P., Manufacturing and Inventory Control: Therese Connell
Composition: Auburn Associates, Inc.
Cover Design: Scott Moden
Cover Image: © Myron Pronyshyn/Shutterstock, Inc.
Printing and Binding: Edwards Brothers Malloy
Cover Printing: Edwards Brothers Malloy

Library of Congress Cataloging-in-Publication Data
Perianesthesia nursing care : a bedside guide for safe recovery / [edited by] Daphne Stannard,
    Dina A. Krenzischek.
        p. ; cm.
    Includes bibliographical references and index.
    ISBN 978-0-7637-6998-7 (pbk.)
    1. Post anesthesia nursing. I. Stannard, Daphne. II. Krenzischek, Dina A.
    [DNLM: 1. Postanesthesia Nursing. WY 161]
    RD51.3.P47 2011
    617'.919—dc22

                                                            2010038300
6048

Printed in the United States of America
17 16 15   10 9 8 7 6 5

TABLE OF CONTENTS

INTRODUCTION

Daphne Stannard & Dina A. Krenzischek

Perianesthesia areas are specialized critical care nursing areas that range from a preoperative (preop) and postanesthesia care unit (PACU) in a free-standing surgical center to one of many large, specialized preop/PACUs in a multicampus medical center. *Peri* means "around" in Greek, and perianesthesia areas wrap themselves around the patient's anesthetic experience in order to safely care for and guide the patient and family through the entire perioperative continuum. The purposes of the perianesthesia area are twofold: to thoroughly prepare the patient, family, and healthcare team *before* the procedure or surgery, and to safely and skillfully recover the patient and care for the family *after* anesthesia and the procedure or surgery.

The vision for this book took hold following a National Conference of the American Society of PeriAnesthesia Nurses (ASPAN). The two editors were discussing the breadth and depth of nursing knowledge and skill necessary to provide excellent care to the wide variety of patients with multiple comorbidities who present for a staggering range of procedures and surgeries on a daily basis. It was at that time that we decided to edit a book designed for any nurse who is caring for the perianesthesia patient and family—be it in a PACU, an intensive care unit (ICU), a procedural recovery area, or on a labor and delivery unit. The book is divided into three sections: core concepts or foundational knowledge that is common to all perianesthesia patients, population specific knowledge, and surgery specific knowledge. While the book is not intended to be encyclopedic or all-encompassing, it is our hope that the majority of common clinical issues and concerns are addressed by our stellar group of contributing authors.

Safety is no accident and providing excellent nursing care is no coincidence. Being able to care for a critically ill phase I recovery patient with an unstable airway in one bed spot, while also caring for a phase II patient who is dressed and in a chair but worried about mobility issues once she gets home is a daily juggle for many perianesthesia nurses. Recognizing the patient and family transitions and deftly providing safe and excellent care requires compassion, specialized knowledge and skills, and exquisite clinical judgment. We hope that this book will be a review for some and an important resource for others.

This book would not be possible without the scores of people from whom we have learned. We would like to honor all of the patients and families that bravely face anesthesia and their procedure or surgery. We have learned much from you and are inspired daily by your hope, confidence, and courage. We salute the nurses who skillfully care for perianesthesia patients and their families. Perianesthesia nursing practice is challenging, sometimes frustrating, but always changing. We are honored to work alongside such amazing colleagues! There are countless administrators, clinicians, and staff who support the safe movement of the patient and family through the perioperative continuum, and while this book is not directly aimed at their practice, safe and excellent patient and family care would not occur without them in any of our settings. We would especially like to thank our contributing authors, who shared their expertise and passion for safe patient and family care, without whom this book would not be possible. Finally, we would like to thank our families: Beau and Dylan Simon and Kurt and Ryan Krenzischek. Their endless love and enthusiastic support made this work a possibility in the first instance and sustained and carried us to the final manuscript!

With love and gratitude,
Daphne and Dina

Donna Beitler, MS, RN, CGRN
Nurse Educator
Department of Medicine
The Johns Hopkins Hospital
Baltimore, MD

Renee Blanding, MD, MPH
Attending Anesthesiologist
    and Medical Director, Operating Room
The Johns Hopkins Bayview Hospital
Baltimore, MD

Joni M. Brady, MSN, RN, CAPA, CLC
Breathline Editor, American Society of
    PeriAnesthesia Nurses
International PeriAnesthesia Consultant
Alexandria, VA

Sarah Brynelson, RN, MS
PACU Educator
UCSF Medical Center
San Francisco, CA

Theresa Clifford, MSN, RN, CPAN
Interim Nurse Manager
Perioperative Services
Mercy Hospital
Portland, ME

Joann Coleman, DNP, RN, MS, ACNP, AOCN
Acute Care Nurse Practitioner
Department of Surgery Oncology
The Johns Hopkins Hospital
Baltimore, MD

Kathy Daley, RN, MSN, CCRN-CMC-CSC, CPAN
Clinical Nurse Specialist Critical Care
Charles George Veterans Administration Medical
    Center
Asheville, NC

Lisa Day, PhD, RN
Assistant Professor
School of Nursing
Duke University
Durham, NC

Kathleen DeLeskey, DNP, RN
Assistant Professor
Lawrence Memorial/Regis College Nursing
Medford, MA

Barbara Godden, MHS, RN, CPAN, CAPA
PACU Clinical Nurse Coordinator
Sky Ridge Medical Center
Lone Tree, CO

Carla Graf, MS, RN, CNS-BC
Geriatric Clinical Nurse Specialist
UCSF Medical Center
San Francisco, CA

Kathleen Gross, MSN, RN-BC, CRN

Gail Gustafson, RN, MSN, CRNP
Nurse Practitioner
Department of Surgery, Cardiology
The Johns Hopkins Hospital
Baltimore, MD

Vallire D. Hooper, PhD, RN, CPAN, FAAN
Manager, Nursing Research
Mission Memorial Hospital
Asheville, NC

Assistant Professor
College of Nursing
Georgia Health Sciences University
Augusta, GA

Erica R. Jancelewicz, RN, BSN
PACU Assistant Patient Care
Manager
UCSF Medical Center
San Francisco, CA

H. Lynn Kane, MSN, MBA, RN, CCRN
Clinical Nurse Specialist, Telemetry
Jefferson Hospital
Philadelphia, PA

Molly M. Killion, RNC-OB, MS, CNS-BC
Perinatal Clinical Nurse Specialist
UCSF Benioff Children's Hospital
San Francisco, CA

Dina A. Krenzischek, PhD, RN, MAS, CPAN, FAAN
Nurse Manager
Perianesthesia Care Units
The Johns Hopkins Hospital
Baltimore, MD

Susan Kulik, MSN, MBA, RN, ONC
Nurse Manager
Department of Surgery, Orthopedic Service
The Johns Hopkins Hospital
Baltimore, MD

Peggy Lang, RN, MSN, ACNP
Nurse Practitioner
Department of Surgery, Thoracic Surgery Service
The Johns Hopkins Hospital
Baltimore, MD

Janet Laughlin, RN, BSN, CPAN
PACU Clinical Nurse III
UCSF Medical Center
San Francisco, CA

Melissa Lee, MS, RN, CNS-BC
Medical/Surgical Clinical Nurse Specialist
UCSF Medical Center
San Francisco, CA

Ruth J. Lee, RN, MS, MB
Nurse Manager
Perianesthesia Care Units
The Johns Hopkins Bayview Hospital
Baltimore, MD

Myrna E. Mamaril, MS, RN, CPAN, CAPA, FAAN
Nurse Manager
Pediatric Same-Day Surgery, Preop, & PACU
The Johns Hopkins Hospital
Baltimore, MD

Carol Maragos, MSN, CRNP, CORLN
Nurse Practitioner
Department of Surgery, EENT Service
The Johns Hopkins Hospital
Baltimore, MD

Maureen F. McLaughlin, MS, RN, CPAN, CAPA
Clinical Educator
PostAnesthesia Care Unit
Lahey Clinic Medical Center
Burlington, MA

Christine Mudge, RN MS PNPc CNN FAAN
Transplant Pediatric Nurse Practitioner
Manager for Pediatric Transplant
Assistant Clinical Professor
University of California
San Francisco Hospital & University
San Francisco, CA

Amy D. Nichols, RN, MBA, CIC
Director
Hospital Epidemiology & Infection Control
UCSF Medical Center
San Francisco, CA

Kim Alexander Noble, PhD, RN, CPAN
Assistant Professor
School of Nursing
Widener University
Philadelphia, PA

Denise O'Brien, MSN, RN, ACNS-BC, CPAN, CAPA, FAAN
Perianesthesia Nurse Clinical Specialist
University of Michigan Hospital
Ann Arbor, MI

Jan Odom-Forren, PhD, RN, CPAN, FAAN
Assistant Professor & Perianesthesia Nursing Consultant
University of Kentucky
Lexington, KY

Chris Pasero, MS, RN-BC, FAAN
Pain Management Educator & Clinical Consultant
El Dorado Hills, CA

Hildy Schell-Chaple, RN, MS, CCNS, CCRN, FAAN
Adult Critical Care Clinical Nurse Specialist
UCSF Medical Center
San Francisco, CA

Lois Schick, MN, MBA, RN, CPAN, CAPA
Perianesthesia Nurse Consultant
Lakewood, CO

Maureen Schnur, MS, RN, CPAN
Director
PACU/Pain Clinic/Preoperative Areas
Faulkner Hospital
Boston, MA

Michele A. Shermak, MD, FACS
Associate Professor
Plastic Surgery
The Johns Hopkins School of Medicine
Baltimore, MD

Daphne Stannard, PhD, RN, CCRN, CCNS, FCCM
Associate Chief Nurse Researcher & Perianesthesia Clinical Nurse Specialist
UCSF Medical Center
San Francisco, CA

Laurel Stocks, RN, MSN, ACNP/BC, CCRN, CCNS
Nurse Practitioner
Department of Anesthesiology, Perianesthesia Care Units
The Johns Hopkins Hospital
Baltimore, MD

Susan Stritzel-Diaz, RN MSN CPNP
Transplant Pediatric Nurse Practitioner
UCSF Medical Center
San Francisco, CA

Deborah Tabulov, RN, CRNP
Nurse Practitioner
Department of Surgery, Vascular Service
The Johns Hopkins Hospital
Baltimore, MD

Candace N. Taylor, RN, BSN, CPAN
PACU Supervisor
Inservice Coordinator
Patient Safety and Security Officer
Cedar Oaks Surgery Center
Warrensburg, MO

John M. Taylor, MD
Assistant Clinical Professor
Anesthesia & Critical Care
UCSF Medical Center
San Francisco, CA

Linda Wilson, PhD, RN. CPAN, CAPA
Assistant Dean of Special Projects, Simulation, and CNE Accreditation
Drexel University
Philadelphia, PA

Pam Windle, MS, RN, NE-BC, CPAN, CAPA, FAAN
Nurse Manager
Perianesthesia Care Units
St. Luke's Hospital
Houston, TX

Susan Wolf, MPAS, MMS, PA-C
Physician Assistant
Opthalmology Department
The Johns Hopkins Hospital
Baltimore, MD

Stephen C. Yang, MD
Chief of Thoracic Surgery
The Johns Hopkins Medical Institutions
Baltimore, MD

Core Concepts

CHAPTER 1

Perianesthesia Organization and Administration

Erica R. Jancelewicz, RN, BSN & Sarah Brynelson, RN, MS

Modern perianesthesia nursing care may involve adult and pediatric phase I and phase II patients, extended care patients, and preoperative patients. Areas of the hospital in which care is provided are often blended units encompassing preoperative and postoperative areas. Therefore, the perianesthesia management team and the overriding institutional organization must be nimble and able to adapt to the rapidly changing clinical environments that characterize perianesthesia care.

1. What is the origin of the postanesthesia care unit (PACU)?

The first public demonstration of the safe use of inhaled anesthesia (in the form of ether) was in 1846 at the Massachusetts General Hospital in Boston (Vandam, 2000); and at the same hospital, a ward was established in 1873 for patients to recover from ether after surgery (Allen & Badgwell, 1996). In the 1940s, during the Second World War, the need for a recovery room was recognized after patients died of respiratory failure after surgery from administration of anesthesia (American Society of PeriAnesthesia Nurses, 2010). Recovery rooms became a specialized area to monitor patients that were physically close to the operating room (OR) and to provide a place that offered safe and competent patient care. Recovery rooms were also needed to separate ward patients from experiencing the sights and sounds of postoperative vomiting and pain from the patients recovering from anesthesia (Barone, Pablo, & Barone, 2003). Today, modern recovery rooms are called Postanesthesia Care Units (PACUs).

2. How are PACUs organized within a facility?

Many PACUs around the country are organized into a perioperative area (including all recovery areas), preoperative holding (preop), and the OR. Other hospitals consolidate the PACU with the critical care areas, and some exclude the OR from the perioperative area. Although the actual location of the care may vary from institution to institution, perianesthesia nursing care may be simply defined as all care that is provided to a patient before and after anesthesia. In contrast, perioperative nursing encompasses all nursing care received before, during, and after a procedure or surgery and comprises all three phases of care—preoperative, intraoperative, and postoperative.

Structuring the facility to include the single category of perioperative services typically means that one director will oversee the different units. This kind of organization usually leads to standardized policies, procedures, and charting methods and can foster better communication and integration between the different areas and their management teams.

3. How many PACU beds are needed?

After a review of the scientific literature, there seems to be controversy as to how many PACU beds a hospital needs to sufficiently service the ORs, and there is no clear consensus on a definition of an ideal PACU layout. After comparing the varied studies that considered the PACU bed to OR ratio, the national average ranges from 1.5:1 to 2:1 (Marcon, Kharraja, Smolski, Luquett, & Viale, 2003).

This range, however, only factors in OR suites and, depending on the facility, more PACU beds may be needed to accommodate the non-OR anesthesia (NORA) cases that require monitored recovery and specialized staff.

4. What is the recommended PACU management structure?

There is little in the literature to support one PACU management team structure over another; however, some principles should guide whatever structure is chosen in any given facility. Although titles vary greatly across the country, there is typically a nurse manager or patient care manager that covers the PACU. The patient care manager may cover a variety of perioperative areas, including preoperative and postoperative or procedural areas, and/or adult or pediatric areas. Patient care managers should be visible to staff to establish trust and to foster regular communication between staff and the management team. Managers may have assistant nurse managers, and if so, this role may be more "frontline" than the patient care manager. Assistant nurse managers may still function as charge nurses, be counted into staffing on certain days, or provide break relief as necessary in addition to their administrative duties. The PACU needs a flexible staffing plan to accommodate patients when they are ready to arrive from the OR, and the assistant manager(s) may be a critical component in providing this flexibility and in enabling the unit to accommodate patients during peak times.

The patient care manager should foster a shared decision-making model to enable a horizontal power structure. In this complex setting, with differing patient populations and variable care needs, establishing a trusting and communicative environment is essential. In a shared decision-making environment, staff nurses are empowered to be active participants in many types of unit decisions, including policies, work-related rules and guidelines, and practice issues. Shared decision making can be facilitated through unit-level committees that focus on different topics, including quality, patient and family care, education, research, and recognition and retention, among others. These committees can be the driving force behind unit-level decisions, assuming the manager allows and encourages this from staff members. With shared decision making, the staff nurse will feel heard, respected by management, and will embrace unit changes more readily (Robertson-Malt & Chapman, 2008).

5. What are the other important leadership roles?

A perianesthesia clinical nurse specialist (CNS) is a treasured resource in perioperative areas. The CNS may function in a full-time or part-time position, may cover multiple units, and may have several managers with whom he or she collaborates. The perianesthesia CNS has multiple roles or domains of practice, including that of clinical expert, educator, researcher, consultant, and liaison (Glover, Newkirk, Cole, Walker & Nader, 2006). As perioperative nurses are required to care for an increasingly wide range of patient types and acuities, the CNS plays a critical role in developing the necessary education, policies, and procedures to support their practice. In addition, the CNS plays a vital role as a liaison between the perianesthesia units and the OR, as well as the surgical units and ICUs. Finally, perianesthesia CNSs also provide a critical link to enhancing communication and collaboration between medical and nursing staff.

The perianesthesia educator role is also advantageous for any facility. The educator is a mentor for staff, working with them side by side to engage them in learning, helping them grow in areas of weakness, and empowering them to become clinical mentors for other staff. The perianesthesia educator may coordinate with the CNS, if available, to facilitate staff education, develop and maintain competencies, and develop and revise new hire orientation programs. The unit educator should spend ample time in direct patient care, alongside the staff members, to assess their educational needs and plan accordingly with classes and/or in-services. In conjunction with the educator and CNS, a perianesthesia patient care manager may also have an assistant patient care manager as part of the administrative team. Hereafter, the term administrative team will be used to refer to the individuals that comprise the perianesthesia nurse management team.

6. What is the role of a charge nurse?

Charge nurses are designated unit leaders, given the authority to "run" a unit for the duration of their shift. Charge nurse responsibilities vary by facility, but, in general, the charge nurse is responsible for ensuring patient flow through the unit by making safe patient–nurse assignments. This is accomplished through communication with procedural or operating areas, hospital bed placement areas, and through regular communication with their supervisors. In addition, the charge nurse may be responsible for coordinating break relief, changes or transfers in patient assignments, and daily unit "chores." Some charge nurses may also be responsible for providing patient care; however, depending on the pace of the unit, patient acuity, and scope of the role, it may be unsafe for patient care and at cross purposes with the overall function of the position to have the charge nurse focusing on patient care in addition to coordinating an entire unit. The charge nurse role is a dynamic position in perianesthesia areas; the constant changes in patient volume, acuity, and in staffing needs requires unique skills that should be mentored by the administrative team and other seasoned charge nurses.

7. How many charge nurses are needed?

Some perianesthesia areas may require more than one charge nurse per day. The preoperative and postoperative areas may each need charge nurses, and if there are separate units for different patient populations, charge nurses may be necessary for each unit to ensure safe patient care and coordination of resources. If the unit has a variety of shifts, or is open all night, there may be more than one charge nurse per day in any given area for different shift coverage. In bigger and busier perianesthesia areas with larger caseloads, having charge nurses that overlap on staggered shifts may be helpful for break relief, assisting staff with difficult patient assignments, and in maintaining unit flow.

8. Should the charge nurse group be limited in size?

Having a small and limited group of charge nurses may provide more reliable leadership on the unit with more consistent practices. There are few studies about the benefits of a smaller, core group of charge nurses versus a larger, more open-ended group of charge nurses. In one facility where a core group of charge nurses was utilized and studied in a nonperioperative setting, the charge nurses evaluated their own leadership skills more highly after becoming core charge nurses. In addition, some of the unit issues related to pharmacy, supplies, information technology, and patient complaints improved, and the job satisfaction scores among the charge nurses improved (Krugman & Smith, 2003).

The disadvantage to a core group of charge nurses may be the limitation this may create for the rest of the staff. Limiting the charge nurse opportunity and responsibility to a small few could be a disincentive for staff members who feel ready to take on this type of leadership but are not given the opportunity. If the core charge nurse model is utilized, the administrative team should monitor the core group members for stress and burnout, because performing this role frequently over time may be overwhelming to some. Additionally, it is important to offer other leadership and professional development opportunities to nurses who are not in the core group (as well as for the charge nurses), and career ladders are one way to foster professional growth and expanded responsibility.

9. What are the American Society of PeriAnesthesia Nurses (ASPAN) standards for staffing ratios in the PACU?

ASPAN standards for staffing ratios state that "[t]wo registered nurses, one of whom is an RN [registered nurse] competent in Phase I postanesthesia nursing, are in the same unit where the patient is receiving Phase I level of care" (American Society of Perianesthesia Nurses, 2008, p. 59). The standards also differentiate between which patients should receive 1:1 or 2:1 nurse-to-patient ratios. ASPAN staffing guidelines were developed in consideration of evidenced-based research, professional opinion, and consensus. Recent evidence suggests that not only must the ASPAN standards factor into staffing guidelines, but the administrative team must also take into account patient acuity, nursing experience and competence, patient complexity, and hours worked (Mamaril, Sullivan, Clifford, Newhouse, & Windle, 2007). It is complicated and challenging to recognize the value of PACU nursing work and "difficult to qualify or quantify the intricate work of providing life-supporting care for recovering the vulnerable anesthetized patient in a fast-paced critical care environment" (Mamaril et al., 2007, p. 394).

10. How do PACU nurses provide safe and competent care to anesthetized patients during the off-hours?

This question seems to be a recurring theme across the country in many PACUs. A high percentage of nurses work some form of off-hour call in their institution, and they consistently encounter situations that are not experienced during a regular work day (Poole, 1996). Regardless of time of day, it is important for facilities to follow the ASPAN *Standards for Perianesthesia Nursing Practice,* as they were written to ensure safe patient care. The standards are updated every 2 years to reflect changing practice and the science that supports the practice.

11. How do PACUs staff for overnight patients?

Patients may spend a night in the PACU at hospitals that provide operations to patients who do not have a room reservation before surgery. Additionally, patients who were previously scheduled to be discharged home from the hospital may be kept longer or may remain in the PACU if surgeons require that specific patients can only be admitted to specific floors. Overnight patients are becoming increasingly more commonplace in many PACUs and hospitals across the country. To meet the inadequate bed situation, some hospitals require floor nurses or ICU (intensive care unit) nurses to "float" to the PACU to provide care to an overnight patient who is recovered (and has met PACU discharge criteria), but who is awaiting a bed. This practice still provides the procedure-specific care that the patient would have received on their indicated floor if the bed would have been available, and does not require the PACU to meet the staffing needs of these recovered patients.

12. How do PACUs deal with delays in patients being admitted from the OR?

The PACU may be unable to admit patients for many reasons; for instance, there may not be enough PACU nurses or bed spaces; patients may be waiting for transport to other units or departments; patients may not be fully recovered from anesthesia; and patients may be waiting for floor, stepdown, or ICU beds. When this happens, the PACU cannot continue to accommodate the flow of the OR schedule, and patients may need to be recovered from anesthesia in the OR under the care of the anesthesia providers. This bottleneck problem leads to dissatisfaction among the physicians, nurses, ancillary staff, as well as patients and their families (Mamaril, 2001). The PACU administrative team may need to make adjustments to the unit to accommodate these delays. Some adjustments include:

- Adjusting PACU nurse schedules each month based on anticipated needs,
- Adjusting PACU nurse schedules the day before but after reviewing the next day's OR schedule,
- Adjusting the staffing schedule the day of surgery,
- Changing the sequencing of the OR schedule to reduce possible PACU admission delays,
- Decreasing the PACU patient length of stay by reducing delays, or
- Redirecting certain patient populations to be recovered elsewhere (Dexter et al., 2005).

While PACU nurses are required to think about safe care for their patients, a patient care manager must listen to the nurses when staffing issues arise and must think critically about taking care of his or her staff (Iacono, 2006).

13. What does it mean to "flex" staff?

PACUs across the country all experience downtime at some point in a given day, and there is much evidence to support the fact that downtime or nonproductive use of staff can be a problem for a PACU budget. A PACU cannot run effectively without enough nurses to cover the patient recoveries or with too many nurses and not enough patients. "Flexing" of staff means being able to look at the unit as a whole and stagger nurses appropriately in order to accommodate changes in PACU arrivals and discharges. Many patient care managers will study the OR caseload the day before and set up a plan for nurses who may voluntarily go home early; they will look at union contracts and/or staffing policies to decide how and when to send nurses home.

14. How do PACUs ensure an adequate skill mix of nurses for all shifts?

Many PACUs require varied or staggered nursing schedules to accommodate the daily OR cases. The PACU administrative team must be aware of the budgetary constraints and the efficiency of the unit. The multiple shifts should be staffed by nurses with varied skills. For example, it is never advisable to place all new or inexperienced hires on the same shift, but rather, it is more prudent to ensure that nurses across the skill-acquisition continuum comprise the staffing for any given shift. Blending skill mix helps to ensure that quality and safe patient care is delivered consistently across all days of the week and all hours that a unit is open. It also creates opportunities for new hires and less experienced staff to learn from the more seasoned staff.

15. Are perioperative assistants needed in the PACU?

Although the title varies from facility to facility, unlicensed personnel or patient care assistants (PCAs) are commonly employed in many hospitals. Either providing direct patient care or care that is more supportive in nature, PCAs perform countless tasks and multiple and indispensable duties. The advantage to having a PCA in the PACU is the potential for reduced PACU turnover time and the creation of a skilled employee that is a combination of a patient transporter and a patient care assistant (Speers & Ziolkowski, 1998). Some hospitals train PCAs to work in the OR and

PACU, whereas other PACUs may share their PCAs with different parts of the hospital, and still other PACUs have dedicated PCA staff.

16. How do PACUs ensure competent nursing staff?

Evaluating nurses' clinical skills, clinical reasoning, and problem-solving abilities should be a continual process in every facility to maintain safe and quality patient care (Burns, 2009). Each facility has its own requirements for annual competency evaluation; this may be addressed through a centralized mechanism that provides annual review days and online modules, or annual competencies may be evaluated at the divisional or unit level.

Hospital-wide competencies may be insufficient for perianesthesia nurses given the specialization of perianesthesia areas. Deciding which skills require a competency is the first step. Then, it is important to determine which competencies need regular or annual review and how the review will be accomplished. In some cases, regulatory and accrediting bodies provide guidance and stipulate which skills require an annual review. But in other cases, the frequency of review may depend on the unit and facility resources, as well as the acuity of the patient population. Low-volume and high-risk clinical skills and reasoning should be reviewed more regularly than high-volume, low-risk clinical skills. Low-volume items need consistent review to maintain a basic level of competency so that if a particular patient need or a device is seen infrequently, the nursing staff is still prepared to competently manage the care when it does arise. In perianesthesia areas where the patient population is vast, there may be several clinical skills that are high risk and low volume and even some that are high risk and high volume. Unit-specific competency completion should be tracked by the perianesthesia educator or administrative team, and made available for charge nurses when they are making patient assignments. A competency grid placed in a charge nurse reference binder can be useful, so that when a particular type of patient that requires a certain competency is expected in the PACU, the charge nurse has a quick reference as to which nurses are competent to care for that type of patient.

In addition to unit-specific competencies, PACUs should require basic life support (BLS) and advanced cardiac life support (ACLS) certification. If the scope of service includes pediatric patients, pediatric advanced life support (PALS) certification should also be maintained by the nursing staff. These certifications assure a unit-wide and standardized competency for patient emergency response.

Perianesthesia nurses can maintain competency through continuing education, specialty certification, BLS, ACLS, and PALS certification. In addition, the department should identify unique clinical skills required for providing safe, quality patient care, and assure competency in these areas through regular review and evaluation of every nurse. Competency review should be mandatory, nonpunitive, and continuous (Burns, 2009). Staff nurses can work together with the administrative team to develop and implement these competency reviews to create a successful program.

17. What does Magnet designation mean and why does it matter?

Magnet designation was developed by the American Nurses Credentialing Center (ANCC) (American Nurses Credentialing Center, 2010) to recognize healthcare organizations that promote nursing excellence. Nurses in Magnet facilities report more support from frontline management, more job satisfaction, and better relationships with other nurses than in facilities without the Magnet designation (Ulrich, Buerhaus, Donelan, Norman, & Dittus, 2007).

18. What are the components of Magnet recognition?

The Magnet Model has five components: (1) transformational leadership; (2) structural empowerment; (3) exemplary professional practice; (4) new knowledge, innovation, and improvements; and (5) empirical quality results. These components encompass the 14 Foundational Forces of Magnetism. Of the 14 forces, the most relevant for management are Force 1 (Quality of Nursing Leadership), Force 3 (Management Style), Force 4 (Personnel Policies and Programs), Force 8 (Consultation and Resources), and Force 9 (Autonomy) (American Nurses Credentialing Center, 2008). These aspects of Magnet are directly influenced by the administrative team.

19. How can the administrative team support the Magnet designation quest or sustain it?

Administrative teams can support Magnet designation through frontline interaction on their given units. In Magnet hospitals, nurses describe several aspects of work-life that are directly influenced by management, including support for education, autonomy, nurse–manager support, and adequate staffing (Kramer, Schmalenberg, & Maguire, 2004). The administrative team can provide paid time off for education, foster-shared decision making, be visible on the unit, and assess and reassess staffing needs to support quality patient care.

20. What is the difference between CPAN and CAPA certification?

The certified postanesthesia nurse (CPAN) and certified ambulatory perianesthesia nurse (CAPA) certifications were developed when surgical, preanesthesia, and postanesthesia patient care moved from the inpatient hospital setting to outpatient clinics or centers (Niebuhr & Muenzen, 2001). CPAN certification examinations were first offered by the American Board of Perianesthesia Nursing Certification (ABPANC) in 1986, and the CAPA certification examination was first offered in 1994. The current versions of these exams were developed after an extensive study conducted by ABPANC in 1999 and 2000. This role delineation study (RDS) was conducted to determine patient needs and nursing knowledge necessary to care for these needs in both ambulatory and inpatient perianesthesia settings. The results of the 1999–2000 RDS determined that patient care needs were the same in ambulatory and inpatient settings, but that they varied in amount of nursing time spent meeting these needs (Niebuhr & Muenzen, 2001). In 2005 and 2006, another RDS was conducted and the examinations were updated. Since 2007, based on the most recent RDS results, the CPAN exam places greater emphasis on behavioral/cognitive and safety patient needs, and the CAPA exam has more emphasis on advocacy needs (Niebuhr & Muenzen, 2008). Both exams include four areas of patient need, physiologic, behavioral, cognitive, and advocacy (American Board of Perianesthesia Nursing Certification, 2009).

21. Who is eligible for CPAN and CAPA certification?

The current requirement to be eligible for either certification is a US registered nursing license and 1800 hours of direct patient care in a perianesthesia setting within the prior 2 years. Nurses that were certified before this requirement and that did not meet it are still eligible for recertification. Nurses may choose to take either exam; however, nurses caring mostly for phase I postanesthesia patients will find the CPAN exam more relevant to their practice, and nurses spending the majority of their time caring for preanesthesia, phase II, and extended care patients will find the CAPA exam more relevant for their practice. Nurses may choose which certification to pursue if they meet the requirements, and may also obtain both certifications (CPAN and CAPA).

22. Why should management support specialty certification?

Specialty nursing certification is an objective measurement of nursing knowledge in a specific area of nursing, and has many benefits for patients, nurses, managers, and the facility. Postanesthesia patients are a vulnerable population and specialty nursing knowledge and skill should be encouraged for the benefit of safe and effective patient care. Additional benefits of specialty certification for nursing staff include an increased sense of professionalism, empowerment, personal satisfaction, and autonomy (Niebuhr & Biel, 2007; Wynd, 2003). Certification is also beneficial for hospitals pursuing Magnet status, as the total number of certified nurses is one element in the Magnet application.

23. How can the management support specialty certification?

The biggest barriers to certification include the cost of taking the exam, lack of rewards, and lack of support (Niebuhr & Biel, 2007). The administrative team can eliminate these barriers and promote specialty certification through financial, award-based, and logistical support.

Financial incentives for staff certification include paying for continuing education hours for certification preparation classes, paying for the certification examination itself, and providing a salary differential for certification once it is achieved.

The administrative team can also support specialty nursing certification by recognizing the certification achievement on a unit level, departmental level, or facility-wide level. Certified employees' names can be engraved onto plaques that are placed in prominent public spaces and nurse achievements, such as certification, should be announced in staff meetings and newsletters. If allowed by the institution, nurses may want their certification listed next to their name on their identification badge.

Logistical support may be provided through coordination of review courses and study sessions by the unit educator or members of the administrative team. Staff should be given access to certification preparation books by having them available for checkout from the unit or facility library.

REFERENCES

Allen, A., & Badgwell, J. M. (1996). The post anesthesia care unit: Unique contribution, unique risk. *Journal of Perianesthesia Nursing*, *11*(4), 248–258.

American Board of Perianesthesia Nursing Certification. (2009). *Determining which exam to take*. Retrieved from http://www.cpancapa.org/certification-difference.html

American Nurses Credentialing Center. (2008). *A new model for ANCC's magnet recognition program* [Brochure]. Retrieved from http://www.nursecredentialing.org/Documents/Magnet/NewModelBrochure.aspx

American Nurses Credentialing Center. (2010). *Magnet program overview*. Retrieved from http://www.nursecredentialing.org/Magnet/ProgramOverview.aspx

American Society of PeriAnesthesia Nurses. (2010). *ASPAN history*. Retrieved from http://www.aspan.org/AboutUs/History/tabid/3146/Default.aspx

American Society of PeriAnesthesia Nurses. (2010). Perianesthesia nursing standards and practice recommendations: 2010–2012. (pp. 59–61). Cherry Hill, NJ: Author.

Barone, C. P., Pablo, C. S., & Barone, G. W. (2003). A history of the PACU. *Journal of Perianesthesia Nursing, 18*(4), 237–241.

Burns, B. (2009). Continuing competency, what's ahead? *The Journal of Perinatal and Neonatal Nursing, 23*(3), 218–227.

Dexter, F., Epstein, R. H., Marcon, E., & de Matta, R. (2005). Strategies to reduce delays in admission into a postanesthesia care unit from operating rooms. *Journal of Perianesthesia Nursing, 20*(2), 92–102.

Glover, D. E., Newkirk, L. E., Cole, L. M., Walker, T. J., & Nader, K. C. (2006). Perioperative clinical nurse specialist role delineation: A systematic review. *Association of Perioperative Registered Nurses Journal, 84*(6), 1017–1029.

Iacono, M. V. (2006). Perianesthesia staffing . . . thinking beyond numbers. *Journal of Perianesthesia Nursing, 21*(5), 346–352.

Kramer, M., Schmalenberg, C., & Maguire, P. (2004). Essentials of a magnetic work environment: Part 3. *Nursing, 2004, 34*(8), 44–47.

Krugman, M., & Smith, V. (2003). Charge nurse leadership development and education. *Journal of Nursing Administration, 33*(5), 284–292.

Mamaril, M. E. (2001). The official ASPAN position: ICU overflow patients in the PACU. *Journal of Perianesthesia Nursing, 16*(4), 274–277.

Mamaril, M. E., Sullivan, E., Clifford T. L., Newhouse R., & Windle, P. E. (2007). Safe staffing for the post anesthesia care unit: Weighing the evidence and identifying the gaps. *Journal of Perianesthesia Nursing, 22*(6), 393–399.

Marcon, E., Kharraja, S., Smolski, N., Luquett, B., and Viale, J. P. (2003). Determining the number of beds in the postanesthesia care unit: A computer simulation flow approach. *Anesthesia & Analgesia, 96,* 1415–1423.

Niebhur, B. S. & Biel, M. (2007). The value of specialty nursing certification. *Nursing Outlook, 55*(4), 176–181.

Niebuhr, B. S., & Muenzen, P. (2001). A study of perianesthesia nursing practice: The foundation for newly revised CPAN and CAPA certification examinations. *Journal of Perianesthesia Nursing, 16*(3), 163–173.

Niebuhr, B. S., & Muenzen, P. (2008). *ABPANC'S 2005–2006 role delineation study: The foundation for the CPAN® and CAPA® certification examinations*. Retrieved from http://www.cpancapa.org/pdf/RDSWhitePapertoBN9-29-08.pdf

Poole, E. L. (1996). Working alone: Can it be done? *Journal of Perianesthesia Nursing, 11*(6), 399–401.

Robertson-Malt, S., & Chapman, Y. (2008). Finding the right direction: The importance of open communication in a governance model of nurse management. *Contemporary Nurse, 29*(1), 60–66.

Speers, A. T., & Ziolkowski, L. (1998). Perioperative assistants are a new resource. *Association of perioperative Registered Nurses Journal, 67*(2), 420–427.

Ulrich, B. T., Buerhaus, P. I., Donelan, K., Norman, L., & Dittus, R. (2007). Magnet status and registered nurse views of the work environment and nursing as a career. *Journal of Nursing Administration, 37*(5), 212–220.

Vandam, L. (2000). History of anesthetic practice (pp. 1–11). In R. Miller (Ed.), *Anesthesia*. Philadelphia: Churchill Livingstone.

Wynd, C. A. (2003). Current factors contributing to professionalism in nursing. *Journal of Professional Nursing, 19*(5), 251–261.

CHAPTER 2

Preanesthesia Care and Preparation of the Patient and Family

Candace N. Taylor, RN, BSN, CPAN

Preanesthesia care begins when the patient is scheduled for surgery. It is the perianesthesia nurse's responsibility to provide care for each patient while maintaining compliance with regulatory and professional agencies. It is the intent of this chapter to outline the concepts of perianesthesia nursing in the preanesthesia setting. The concept is to include the patient and his or her family in the preoperative setting, as well as collaborating with the surgeon, anesthesia provider, and surgical staff.

PREOPERATIVE ASSESSMENT

1. What is the history of the preoperative assessment/nursing specialty?

Historically, patients have been assessed by the anesthesia provider the day of or the day before surgery. If significant comorbidities were identified, this often resulted in the delay or cancellation of surgery. This late delay is stressful to the patient, as well as frustrating to the surgeon and perioperative staff. According to Anderson and Hames (2009), the use of nurse-led preadmission testing clinics enable staff to manage any comorbidities, thereby increasing patient satisfaction, ensuring safe quality patient care, and decreasing the number of cancellations.

2. Are there advantages to having dedicated preoperative/postanesthesia care unit nurses versus operating room nurses conducting the preoperative assessment?

Whereas the preoperative/postanesthesia care unit (PACU) nurse understands the science of the

perianesthesia experience, the operating room (OR) nurse understands the science of the intraoperative experience. Both perianesthesia and intraoperative perspectives gives nurses the ability to communicate different aspects of the surgical experience to patients and their families. No matter which department oversees the preoperative assessment screening, the policies and procedures should be under the direction of the anesthesia department.

3. What are the goals of the preoperative assessment?

According to the Institute for Clinical Systems Improvement (2008), the goals of the preoperative assessment include decreased morbidity and mortality due to surgery, elimination of canceled or delayed surgical procedures, reduction of unnecessary diagnostic testing, and appropriate management of patients' comorbidities. The preoperative assessment, whether for a minor noninvasive or major surgical procedure, is important for the preparation of the patient—both physically and psychologically. Preparing a patient preoperatively will result in better surgical outcomes.

4. What information should the preoperative assessment include?

The preoperative assessment should include a history and physical examination that includes the patient's surgical and anesthesia background. The patient should be assessed for any family history of anesthetic complications such as malignant hyperthermia (MH). Also included should be a review of the complete medication list, which includes allergies and use of prescription and nonprescription medications, herbal and dietary supplements, history of tobacco use, history of alcohol or illicit drug use, and any medical conditions. Patients should be questioned regarding dentures, loose teeth, caps, or crowns. Height and weight should be noted for the calculation of anesthetics. To ensure cultural sensitivity, patients should be assessed for cultural beliefs (Anderson & Hames, 2008). Safety needs should be assessed to include any sensory limitations, the cognitive ability of patient and caregiver, the home use of noninvasive positive pressure ventilation (i.e., continuous positive airway pressure device or CPAP), and psychosocial family status (American Society of PeriAnesthesia Nurses [ASPAN], 2010).

5. How might the above information change the plan of care for the patient?

The above information helps with the development of the plan of care for the patient. The results of the preanesthesia assessment will help the involved nurses better care for the patient and family, and will also enable the anesthesia provider to determine premedications needed, the type of anesthesia required for the procedure, and as well as any potential risks for that patient.

6. What is the American Society of Anesthesiologists' classification?

The American Society of Anesthesiologists (ASA) uses a classification system to describe the overall physical status of a patient. This classification system correlates with patient outcomes. The classifications are labeled 1 through 5 with a class 6 added for organ donation. For any class, an E is added to identify an emergency procedure (see Table 2-1).

7. When should preoperative laboratory tests such as ECG or chest x-rays be ordered?

Since evidence shows that routine tests rarely change the plan of care for a surgical patient, routine preoperative laboratory testing is not recommended. All testing should be related to patient history and symptoms (see Table 2-2). Policies and procedures should be in place in all facilities to determine preoperative and preprocedure laboratory testing (Anderson & Hames, 2008).

TABLE 2-1. ASA physical status classification

Classification	Description
ASA-1	Healthy
ASA-2	Mild systemic disease with no function limitations. Examples: hypertension, diabetes mellitus, chronic bronchitis, morbid obesity, extreme ages
ASA-3	Severe systemic disease with functional limitations. Examples: poorly controlled hypertension, diabetes mellitus with vascular complications, angina pectoris, previous myocardial infarction, pulmonary disease that limits activity
ASA-4	Severe systemic disease with a constant threat to life. Examples: congestive heart failure, unstable angina pectoris, advanced pulmonary, renal or hepatic dysfunction
ASA-5	Patient is not expected to survive without the operation. Examples: ruptured abdominal aneurysm, pulmonary embolus, head injury with increased intracranial pressure
ASA-6	Declared brain dead, organs are removed for donor purposes.
Emergency Operation (E)	Emergency operation is required. Example: healthy 39-year-old woman who requires dilatation and curettage for moderate but persistent vaginal bleeding (ASA-1E)

Modified from Anderson and Hames, 2008.

TABLE 2-2. Recommended preoperative testing

ECG	Cardiac and circulatory disease, respiratory disease (should be within 6 months of planned procedure)
Chest x-ray	Chronic lung disease, history of congestive heart failure (should be within 6 months of planned procedure)
Pulmonary function tests	Reactive airway disease, chronic lung disease, restrictive lung disease
Hgb/Hct	Anemia, bleeding disorder (should be done within 1 month of procedure)
Coagulation studies	Bleeding disorders, liver dysfunction, anticoagulants therapy (should be no more than 1 week prior to procedure)
Serum chemistry	Endocrine disorders, medications, renal disease
Pregnancy test	Uncertain pregnancy history, history suggestive of current pregnancy (should be done according to facility policy)

Modified from Swank "Preanesthesia Evaluation" in Duke, 2006.

8. Should pregnancy testing be included with preoperative laboratory testing?

Controversy surrounding the patient's right to privacy and choice makes testing for pregnancy a delicate subject in many surgical centers. Preoperative pregnancy testing should be done according to the facility's policies and procedures.

9. When should a patient begin smoking cessation prior to surgery?

Smoking increases postoperative risk of pulmonary complications, wound dehiscence, wound infections, and delayed healing. There is also an increased risk for perianesthesia respiratory and cardiac complications for the smoking patient. When and for how long cessation of smoking should occur is debatable, but all cessation improves patient risk. It is acceptable to strongly encourage complete smoking cessation to the patient, while educating him or her on the risks of smoking related to the procedure planned. Recommended time of cessation ranges from 12 hours to several weeks preoperatively with complete cessation being optimal.

PREOPERATIVE INSTRUCTIONS

10. What are the fasting recommendations?

Historically, fasting recommendations mandated that the patient should have nothing by mouth (NPO) after midnight prior to the day of surgery. This recommendation was based on the premise that minimizing gastric contents would decrease the patient's risk for pulmonary aspiration during induction. Since gastric emptying differs for solid food and liquids, the recommendation for fasting is now differentiated (see Table 2-3). These recommendations are based on healthy patients undergoing elective surgery and do not guarantee gastric emptying (Dotson, Wiener-Kronish, & Ajayi, 2007).

TABLE 2-3. Fasting recommendations for reducing pulmonary aspiration risk

Ingested material	Minimum fasting period
Clear liquids (water, pulp-free juice, carbonated beverages, clear tea, black coffee)	2 hours
Nonclear liquids (breast milk, Jell-O)	4 hours
Infant formula	6 hours
Nonhuman milk	6 hours
Light meal (dry toast, crackers, clear liquids)	6 hours
Normal meal (fried or fatty foods, meat)	8 hours

Modified from Dotson, Wiener-Kronish, and Ajayi, 2007.

11. Which medications should a patient take on the morning of surgery?

With the new recommendations for fasting prior to surgery, it is acceptable to have the patient take their medications with a sip of water (up to 150 ml) within the hour leading up to administration of anesthesia (Dotson et al., 2007). This recommendation should be part of the preoperative teaching and approved by the anesthesia department at the facility.

12. Which medications or herbs should be held prior to surgery and for how long?

Holding medications is at the discretion of the surgeon and anesthesia provider. It is typically recommended to hold thrombolytic medications 5–10 days prior to the day of the procedure. Because of differing medical conditions, the amount of time that this medication can be held should be approved by the patient's primary care provider and/or cardiologist.

Many patients are now utilizing complimentary medications. All herbal supplements have different side effects and are recommended to be held at individual increments ranging from 24 hours to 2 weeks prior to the day of surgery (Goodwin & Dierenfield, 2010).

PREPARING THE PATIENT THE DAY OF SURGERY

13. What should the patient expect on the day of surgery?

The patient should expect that his or her preoperative assessment and any relevant medical conditions will be reviewed. Current pain and comfort will be assessed, as well as any relevant preoperative emotional, safety, and psychosocial needs. The patient's identification and expected procedure will be identified. Any presurgical preparation will be performed and administered (e.g., bowel prep, hair removal, appropriate skin scrub, among others). Any procedural teaching and discharge planning will be discussed to ensure that the patient and family are knowledgeable for aftercare. The patient should be prepared to have someone drive him or her home and stay for the first 24 hours postoperatively. Since there is an expectation of having a responsible adult at home with the patient for the first 24 hours postoperatively, the family should be included during procedural teaching and discharge planning (ASPAN, 2008).

14. What information should be included in discharge instructions?

It has been found that preoperative patient teaching decreases patient anxiety and postoperative

pain, reduces length of stay, and increases patient satisfaction. Discharge instructions should relate to the procedure being performed and the type of anesthesia being administered. When performing patient education, the nurse should speak clearly, avoiding the use of medical jargon, and include active listening. Instructions should include verbal as well as written instructions to ensure understanding and knowledge retention (Joanna Briggs Institute, 2000). When discharge instructions are given during the preanesthesia assessment, they should include the expected length of stay at the facility (i.e., day surgery vs inpatient stay).

Prior to discharge, the patient and caregiver should be knowledgeable about the care of the patient at home. Instructions related to anesthesia include dietary restrictions related to postoperative nausea and vomiting (PONV), activity restrictions related to the prolonged sedative effects of anesthesia, and any potential complications. Discharge instructions related to the surgery should include any dietary restrictions, activity limitations (e.g., when to return to work, resume exercise among other things), what type and how long the patient might experience pain, follow-up therapy/visits, and when the patient should contact the physician (e.g., fever, pain not relieved by pain medication, drainage from incision). The patient should also be given instructions on incision care.

If the facility performs a postoperative phone call, the patient should be notified prior to discharge. A form can be filled out by the patient giving the facility permission to call, as well as the preferred phone number and contact names.

15. Who is responsible for informed consent?

Informed consent is a process whereby the patient is made fully aware of the procedure being performed, the risks and benefits, side effects, and alternative treatments. The patient should have all questions answered. This process gives the patient the opportunity to be involved in his or her care. The responsibility for providing informed consent lies with the surgeon for the procedure and the anesthesia provider for the anesthesia. As the patient advocate, the preanesthesia nurse and the intraoperative nurse should review the consent and verify with the patient the procedure being performed (Hamlin & Davies, 2008).

16. How do the The Joint Commission regulations on time-out/hands-free report affect the preoperative area?

Patient safety begins when the patient's procedure or surgery is scheduled and continues throughout the perianesthesia process. According to The Joint Commission (TJC) *National Patient Safety Goals* (2010), safety can be enhanced through proper identification of the patient, appropriate procedures, and ensuring the correct site of the procedure. This can be accomplished through hands-free report at the bedside with the patient, as well as with time-out prior to incision with all caregivers involved. When a facility implements a protocol that promotes teamwork, the patient and all involved staff are empowered to protect and promote patient safety.

PATIENTS WITH SPECIAL NEEDS

17. What are some special considerations for the patient with renal failure?

Patients with end-stage renal failure are unable to eliminate waste products and maintain fluid and electrolyte balance. Special considerations should include careful intake and output with possible fluid restriction and the use of 0.9% normal saline or 5% dextrose in 0.45% normal saline IV solutions to decrease the risk of acidosis that can occur when using lactated ringers IV solution. The preanesthesia nurse should obtain a weight, determine the date of the last dialysis, assess renal function and electrolytes (potassium, blood urea nitrogen (BUN), serum creatinine, and urinalysis), avoid the use of the arteriovenous arm for blood pressures or venipunctures, and avoid nephrotoxic drugs. Renal failure patients are at increased risk for infection, electrolyte imbalance, and fluid retention (Schick, 2010).

18. Should there be special instructions for the diabetic patient?

Patients with diabetes should be assessed for average home glucose levels via finger sticks, diet followed, and diabetic medications used (including the route, dose, and schedule.) The current preoperative glucose goal for insulin-dependent patients is less than 200 mg/dL. A diabetic patient plan should be implemented at the facility to safely care for all diabetic patients. When caring for patients on insulin pumps, the nurse needs to follow facility protocols and consider consultation with the patient's endocrinologist. Patients should be instructed to handle any symptomatic hypoglycemia the morning of surgery (Power & Ostrow, 2008).

19. How do you prepare for a patient in precautions or isolation?

The nurse should determine why the patient has precautions or is in isolation and be prepared for the related disease process. Isolation is the process

used for patients that need special precautions related to an infectious disease. It is also used for patients that may need protection from bacteria or viruses, such as patients with neutropenia. Understanding the three elements needed for the transmission of disease is the nurse's first line of defense in preparing for the patient in isolation. These three elements are: a source of infection, a susceptible host with a portal for entry, and a mode of transmission. Nurses should never underestimate the power of good hand washing to eliminate the mode of transmission (Siegel et al., 2007).

20. What are the Surgical Care Improvement Project guidelines related to prewarming patients for surgery?

The Surgical Care Improvement Project (SCIP) is a national quality partnership of organizations that are focused on the improvement of surgical care and reduction of surgical complications. The goal of SCIP is to reduce by 25% the incidence of surgical complications nationally by 2010. The theory behind prewarming patients is that hypothermia increases the risk for surgical site infections (SSIs). The SCIP Infection 10 guidelines direct providers to decrease hypothermia as a way to decrease SSIs. Hypothermia reduces tissue oxygen tension by vasoconstriction, reduces leukocyte superoxide production, and increases bleeding and blood transfusion requirements. All of these factors have been shown to be statistically significant in causing greater SSI risk. This guideline calls for "at least one body temperature equal to or greater than 96.8°F (36°C) recorded within the 30 minutes immediately prior to or the 15 minutes immediately after anesthesia end time" (Centers for Medicare and Medicaid Services, 2009). Given the emphasis on normothermia in the immediate postoperative phase, it is prudent to prewarm select patients in the preoperative area.

REFERENCES

American Society of Perianesthesia Nurses. (2010). Perianesthesia nursing standards and practice recommendations: 2010–2012. Cherry Hill, NJ: Author.

Anderson, L., & Hames, P. (2008). Preadmission and preoperative patient care. In L. Hamlin, M. Richardson-Tench, & M. Davies (Eds.), *Perioperative nursing: An introductory text*. Chatswood, NSW: Elsevier Australia.

Centers for Medicare and Medicaid Services. (2009). *Fact sheet: Medicare adds quality measures for reporting by acute care hospitals for inpatients stay in FY 2010*. Retrieved from www.cms.hhs.gov

Dotson, R., Wiener-Kronish, J. P., & Ajayi, T. (2007). Preoperative evaluation and medication. In R. K.

Stoelting & R. D. Miller (Eds.), *Basics of anesthesia* (pp. 157–177). Philadelphia: Elsevier.

Duke, J. (Ed). (2006). *Anesthesia secrets* (3rd ed.). Philadelphia: Elsevier.

Goodwin, S., & Dierenfield, J. (2010). Complementary therapies. In L. Schick & P. Windle (Eds.), *Perianesthesia nursing core curriculum: Preprocedure, phase I and phase II PACU nursing*. St. Louis, MO: Saunders Elsevier.

Hamlin, L., & Davies, M. (2009). Medicolegal aspects of perioperative nursing practice. In L. Hamlin, M. Richardson-Tench, & M. Davies (Eds.), *Perioperative nursing: An introductory text*. Chatswood, NSW: Elsevier Australia.

Institute for Clinical Systems Improvement. (2008, July). *Preoperative evaluation*. Retrieved from http://www .guideline.gov/summary/summary.aspx?ss=15&doc_ id=12973&string=6682

Joanna Briggs Institute. (2000). Knowledge retention from pre-operative patient information. In *Best practices: Evidence based practice information sheets for health professionals, 4*(6), 1329–1874. Retrieved from http://www.joannabriggs.net.au

Power, M., & Ostrow, C. L. (2008). Preoperative diabetes management protocol for adult outpatients. *Journal of Perianesthesia Nursing, 23*(6), 371–378.

Schick, L. (2010). Preexisting medical conditions. In L. Schick & P. Windle (Eds.), *Perianesthesia nursing core curriculum: Preprocedure, phase I and phase II PACU nursing*. St. Louis, MO: Saunders Elsevier.

Seigel, J. D., Rhinehart, E., Jackson, M., Chiarello, L., and the Healthcare Infection Control Practices Advisory Committee. (2007). *2007 Guideline for isolation precautions: Preventing transmission of infectious agents in healthcare setting*. Retrieved from http://www .cdc.gov/ncidod/dhqp/pdf/isolation2007.pdf

The Joint Commission. (2010). *National patient safety goals*. Retrieved from http://www.jointcommission.org

CHAPTER 3

Phase I and Phase II Recovery

Theresa Clifford, MSN, RN, CPAN

As early as 1751 at the Newcastle Infirmary in Newcastle, England, rooms were reserved for patients who had undergone major surgery or who were critically ill. Over 100 years later, Florence Nightingale prepared separate rooms for patients who were experiencing the immediate effects of anesthesia. By the 20th century, there were records of recovery rooms at Boston City Hospital in Massachusetts, Johns Hopkins Hospital in Maryland, Cook County Hospital in Illinois, and New Britain General Hospital in Connecticut (Barone, Pablo, & Barone, 2003).

By the late 1940s, the value of dedicated recovery rooms was gaining acceptance. An anesthesia study commission of the Philadelphia County Medical Society reported that postoperative nursing care could have eliminated nearly one third of preventable postsurgical deaths during an 11-year period (Ruth, Haugen, & Grove, 1947).

1. How has the scope of perianesthesia services evolved?

The scope of perianesthesia services has expanded over the years in a number of ways. Advances in technology have allowed for more complex procedures to be done on an outpatient basis. Advances in the development of anesthesia medications have allowed for more rapid induction and less recovery time. In addition, there has been a vast increase in the volume of diagnostic procedures being done using a range of anesthesia techniques requiring close postprocedure monitoring.

PHASE I LEVEL OF CARE

2. How is phase I recovery defined?

Phase I is the level of care in which close monitoring is required and basic life-sustaining needs are of the highest priority (American Society of PeriAnesthesia Nurses [ASPAN], 2010). During this phase of care, perianesthesia nurses conduct assessments, interventions, and monitoring to maintain airway patency, hemodynamic stability, pain management, fluid management, and other aspects of patient care. The primary goal is to facilitate the transition of the patient from this level of care to phase II level of care, an inpatient setting, or to an intensive care setting for continued care.

3. What are the admission assessment recommendations for phase I level of care?

There are multiple and concurrent assessments that occur upon admission to the phase I level of care (ASPAN, 2010). A transfer of care report is delivered by the transferring provider. This report may include, but is not limited to, information regarding preoperative history, type and length of anesthesia, medications administered, type of procedure, relevant fluid status, and any actual or potential complications. The actual physical assessment of the patient includes vital signs, pain level, neurologic and neurovascular status, sensory motor status, integumentary and wound status, fluid status, and assessments specific to the actual procedure.

4. What are the most common patient care priorities during phase I level of care?

The first priority for patient care in phase I level of care is the establishment and maintenance of a stable airway with adequate ventilatory support. Determination of hemodynamic stability and the initiation of any interventions to support cardiovascular function is also a priority. Another clinical priority in phase I is the provision of adequate pain and comfort measures and the evaluation of the effectiveness of any pharmacologic or nonpharmacologic interventions. An additional main concern is related to the actual impact of the surgical procedure and assessment of wound integrity.

5. What are some common potential complications during phase I level of care?

Complications associated with phase I level of care include airway compromise, cardiovascular depression, pain, nausea, vomiting, delirium, and maintenance of normothermia.

6. How long does phase I last?

Determining when the patient is ready to move from one phase of perianesthesia care to the next is best determined by assessing the wide variety of reactions and responses to the administration of anesthesia, as well as the reactions and responses to the surgical/procedural experience. In addition to the individuality of patients, there are a number of factors that impact the overall readiness to move (Clifford, 2009). These may include variables such as practitioner preference in anesthetic choices, the need for preoperative anxiolytics, a history of prolonged emergence, and the presence of preexisting medical conditions. The decision to move a patient from one level of care to the next should be based on clinical assessments and desired patient outcomes and criteria. The ASPAN Standards for Perianesthesia Nursing Practice provide comprehensive lists of assessment criteria that can be used for discharge from phase I and phase II (ASPAN, 2010).

7. What are the discharge assessment recommendations for phase I level of care?

Patients are generally assessed prior to discharge from phase I level of care to determine the following: adequacy of airway and ventilatory status, cardiac and hemodynamic stability, normothermia, managed pain and comfort, integrity of surgical wound and dressings, and fluid balances.

8. What are the staffing recommendations for phase I level of care?

According to the ASPAN Standards for Perianesthesia Nursing Practice, it is recommended that two registered nurses, one of whom is a nurse competent in phase I level of care, should be in the same unit where a patient is receiving phase I level of care (ASPAN, 2010). In general, one nurse can provide care to two patients who are described as follows: one unconscious, stable, without artificial airway, and over the age of 8 years and one conscious, stable, and free of complications, or two conscious, stable, and free of complications or two conscious, stable, 8 years of age and under, with family or competent support staff present (ASPAN, 2010). A patient–nurse ratio of one to one occurs at the time of admission until the patient is thoroughly assessed and determined to be stable, or if the patient has an unstable airway, or if the patient is 8 years of age and under and unconscious. The most seriously ill patients, those that are critically ill and unstable, require two nurses for safe care.

9. What are equipment recommendations for phase I level of care?

Each patient care area where phase I care is provided should have, but is not limited to, the following equipment: general stock supplies for patient care, including dressings; supplies for emergency and preemptive bedside response, including oxygen delivery devices, airways, and suction; equipment for measuring vital signs and cardiovascular monitoring; stock medications and intravenous fluids; patient warming devices; adequately stocked age-specific emergency carts; and personal protective equipment (ASPAN, 2010).

PHASE II LEVEL OF CARE

10. How is phase II recovery defined?

Phase II is the level of care in which clinical care and strategic planning are aimed at preparing the patient for return home or for transition to extended care for further observation.

11. What is the difference between phase I and phase II?

Phase I describes the level of care provided when a patient is emerging from surgical, diagnostic, or interventional procedures requiring the administration of general or regional anesthesia or moderate sedation. The primary goals of nursing care during phase I include the establishment and maintenance of a stable airway; hemodynamic stability, including blood pressure and heart rate; fluid resuscitation; pain management; nausea and vomiting management; normothermia management; and assessment for wound integrity and bleeding. "Constant vigilance is required during this phase" (Clifford, 2009, p. 409–410).

Phase II describes the level of care provided when the patient is being prepared for discharge to home or an extended care environment. In this phase, the patient has a stable airway with good ventilatory status on room air (unless baseline status requires supplemental oxygen at home), satisfactory pain management (as defined by the patient), satisfactory control of postoperative nausea and vomiting, appropriate ambulatory ability for procedure and baseline, among other things (Clifford, 2009).

12. What are the admission assessment recommendations for phase II level of care?

Upon transfer to phase II level of care, a transfer of care report is delivered by the transferring provider. This report may include, but is not limited to, information regarding preoperative history; type and length of anesthesia; medications administered by anesthesia providers; and, during phase I level of care, type of procedure, relevant fluid status, and any actual or potential complications. The actual physical assessment of the patient includes vital signs, pain level, neurologic and neurovascular status, sensory motor status, integumentary and wound status, fluid status, and assessments specific to the actual procedure.

13. What are the most common patient care priorities during phase II level of care?

The focus of care during phase II is preparation of the patient for returning home or for transitioning to extended care for further observation. Adequate patient knowledge for continued care at home requires thorough patient/family teaching and documentation of learning regarding discharge instructions.

14. What are some common potential complications during phase II level of care?

Common issues requiring interventions during phase II level of care include pain and nausea. Prolonged drowsiness may also occur, as well as a persistent sore throat.

15. What are the discharge assessment recommendations for phase II level of care?

Patients are generally assessed prior to discharge from phase I level of care to determine the

following: adequacy of pain and comfort interventions, hemodynamic stability, integrity of surgical wounds and dressings, safe transportation from the facility, and knowledge of discharge instructions.

16. How is "safe transportation" defined?

It is possible that, despite meeting the criteria for being discharged home, ambulatory surgery patients may experience varying degrees of sedation and psychomotor impairment following anesthesia. State regulatory agencies, accrediting organizations, and professional medical and nursing associations suggest that ambulatory surgery patients have a responsible person accompany him or her home and stay overnight. A responsible adult can function to ensure that the patient is transported home safely and the patient can be assisted should minor issues related to pain or vomiting arise.

17. What are the staffing recommendations for phase II level of care?

According to the ASPAN Standards for Perianesthesia Nursing Practice, two competent personnel, one of whom is a registered nurse competent in phase II level of care, are in the same unit where a patient is receiving phase II level of care (ASPAN, 2010). In general, one nurse can provide care to three patients who are described as follows: over 8 years of age, or under 8 years of age with family present. A patient–nurse ratio of one nurse to two patients is possible when one patient is 8 years of age and under without family or support staff present and during initial admission of the patient postprocedure. If any patient should become unstable and require transfer to a higher level of care, the staffing should allow for one nurse to care for one patient.

18. What are equipment recommendations for phase II level of care?

Each patient care area where phase II care is provided should have, but is not limited to, the following equipment: general stock supplies for patient care including dressings; supplies for emergency and preemptive bedside response, including oxygen delivery devices, airways, and suction; equipment for measuring vital signs; stock medications and intravenous fluids; patient warming devices; adequately stocked age-specific emergency carts; and personal protective equipment (ASPAN, 2010). In addition, the unit should have adequate supplies for transferring the patient from the unit.

19. What does the term "blended unit" mean?

A "blended unit" is a unit that cares for patients who are preparing for surgery (preoperative phase), recovering from surgery (phase I and/or phase II), and/or who have recovered from surgery and are waiting for an inpatient bed. As a result of the expanding scope of services provided by postanesthesia care units, patients arriving in postanesthesia care units are no longer the traditional postsurgical patient. It is not uncommon to find patients in various stages of recovery from various levels of anesthetics administered for the purpose of interventional or diagnostic radiologic procedures, from sedation provided for endoscopic or colonoscopic exams, or for postprocedural monitoring.

REFERENCES

American Society of Perianesthesia Nurses. (2010). Perianesthesia nursing Standards and practice recommendations: 2010–2012. Cherry Hill, NJ: Author.

Barone, C. P., Pablo, C. S., & Barone, G. W. (2003). A history of the PACU. *Journal of PeriAnesthesia Nursing, 18*(4), 237–241.

Clifford, T. (2009). Practice corner. *Journal of PeriAnesthesia Nursing, 24*(6), 409–410.

Ruth, H., Haugen, F., & Grove, D. D. (1947). Anesthesia study commission. *Journal of the American Medical Association, 135*(14), 881–884.

CHAPTER 4

Airway Issues

Barbara Godden, MHS, RN, CPAN, CAPA

Airway management is the core of postanesthesia nursing. The care is back to basics with the ABCs. There is a saying among PACU (postanesthesia care unit) nurses that "if you don't have A, don't worry about B and C." This is the essence of what perianesthesia nurses do, and it is critical to understand airway concepts and management and be competent in this important aspect of our practice. The patient requires constant nurse presence and observation while awakening from anesthesia and until the patient has a stable and secure airway.

1. What are the significant anatomical and physiological components of the respiratory system?

The airway system consists of the nose, pharynx, larynx, trachea, bronchial trees, the lungs, and the diaphragm.

- Nose: The nose is where the air comes in, is filtered, and humidified. The nose is lined with cilia, which allow secretions to be moved in or out of the pharynx.
- Pharynx: The pharynx consists of the back of the nasal and oral cavity. The pharynx includes the nasopharynx, the oropharynx, and the laryngopharynx, and is often referred to as the upper airway.
- Larynx: The larynx connects the upper and lower airways and consists of ligaments and muscles along the cervical vertebrae. It is cylinder-shaped in adults. The vocal cords, thyroid cartilage (or Adam's apple), the cricoid cartilage, cricothyroid membrane, epiglottis,

and the glottis are part of the larynx. The vocal cords consist of the false vocal cords (or the supraglottis) and the true vocal cords. The space between the true vocal cords is the glottis. The muscles of the larynx are important to swallowing, respiration, and vocalization.

- Trachea: The trachea is a long tube that connects the larynx to the bronchi. The trachea is surrounded by 16 to 20 cartilaginous rings, which prevent collapse of the trachea, and is lined with cilia, which facilitate movement of secretions and foreign substances. The carina is at the lower end of the trachea and is the bifurcation point for the right and left bronchi. The carina is an important landmark for endotracheal intubation. The endotracheal tube (ETT) in the adult should be at the proximal point of the carina.
- Lungs and Bronchial Trees: At the distal end of the trachea, or carina, is the bronchial tree. The bronchi bifurcate into the left and right bronchial trees. The left bronchus veers off the trachea at a 40° angle for males and at a 50° angle for females. The right bronchus veers off the trachea at a 20° angle for both males and females. When intubating a patient, because of the straighter angle on the right side, it is easier to misplace the ETT down the right bronchus. When breath sounds are absent on the left side, the ETT down the right main stem is the most likely cause. In this situation, the ETT needs to be pulled back in order to facilitate ventilation in

both lungs. The right lung is also more at risk for aspiration because of the straighter angle of the bronchus. The right and left bronchi further bifurcate into smaller bronchioles, at the end of which are the alveolar ducts and the alveoli. The alveoli are the primary gas exchange units of the lung. This is where oxygen enters the blood and carbon dioxide is removed. The right lung has three lobes: the right upper lobe, the right middle lobe, and the right lower lobe. The left lung has two lobes: the left upper lobe and the left lower lobe. The lungs are contained in the visceral pleura, a thin membranous sac. The parietal pleura line the chest wall. Viscous fluid lines the area between these two membranes.

- Diaphragm: The diaphragm is a dome-shaped muscle that separates the thoracic and abdominal cavities. This is the major muscle of inspiration. The phrenic nerve innervates the diaphragm (Drain & Odom-Forren, 2009; Schick & Windle, 2010).

2. How does the anatomy of the pediatric airway differ from that of the adult?

Important differences in the pediatric airway:

- Airway is smaller and shorter than in adults.
- Tongue is larger than in adults.
- Larynx is higher/more toward the head and is funnel-shaped.
- Epiglottis is long, floppy, and narrowed.
- Vocal cords are attached more anterior and lower than in adults.
- Narrowest part of the airway is at the cricoid cartilage because of the funnel shape.
- Airway edema in an infant or child creates a greater amount of airway resistance than in adults because of the smaller diameter and the greater percentage of edema in relationship to the overall diameter (American Heart Association, 2006).

3. What are the critical physiologic concepts of the respiratory system?

The physiology of the respiratory system is complex. Some critical concepts are:

- Lung capacity and mechanical function of the lungs: Lungs are at their greatest capacity with inspiration. The lungs have elastic recoil, which means that they will spring back into their smallest position after being stretched through inspiration. Expiration is passive.

- Pulmonary circulation: Takes unoxygenated blood back to the lungs for oxygenation, which takes place at the alveolar membrane.
- The nervous system controls much of the respiratory system, including the respiratory center in the brain, central peripheral chemoreceptors, and the autonomic nervous system. These systems control the inspiration and expiration phases of respiration.
- Mechanics of gas exchange include ventilation, diffusion, and perfusion.

4. What is oxygenation?

Oxygenation is the process of oxygen combining with hemoglobin. It refers to how well the body is using oxygen.

5. What is ventilation?

Ventilation is the mechanical movement of gases in and out of the lungs, between the alveoli and the atmosphere.

6. What are respirations?

Respirations are the exchange of oxygen and carbon dioxide between the body's cells during cellular metabolism. Respiratory rate is actually a ventilatory rate.

7. What is hypoxia?

Hypoxia is a deficiency of oxygen at the cellular level in the tissues.

8. What is hypoxemia?

Hypoxemia is a deficiency of oxygen in the arterial blood.

9. What is hypercarbia?

Hypercarbia is elevated carbon dioxide levels in the blood, or respiratory acidosis. The easiest way to decrease carbon dioxide is to have the patient breathe deeply to increase ventilation and oxygenation. Hypercarbia is also called hypercapnia (Anderson, 1998).

10. What is the stir-up regimen?

The stir-up regimen involves using verbiage, coughing, deep breathing, and mobilization to help a patient awaken from anesthesia. Gentle statements to the patient regarding where they are and what time it is help in assimilating the patient to the present. Regular deep breathing in through the nose and out through the mouth as well as coughing also hasten the elimination of anesthesia. Adequate pain management, gentle encouragement to the patient to move, and raising the head of the bed all help to arouse the patient and are part of the stir-up regimen. The stir-up regimen is an important part of postanesthesia care to help prevent complications, including atelectasis and venous stasis (Drain & Odom-Forren, 2009).

11. When do you use heated oxygen as opposed to cool mist?

Heated oxygen is useful for hypothermic patients, those with upper airway inflammation, and to liquefy thick pulmonary secretions. A heated collar can be applied to many different types of oxygen delivery devices (see Table 4-1). Cool mist is helpful for patients who have had a nasal or oral procedure. Cooling soothes the area of the procedure and provides comfort.

12. When do you use albuterol as opposed to racemic epinephrine?

Albuterol is a bronchodilator and is useful for patients who are exhibiting signs of reversible obstructive airway disease. These patients may sound congested or have course breath sounds (see Table 4-2), and an albuterol nebulizer treatment often clears the bronchial passageways and allows for better oxygenation and ventilation.

Racemic epinephrine is also used for bronchospasms, but often these bronchospasms are of a more acute nature and may include hypersensitivity reactions and anaphylaxis. The patient may have difficulty breathing due to the type of surgery or edema from intubation or from the surgery itself. Racemic epinephrine may be given along with dexamethasone for the treatment of swelling and edema.

13. How do I administer a nebulizer treatment?

To administer a nebulizer treatment, obtain a small volume jet nebulizer. Get the ordered medication from the medication-dispensing machine. Pour the medicine into the reservoir and connect it to an oxygen source. Depending on the medication, one may need to dilute it with sterile normal saline. Position the patient in Fowler's or semi-Fowler's position. Give the patient the mouthpiece (or face mask if the patient is unable to hold the mouthpiece) and have the patient breathe slowly and regularly. The oxygen flow rate for a nebulizer treatment should be at least 6 to 8 L/min. If the patient is ventilated, a nebulized treatment can also be administered through the ventilator circuit.

14. What assessments are necessary when a patient arrives in the PACU?

- Inspect the chest.
- Note rise and fall of the chest wall.
- Assess chest for depth of respirations, paradoxical movement, and symmetry of respirations.
- Note any nasal flaring, tracheal deviation, or chest deformities.
- Note use of accessory muscles.
- Note any cough.

TABLE 4-1. Common oxygen delivery devices

Delivery method	Oxygen levels	Flow rate	Comments
Nasal cannula	24–44%	1–6 L/min	Causes nasal irritation if greater than 6 L/min
Simple face mask	40–60%	5–10 L/min	Need at least 5 L to prevent buildup of CO_2
Face tent/Mist mask	70%	8–10 L/min	Useful if extra humidity is needed
Venturi mask	24–55%	2–14 L/min	
Non-rebreather (NRB)	80–100%	10–15 L/min	Need increased flow rate to prevent buildup of CO_2 and prevent collapse of bag on inspiration
T-Piece/Blowby	21–100%	2–10 L/min	Helpful for weaning from ventilator
Trach collar	28–98%	>8 L/min	
Mechanical ventilator	21–100%	Per ventilator settings	All adjustable settings

TABLE 4-2. Breath sounds

Breath sound	Descriptors
Clear	Breathing with no extraneous noises. Air movement is regular and without great effort.
Course	Noisy breath sounds.
Bronchial sounds	Normal high-pitched sounds heard over the trachea and bronchi. Expiration is equal to inspiration. If heard in the lungs, this usually indicates consolidation.
Bronchovesicular sounds	Normal sounds over the bronchial tubes and the alveoli. Muffled quality; medium pitched. Inspiratory phase is equal to expiratory phase.
Vesicular sounds	Low-pitched sounds normally heard in the periphery of the lungs. Inspiratory phase is greater than expiratory phase.
Rhonchi	Abnormal sounds, indicating obstruction. Described as continuous rumbling, more pronounced on expiration. Usually clear with coughing.
Crackles	Abnormal breath sounds heard on inspiration. Characterized by discontinuous bubbling noises. Fine crackles have a crackling or popping sound caused by air entering the distal bronchioles or alveoli. These sounds are heard in congestive heart failure and pneumonia. Course crackles originate in the larger bronchi and have a lower pitch. Crackles (previously called rales) generally do not clear with coughing.
Wheezes	Abnormal breath sounds. Can be high pitched or low pitched. Musical quality. Caused by a high velocity flow of air through a narrow passageway. Can be heard during inspiration or expiration. Can be the result of a bronchospasm, obstruction, inflammation, asthma or chronic bronchitis, or a bronchogenic lesion.
Rubs	Grating sound of inflamed pleural membranes heard at the end of inspiration.
Voice sounds	Amplified sounds of the voice heard through the chest. May indicate areas of density or atelectasis.

- Listen to respirations without a stethoscope.
- Auscultate breath sounds in all lobes (see Table 4-3) (American Society of PeriAnesthesia Nurses, 2010).

15. What is SpO_2?

SpO_2 is a noninvasive measurement of arterial oxygen saturation. It is also called pulse oximetry. The sensors in the probe emit wavelengths of light that are selectively absorbed by oxyhemoglobin and reduced hemoglobin.

16. What factors influence the accuracy of measuring SpO_2 or pulse oximetry?

- Incorrect fit of the pulse oximeter probe
- Dark fingernail polish
- Hypothermia
- Hypotension
- Vasoconstriction
- Anemia
- Carboxyhemoglobinemia
- Motion and light artifact

Pulse oximetry measurements strongly correlate with the oxygen dissociation curve, but should not be the only indicator to evaluate ventilatory effectiveness. Other assessments, including assessment of the color of lips and nail beds and restlessness should be used to evaluate a patient's ventilation and oxygenation. Restlessness and disorientation are often classic signs of hypoventilation (Drain & Odom-Forren, 2009).

17. What is the oxygen dissociation curve?

The oxygen dissociation curve is a grid with oxygen saturation (SpO_2) on the left of the grid, and arterial oxygen (PaO_2) on the bottom of the curve. The key concept is that, with an SpO_2 of 90–100%, the patient has a correlating PaO_2 of

80–100%. Once the patient's SpO_2 drops to below 90%, the curve quickly decreases and the PaO_2 quickly decreases as well. The decrease is even more dramatic after the patient's pulse oximetry reading falls below 80%. In this case, the deterioration of the PaO_2 drops quickly to 50% and below.

Other factors that influence the curve are pH, temperature, and carbon dioxide pressure, which, when abnormal, can shift the curve to the right or to the left. Events that shift the curve to the left (such as acidosis and hyperthermia) affect tissue oxygenation because oxygen is more tightly bound to the hemoglobin and PaO_2 must decrease to a lower than normal level before oxygen is released from hemoglobin and is available to tissues. Events that shift the curve to the right (such as alkalosis and hypothermia) facilitate tissue oxygenation by permitting larger amounts of oxygen to dissociate from hemoglobin in the tissues (Drain & Odom-Forren, 2009; Schick & Windle, 2010; Stillwell, 2002).

18. When is a chin lift necessary?

- Decreased ventilation or air movement in and out of the lungs.

- Decreased oxygenation as evidenced by pulse oximetry. If a patient is using supplemental oxygen, saturations should be 98–100% unless the patient has underlying lung disease. If a patient has an oxygen delivery device in place, and oxygen saturations are in the low 90s, a chin lift will be necessary.

- Snoring is a sign of partial obstruction and requires a chin lift if the patient is still unconscious. If the patient is conscious, frequent deep breathing should be encouraged in through the nose and out through the mouth.

19. When is a jaw thrust necessary?

A jaw thrust is necessary when a chin lift is insufficient to obtain adequate ventilation and increased oxygen saturations.

20. What is end tidal carbon dioxide ($ETCO_2$)?

End-tidal carbon dioxide ($ETCO_2$) is a measurement of alveolar carbon dioxide at the end of expiration.

21. What is capnography and when is it helpful?

Capnography is an assessment tool that measures a patient's $ETCO_2$. Cardiac monitor software or separate instruments can display both a number and a waveform. It can be monitored via a special oxygen cannula or via an endotracheal tube.

Because capnography measures ventilation directly at the alveoli level, it provides earlier detection of ventilation and oxygenation issues. Deterioration in a patient will manifest itself 2–3 minutes earlier in a patient with capnography than with pulse oximetry (Stoelting & Miller, 2007).

22. What is an oral airway, and what function does it play?

An oral airway is a hard plastic device that can be inserted into the oral cavity. Oral airways are helpful when there is a soft tissue obstruction, such as the tongue, that is interfering with adequate ventilation. Oral airways are also helpful in preventing a patient from biting down on an ETT or laryngeal mask airway (LMA). Patients with a gag reflex do not generally tolerate an oral airway. The appropriate size of an oral airway should be used for maximum effectiveness. The size is measured by placing the airway along the cheek and should be the length from the corner of the mouth to the tragus of the ear. The airway is inserted upside down into the corner of the mouth, and then rotating it right side up over the tongue. A nurse should never leave the bedside if a patient has an oral airway in place, because vomiting, aspiration, and laryngospasm may occur if the patient begins waking and has return of their gag reflex while the oral airway is in place.

23. When would a nasal airway be used instead of an oral airway?

A nasal airway is useful for a patient that has a gag reflex, but continues to have a soft tissue obstruction, such as the tongue or collapse of soft tissue in the pharynx that is limiting ventilation. Nasal airways are better tolerated if the patient is semiconscious. To obtain the correct size, place the airway externally and measure from the proximal end of the nares and the other end at the tragus of the ear. Use lubricant to avoid nasal trauma.

24. What is a laryngeal mask airway (LMA), and in what situations is it used?

A laryngeal mask airway (LMA) is a substitute for an endotracheal tube when aspiration is less of a risk. The LMA does not go into the trachea, but covers the back of the throat and seals the area with an inflated cuff. The cuff of an LMA requires a 60-ml syringe (Stoelting & Miller, 2007).

25. What is an endotracheal tube (ETT), and is what situations is it used?

An endotracheal tube is an airway device that ensures an unobstructed airway. It is useful when there is a risk of aspiration, to facilitate mechanical ventilation, for suctioning, and to ensure a patent airway with increased airway edema. The cuff of an ETT requires a 10-ml syringe (Stoelting & Miller, 2007).

26. What are the risks associated with endotracheal intubation?

- Postextubation laryngeal edema
- Negative pressure pulmonary edema
- Bronchospasm
- Hoarseness or pharyngitis
- Tachycardia
- Hypertension

27. When is it necessary to reintubate a patient in the PACU?

Reintubating a patient is necessary if any of the following conditions occur:

- Decreased ability to maintain oxygenation
- Decreased ability to maintain a patent airway even with chin lift or jaw thrust
- Increased work of breathing as indicated by struggling chest movements
- Tachypnea
- "Fishlike" or "floppy" respiratory effort
- Diminished breath sounds
- Diminished level of consciousness

28. What supplies are needed when intubating a patient?

- Endotracheal tubes of appropriate sizes
- Laryngoscope handle, with straight and curved blades
- Stylet
- Water-soluble lubricant
- Suction equipment
- Bag valve mask
- Oxygen source
- Stethoscope
- Drugs as requested by anesthesia provider (e.g., midazolam, muscle relaxant)
- Ventilator if requested

29. What is the role of the PACU nurse in intubation?

- Assist in gathering supplies and drugs as requested
- Monitor vital signs preintubation and postintubation

- Administer drugs as requested and according to facility policy
- Apply cricoid pressure as requested by the anesthesia provider
- Assist in bag valve mask/hyperventilating the patient as needed
- Auscultate breath sounds for proper tube placement
- Secure the endotracheal tube (American Society of PeriAnesthesia Nurses, 2009)

30. What is cricoid pressure?

Cricoid pressure is a technique to decrease the risk of aspiration during intubation. Prior to and during intubation, pressure is applied against the cricoid cartilage at the sixth cervical vertebrae. This compresses the esophagus and prevents passive aspiration of stomach contents. This technique is also called Sellick's maneuver.

31. What criteria and assessments are necessary to determine whether a patient is ready to be extubated?

- Patient is awake or awakening
- Spontaneous respirations
- No respiratory distress
- Ability to keep eyes open
- Ability to sustain head lift for more than 5 seconds
- Equal and strong hand grasps
- Return of protective reflexes (e.g., swallowing, lid reflex)
- Moving all extremities

32. How do I extubate a patient?

- Assess patient for extubation using previous criteria.
- Gather equipment for extubation (suction, 10-ml syringe or 60-ml syringe, bag valve mask, and oxygen delivery device to use after extubation).
- Suction patient per ETT/LMA and orally if indicated by assessing the patient for secretions.
- Connect 10-ml syringe to ETT balloon tag or 60-ml syringe to LMA balloon tag.
- Deflate balloon until no further air comes out of the balloon.
- Have patient take a deep breath and pull the tube gently as patient exhales. Extubation should occur on expiration versus inspiration, as this allows any secretions on the end of

tube to come out with the tube rather than
going back into the lungs.

- Apply alternate airway delivery device (simple
  mask or nasal cannula) (American Society of
  PeriAnesthesia Nurses, 2009).

33. What is a cricothyrotomy?

A cricothyrotomy is a procedure in which a large
bore needle is used to make a puncture wound
into the cricothyroid membrane for immediate
access to the airway. It is an emergency situation,
and cricothyrotomy trays should be kept in the
PACU (Drain & Odom-Forren, 2009).

34. What is an airway obstruction?

An airway obstruction occurs any time something
occludes the airway, causing hypoxia, hypoventilation, and apnea. Most often the cause is the tongue
or the collapse of soft tissue in the pharynx. This is
a postanesthesia emergency and requires immediate intervention with a chin lift, jaw thrust, repositioning, and/or reintubation. Snoring is a sign of
partial obstruction; it does not mean that the patient is sleeping. Snoring requires an immediate
chin lift or some other means of relieving the obstruction so that adequate ventilation can occur. If
the patient is conscious, deep breathing and coughing should be encouraged.

35. What is a bronchospasm?

A bronchospasm is a narrowing or constriction of
the bronchi or bronchioles. This may be the result
of asthma, an allergic reaction or histamine release,
aspiration, tobacco use, or pulmonary edema. Signs
and symptoms include a cough, dyspnea, tachypnea,
expiratory wheezing, and use of accessory muscles.

36. What is a laryngospasm?

A laryngospasm is a partial or complete closing of
the vocal cords. It can be caused by secretions or
irritation of the vocal cords during emergence and/
or extubation. Signs and symptoms for a partial
laryngospasm include high-pitched inspiratory
stridor, often described as crowing; wheezing;
paradoxical chest and/or abdominal movements;
and decreased ventilation. In a complete laryngospasm, there is silence, a total absence of ventilation,
and paradoxical chest and/or abdominal movements. The patient may also exhibit facial expressions of anxiety and terror.

37. How do I treat a laryngospasm?

A partial laryngospasm is treated with basic airway
management, including a chin lift or jaw thrust,
gentle suctioning if appropriate, or positive pressure ventilation with a bag valve mask. Sometimes
midazolam will help relax the patient enough to
break the spasm. A complete laryngospasm is
treated with 100% positive pressure with a bag
valve mask. If this is unsuccessful, 0.1–0.2 mg/kg
of succinylcholine may be given to break the
spasm. If succinylcholine is given, the patient
should be bagged for 5–10 minutes until the
succinylcholine wears off. If a complete laryngospasm occurs, the patient may need to be
reintubated.

38. What is negative pressure pulmonary edema?

Negative pressure pulmonary edema is pulmonary
edema that does not have a cardiac component as
its cause. Rather, the cause can be an upper airway
obstruction, a bolus dose of naloxone, postextubation laryngospasm, or incomplete reversal of a

TABLE 4-3. Cough, chest noise, or breathing patterns

Cough, chest noise, or breathing pattern	Descriptors
Barking	Croupy, resonant cough, inspiratory stridor, usually from upper airway inflammation
Asthmatic	Wheezing, prolonged expiration, irritative and wheezing cough, retraction of sternocleidomastoid, suprasternal, intercostal, and substernal muscles in severe attacks
Chronic obstructive pulmonary disease	Chronic cough, difficulty with inspiration and expiration, but more so with expiration
Fremitus	Quivering vibration of the chest that can be palpated
Subcutaneous emphysema	Free air or gas that has migrated to the chest and neck; produces a palpable crackling or popping sound.

muscle relaxant. The signs and symptoms result from the patient attempting to clear the obstruction, which generates high negative intrapleural pressure. The classic sign is pink, frothy sputum. Other signs and symptoms are restlessness, wheezing, and severe respiratory distress. Oxygen saturations can decrease to 70% or lower. Treatment involves improving ventilation with a non-rebreather, and can include bag valve mask and reintubation if the symptoms are not relieved quickly. Furosemide and morphine may be given, and a chest x-ray is obtained. The chest x-ray will show signs of pulmonary edema and often has a cracked glass appearance. The patient usually requires an overnight stay in the intensive care unit (ICU) (Drain & Odom-Forren, 2009; Schick & Windle, 2010).

39. What is obstructive sleep apnea, and what care considerations are necessary?

Obstructive sleep apnea is a physiological condition in which a part of the posterior pharynx collapses, leading to obstruction of the airway. The obstruction creates periods of apnea, leading to decreased oxygen levels, increased carbon dioxide, and decreased pH. This causes an awakening from sleep, breathing resumes, and the patient goes back to sleep. The pharynx collapses again during sleep, causing the cycle to start over again.

Care considerations include basic airway management, careful monitoring and assessment with any sedation, avoiding the supine position, and supplemental oxygen. These patients may require extended observation in the PACU. If patients have known obstructive sleep apnea and use a CPAP machine at home, CPAP may be required in the PACU.

40. What is aspiration?

Aspiration is inhalation of gastric contents into the lungs. It is more common with "full-stomach" patients, including inadequate amount of NPO ("nothing by mouth") time, obesity, pregnancy, trauma patients, patients with hiatal hernias, gastroparesis, upper abdominal surgeries, and can also occur with inhalation of blood or a foreign body, such as loose teeth. The patient should be assessed for oxygenation, dyspnea, abnormal breath sounds, coughing, bronchospasms, and hemodynamic changes.

Treatment includes obtaining a chest x-ray, ensuring the patient is oxygenated and ventilating well, providing humidified oxygen, and frequent assessment. Steroids, antibiotics, antacids, antiemetics, and H_2 receptors may be considered.

The right lung is more susceptible to aspiration because of the straighter angle of the right main stem bronchus.

41. What is atelectasis?

Atelectasis is collapse of the alveoli, which then prevents adequate respiratory exchange of oxygen and carbon dioxide. The atelectasis can be either compression atelectasis or absorption atelectasis. Compression atelectasis is caused by external pressure exerted on the lung, such as a tumor, fluid, air in the pleural space, or abdominal distention that presses up against the lung. Absorption atelectasis is caused by removal of air from the alveoli, which is absorbed into the bloodstream. This can be from inhalation of oxygen or anesthetic gases, which are quickly absorbed into the bloodstream, leading to collapse of the alveoli, especially in the dependent portion of the lung. Secretions also tend to pool in the dependent portions of the lungs, putting the patient at risk for infection and pneumonia. Treatment and prevention of atelectasis includes encouraging the patient to breathe deeply and cough, changing the patient's position, and early ambulation. Deep breathing and coughing are important because they promote clearance of secretions through the cilia, redistribute surfactant, and open up the obstructed alveoli (Drain & Odom-Forren, 2009; Stillwell, 2002).

42. What is subglottic edema?

Subglottic edema is usually seen in young children. This most often occurs after a traumatic intubation, coughing with the tube still in place, surgery of the head or neck, and long procedures. Signs and symptoms include stridor, crowing respirations, and rocking chest movements. Treatment should include humidified oxygen, racemic epinephrine nebulizer treatment, and drugs such as dexamethasone for the edema, and benzodiazepines or opioid treatment to calm the patient (Drain & Odom-Forren, 2009).

43. What is status asthmaticus?

Status asthmaticus is an acute, prolonged, and very severe asthma attack. It is a result of ongoing bronchospasms, edema, and mucous plugs, which cause a severe decrease in the diameter of the bronchioles. These attacks may be fatal if not treated immediately and aggressively. Treatment includes oxygen, bronchodilators intravenously or via aerosol inhalation, corticosteroids, sedation, and, often, positive pressure ventilation (Anderson, 1998).

44. What is chronic obstructive pulmonary disease (COPD), and how is care altered for these patients?

Chronic obstructive pulmonary disease (COPD) is a breathing disorder characterized by progressive obstruction of airflow. It is not generally reversible. COPD includes emphysema and chronic bronchitis. In emphysema, the small bronchioles and the alveoli walls are destroyed. This leads to impaired gas exchange. Emphysema is often accompanied by chronic bronchitis, inflammation of the bronchioles, and a chronic productive cough. There is prolonged expiratory time and breath sounds are diminished. In the early stages of COPD, patients have mild hypoxemia. In later stages, the hypoxemia is greater along with hypercapnia. With chronic elevation of CO_2, the central chemoreceptors no longer act as the stimulus to breathe. Rather, the peripheral chemoreceptors take over and do not stimulate the patient to breathe if the PaO_2 is much over 60 mm Hg. If oxygen therapy causes the PaO_2 to increase over 60, the CO_2 increases and apnea results. Hypoxia is what stimulates breathing in patients with COPD. Therefore, high flow oxygen may diminish a patient's stimulus to breathe (Stoelting & Miller, 2007).

45. What is a pulmonary embolus?

A pulmonary embolus is an occlusion in the pulmonary vascular bed. The cause can be a blood clot, a tissue fragment, venous stasis, a fat embolism that has traveled to the lungs, an air bubble, or a hypercoagulability condition. The risk of clot formation increases whenever there is vessel damage (such as with surgery), venous stasis, and decreased mobility. A clot becomes a pulmonary embolus when it breaks off from the site of formation and travels to the lungs. Signs and symptoms are sudden onset of chest pain, tachypnea, tachycardia, agitation and restlessness, hypoxia, and often hemoptysis. Treatment includes correcting the hemodynamic instability, oxygenating the patient, anticoagulation, elastic stockings or sequential compression devices, and early mobility.

46. What is a pneumothorax?

A pneumothorax is entry of air into the pleural space. Air enters the space and destroys the negative pressure of the pleural space. A pneumothorax can be caused by a thoracotomy procedure; placement of a central line; or it can be a complication of an interscalene, intercostal, or brachial plexus block. The signs and symptoms include chest pain, absence of breath sounds on the affected side, and dyspnea. Treatment involves getting the lung reinflated with a chest tube, elevating the patient's head of bed, and ensuring adequate oxygenation.

REFERENCES

American Heart Association. (2006). *Pediatric advanced life support*. Dallas, TX: Author.

American Society of PeriAnesthesia Nurses. (2009). *Competency based orientation and credentialing program for the registered nurse in the perianesthesia setting*. Cherry Hill, NJ: Author.

American Society of PeriAnesthesia Nurses. (2010). Perianesthesia nursing standards and practice recommendations: 2010–2012. Cherry Hill, NJ: Author.

Anderson, K. N. (1998). *Mosby's medical, nursing, & allied health dictionary* (5th ed.). St. Louis, MO: Mosby.

Drain, C. B., & Odom-Forren, J. (2009). *Perianesthesia nursing: A critical care approach* (5th ed.). St. Louis, MO: Saunders.

Schick, L., & Windle, P. E. (2010). *PeriAnesthesia nursing core curriculum: Preprocedure, phase I and phase II PACU nursing* (2nd ed.). St. Louis, MO: Saunders.

Stillwell, S. B. (2002). *Critical care nursing reference* (3rd ed.). St. Louis: Mosby.

Stoelting, R. K., & Miller, R. D. (2007). *Basics of anesthesia* (5th ed.). Philadelphia: Churchill Livingstone Elsevier.

CHAPTER 5

Pain Management

Chris Pasero, MS, RN-BC, FAAN

Perianesthesia nurses have an active and pivotal role in the management of pain. They teach patients about the pain experience before surgery and are the first defense in preventing and fighting pain after surgery. They are the patient's advocate when adjustments in the treatment plan must be made to optimize pain relief. This chapter discusses the types of pain seen in the perioperative setting and the analgesics used to treat patients. Practical tips on the management of patients who are opioid tolerant, those with chronic (persistent) pain, and patients with addictive disease are provided. The importance of providing both effective and safe pain relief is emphasized throughout the chapter.

1. What is the definition of pain?

The International Association for the Study of Pain (IASP) (1994) and the American Pain Society (APS) (2008) define pain as "an unpleasant sensory and emotional experience associated with actual or potential tissue damage, or described in terms of such damage." This definition describes pain as a complex phenomenon with multiple components that impacts a person's psychosocial and physical functioning (McCaffery, Herr, & Pasero, 2011). The accepted clinical definition of pain, which was proposed by Margo McCaffery in 1968 and is now accepted worldwide, reinforces that pain is a highly personal and subjective experience: "Pain is whatever the experiencing person says it is, existing whenever he says it does" (McCaffery, 1968).

2. What is the difference between acute pain and chronic (persistent) pain?

Acute pain follows tissue damage (e.g., surgery) with a distinct onset and relatively brief duration that subsides as healing takes place (Vadivelu, Whitney, & Sinatra, 2009). Chronic pain persists beyond the expected period of healing, which explains why it is also called persistent pain (Pasero & Portenoy, 2011). It can occur from multiple causes (e.g., cancer, noncancer), may have a gradual or distinct onset, is often refractory to treatment, and serves no useful purpose (Vadivelu et al., 2009).

3. What is the difference between nociceptive pain and neuropathic pain?

Nociception refers to the normal functioning of physiologic systems that leads to the perception of noxious stimuli as being painful (Pasero & Portenoy, 2011). In short, it means "normal" pain transmission occurs when tissue damage (e.g., surgical incision) produces enough noxious stimuli to activate free nerve endings (nociceptors) and initiate the transmission of pain. Somatic (bone) and visceral (organ) pain are types of nociceptive pain. In contrast to nociceptive pain, neuropathic pain is sustained by the abnormal processing of stimuli from the peripheral or central nervous system or both (Pasero & Portenoy, 2011).

4. What is the best way to assess pain in patients who can report pain in the postanesthesia care unit (PACU)?

The gold standard of pain assessment is the report of pain by patients who are capable of doing so (American Pain Society [APS], 2008; McCaffery et al., 2011). A comprehensive assessment includes the patient's description of the pain, including its location, duration, what aggravates and relieves it, and its intensity. Pain intensity is rated by the patient using a reliable and valid pain assessment tool, such as the 0 to 10 numerical pain rating scale (NRS), Wong-Baker FACES scale, or the Faces Pain Scale–Revised (FPS-R) (www.painsourcebook.ca) (McCaffery et al., 2011). Some patients prefer a verbal descriptor scale (VDS), which uses words that correlate with the NRS, such as no pain (0), mild pain (1–3), moderate pain (4–6), or severe pain (7–10).

5. What is the best way to assess pain in patients who cannot report pain in the PACU?

Many patients in the PACU are unable to provide a report of their pain because they are sedated from anesthesia and/or other drugs given during surgery. Some may be cognitively impaired or critically ill (e.g., intubated, unresponsive), and some may be too young (e.g., infants, small children) to report their pain using customary self-report pain assessment tools. These patients are collectively referred to as "nonverbal" patients (Herr et al., 2006). When patients are unable to report pain using traditional methods, an alternative approach based on the Hierarchy of Importance of Pain Measures (McCaffery & Pasero, 1999) is recommended (Herr et al., 2006; McCaffery et al., 2011; Pasero, 2009a). The key components of the hierarchy are to (1) attempt to obtain self-report; (2) consider underlying pathology or conditions and procedures that might be painful (e.g., surgery); (3) observe behaviors; (4) evaluate physiologic indicators; and (5) conduct an analgesic trial (see Table 5-1).

6. Is it acceptable to assume that pain is present in patients who cannot report pain after surgery?

When a self-report cannot be obtained, the Hierarchy of Importance of Pain Measures (Table 5-1) directs the clinician to consider the presence of a potentially painful condition (e.g., surgery) or pathology (e.g., cancer). When such conditions exist, nurses should assume that pain is present and should provide appropriate treatment, such as the administration of starting doses of analgesics. This

TABLE 5-1. Hierarchy of importance of pain measures

1. Attempt to obtain the patient's self-report, the single most reliable indicator of pain.
2. Consider the patient's condition or exposure to a procedure that is thought to be painful. If appropriate, assume pain is present (APP); if approved by institution policy and procedure, document APP.
3. Observe behavioral signs (e.g., facial expressions, crying, restlessness, and changes in activity). • A surrogate who knows the patient (e.g., parent, spouse, caregiver) may be able to provide information about underlying painful pathology or behaviors that may indicate pain.
4. Evaluate physiologic indicators with the understanding that they are the least sensitive indicators of pain and may signal the existence of conditions other than pain or a lack of it (e.g., hypovolemia, blood loss).
5. Conduct an analgesic trial to confirm the presence of pain and to establish a basis for developing a treatment plan if pain is thought to be present.

From Herr et al., 2006; McCaffery, Herr, and Pasero, 2011; and McCaffery and Pasero, 1999.

action is commonplace in PACUs where nurses appropriately assume surgery is painful and administer analgesics, regardless of the patient's ability to report pain (Pasero, 2009a).

Nurses should never presume that patients cannot feel pain and should realize that medications such as neuromuscular blocking agents, propofol (Diprivan), and midazolam (Versed), do not produce analgesia (Pasero, Quinn, Portenoy, McCaffery, & Rizos, 2011). When pain is assumed to be present, the condition thought to be present is documented, and, when approved by institutional policy and procedure, the abbreviation APP (assume pain present) may be used (McCaffery, 2011, 2001; Pasero & McCaffery, 2002).

7. Are behaviors reliable indicators of pain?

Patients' behaviors may provide clues about whether or not they have pain. For example, facial expressions, restlessness, bracing, and changes in activity have been shown to be indicators of pain in nonverbal patients (Gelinas, Fillion, Puntillo, Viens,

& Fortier, 2006; Hadjistavropoulos et al., 2007; Herr et al., 2006; McCaffery et al., 2011; Pasero, 2009a).

There are a number of behavioral pain assessment tools that have been tested in patients who cannot report pain; for example, the Critical Care Observation Tool (CPOT) for patients who are critically ill (Gelinas et al., 2006; Gelinas, Harel, Fillion, Puntillo, & Johnston, 2009; Gelinas & Johnston, 2007). Although behavioral pain assessment tools help to determine if patients have pain, a limitation of many of them is that they designate specific behaviors, such as body movements and muscle tension, which must be observed and scored depending on the extent to which the behaviors are present. Appropriate use of these tools requires nurses to carefully evaluate each patient's ability to respond with the requisite behaviors specified by the tool to prevent undertreatment of pain (Pasero, 2009a). For example, tools that require assessment of body movement are not appropriate for use in patients who cannot move, such as those receiving a neuromuscular blocking agent. In such patients, the recommended approach is to assume pain is present (see Table 5-1) and provide recommended doses of analgesics. This assumption can be justified by research that has shown that endotracheal intubation, ventilation, and suctioning—all required in patients receiving a neuromuscular blocking agent—are painful (Puntillo et al., 2001; Stanik-Hutt, Soeken, Belcher, Fontaine, & Gift, 2001).

8. Is a behavioral pain score the same as a pain intensity rating?

A common pitfall of using behavioral pain assessment tools is the tendency of clinicians to draw conclusions about the intensity of a patient's pain based on the behavioral score the tool yields (Pasero, 2009a). There is no research that shows that a certain behavior or number of behaviors indicate a certain pain intensity. For example, one patient may lie completely still and quiet, and another may grimace and be restless, but both may be experiencing severe pain. It is essential that nurses use behavioral tools to help determine the presence of pain and to guide treatment with the understanding that behavioral tools are *not* pain intensity rating scales. If a patient cannot report pain intensity, the exact intensity of the pain cannot be known (Pasero & McCaffery, 2005a).

9. Are physiologic parameters, such as blood pressure and pulse, reliable indicators of pain?

Although nurses often rely on physiologic indicators such as an elevated heart rate or blood

pressure when assessing pain, these parameters are not considered good indicators of pain (McCaffery et al., 2011). Research has shown that vital signs are not consistent with pain and such indicators should be used with caution (Arbour & Gelinas, 2009; Gelinas & Arbour, 2009). Increases in heart rate or blood pressure may occur with sudden, severe pain; however, the human body seeks equilibrium and quickly adapts (Pasero, 2009a). In addition, other factors such as hypovolemia, hypothermia, and some anesthetics may influence vital signs.

10. Should patients be asked to establish a pain rating goal preoperatively?

Prior to surgery, patients should be told by their surgeon and preadmission nurses about the functional goals of postoperative care and the importance of being comfortable enough to accomplish those goals with relative ease. For example, patients need to breathe deeply, cough, and ambulate or participate in physical therapy during the postoperative period. It is important to remind patients when establishing a pain rating goal (also called comfort-function goal) that pain ratings above a 3/10 have been found to interfere with optimal activity (McCaffery et al., 2011). Although it is not always possible to achieve a patient's pain rating goal in the short time a patient is in the PACU, the goal provides direction for pain treatment during the continuum of care.

11. Should the criteria for discharge from the PACU include the requirement that patients must achieve their pain rating goal?

The quality of patients' pain control should be addressed when they are discharged from one clinical area to another. Many short stay units, outpatient surgery units, and PACUs establish the criterion that patients must achieve a pain rating of 4/10 or better before discharge; however, the expectation that all patients must be discharged from these areas with pain ratings below an arbitrary number is unrealistic and can lead to the unsafe administration of further opioid doses to patients who are excessively sedated, which is widely discouraged (Blumstein & Moore, 2003; Lucas, Vlahos, & Ledgerwood, 2007; Vila et al., 2005). Instead, achieving optimal pain relief is best viewed on a continuum with the primary objective being to provide both effective and safe analgesia (Pasero, Quinn et al., 2011). Optimal pain relief is the responsibility of every member of the healthcare team and begins with analgesic titration in the PACU followed by continued prompt assessment and analgesic administration after discharge from the PACU to achieve pain ratings that allow patients to meet their functional goals with relative ease.

Although it may not always be possible to achieve a patient's pain rating goal within the short time the patient is in an area like the PACU, this goal provides direction for ongoing analgesic care. Important information to give to the nurse that is assuming care of the patient on the clinical unit is the patient's pain rating goal, how close the patient is to achieving it, what has been done thus far to achieve it (analgesics and doses), and how well the patient has tolerated analgesic administration (adverse effects).

12. What is the recommended approach for the management of pain in the immediate postoperative period?

Pain is a complex phenomenon involving multiple underlying mechanisms. These characteristics mandate the use of more than one analgesic, sometimes provided by more than one route of administration, to manage immediate and ongoing postoperative pain. Guidelines recommend the use of multimodal analgesia as a means of reducing postoperative opioid doses and preventing clinically significant opioid-induced adverse effects (American Society of Anesthesiologists, 2004. For example, numerous studies have demonstrated that the combination of nonopioids (e.g., acetaminophen and nonsteroidal anti-inflammatory drugs [NSAIDs]) with other analgesics (e.g., opioids and local anesthetics) can produce better analgesia with fewer adverse effects than any single analgesic administered alone (Jorgensen, Wetterslev, Møiniche, & Dahl, 2000; Marret, Kurdi, Zufferey, & Bonnet, 2005; Meek, 2004; Pouzeratte et al., 2001; Schug & Manopas, 2007; Vascello & McQuillan, 2006). Nonpharmacologic approaches such as proper positioning and the application of heat or cold should be added to complement the pharmacologic treatment plan.

13. What is the difference between multimodal analgesia and polypharmacy, and how can the risks associated with polypharmacy be minimized?

The term polypharmacy carries a negative connotation, in contrast to multimodal therapy or combination therapy. Whereas multimodal therapy is based on rational combinations of analgesics with differing underlying mechanisms to achieve the greatest benefit in pain control, polypharmacy suggests the use of drug combinations that are irrational and less effective or less safe than would be a regimen that had fewer or different agents (Pasero & Portenoy, 2011). For example, combining two NSAIDs in a treatment plan is not advised, as this is unlikely to improve analgesia and would increase

the patient's risk of GI toxicity (Pasero, Portenoy, & McCaffery, 2011). Important principles of safe drug administration are to be aware of the potential for interactions specific to each analgesic and to avoid unnecessary duplicate prescribing that can lead to toxicities (Hanks, Roberts, & Davies, 2004).

14. What is preemptive analgesia and does it work?

In the scientific literature, the term "preemptive analgesia" is used when discussing research that compares the effects of preoperative administration of a single (most often) analgesic intervention, such as local anesthetic surgical site infiltration or oral opioid administration, with the effects of this same intervention administered immediately after surgery on the intensity of postoperative pain. Many clinicians have proposed that a more appropriate term and approach in the clinical setting is "protective analgesia," whereby aggressive and sustained multimodal interventions are initiated preoperatively and continued throughout the intraoperative and postoperative periods (Møiniche, Kehlet, & Dahl, 2002; Dahl & Møiniche, 2004). Consistent with this strategy are the goals of immediate postoperative pain reduction and prevention of postsurgical pain syndromes (Kelly, Ahmad, & Brull, 2001). In addition, the initiation of multimodal analgesic interventions preoperatively or as soon as possible postoperatively facilitates the administration of the lowest effective analgesic doses during the critical immediate postoperative period when patients are likely to experience both excessive sedation from anesthetics and other drugs and severe pain (Pasero, Quinn et al, 2011).

15. What are the primary pharmacologic strategies for the management of postoperative pain?

There are a number of pharmacologic strategies for the management of postoperative pain, and all involve the administration of one or more of the most common types of analgesics used in the postoperative period:

- Nonopioids, including acetaminophen and the NSAIDs (e.g., IV ketorolac or ibuprofen; oral or rectal celecoxib, ibuprofen, or naproxen)
- Opioids, including the first-line options, fentanyl, hydromorphone, morphine, and oxycodone
- Local anesthetics, most often bupivacaine and ropivacaine, used alone for peripheral nerve blocks or in combination with opioids for epidural analgesia
- Anticonvulsants, including gabapentin and pregabalin

A variety of routes of administration are used to deliver analgesics in the perioperative setting as well. Many of the methods used to manage postoperative pain are accomplished via catheter techniques such as epidural analgesia and continuous peripheral nerve block infusions. Nurses play a key and extensive role in the successful management of these therapies, and the American Society for Pain Management Nursing (ASPMN) provides guidelines for care (Pasero, Eksterowicz, Primeau, & Cowley, 2007).

16. Which first-line opioid is best to treat immediate postoperative pain and is there value in using more than one for this type of pain?

The mu-agonist opioids, morphine, hydromorphone, and fentanyl, are the most commonly used for initial IV titration for the treatment of postoperative pain. Important patient characteristics to consider when selecting an opioid include previous exposure and tolerance of opioids, current organ function, and hemodynamic stability. For example, fentanyl is favored in patients with any type of end-organ failure. It also produces minimal hemodynamic effects, which adds to its appeal in patients with unstable blood pressure (Pasero, Quinn et al., 2011).

In addition to patient characteristics, the pharmacokinetics of the opioid and the goals of treatment are considered when deciding which opioid is best for titration in a particular patient (Pasero, Quinn et al., 2011). Whereas morphine requires several minutes (15–30) to cross the blood–brain barrier and yield peak effects after IV administration, the more lipophilic opioids, such as fentanyl, cross very quickly and produce peak effects almost immediately when given intravenously. Hydromorphone is less hydrophilic than morphine and so has an intermediate onset (see Table 5-2).

Fentanyl tends to be a first-choice opioid for procedural pain and is a logical selection in ambulatory surgery PACU where the goal is to transition the patient quickly to the oral analgesic that the patient will take after discharge. For patients who have undergone major surgery, some PACU nurses like to administer a few doses of fentanyl and then follow with either hydromorphone or morphine for longer-lasting analgesia. However, although it makes sense to use a fast-onset opioid such as fentanyl in patients presenting with severe, escalating pain, it may not be necessary and can complicate the assessment process in those with less severe pain; when opioids are combined and adverse effects occur it is difficult to interpret which one might be the culprit. Therefore, a general principle of initial titration in patients with acute pain is to keep in mind the patients' ongoing pain treatment plan. As an example, consider the patient who is admitted to the PACU and will have hydromorphone IV patient-controlled analgesia (PCA) for ongoing postoperative pain management. Unless the patient has severe, rapidly escalating pain on admission, it makes sense to begin titration with hydromorphone so that the effects (both pain relief and adverse effects) of the drug that will be used by PCA can be evaluated more easily.

17. What is the correct way to titrate IV opioid analgesics?

Considerable variation exists in the amount of opioid individuals require for comfort (APS, 2008). For example, research has established that as much as a 10-fold difference exists among patients in opioid requirements during the postoperative period (Myles, 2004). At all times, nurses must strive to achieve a balance between pain relief and adverse effects (Hanks, Cherny, & Fallon, 2004).

TABLE 5-2. First-line IV opioids administered for postoperative pain management: pharmacokinetic information

Opioid	Onset (min)	Peak (min)[1]	Duration (hrs)[2]	Half-life (hrs)
Morphine	5–10	15–30	3–4	2–4
Hydromorphone	5	15–30	3–4	2–3
Fentanyl	3–5	15–30	2	3–4

[1] Of all of the routes of administration, IV produces the highest peak concentration of the drug, and the peak concentration is associated with the highest level of toxicity (e.g., sedation). To decrease the peak effect and lower the level of toxicity, IV boluses may be administered more slowly or smaller doses may be administered more often.

[2] Duration of analgesia is dose dependent; the higher the dose, usually the longer the duration.

From Pasero, Quinn, Portenoy, McCaffery, and Rizos, 2011.

The goal of titration is to use the smallest dose that provides satisfactory analgesia with the fewest adverse effects (Pasero, Quinn et al., 2011).

In opioid-naïve patients with moderate to severe pain, recommended starting IV doses are given (e.g., 2–3 mg of morphine, 0.4 mg of hydromorphone, or 25–50 mcg of fentanyl) (APS, 2008). When an increase in the opioid dose is necessary and safe, many clinicians increase by percentages. When a slight improvement in analgesia is needed, a 25% increase in the opioid dose may be sufficient; for a moderate effect, a 50% increase; and for a strong effect, such as for the treatment of continued severe pain, a 100% increase may be indicated (Pasero, Quinn et al., 2011). The time that the dose should be increased is determined by considering the peak effect of the opioid. The frequency of IV opioid doses during initial titration may be as often as every 5 to 15 minutes (see Table 5-2). The patient must be observed closely for adverse effects (Aubrun, Monsel, Langeron, Coriat, & Riou, 2001; Lvovschi et al., 2008). Conservative initial opioid doses along with careful monitoring during titration are recommended in the older adult population (APS, 2008; Keïta, Tubach, Maalouli, Desmonts, & Mantz, 2008; Pasero, Quinn et al., 2011); however, doses should be increased based on patient response rather than a specific age.

Doses should *not* be increased in patients who are excessively sedated (e.g., unable to keep eyes open and falling asleep mid-sentence). In such cases, nonopioid analgesics should be added or increased (e.g., full doses of an NSAID and acetaminophen). As noted, it may not be possible to achieve optimal pain control in the PACU for all patients; the process is viewed as occurring on a continuum (Pasero, Quinn et al., 2011). Insuring safe pain management is a primary objective.

18. Is there a predictable relationship between pain intensity and opioid dose requirement?

Research has shown that the relationship between pain intensity scores and dose requirements during and after titration in postoperative patients is not linear, suggesting that many factors influence pain and its relief, and that there is no specific dose that will relieve pain of a specific intensity (Aubrun & Riou, 2004). Research underscores the importance of individualized selection of analgesic doses and systematic assessment of response during titration (Aubrun, Langeron, Quesnel, Coriat, & Riou, 2003). Dosing to a specific pain intensity (e.g., set orders that mandate 2 mg of IV morphine for pain ratings of 1–3 on a scale of 0–10; 4 mg for pain

ratings of 4–6; and 6 mg for pain ratings of 7–10) can be very dangerous and is strongly discouraged (Pasero, Quinn et al., 2011; Vila et al., 2005). Many factors, such as sedation level, respiratory status, and previous analgesic and sedative intake, in addition to pain intensity must be considered when selecting an opioid dose.

19. Why are anticonvulsants used to treat postoperative pain?

Anticonvulsants are added to multimodal pain treatment plans to improve postoperative analgesia and prevent persistent neuropathic postsurgical pain; for example, following thoracotomy, mastectomy, hernia repair, limb amputation, abdominal hysterectomy, and cholecystectomy (Brogly et al., 2008; Buvanendran et al., 2010; Ho, Gan, & Habib, 2006; Tiippana, Hamunen, Kontinen, & Kalso, 2007). In addition, as part of a multimodal treatment plan, anticonvulsants can reduce opioid and nonopioid dose requirements and related adverse effects (Azer, Abdelhalim, & Elsayed, 2006; Gilron, 2006; Hurley, Cohen, Williams, Rowlingson, & Wu, 2006; Murcia Sanchez, Orts Castro, Perez Doblado, & Perez-Cerda, 2006; Peng, Wijeysundera, & Li, 2007; Seib & Paul, 2006).

20. Is the rectal route an acceptable route for analgesic administration in the perioperative setting?

The rectal route for analgesic administration has a long history of safety in children undergoing surgery and is also an attractive alternative when oral or parenteral analgesics are not an option in patients of any age (Pasero, 2010). Although all of the first-line opioids can be given intravenously, there are currently only three IV nonopioid analgesic formulations available in the United States: acetaminophen, ketorolac, and ibuprofen (IV indomethacin is used primarily for closure of patent ductus arteriosus). Postoperative nausea and vomiting and NPO status limit the usefulness of the oral route of administration in many patients.

Given the lack of available parenteral nonopioids and the constraints of the oral route in the immediate postoperative period, the use of the rectal route to administer nonopioids is a particularly effective strategy for reducing postoperative opioid doses and for preventing clinically significant opioid-induced adverse effects. Several studies have shown improved pain relief and reductions in opioid consumption with rectal nonopioid analgesics alone (Achariyapota & Titapant, 2008; Bahar, Jangjoo, Soltani, Armand, & Mozaffari, 2010; Ng, Parker, Toogood, Cotton, & Smith, 2002; Siddik, Aouad, Jalbout, Rizk, Kamar, & Baraka, 2001). Other studies have demonstrated highly effective pain control with combinations of rectal acetaminophen and various NSAIDs or other analgesics (Bannwarth & Pehourcq, 2003; Carli et al., 2002; Ng, Swami, Smith, & Emembolu, 2008; Romsing, Møiniche, & Dahl, 2002). The nonopioids, acetaminophen, aspirin, and indomethacin, are available commercially in rectal formulations; however, any of the oral nonopioids can be administered rectally, either by inserting the intact tablet or by placing the intact or crushed tablet in a gelatin capsule for insertion. This can be done preoperatively or as soon as possible in the PACU.

21. What are the patient selection criteria for using patient-controlled analgesia (PCA)?

A number of factors need to be considered in determining whether a patient is a candidate for PCA therapy. The most important factor is that the patient must be able to understand the relationship between pain, pushing the PCA button, and pain relief (Pasero, Quinn et al., 2011). When PCA is warranted, patients should be carefully screened for their cognitive and physical ability to manage their pain by that method. Clinicians often hesitate to prescribe PCA for children, believing that they are too young to understand the concept of PCA and how to use the pump appropriately. However, PCA has been used effectively and safely in developmentally normal children as young as 4 years old (Wellington & Chia, 2009). IV PCAs have been shown for many years to be safe in older patients (Gagliese, Gauthier, Macpherson, Jovellanos, & Chan, 2008), but providers often do not prescribe it for fear of producing confusion in these patients. Although the opioid (by whatever approach it is delivered) can contribute to confusion, the factors that may be responsible for postoperative confusion are numerous (Bagri, Rico, & Ruiz, 2008; Redelmeier, 2007; Sharma et al., 2005; Zakriya et al., 2002), and its development should not be assumed to be related to either the drug or the delivery approach. For example, the presence of postoperative pain and increased intensity of postoperative pain have been found to be independent predictors of postoperative delirium (Vaurio, Sands, Wang, Mullen, & Leung, 2006).

22. Should IV PCA therapy be initiated in the PACU?

When IV PCA is prescribed for postoperative patients, it should be initiated whenever possible in the PACU. This allows the healthcare team to evaluate patient response to the therapy early in the postoperative course and prevents delays in analgesia (analgesic gaps) on the clinical nursing unit (Pasero, Quinn et al., 2011). A particularly dangerous scenario to avoid is that of patients receiving IM opioid injections on the clinical unit while waiting for IV PCA to be initiated.

The PACU nurse can save time by using the PCA pump to administer loading doses to establish satisfactory analgesia. Then the PCA button should be given to patients as soon as they are awake and alert enough to manage their own pain. At that time, pain management plans can be reviewed with patients, including what action to take when pain relief is inadequate. PACU nurses can reinforce the safety mechanisms of the PCA pump and how to correctly use the PCA button, reminding patients that it is for their use only.

23. What methods are used to administer intraspinal (epidural, intrathecal) analgesia?

The three methods for administering intraspinal analgesia are: (1) bolus (administered by the clinician), (2) continuous infusion or basal rate (administered by a pump), and (3) patient-controlled epidural analgesia (PCEA) (administered by the patient using a pump).

For some surgical procedures, a single intraspinal morphine bolus provides sufficient pain control for several hours. For example, an epidural or intrathecal bolus of morphine often is administered to manage pain that does not warrant the placement of a catheter, such as after cesarean section and some gynecologic, orthopedic, and urologic procedures (Dabu-Bondoc, Franco, & Sinatra, 2009). A single epidural morphine dose is capable of providing analgesia for 24 to 48 hours depending on the formulation used. Single bolusing is also used when indwelling epidural catheters are contraindicated such as in some patients who require anticoagulant therapy (Dabu-Bondoc et al., 2009).

Analgesic infusion pumps are used to deliver continuous epidural analgesic infusions (basal rate). Supplemental bolus doses are prescribed for breakthrough pain and can be administered using the clinician-administered bolus mode available on most infusion pumps.

PCEA permits patients to treat their pain by self-administering doses of epidural analgesics to meet their individual analgesic requirements. When PCEA is administered, a basal rate usually provides most of the patient's analgesic requirement and the PCEA bolus doses are used to manage breakthrough pain. If a basal rate is not provided, it is especially important to remind patients to "stay on top of the pain" by maintaining a steady neuraxial analgesic level and self-administering bolus doses before the pain is severe and out of control.

24. What is extended-release epidural morphine?

Extended-release epidural morphine (EREM; DepoDur) is distinguished from conventional epidural morphine (e.g., Astramorph, Duramorph) by its unique delivery system called DepoFoam, which consists of multiple microscopic, liposomal particles (Pasero & McCaffery, 2005b). The liposomes contain aqueous chambers that encapsulate preservative-free morphine (Carvalho et al., 2005). After an epidural injection, the liposomes slowly release morphine over a period of 48 hours by erosion or reorganization of the lipid membranes (Heitz & Viscusi, 2009). Primary advantages of this formulation are that it allows up to 48 hours of pain relief without the use of an indwelling catheter, which can pose a risk of infection, impede mobility, and raise concerns about postoperative anticoagulant therapy (Pasero & McCaffery, 2005b; Viscusi et al., 2005). Further, problems with infusion device programming errors are eliminated with this approach.

25. What is a continuous peripheral nerve block?

A continuous peripheral nerve block (also called perineural regional analgesia) involves the establishment of an initial local anesthetic block, followed by the placement of a catheter through which an infusion of local anesthetic is administered continuously, with or without PCA capability. When PCA capability is added, this is referred to as PCRA (patient-controlled regional analgesia). Supplemental opioid or nonopioid–opioid analgesia is provided for breakthrough pain when continuous infusion only is used. In the acute pain setting, the therapy typically is continued during the first 24 to 72 hours postoperatively, depending on the type of surgery. Recent advances in operator skill and catheters and infusion devices made specifically for continuous peripheral nerve block have resulted in the widespread use of this technique for a variety of types of pain, particularly surgical pain, in both inpatient and outpatient settings.

26. What is a continuous local anesthetic wound infusion?

Continuous local anesthetic wound infusions involve the surgeon's placement of a catheter subcutaneously into the surgical wound at the end of the surgical procedure to be used for continuous infusion of local anesthetics, such as bupivacaine or ropivacaine, to control postoperative pain (Rawal, 2007). Just as with continuous peripheral nerve blocks, supplemental opioid or nonopioid–opioid combination analgesics should be provided in addition to this therapy.

27. How should the effectiveness of the pain treatment plan be evaluated?

Systematic reassessment is essential to determine the effectiveness and safety of the pain treatment plan. The pain rating scale is the primary tool used in the postoperative setting to evaluate effectiveness, allowing nurses to compare the intensity of pain before and after analgesic interventions. The frequency with which pain ratings are obtained depends on the situation. Guidelines recommend that, at a minimum, pain should be assessed during the initial encounter and then reassessed and documented at regular intervals after a management plan is initiated, with each new report of pain, and at an appropriate interval after intervention (APS, 2008; McCaffery et al., 2011; APS, 2005). For example, pain ratings every 5 to 15 minutes may be appropriate during IV opioid titration for severe pain in the PACU.

Reassessment also includes evaluating patients for the presence and severity of adverse effects from pain treatment interventions and determining the need to treat adverse effects or perhaps change the pain management plan (Pasero, Quinn et al., 2011). Patient safety is a primary concern. In all cases, adjustments in the treatment plan are individualized according to the patient response (both to pain relief *and* adverse effects).

28. What should be done if the pain treatment plan is not effective?

As the patient's primary pain manager, the nurse is responsible for advocating for changes to the treatment plan when what has been prescribed is not effective or if treatment results in unmanageable and intolerable adverse effects or the potential for such. For example, to prevent clinically significant opioid-induced respiratory depression, the nurse must advocate for adding or increasing the dose of nonopioid analgesics (acetaminophen or an NSAID) rather than administering increased opioid doses to a patient who is both excessively sedated and in severe pain.

29. What is the relationship between anxiety and pain, and how are they differentiated and treated?

When the physical cause of pain is unknown or seems insufficient to account for the severity of pain that the patient reports, clinicians sometimes attribute the pain to the patient's emotional state and cease treating it. However, evidence that anxiety increases pain is limited, and a cause and effect relationship is unclear (McCaffery et al., 2011). It is difficult to know if anxiety causes pain or if anxiety is the result of pain. The belief that anxiety causes pain is reflected in the common practice of combining anxiolytics and opioids, but a major problem with the administration of benzodiazepines in the perioperative period is that they increase the risk of sedation and respiratory depression and the dose of opioid that may be safely administered to the patient to relieve pain must be limited (APS, 2008).

There is no doubt that pain results in considerable distress for many patients. Until the relationship between pain and anxiety is clarified, the most practical initial approach to patients who are both in pain and anxious is to assume that pain causes this emotional response rather than to assume that the emotional response causes or intensifies pain (McCaffery et al., 2011). Anxiety appears to be a normal response to pain. When the patient is both in pain and anxious, initial interventions should be aimed at reducing the pain. Analgesic titration should precede treatment with benzodiazepines in anxious patients with pain. Pain relief may well reduce the anxiety and avoid the need for a benzodiazepine and the potential for increased sedation (McCaffery et al., 2011).

30. What is the difference between an opioid-tolerant patient and one who is opioid-naïve?

The terms opioid-tolerant and opioid-naïve are used to distinguish between patients who have, or have not, respectively, been taking opioid drugs regularly. An opioid-tolerant person has taken opioids long enough at doses high enough to develop tolerance to many of the effects of an opioid, including analgesia and sedation (Pasero, Quinn et al., 2011). There is great variation among individuals, however, with some not developing tolerance at all (Webster & Dove, 2007). Therefore, it is difficult to determine if and when an individual on regular doses of opioids has become tolerant. Consequently, there is no widely accepted definition for classifying a patient as opioid-tolerant (Patanwala, Jarzyna, Miller, & Erstad, 2008). However, clinicians appear to agree that if a patient has been on long-term opioid therapy, opioid tolerance should be expected (APS, 2005). By convention, many clinicians consider a patient who has used opioids regularly for approximately 7 days or more to be opioid-tolerant (Pasero, Quinn et al., 2011).

31. What is the difference between opioid addiction, physical dependence, and tolerance?

The terms physical dependence and tolerance often are confused with addiction, so clarification of terms is important (McCaffery et al., 2011). The definitions proposed in a 2001 consensus statement by the American Academy of Pain Medicine (AAPM), the American Pain Society (APS), and the American Society of Addiction Medicine (ASAM) are as follows:

- *Physical dependence* is a normal response that occurs with repeated administration of an opioid for more than 2 weeks and cannot be equated with addictive disease. It is manifested by the occurrence of withdrawal symptoms when the opioid is suddenly stopped or rapidly reduced or an antagonist such as naloxone is given. Withdrawal symptoms may be suppressed by the natural, gradual reduction of the opioid as pain decreases or by gradual, systematic reduction, referred to as tapering (ASAM, 2001).

- *Tolerance* is also a normal response that occurs with regular administration of an opioid and consists of a decrease in one or more effects of the opioid (e.g., decreased analgesia, sedation, or respiratory depression). It cannot be equated with addictive disease. Tolerance to analgesia usually occurs in the first days to 2 weeks of opioid therapy but is uncommon after that. It may be treated with increases in dose. However, disease progression, not tolerance to analgesia, appears to be the reason for most dose escalations. Stable pain usually results in stable doses. Thus, tolerance poses very few clinical problems (ASAM, 2001).

- *Opioid addiction,* or addictive disease, is a chronic neurologic and biologic disease. Its development and manifestations are influenced by genetic, psychosocial, and environmental factors. No single cause of addiction, such as taking an opioid for pain relief, has been found. It is characterized by behaviors that include one or more of the following: impaired control over drug use, compulsive use, continued use despite harm, and craving (ASAM, 2001).

The consensus statement reinforces an important message—that taking opioids for pain relief is not addiction, no matter how long a person takes opioids or at what doses. Individuals taking opioid drugs for relief of pain are using them therapeutically.

32. What is pseudoaddiction?

Pseudoaddiction, as the name implies, is a mistaken diagnosis of addictive disease. The term was first used and the behaviors described in a case report by Weissman and Haddox (1989). When a patient's pain is not well controlled, the patient may begin to manifest symptoms suggestive of addictive disease.

In an effort to obtain adequate pain relief, the patient may respond with demanding behavior, escalating demands for more or different medications, repeated requests for opioids on time or before the prescribed interval between doses has elapsed, and frequent visits to the emergency department. As an example, patients who receive opioid doses that are too low or at intervals greater than the opioid's duration of action may understandably try to manipulate the staff into giving them more analgesic. Pain relief typically eliminates these behaviors and is often accomplished by increasing opioid doses, decreasing intervals between doses, or providing an extra prescription in case it is needed.

33. What is the risk of opioid addiction when opioids are taken for pain relief?

The incidence of addiction as a result of taking an opioid for therapeutic reasons, such as postoperative pain management, is thought to be quite rare (Jackson, 2009). Research on long-term opioid use is limited (Pasero, Quinn et al., 2011). An evidence-based review of all available studies on the development of addiction and aberrant drug-related behaviors in patients with persistent noncancer pain being treated with opioids calculated the percentage of abuse and/or addiction following opioid therapy to be 0.19% (Fishbain, Cole, Lewis, Rosomoff, & Rosomoff, 2008). These data are reassuring, suggesting that patients with no past or present history of abuse or addiction usually remain responsible medication users over time. Similarly, a registry study of patients who were treated with modified-release oxycodone and followed for up to 3 years after participating in a clinical trial also showed a very low occurrence of problematic drug-related behavior—of the 227 patients studied, there were just 6 cases of misuse and no cases of new addiction (Portenoy et al., 2007). Again, this number is very reassuring in terms of the rate of iatrogenic addiction among those with no history of abuse.

34. What can be done to improve pain management in the postoperative patient with underlying persistent (chronic) pain?

A general principle of perioperative care is to optimize the patient's condition, including the management of persistent pain, prior to a surgical procedure (Pasero, Quinn et al., 2011). If preexisting pain is poorly controlled preoperatively, the primary care provider or anesthesiologist should be contacted for appropriate orders.

A multimodal postoperative pain treatment plan, initiated preoperatively whenever possible, is essential in patients with underlying persistent pain. The American Society of Anesthesiologists (ASA, 2004) recommends the continuation of opioid analgesics to prevent opioid withdrawal syndrome in patients who take them preoperatively for preexistent pain. Other clinicians provide similar recommendations (Ashraf, Wong, Ronayne, & Williams, 2004). It is important to remember that patients who have been taking opioids on a long-term basis preoperatively are likely to be opioid tolerant and require higher postoperative opioid doses than opioid-naïve patients. Although most of the nonselective NSAIDs (e.g., ibuprofen, naproxen) should be discontinued prior to surgery if bleeding is a concern, some nonselective NSAIDs (nabumetone, meloxicam, choline magnesium trisalicylate, magnesium salicylate, and salsalate) and the COX-2 selective NSAID celecoxib have no effect on bleeding time and may be continued throughout the perioperative period (Ashraf et al., 2004). Anticonvulsants and antidepressants, which are often administered for treatment of persistent neuropathic pain, should also be continued if taken preoperatively.

35. What can be done to improve the pain experience for the opioid-tolerant patient undergoing surgery?

Clinicians unfamiliar with caring for opioid-tolerant patients are likely to be fearful of the high doses often required by patients who are opioid tolerant, and as a result, the patient may be underdosed. Tolerance to the adverse effects of opioids develops more rapidly than to analgesia, meaning that opioids may be safely titrated to relatively high doses to provide adequate analgesia (Mehta & Langford, 2006). Most importantly, although respiratory depression can occur in opioid tolerant patients, the occurrence is rare when doses are carefully titrated and the patient is monitored appropriately for effect.

Unfortunately, there are no evidence-based guidelines for predicting postoperative opioid requirements on the basis of the opioid dose consumed before surgery. One suggestion is to expect opioid requirements postoperatively in the opioid-tolerant patient to be two to four times the dose required in an opioid-naïve person (Carroll, Angst, & Clark, 2004); however, individualization of care is essential to ensure patient safety (Pasero, Quinn et al., 2011).

36. How should postoperative pain be treated in a patient with addictive disease?

Opioids, if they are appropriate, should not be withheld from patients with pain who also have addictive disease (May, White, Leonard-White, Warltier, & Pagel, 2001; Mitra & Sinatra, 2004). The acute setting is not the optimal time to attempt detoxification or rehabilitation of a patient who is abusing opioids or other substances (Mitra & Sinatra, 2004). Clinicians often fear that by providing opioids for pain they are feeding the addiction; however, no research shows that providing opioid analgesics to a person with addictive disease will worsen the disease. Conversely, there is no research to show that withholding opioid analgesics when needed will increase the likelihood of recovery (Compton, 1999). In fact, withholding opioids in this situation may cause significant pain, increasing the patient's level of stress, and may lead to increased craving for drugs of abuse. The patient may make efforts to obtain the drug that has been abused, or a patient in recovery may relapse. In the inpatient setting, the patient may make efforts to bring in illicit drugs. Clearly, on many levels, providing pain relief to the patient with addictive disease, even when it includes opioids, is preferable to withholding opioids (Pasero, Quinn et al., 2011).

An excellent resource for pain management in the patient with pain and addictive disease was developed by the American Society for Pain Management Nursing (ASPMN): ASPMN Position Statement: Pain Management in Patients with Addictive Disease, available at http://www.aspmn.org. It covers patients actively using alcohol or other drugs, patients in recovery, and those receiving medical management for opioid addictive disease. The ASPMN paper states a belief that is crucial for clinicians to adopt: "patients with addictive disease and pain have the right to be treated with dignity, respect, and the same quality of pain assessment and management as all other patients" (ASPMN, 2002), (p. 1). It is a quote worth posting for all to see, including clinicians, patients, and families (Pasero, Quinn et al., 2011).

37. What are the most common adverse effects of NSAIDs in the perioperative setting and what approaches are used to minimize and manage them?

The most common adverse effects of NSAIDs involve the GI system. NSAID-induced GI toxicity usually is addressed in the literature as an adverse effect resulting from long-term NSAID use; however, GI ulceration can occur with short-term perioperative administration as well (Schug & Manopas, 2007). This is particularly true in individuals with elevated risk for GI toxicity, such as older adults and those with a previous GI complication. The use of the least ulcerogenic nonselective NSAID or a COX-2 selective NSAID if not contraindicated by cardiovascular risk is encouraged. The lowest effective NSAID dose for the shortest period of time necessary is also recommended (Pasero, Portenoy et al., 2011).

The possibility of increased bleeding time is of special concern when NSAIDs are used for postoperative pain. Aspirin has an irreversible effect on platelets and will increase bleeding time for up to 7 days after the last dose (i.e., until the damaged platelets are replaced by new ones). For that reason, aspirin therapy is usually discontinued 1 week or more before surgery, and aspirin is not recommended for perioperative analgesic use (Ashraf et al., 2004). Other nonselective NSAIDs are also sometimes withheld during the perioperative period because of their tendency to prolong bleeding time. However, the nonselective NSAIDs nabumetone, meloxicam, choline magnesium trisalicylate, magnesium salicylate, and salsalate and the COX-2 selective NSAID celecoxib have no effect on bleeding time and should be considered instead (Visser & Goucke, 2008).

Shortly after the release of the COX-2 selective NSAIDs, studies revealed an association between the perioperative use of valdecoxib and an increase in adverse cardiovascular events (e.g., myocardial infarction, stroke, pulmonary embolism) in patients who had undergone high-risk cardiac surgery (Nussmeier et al., 2005; Ott et al., 2003). The general recommendation is to avoid the perioperative use of NSAIDs following high-risk, open heart surgery (United States Food and Drug Administration [USFDA], 2007).

Adverse renal effects are relatively rare in otherwise healthy individuals who are given NSAIDs during the perioperative period (Lee, Cooper, Craig, Knight, & Keneally, 2007). In contrast, individuals with acute or chronic volume depletion or hypotension depend on prostaglandin synthesis to maintain adequate renal blood flow ("prostaglandin dependence") (Helstrom & Rosow, 2006), and NSAID inhibition of prostaglandin synthesis in such patients can cause acute renal ischemia and acute renal failure (ARF) (Helstrom & Rosow, 2006). ARF, as a result of hypovolemia, is usually reversed when the NSAID is stopped and volume is replenished (Miyoshi, 2001), but it underscores the importance of adequate hydration and maintenance of acceptable BP before and during NSAID administration.

Patients at increased risk for perioperative ARF and who might be more susceptible to NSAID-induced renal injury include those with cardiac failure, liver cirrhosis, ascites, diabetes, preexisting hypertension, and patients being treated with ACE inhibitors (Forrest et al., 2002; Helstrom & Rosow, 2006; Launay-Vacher et al., 2005). Other risk factors are preexisting renal impairment, advanced age, and left ventricular dysfunction (Helstrom & Rosow, 2006). It is generally recommended that NSAIDs be avoided in patients with chronic renal failure and in any patient with a creatinine clearance below 30 mL/min (Laine, White, Rostom, & Hochberg, 2008; Launay-Vacher et al., 2005). Acetaminophen and opioids (e.g., fentanyl) are better choices in these patients.

38. What are the adverse effects of local anesthetics?

The use of local anesthetics for postoperative pain is most often in combination with opioids for epidural analgesia or alone for continuous peripheral nerve block. The doses of local anesthetic used for these methods rarely result in blood concentrations sufficient to cause systemic effects. However, vascular uptake or injection or infusion of local anesthetic directly into the systemic circulation can result in adverse reactions related to high blood levels of local anesthetic, although there are reports of no adverse effects following accidental IV infusion of epidural doses of local anesthetics (Allegri et al., 2009). Central nervous system signs of systemic toxicity include ringing in ears, metallic taste, slow speech, confusion, irritability, twitching, and seizures. Signs of cardiotoxicity include circumoral tingling and numbness, bradycardia, cardiac dysrhythmias, acidosis, and cardiovascular collapse (Covino & Wildsmith, 1998). Patients receiving local anesthetics should be evaluated systematically for these signs, and those who receive continuous peripheral nerve block in the home setting must be given verbal and written instructions that include the signs and symptoms of adverse effects, and what to do if detected.

39. What are the most common adverse effects of opioid analgesics in the perioperative setting and what approaches are used to minimize and manage them?

The most common opioid adverse effects are postoperative nausea and vomiting (PONV), pruritus, hypotension, and sedation. Respiratory depression is less common but the most feared of the opioid adverse effects. The adverse effects of opioids are dose dependent. Thus, the single most effective, safest, and least expensive treatment is to decrease the opioid dose (Pasero, Quinn et al., 2011). Decreasing the opioid dose is facilitated by adding or increasing the dose of a nonopioid, such as an NSAID or acetaminophen, and using local anesthetics for peripheral nerve blocks or adding a

local anesthetic to the epidural opioid solution to provide additional pain relief.

Consensus guidelines present a number of recommendations for the management of PONV (Gan et al., 2003, 2007). Algorithms that incorporate guideline recommendations are available (American Society of PeriAnesthesia Nurses, 2006; Gan et al., 2007). Key points are to identify patients at high risk for PONV (e.g., females, those with a prior history of motion sickness or PONV, nonsmokers, and those who use postoperative opioids); reduce baseline risk factors (e.g., implement multimodal analgesic strategies); and administer PONV prophylaxis for patients with a moderate-to-high risk. Prophylactic antiemetic treatment is not recommended in low-risk patients; however, antiemetic treatment is provided in those who develop PONV and did not receive prophylaxis or in whom prophylaxis failed (Gan et al., 2003, 2007).

Pruritus (itching) is an adverse effect, not an allergic reaction to opioids (Ho & Gan, 2009). A number of treatments are used in an effort to relieve itching, and there is no consensus on which method is most effective. Although they are widely used, there is no strong evidence that antihistamines, such as diphenhydramine (Benadryl), relieve opioid-induced pruritus (Grape & Schug, 2008). Patients may report being less bothered by itching after taking an antihistamine, but this is likely the result of sedating effects (Ho & Gan, 2009). Sedation can be problematic in those already at risk for excessive sedation, such as postoperative patients, as this can lead to life-threatening respiratory depression (Anwari & Iqbal, 2003). Thus, careful monitoring of sedation levels is recommended when antihistamines are combined with opioid administration, and they should not be administered if patients are excessively sedated.

Opioid antagonists (e.g., naloxone [Narcan]) and agonist-antagonists (e.g., nalbuphine [Nubain]) are sometimes used to treat pruritus; however, this practice risks reversal of analgesia if the administered doses are too high. Pain must be monitored closely when opioid antagonists are used. Numerous studies have shown that serotonin receptor antagonists, such as ondansetron, dolasetron, and granisetron, prevent pruritus caused by intraspinal opioids (Charuluxananan, Somboonviboon, Kyokong, & Nimcharoendee, 2000; Gurkan & Toker, 2002; Henry, Tetzlaff, & Steckner, 2002; Iatrou et al., 2005; Pirat, Tuncay, Torgay, Candan, & Arslan, 2005). A common clinical observation is that postoperative patients with opioid-induced pruritus also have well-controlled pain, tolerate a small reduction in opioid dose without any loss of analgesia, and experience a significant reduction or resolution of their pruritus (Pasero, Quinn et al., 2011). This should be considered prior to or in conjunction with pharmacologic treatment.

Although the opioid doses commonly used for pain management rarely cause hypotension (Ho & Gan, 2009), when it does occur, it is more likely to be in individuals with high sympathetic tone, such as those with pain or poor cardiac function, or in patients who are hypovolemic. In fact, addressing pain is important because pain may be contributing to hemodynamic instability. In other words, opioids should not be withheld for fear of causing hypotension. When hypotension is a concern, it can be minimized by administering the opioid slowly, keeping the patient supine, and optimizing intravascular volume (Harris & Kotob, 2006; Ho & Gan, 2009). Therapy can begin with a small dose while closely observing patient response. Administration of opioids via slow IV infusion may be appropriate in some patients (Harris & Kotob, 2006).

40. Are there any long-term adverse effects of opioid analgesics?

Surprisingly, little is known about the long-term effects of opioid analgesics; most of the literature that exists discusses the effects of chronic opioid use in individuals with persistent pain (Pasero, Quinn et al., 2011). The effect of opioids on immune function has been studied in animals and in humans in the absence of pain and has been found to suppress immune function; however, in the presence of acute pain, opioid administration in analgesic doses seems to be protective (Page, 2005). Much less is known about the effect on the immune system of prolonged opioid administration in the presence of persistent pain. It is well-known that pain itself suppresses immune function; opioids in analgesic doses could provide relief of pain and thereby provide some relief of the immune suppression of pain (Page, 2005).

Negative effects of opioids on the endocrine system have been known for years, but little has been written about this (Pasero, Quinn et al., 2011). Most of the literature concerns opioid-induced hypogonadism, which is probably common in both male and female patients on long-term opioid therapy (Katz & Mazer, 2009). No standards for laboratory monitoring exist but recommendations include testing for total and free testosterone (especially in men) and monitoring bone density. Symptoms include decreased libido, erectile dysfunction in men, depression, anxiety, and fatigue. Of course, these symptoms may be due to many

other causes, such as pain itself. Treatment considerations include opioid rotation (switching to another opioid) and testosterone supplementation. Based on available information, it is not reasonable to withhold opioid therapy because of concerns about endocrine effects of long-term opioid use. These can be monitored and treated.

41. How should sedation be assessed during opioid administration?

The observation that excessive sedation precedes opioid-induced respiratory depression (Abou Hammoud et al., 2009) indicates that systematic sedation assessment is an essential aspect of the care of opioid-naïve patients receiving opioid therapy (Nisbet & Mooney-Cotter, 2009; Pasero, 2009b). The importance of monitoring sedation to prevent clinically significant respiratory depression cannot be overemphasized.

Nursing assessment of opioid-induced sedation is convenient, inexpensive, and takes minimal time to perform (Pasero, 2009b). PACU nurses often use scoring systems (e.g., Aldrete) that include level of consciousness to determine readiness for discharge, which is acceptable; however, a simple, easy-to-understand sedation scale that includes what should be done at each level of sedation should be used for ongoing assessment of opioid-induced sedation after the patient has been transferred to the clinical unit. The use of such a scale will help to enhance accuracy and consistency of assessment and treatment, will help to monitor trends, and will help to communicate effectively between members of the healthcare team. A commonly used sedation scale on clinical units is the Pasero Opioid-Induced Sedation Scale (POSS) (Box 5-1). Note that the POSS links nursing interventions to the various levels of sedation. Research has shown that nurses find this approach helpful in making the appropriate decisions on how to proceed with opioid treatment (Nisbet & Mooney-Cotter, 2009).

42. Does a patient's level of sedation correspond with pain relief?

The presence of sedation does not necessarily mean that patients are comfortable, and despite being excessively sedated, some patients will report pain (Pasero, Quinn et al., 2011). Further, sleep during opioid titration is not normal sleep but primarily the result of the sedative effects of the opioid (Paqueron et al., 2002). Opioid doses should *not* be increased (titration should be stopped) in patients who are excessively sedated. A multimodal approach that administers both acetaminophen and an NSAID preoperatively, or, at the latest, on

BOX 5-1. Pasero Opioid-Induced Sedation Scale (POSS) With Interventions[1]

S = Sleep, easy to arouse
  Acceptable; no action necessary; may increase opioid dose if needed.
1 = Awake and alert
  Acceptable; no action necessary; may increase opioid dose if needed.
2 = Slightly drowsy, easily aroused
  Acceptable; no action necessary; may increase opioid dose if needed.
3 = Frequently drowsy, arousable, drifts off to sleep during conversation
  Unacceptable; monitor respiratory status and sedation level closely until sedation level is stable at less than 3 and respiratory status is satisfactory; decrease opioid dose 25–50%[2] or notify primary[3] or anesthesia provider for orders; consider administering a nonsedating, opioid-sparing nonopioid, such as acetaminophen or a NSAID, if not contraindicated; ask patient to take deep breaths every 15–30 minutes.
4 = Somnolent, minimal or no response to verbal and physical stimulation
  Unacceptable; stop opioid; consider administering naloxone[4,5]; call Rapid Response Team (Code Blue); stay with patient, stimulate, and support respiration as indicated by patient status; notify primary[3] or anesthesia provider; monitor respiratory status and sedation level closely until sedation level is stable at less than 3 and respiratory status is satisfactory.

[1] Copyright 1994, Chris Pasero. Used with permission. Reliability and validity information for the POSS can be found in Nisbet & Mooney-Cotter, 2009.
[2] Opioid analgesic orders or a hospital protocol should include the expectation that a nurse will decrease the opioid dose if a patient is excessively sedated.
[3] For example, the physician, nurse practitioner, advanced practice nurse, or physician assistant responsible for the pain management prescription.
[4] For adults experiencing respiratory depression, mix 0.4 mg of naloxone and 10 mL of normal saline in syringe and administer this dilute solution very slowly (0.5 mL over 2 minutes) while observing the patient's response (titrate to effect).
[5] Hospital protocols should include the expectation that a nurse will administer naloxone to any patient suspected of having life-threatening, opioid-induced sedation and respiratory depression.

admission to the PACU, will facilitate the management of pain in these high-risk and challenging patients.

43. How can clinically significant opioid-induced respiratory depression be prevented?

Clinically significant opioid-induced respiratory depression can be prevented by careful opioid titration and close monitoring by the nurse of sedation and respiratory status (Pasero, 2009b). Opioid-induced sedation and respiratory depression are dose-related, suggesting that opioid orders and hospital protocols should include the expectation that nurses will stop titration or promptly decrease the opioid dose whenever excessive sedation is detected. Routine administration of nonsedating analgesics as part of a multimodal approach initiated preoperatively or as soon as the patient is started on opioid therapy is essential to help prevent excessive sedation from occurring later in the course of care (Pasero, Quinn et al., 2011). In all patients with elevated risk, starting opioid doses should be decreased 25–50%. Continuous mechanical monitoring (e.g., pulse oximetry or

capnography [$ETCO_2$]) may also be indicated in some patients with high risk factors (Box 2).

44. What is the correct technique for administering naloxone to reverse opioid-induced respiratory depression?

If it is necessary to use naloxone to reverse clinically significant respiratory depression, it should be titrated very carefully (APS, 2008). Sometimes, more than one dose of naloxone is necessary because naloxone has a shorter duration (1 hour in most patients) than most opioids; however, giving too much naloxone or giving it too fast can precipitate severe pain that is extremely difficult to control and can increase sympathetic activity leading to hypertension, tachycardia, ventricular dysrhythmias, pulmonary edema, and cardiac arrest (Brimacombe, Archdeacon, Newell, & Martin, 1991; O'Malley-Dafner & Davies, 2000). Hospital protocols and opioid orders should include the expectation that nurses will administer naloxone in accordance with the procedure described in the footnotes of Box 1 whenever a patient is found to have clinically significant opioid-induced

BOX 5-2. Risk Factors for Opioid-Induced Respiratory Depression

---

Patient may have any one or more of the following to be considered high risk:
- Opioid naïvety (patients who have not been taking regular daily doses of opioids for several days)
- Older age (e.g., ≥65 years[1])
- Obesity (e.g., BMI ≥35 kg/m²)
- Obstructive sleep apnea (OSA)[2]
- History of snoring or witnessed apneas[2]
- Excessive daytime sleepiness[2]
- Preexisting pulmonary disease or dysfunction (e.g., chronic obstructive pulmonary disease [COPD])
- Major organ failure
- Smoker
- American Society of Anesthesiologists (ASA) Patient Status Classification 3, 4, or 5 in surgical patients (level determined by anesthesia provider preoperatively)
  - Classification 3: A patient that has a severe systemic disease.
  - Classification 4: A patient with severe systemic disease that is a constant threat to life.
  - Classification 5: A moribund patient who is not expected to survive without the operation.
- Increased opioid dose requirement
  - Opioid-naïve patients who require more than 10 mg morphine equivalent in a short period of time (e.g., in the PACU)[3,4]
  - Opioid-tolerant patients who are given a significant amount of opioid in addition to their usual amount, such as the patient who takes an opioid analgesic preoperatively for persistent pain and receives several IV opioid bolus doses in the PACU followed by high-dose IV PCA for ongoing acute postoperative pain[4]
- Pain is controlled after a period of poor control
- Prolonged surgery
- Thoracic and other large incisions that may interfere with adequate ventilation
- Concomitant administration of sedating agents, such as benzodiazepines, anxiolytics, or antihistamines
- Large single bolus techniques (e.g., single-injection neuraxial morphine)
- Continuous opioid infusion in opioid-naïve patients (e.g., IV PCA with basal rate [background infusion] or epidural continuous infusion)
- Naloxone administration: Patients who are given naloxone for clinically significant respiratory depression are at risk for repeated respiratory depression; another dose of naloxone may be needed as early as 30 minutes after the first dose because the duration of naloxone is shorter than the duration of most opioids.

Copyright 2010, Chris Pasero. Used with permission.

[1] There is no consensus on what age constitutes "older;" some cite it as over 65 years and others cite it as over 75 years. It is important to consider the patient's general health and condition in addition to age.

[2] Most people with OSA do not know they have the condition; therefore, all patients and particularly their family members should be asked on admission if the patient snores or has apneic episodes during sleep or is excessively sleepy during the day. Other risk factors for OSA should be assessed as well (ASA, 2006).

[3] Patients who require 20 mg or more of morphine are at very high risk for opioid-induced sedation and clinically significant respiratory depression (Abou Hammoud et al., 2009).

[4] It is recommended that patients be watched closely for at least 3 hours past the peak concentration of the last opioid dose (APS, 2008).

Reference: Opioid analgesics. In C. Pasero & M. McCaffery, *Pain assessment and pharmacologic management.* St. Louis, MO: Mosby.

respiratory depression. In physically dependent patients, withdrawal syndrome can be precipitated by naloxone administration; patients who have been receiving opioids for more than 1 week may be exquisitely sensitive to antagonists (APS, 2008).

45. What information about pain control should be included in handoff communication?

A comprehensive report about the patient's pain and measures that have been taken to get it under control in addition to the customary information about the patient's surgical procedure and general condition is essential to communicate when care is transferred from one nurse to another. If indicated, it is important to include the patient's risk factors for respiratory depression (Box 2). For example, high opioid doses intraoperatively or in the PACU, a history of snoring or apnea, and prolonged surgery are significant risk factors and should be included in the report, so that the nurse on the clinical unit can prepare for appropriate close monitoring of the patient. It may be necessary in some cases to arrange transfer to a unit that can provide the needed monitoring if it is discovered that the intended clinical unit is unable to provide it.

Complete pain control on admission to the clinical unit for all patients is an unrealistic and dangerous expectation. All team members must appreciate that it may take time after transfer to the clinical unit to establish optimal pain control in patients who had severe pain on admission to the PACU; the primary objective is to provide both effective and safe analgesia (Pasero, Quinn et al., 2010). The PACU nurse should inform the nurse assuming care of the patient on the clinical unit about the patient's pain rating goal, how close the patient is to achieving it, what has been done thus far to achieve it (e.g., analgesics, doses, and time of administration), and how well the patient has tolerated analgesic administration (adverse effects).

REFERENCES

Abou Hammoud, H., Simon, N., Urien, S., Riou, B., Lechat, P., Aubrun, F. (2009). Intravenous morphine titration in immediate postoperative pain management: Population kinetic-pharmacodynamic and logistic regression analysis. *Pain, 144*(1–2), 139–146.

Achariyapota, V., & Titapant, V. (2008). Relieving perineal pain after perineorrhaphy by diclofenac rectal suppositories: A randomized double-blinded placebo-controlled trial. *Journal of the Medical Association of Thailand, 91*(6), 799–804.

Allegri, M., Baldi, C., Pitino, E., Cusato, M., Regazzi, M., & Braschi, A. (2009). An accidental intravenous infusion of ropivacaine without any adverse effects. *Journal of Clinical Anesthesia, 21*(4), 312–313.

American Pain Society. (2005). *Guideline for the management of cancer pain in adults and children.* Glenview, IL: Author.

American Pain Society. (2008). *Principles of analgesic use in the treatment of acute pain and cancer pain* (6th ed.). Glenview, IL: American Pain Society.

American Society for Pain Management Nursing (ASPMN). (2002). ASPMN position statement: Pain management in patients with addictive disease. Lenexa, KS: ASPMN. Retrieved form http://ASPMN.org

American Society of Addiction Medicine. (2001). Definitions related to the use of opioids for the treatment of pain: Consensus statement of the American Academy of Pain Medicine, the American Pain Society, and the American Society of Addiction Medicine. Retrieved from http://www.asam.org/DefinitionsRelatedtoUseofOpioidsforTreatmentofPain.html

American Society of Anesthesiologists. (2004). Practice guidelines for acute pain management in the perioperative setting. *Anesthesiology, 100*(6), 1573–1581.

American Society of Anesthesiologists. (2006). Practice guidelines for the perioperative management of patients with obstructive sleep apnea. *Anesthesiology, 104*(5), 1081–1093.

American Society of PeriAnesthesia Nurses. (2006). ASPAN's evidence-based clinical practice guideline for the prevention and/or management of PONV/PDNV. *Journal of Perianesthesia Nursing, 21*(4), 230–250.

Anwari, J. S., & Iqbal, S. (2003). Antihistamines and potentiation of opioid induced sedation and respiratory depression. *Anaesthesia, 58*(5), 494–495.

Arbour, C., & Gelinas, C. (2009). Are vital signs valid indicators of pain in postoperative cardiac surgery ICU adults? *Intensive & Critical Care Nursing, 26*(2), 83–90.

Ashraf, W., Wong, D. T., Ronayne, M., & Williams, D. (2004). Guidelines for preoperative administration of patients' home medications. *Journal of Perianesthesia Nursing, 19*(4), 228–233.

Aubrun, F., Langeron, O., Quesnel, C., Saillant, G., Coriat, P., & Riou, B. (2003). Relationships between measurement of pain using visual analog score and morphine requirements during postoperative intravenous morphine titration. *Anesthesiology, 98*(6), 1415–1421.

Aubrun, F., Monsel, S., Langeron, O., Coriat, P., & Riou, B. (2002). Postoperative titration of intravenous morphine in the elderly patient. *Anesthesiology, 96*(1), 17–23.

Aubrun, F., & Riou, B. (2004). In reply to correspondence. *Anesthesiology, 100*(3), 745.

Azer, M. S., Abdelhalim, S. M., & Elsayed, G. G. (2006). Preemptive use of pregabalin in postamputation limb pain in cancer hospital: A randomized, double-blind, placebo-controlled, double dose study. *European Journal of Pain, 10*(1), S98.

Bagri, A. S., Rico, A., & Ruiz, J. G. (2008). Evaluation and management of the elderly patient at risk for postoperative delirium. *Clinics in Geriatric Medicine, 24*(4), 667–686.

Bahar, M. M., Jangjoo, A., Soltani, E., Armand, M., & Mozaffari, S. (2010). Effect of preoperative rectal indomethacin on postoperative pain reduction after open cholecystectomy. *Journal of Perianesthesia Nursing, 25*(1), 3–6.

Bannwarth, B., & Pehourcq, F. (2003). Pharmacologic basis for using paracetamol: Pharmacokinetics and pharmacodynamic issues. *Drugs, 63*(2), 5–13.

Blumstein, H. A., & Moore, D. (2003). Visual analog pain scores do not define desire for analgesia in patients with acute pain. *Academic Emergency Medicine, 10*(3), 211–214.

Brimacombe, J., Archdeacon, J., Newell, S., & Martin, J. (1991). Two cases of naloxone-induced pulmonary oedema: The possible use of phentolamine in management. *Anesthesia Intensive Care, 19*(4), 578–580.

Brogly, N., Wattier, J. M., Andrieu, G., Peres, D., Robin, E., Kipnis, E., et al. (2008). Gabapentin attenuates late but not early postoperative pain after thyroidectomy with superficial cervical plexus block. *Anesthesia & Analgesia, 107*(5), 1720–1725.

Buvanendran, A., Kroin, J. S., Della Valle, C. J., Kari, M., Moric, M., & Tuman, K. J. (2010). Perioperative oral pregabalin reduces chronic pain after total knee arthroplasty: A prospective, randomized, controlled trial. *Anesthesia & Analgesia, 110*(1), 199–207.

Carli, F., Mayo, N., Klubien, K., Schricker, T., Trudel, J., & Belliveau, P. (2002). Epidural analgesia enhances functional exercise capacity and health-related quality of life after colonic surgery. *Anesthesiology, 97*(3), 540–549.

Carroll, I. R., Angst, M. S., & Clark, J. F. (2004). Management of perioperative pain in patients chronically consuming opioids. *Regional Anesthesia Pain Medicine, 29*(6), 576–591.

Carvalho, B., Riley, E., Cohen, S. E., Gambling, D., Palmer, C., Huffnagle, H. J., et al. (2005). Single-dose, sustained-release epidural morphine in the management of postoperative pain after elective cesarean delivery: Results of a multicenter randomized controlled study. *Anesthesia & Analgesia, 100*(4), 1150–1158.

Charuluxananan, S., Somboonviboon, W., Kyokong, O., & Nimcharoendee, K. (2000). Ondansetron for treatment of intrathecal morphine-induced pruritus after cesarean delivery. *Regional Anesthesia Pain Medicine, 25*(5), 535–539.

Compton, P. (1999). Substance abuse. In M. McCaffery & C. Pasero (Eds.), *Pain: Clinical manual* (2nd ed., pp. 429–466). St. Louis, MO: Mosby.

Covino, B. G., & Wildsmith, J. A. W. (1998). Clinical pharmacology of local anesthetic agents. In M. J. Cousins & P. O. Bridenbaugh (Eds.), *Neural blockade in clinical anesthesia and management of pain* (pp. 97–128). Philadelphia: Lippincott.

Dabu-Bondoc, S., Franco, S. A., & Sinatra, R. S. (2009). Neuraxial analgesia with hydromorphone, morphine, and fentanyl: Dosing and safety guidelines. In R. S. Sinatra, O. A. de Leon-Casasola, B. Ginsberg, & E. R. Viscusi (Eds.), *Acute pain management* (pp. 230–244). Cambridge, NY: Cambridge University Press.

Dahl, J. B., & Møiniche, S. (2004). Pre-emptive analgesia. *British Medical Bulletin, 71*(1), 13–27.

Fishbain, D. A., Cole, B., Lewis, J., Rosomoff, H. L, & Rosomoff, R. S. (2008). What percentage of chronic nonmalignant pain patients exposed to chronic opioid analgesic therapy develop abuse/addiction and/or aberrant drug-related behaviors? A structured evidence-based review. *Pain Medicine, 9*(4), 444–459.

Forrest, J. B., Camu, F., Greer, I. A., Kehlet, H., Abdalla, M., Bonnet, F., et al. (2002). Ketorolac, diclofenac, and ketoprofen are equally safe for pain relief after major surgery. *British Journal of Anaesthesia, 88*(2), 227–233.

Gagliese, L., Gauthier, L. R., Macpherson, A. K., Jovellanos, M., & Chan, V. W. (2008). Correlates of postoperative pain and intravenous patient-controlled analgesia use in younger and older surgical patients. *Pain Medicine, 9*(3), 299–314.

Gan, T. J., Meyer, T., Apfel, C. C., Chung, F., Davis, P. J., Eubanks, S., et al. (2003). Consensus guidelines for managing postoperative nausea and vomiting. *Anesthesia & Analgesia, 97*(1), 62–71.

Gan, T. J, Meyer, T., Apfel, C. C., Chung, F., Davis, P. J., Habib, A. S., et al. (2007). Society for Ambulatory Anesthesia guidelines for the management of postoperative nausea and vomiting. *Anesthesia & Analgesia, 105*(6), 1615–1628.

Gelinas, C., & Arbour, C. (2009). Behavioral and physiologic indicators during a nociceptive procedure in conscious and unconscious mechanically-ventilated adults: Similar or different? *Journal of Critical Care, 24*(4), e7–17.

Gelinas, C., Fillion, L., Puntillo, K. A., Viens, C., & Fortier, M. (2006). Validation of critical-care pain observation tool. *American Journal of Critical Care, 15*(4), 420–427.

Gelinas, C., Harel, F., Fillion, L., Puntillo, K. A., & Johnston, C. (2009). Sensitivity and specificity of the critical-care pain observation tool for the detection of pain in intubated adults after cardiac surgery. *Journal of Pain Symptom Management, 37*(1), 58–67.

Gelinas, C., & Johnston, C. (2007). Pain assessment in the critically ill ventilated adult: Validation of the CPOT. *Clinical Journal of Pain, 23*(6), 497–505.

Gilron, I. (2006). Review article: The role of anticonvulsant drugs in postoperative pain management: A bench-to-bed-side perspective. *Canadian Journal of Anesthesia, 53*(6), 562–571.

Grape, S., & Schug, S. A. (2008). Epidural and spinal analgesia. In P .E. Macintyre, S. M. Walker, & D. J. Rowbotham (Eds.), *Clinical pain management. Acute pain* (pp. 255–270). London: Hodder Arnold.

Gurkan, Y., & Toker, K. (2002). Prophylactic ondansetron reduces the incidence of intrathecal fentanyl-induced pruritus. *Anesthesia & Analgesia, 96*(6), 1763–1766.

Hadjistavropolous, T., Herr, K., Turk, D., Fine, P. G., Dworkin, R. H., Helme, R., et al. (2007). An interdisciplinary expert consensus statement on assessment of pain in older persons. *Clinical Journal of Pain, 23*(1), S1–S43.

Hanks, G., Cherny, N. I., & Fallon, M. (2004). Opioid analgesic therapy. In D. Doyle, G. Hanks, N. I. Cherny, & K. Calman (Eds.), *Oxford textbook of palliative medicine* (3rd ed., pp. 316–341). New York: Oxford Press.

Hanks, G., Roberts, C. J. C., & Davies, A. N. (2004). Principles of drug use in palliative medicine. In D. Doyle, G. Hanks, N. I. Cherny, & K. Calman (Eds.), *Oxford textbook of palliative medicine* (3rd ed., pp. 213–225). New York: Oxford Press.

Harris, J. D., & Kotob, F. (2006). In O. A. de Leon-Casasola (Ed.), *Cancer pain. Pharmacological, interventional and palliative care approaches* (pp. 207–234). Philadelphia: Saunders Elsevier.

Heitz, J. W., & Viscusi E. R. (2009). Novel analgesic drug delivery systems for acute pain management. In R. S. Sinatra, O. A. de Leon-Casasola, B. Ginsberg, & E. R. Viscusi (Eds.), *Acute pain management* (pp. 323–331). Cambridge, NY: Cambridge University Press.

Helstrom, J., & Rosow, C. E. (2006). Nonsteroidal anti-inflammatory drugs in postoperative pain. In G. Shorten, D. B. Carr, D. Harmon, M. M. Puig, & J. Browne (Eds.), *Postoperative pain management: An evidence-based guide to practice* (pp. 161–181). Philadelphia: Saunders Elsevier.

Henry, A., Tetzlaff, J. E., & Steckner, K. (2002). Ondansetron is effective in treatment of pruritus after intrathecal fentanyl. *Regional Anesthesia & Pain Medicine, 27*(5), 538–539.

Herr, K., Coyne, P. J., Key, T., Manworren, R., McCaffery, M., Merkel, S., et al. (2006). Pain assessment in the nonverbal patient: Position statement with clinical practice recommendations. *Pain Management Nursing, 7*(2), 44–52.

Ho, K. T., & Gan, T. J. (2009). Opioid-related adverse effects and treatment options. In R. S. Sinatra, O. A. de Leon-Casasola, B. Ginsberg, & E. R. Viscusi (Eds.), *Acute pain management* (pp. 406–415). Cambridge, NY: Cambridge University Press.

Ho, K. Y., Gan, T. J., & Habib, A. S. (2006). Gabapentin and postoperative pain—a systematic review of randomized controlled trials. *Pain, 126*(1–3), 91–101.

Hurley, R. W., Cohen, S. P., Williams, K. A., Rowlingson, A. J., & Wu, C. L. (2006). The analgesic effects of perioperative gabapentin on postoperative pain: A meta-analysis. *Regional Anesthesia & Pain Medicine, 31*(3), 237–247.

Iatrou, C. A., Dragoumanis, C. K., Vogiatzaki, T. D., Vretzakis, G. I., Simopoulos, C. E., & Dimitriou, V. K. (2005). Prophylactic intravenous ondansetron and dolasetron in intrathecal morphine-induced pruritus: A randomized, double-blinded, placebo-controlled study. *Anesthesia & Analgesia, 101*(5), 1516–1520.

International Association for the Study of Pain. (1994). Part III: Pain terms, a current list with definitions and notes on usage. In H. Merskey & N. Bodduk (Eds.), *Classifications of chronic pain* (2nd ed., pp. 209–214). Seattle, WA: IASP Press. Retrieved from http://www.iasp-pain.org/AM/Template.cfm?Section=Pain_Defi...isplay.cfm&ContentID=1728

Jackson, K. C. (2009). Opioid pharmacology. In H. S. Smith (Ed.), *Current therapy in pain* (pp. 78–84). Philadelphia: Saunders Elsevier.

Jorgensen, H., Wetterslev, J., Møiniche, S., & Dahl, J. B. (2000). Epidural local anaesthetics versus opioid-based analgesic regimens for postoperative gastrointestinal paralysis, PONV and pain after abdominal surgery. *Cochrane Database of Systematic Reviews, 1*, CD001893. doi: 10.1002/14651858.CD001893

Katz, N., & Mazer, N. A. (2009). The impact of opioids on the endocrine system. *Clinical Journal of Pain, 25*(2), 170–175.

Keïta, H., Tubach, F., Maalouli, J., Desmonts, J. M., & Mantz, J. (2008). Age-adapted morphine titration produces equivalent analgesia and adverse effects in younger and older patients. *European Journal of Anaesthesiology, 25*(5), 352–356.

Kelly, D. J., Ahmad, M., & Brull, S. J. (2001). Preemptive analgesia II: Recent advances and current trends. *Canadian Journal of Anesthesia, 48*(11), 1091–1101.

Laine, L., White, W. B., Rostom, A., & Hochberg, M. (2008). COX-2 selective inhibitors in the treatment of osteoarthritis. *Seminars in Arthritis & Rheumatism, 38*(3), 165–187.

Launay-Vacher, V., Karie, S., Fau, J. B., Izzedine, H., & Deray, G. (2005). Treatment of pain in patients with renal insufficiency: The World Health Organization three-step ladder adapted. *The Journal of Pain, 6*(3), 137–148.

Lee, A., Cooper, M. G., Craig, J. C., Knight, J. F., & Keneally, J. P. (2007). Effects of nonsteroidal anti-inflammatory drugs on postoperative renal function in adults with normal renal function. *Cochrane Database of Systematic Reviews, 2*, CD002765. doi: 10.1002/14651858.CD002765.pub3

Lucas, C. E., Vlahos, A. L., Ledgerwood, A. M. (2007). Kindness kills: The negative impact of pain as the fifth vital sign. *Journal of American College of Surgeons, 205*(1), 101–107.

Lvovschi, V., Aubrun, F., Bonnet, P., Bouchara, A., Bendahou, M., Humbert, B., et al. (2008). Intravenous morphine titration to treat severe pain in the ED. *American Journal of Emergency Medicine, 26*(4), 676–682.

Marret, E., Kurdi, O., Zufferey, P., & Bonnet, F. (2005). Effects of nonsteroidal antiinflammatory drugs on patient-controlled analgesia morphine side effects. *Anesthesiology, 102*(6), 1249–1260.

May, J. A., White, H. C., Leonard-White, A., Warltier, D. C., & Pagel, P. S. (2001). The patient recovering from alcohol or drug addiction: Special issues for the anesthesiologist. *Anesthesia & Analgesia, 92*(6), 1601–1608.

McCaffery, M. (1968). *Nursing Practice Theories Related to Cognition, Bodily Pain, and Man-environment Interactions.* Los Angeles: University of California, Los Angeles.

McCaffery, M., Herr, K., & Pasero, C. (2011). Assessment: Basic problems, misconceptions, and practical tools. In C. Pasero & M. McCaffery, *Pain assessment and pharmacologic management* (pp. 13–177). St. Louis: Mosby.

McCaffery, M., & Pasero, C. (1999). Assessment: Underlying complexities, misconceptions, and practical tools. In M. McCaffery & C. Pasero (Eds.), *Pain: Clinical manual* (2nd ed., pp. 35–102). St. Louis, MO: Mosby.

Meek, T. (2004). Epidural anaesthesia and analgesia in major surgery. *Current Anaesthesia & Critical Care, 15*(4–5), 239–246.

Mehta, V., & Langford, R. M. (2006). Acute pain management for opioid dependent patients. *Anaesthesia, 61*(3), 269–276.

Mitra, S., & Sinatra, R. S. (2004). Perioperative management of acute pain in the opioid dependent patient. *Anesthesiology, 101*(1), 212–227.

Miyoshi, H. R. (2001). Systemic nonopioid analgesics. In J. D. Loeser, S. H. Butler, & C. R. Chapman (Eds.), *Bonica's management of pain* (3rd ed., pp. 1667–1681). Philadelphia: Lippincott Williams & Wilkins.

Møiniche, S., Kehlet, H., & Dahl, J. B. (2002). A qualitative and quantitative systematic review of preemptive analgesia for postoperative pain relief. *Anesthesiology, 96*(3), 725–741.

Murcia Sanchez, E., Orts Castro, A., Perez Doblado, P., & Perez-Cerda, F. (2006). Pre-emptive analgesia with pregabalin in laparascopic cholecystectomy. *European Journal of Pain, 10*(1), S198.

Myles, P. S. (2004). The pain visual analog scale: Linear or nonlinear? *Anesthesiology, 100*(3), 744.

Ng, A., Parker, J., Toogood, L., Cotton, B. R., & Smith, G. (2002). Does the opioid-sparing effect of rectal diclofenac following total abdominal hysterectomy benefit the patient? *British Journal of Anaesthesia, 88*(5), 714–716.

Ng, A., Swami, A., Smith, G., & Emembolu, J. (2008). Early analgesic effects of intravenous parecoxib and rectal diclofenac following laparoscopic sterilization: A double-blind, double-dummy randomized controlled trial. *Journal of Opioid Management, 4*(1), 49–53.

Nisbet, A. T., & Mooney-Cotter, F. (2009). Selected scales for reporting opioid-induced sedation. *Pain Management Nursing, 10*(3), 154–164.

Nussmeier, N. A., Whelton, A. A., Brown, M. T., Langford, R. M., Hoeft, A., Parlow, J. L., et al. (2005). Complications of the COX-2 inhibitors parecoxib and valdecoxib after cardiac surgery. *New England Journal of Medicine, 352*(11), 1081–1091.

O'Malley-Dafner, L., & Davies, P. (2000). Naloxone-induced pulmonary edema. *American Journal of Nursing, 100*(11), 24AA–24JJ.

Ott, E., Nussmeier, N. A., Duke, P. C., Feneck, R. O., Alston, R. P., Snabes, M. C., et al. (2003). Efficacy and safety of the cyclooxygenase 2 inhibitors parecoxib and valdecoxib in patients undergoing coronary artery bypass surgery. *The Journal of Thoracic & Cardiovascular Surgery, 125*(6), 1481–1492.

Page, G. (2005). Immunologic effects of opioids in the presence or absence of pain. *Journal of Pain & Symptom Management, 29*(5), S25–S31.

Paqueron, X., Lumbroso, A., Mergoni, P., Aubrun, F., Langeron, O., Coriat, P., et al. (2002). Is morphine-induced sedation synonymous with analgesia during intravenous morphine titration? *British Journal of Anaesthesia, 89*(5), 687–701.

Pasero, C. (2009a). Challenges in pain assessment. *Journal of Perianesthesia Nursing, 24*(1), 50–54.

Pasero, C. (2009b). Assessment of sedation during opioid administration for pain management. *Journal of Perianesthesia Nursing, 24*(3), 186–190.

Pasero, C. (2010). Perioperative rectal administration of nonopioid analgesics. *Journal of Perianesthesia Nursing, 25*(1), 5–6.

Pasero, C., Eksterowicz, N., Primeau, M., & Cowley, C. (2007). ASPMN position statement: Registered nurse management and monitoring of analgesia by catheter techniques. *Pain Management Nursing, 8*(2), 48–54.

Pasero, C., & McCaffery, M. (2002). Pain in the critically ill. *Americal Journal of Nursing, 102*(1), 59–60.

Pasero, C., & McCaffery, M. (2005a). No self report means no pain intensity. *Americal Journal of Nursing, 105*(10), 50–53.

Pasero, C., & McCaffery, M. (2005b). Extended-release epidural morphine: DepoDur. *Journal of Perianesthesia Nursing, 20*(5), 345–350.

Pasero, C., & Portenoy, R. K. (2011). Neurophysiology of pain and analgesia and the pathophysiology of neuropathic pain. In C. Pasero & M. McCaffery (Eds.), *Pain assessment and pharmacologic management* (pp. 1–12). St. Louis, MO: Mosby.

Pasero, C., Portenoy, R. K., & McCaffery, M. (2011). Nonopioid analgesics. In C. Pasero & M. McCaffery (Eds.), *Pain assessment and pharmacologic management* (pp. 177–276). St. Louis, MO: Mosby.

Pasero, C., Quinn, T. E., Portenoy, R. K., McCaffery, M., & Rizos, A. (2011). Opioid analgesics. In C. Pasero & M. McCaffery (Eds.), *Pain assessment and pharmacologic management* (pp. 277–622). St. Louis, MO: Mosby.

Patanwala, A. E., Jarzyna, D. L., Miller, M. D., & Erstad, B. (2008). Comparison of opioid requirements and analgesic response in opioid-tolerant versus opioid-naïve patients after total knee arthroplasty. *Pharmacotherapy, 28*(12), 1453–1460.

Peng, P. W. H., Wijeysundera, D. N., & Li, C. C. F. (2007). Use of gabapentin for perioperative pain control—a meta-analysis. *Pain Research & Management, 12*(2), 85–91.

Pirat, A., Tuncay, S. F., Torga, A., Candan, S., Arslan, G. (2005). Ondansetron, orally disintegrating tablets versus intravenous injection for prevention of intrathecal morphine-induced nausea, vomiting and pruritus in young males. *Anesthesia & Analgesia, 101*(5), 1330–1336.

Portenoy, R. K., Farrar, J. T., Backonja, M. M., Cleeland, C. S., Yang, K., Friedman, M., et al. (2007). Long-term use of controlled-release oxycodone for noncancer pain: Results of a 3-year registry study. *The Clinical Journal of Pain, 23*(4), 287–299.

Pouzeratte, Y., Delay, J. M., Brunat, G., Boccara, G., Vergne, C., Jaber, S., et al. (2001). Patient-controlled epidural analgesia after abdominal surgery: Ropivacaine versus bupivacaine. *Anesthesia & Analgesia, 93*(6), 1587–1592.

Puntillo, K. A., White, C., Morris, A. B., Perdue, S. T., Stanik-Hutt, J. A., Thompson, C. L., et al. (2001). Patients' perceptions and responses to procedural pain: Results from Thunder Project II. *Americal Journal of Critical Care, 10*(4), 238–251.

Rawal N. (2007). Postoperative pain relief using regional anaesthesia. *Current Anaesthesia & Critical Care, 18*(3), 140–148.

Redelmeier, D. (2007). New thinking about postoperative delirium. *Canadian Medical Association Journal, 177*(4), 424.

Romsing, J., Møiniche, S., & Dahl, J. B. (2002). Rectal and parenteral paracetamol, and paracetamol in combination with NSAIDs, for postoperative analgesia. *British Journal of Anaesthesia, 88*(2), 215–226.

Schug, S. A., & Manopas, A. (2007). Update on the role of non-opioids for postoperative pain treatment. *Best Practice & Research. Clinical Anesthesiology, 21*(1), 15–30.

Seib, R. K., & Paul, J. E. (2006). Preoperative gabapentin for postoperative analgesia: A meta-analysis. *Canadian Journal of Anaesthesia, 53*(5), 461–469.

Sharma, P. T., Sieber, F. E., Zakriya, K. J., Pauldine, R. W., Gerold, K. B., Hang, J., et al. (2005). Recovery room delirium predicts postoperative delirium after hip-fracture repair. *Anesthesia & Analgesia, 101*(4), 1215–1220.

Siddik, S. M., Aouad, M. T., Jalbout, M. I., Rizk, L. B., Kamar, G. H., & Baraka, A. S. (2001). Diclofenac and/or propacetamol for postoperative pain management after Cesarean delivery in patients receiving patient controlled analgesia morphine. *Regional Anesthesia Pain Medicine, 26*(4), 310–315.

Stanik-Hutt, J. A., Soeken, K. L., Belcher, A. E., Fontaine, D. K., & Gift, A. G. (2001). Pain experiences of the traumatically injured in a critical care setting. *American Journal of Critical Care, 10*(4), 252–259.

Tiippana, E. M., Hamunen, K., Kontinen, V. K., & Kalso, E. (2007). Do surgical patients benefit from perioperative gabapentin/pregabalin? A systematic review of efficacy and safety. *Anesthesia & Analgesia, 104*(6), 1545–1556.

United States Food and Drug Administration. (2007). *Medication guide for non-steroidal anti-inflammatory drugs (NSAIDs).* Retrieved from http://www.fda.gov/cder/drug/infopage/COX2/NSAIDmedguide.htm

Vadivelu, N., Whitney, C. J., & Sinatra, R. S. (2009). Pain pathways and acute pain processing. In R. S. Sinatra, O. A. de Leon-Casasola, B. Ginsberg, & E. R. Viscusi (Eds.), *Acute pain management* (pp. 3–20). Cambridge, NY: Cambridge University Press.

Vascello, L., & McQuillan, R. J. (2006). Opioid analgesics and routes of administration. In O. A. de Leon-Casasola (Ed.), *Cancer pain. Pharmacological, interventional and palliative care approaches* (pp. 171–193). Philadelphia: Saunders Elsevier.

Vaurio, L. E., Sands, L. P., Wang, Y., Mullen, E. A., & Leung, J. M. (2006). Postoperative delirium: The importance of pain and pain management. *Anesthesia & Analgesia, 102*(4), 1267–1273.

Vila, H., Smith, R. A., Augustyniak, M. J., Nagl, P. A., Soto, R. G., Ross, T. W., et al. (2005). The efficacy and safety of pain management before and after implementation of hospital-wide pain management standards: Is patient safety compromised by treatment based solely on numerical pain ratings? *Anesthesia & Analgesia, 101*(2), 474–480.

Viscusi, E. R., Martin, G., Hartrick, C. T., Singla, N., Manvelian, G., & EREM Study Group. (2005). Forty-eight hours of postoperative pain relief after total hip arthroplasty with a novel, extended-release epidural morphine formulation. *Anesthesiology, 102*(5), 1014–1022.

Visser, E. J., & Goucke, C. R. (2008). Acute pain and medical disorders. In P. E. Macintyre, S. M. Walker, & D. J. Rowbotham (Eds.), *Clinical pain management: Acute pain* (2nd ed., pp. 410–429). London: Hodder Arnold.

Webster, L. R., & Dove, B. (2007). *Avoiding opioid abuse while managing pain.* North Branch, MN: Sunrise River Press.

Weissman, D. E., & Haddox, J. D. (1989). Opioid pseudo-addiction—an iatrogenic syndrome. *Pain, 36*(3), 363–366.

Wellington, J., & Chia Y. Y. (2009). Patient variables influencing acute pain management. In R. S. Sinatra, O. A. de Leon-Casasola, B. Ginsberg, & E. R. Viscusi (Eds.), *Acute pain management* (pp. 33–40). Cambridge, NY: Cambridge University Press.

Zakriya, K. J., Christmas, C., Wenz, J. F., Franckowiak, S., Anderson, R., & Sieber, F. E. (2002). Preoperative factors associated with postoperative change in confusion assessment method score in hip fracture patients. *Anesthesia & Analgesia, 94*(6), 1628–1632.

CHAPTER 6

Postoperative and Postdischarge Nausea and Vomiting

Jan Odom-Forren, PhD, RN, CPAN, FAAN

Postoperative nausea and vomiting (PONV) affects 20–30% of patients undergoing surgery, and the possibility of occurrence can be as high as 70–80% for high-risk patients (Apfel, Laara, Koivuranta, Greim, & Roewer, 1999). When one considers that millions of patients undergo surgical procedures each year, this translates into a significant problem for patients who experience the symptoms. PONV can lead to patient dissatisfaction with care, dehydration and electrolyte disturbance, wound tears, and patient discomfort. Postdischarge nausea and vomiting (PDNV) also affects up to 30% of patients after outpatient surgery with some patients experiencing PDNV for up to 7 days (Odom-Forren, 2009).

1. What is PONV?

PONV is nausea and/or vomiting that takes place within the first 24 hours after a surgical procedure (American Society of PeriAnesthesia Nurses [ASPAN], 2006). PONV can be further delineated, with early PONV, which occurs within 2–6 hours after surgery; late PONV, which occurs 6–24 hours after surgery; and delayed PONV, which occurs beyond 24 hours in the inpatient setting.

2. What is PDNV?

PDNV is nausea and/or vomiting that occurs after discharge from the healthcare facility following outpatient surgery. PDNV can occur in the car on the way home or while at home. Delayed PDNV occurs beyond the initial 24 hours after discharge (ASPAN, 2006).

3. How prevalent is PONV and PDNV?

PONV affects 20–30% of patients undergoing surgery, and the possibility of occurrence can be as high as 70–80% for high-risk patients (Apfel et al., 1999). PDNV affects up to one third of outpatients after leaving the healthcare facility, with some patients experiencing symptoms until the 7th postoperative day (Odom-Forren, 2009).

4. What are risk factors for PONV?

Risk factors for PONV can be divided into three categories: patient-specific, anesthetic-related, and surgery-related (Murphy, Hooper, Sullivan, Clifford, & Apfel, 2006). See Box 6-1.

Gender is an independent predictor of PONV. Females are two to three times as likely as males to suffer from PONV, although this difference does not show up until after a female has experienced puberty. Other independent predictors for PONV include nonsmoking and a history of PONV or motion sickness. Further associated factors are migraine headaches, health status as defined by the American Society of Anesthesiologists (ASA) patient classification system, and anxiety (ASPAN, 2006; Apfel et al., 1999; Gan et al., 2007; Murphy et al., 2006). The use of volatile anesthetic agents contributes to vomiting in the postanesthesia care unit (PACU) and PONV occurs twice as often with inhalation anesthetics as with propofol (Verheecke, 2003). When regional anesthesia is used, the risk of PONV significantly decreases. Postoperative use of opioids is correlated to PONV, but intraoperative

BOX 6-1. Primary Risk Factors Associated with PONV

Patient specific:
Female gender
Nonsmoker
History of PONV
History of motion sickness
Age

Anesthesia related:
Use of volatile anesthetics
Use of nitrous oxide
Postoperative use of opioids

Surgery related:
Duration of surgery
Type of surgery

Source: ASPAN, 2006; Gan et al., 2007; Murphy et al., 2006.

use of opioids is not as well understood (Murphy et al., 2006).

The duration of surgery is associated with the incidence of PONV, possibly due to the fact that longer procedures mean a longer exposure to volatile anesthetics and a larger dose of opioids intraoperatively. The type of surgery has been linked to PONV, although there is conflicting evidence regarding the site and type of surgery (Gan et al., 2007; Murphy et al., 2006). In one recent study, investigators discovered that patients undergoing neurologic, head or neck, and abdominal surgeries required antiemetic administration significantly more often than integumentary, musculoskeletal, and superficial surgeries (Ruiz et al., 2010).

Associated risks for PONV during the immediate postoperative period are pain, movement, hypotension, and blood in the stomach due to oropharyngeal bleeding or gastrointestinal procedures (Fetzer, 2010).

5. What are risk factors for PDNV?

It is presumed that risk factors for PDNV are similar to those for PONV (Murphy et al., 2006). In recent studies, researchers noted that gender, use of postoperative opioids in the PACU, PONV in the PACU, and a history of PONV were all related to the presence of PDNV (Apfel, Philip, Stader, Leslie, & Kovac, 2009; Odom-Forren, 2009).

6. What are the consequences of PONV and PDNV?

The consequences of PONV include minor symptoms such as fatigue and delay of oral nutrition. Other more serious symptoms include wound disruption, dehydration, aspiration, increased

intracranial pressure, and increased ocular pressures. PONV also contributes to poor pain management when the patient is unable to tolerate oral pain medication or refuses to take pain medication because of fear that it is the source of the PONV. Increased costs have been associated with PONV due to delayed discharge from the PACU, costs of treatment, and readmission (Fetzer, 2010). The presence of PONV can also decrease patient satisfaction with care. Consequences of PDNV have included the inability to resume normal activities of daily living, readmission to the healthcare facility, inability to eat or drink, decreased patient satisfaction with care, and inability to return to work in a timely manner. Some patients also stop taking pain medications after discharge when they believe the medications are the source of the PDNV (Fetzer, Hand, Bouchard, Smith, & Jenkins, 2005; Odom-Forren, 2009).

7. How do you assess the risk of PONV preoperatively?

National guidelines suggest that one of two risk assessment instruments can be used to assess the risk of PONV before surgery (ASPAN, 2006). The Apfel Simplified Risk Assessment Tool scores four risk factors: female gender, nonsmoking status, history of motion sickness or PONV, and use of postoperative opioids. The Koivuranta Risk Assessment Tool scores one point for each of five factors: female gender, history of PONV, history of motion sickness, nonsmoker, and surgery lasting more than 60 minutes. The risk of PONV is associated with the scores of the Apfel and Koivuranta risk assessment tools. The patient's risk for PONV increases with the number of risk factors present. Risk factors should be assessed before surgery and then management planned based on the number of risk factors and the risk of PONV (Odom-Forren, 2009). See Box 6-2.

8. What are the recommendations for preoperative antiemetic prophylaxis?

The ASPAN guideline for management of PONV and PDNV states that each patient should be assessed for risk factors that are then documented and communicated to the anesthesia team. Planning the patient's prophylaxis based on his or her risk for developing PONV is the next step. Patients with no risk factors should require no prophylactic treatment. Those patients who are at risk should have considerations for prophylaxis that include anesthesia options such as total intravenous anesthesia (TIVA), blocks, nonsteroidal anti-inflammatory drugs (NSAIDs); pharmacologic considerations; and other considerations such as hydration, multimodal pain management, and acustimulation (ASPAN, 2006).

BOX 6-2. PONV Risk Assessment Tools

Apfel Risk Assessment Tool		
Risk Assessment Score	*Risk of PONV*	
0	10%	
1	21%	
2	39%	
3	61%	
4	79%	

Koivuranta Risk Assessment Tool		
Risk Assessment Score	*Risk of PON*	*Risk of POV*
0	17%	7%
1	18%	7%
2	42%	17%
3	54%	25%
4	47%	38%
5	87%	61%

Source: Apfel, et al., 1999; Koivuranta, Laara, Snare, & Alahuhta, 1997

9. What is the anatomy and physiology of nausea and vomiting?

Nausea and vomiting are coordinated by the vomiting center located in the lateral reticular formation of the medulla oblongata of the brain. It is located near the nucleus tractus solitarius and dorsal motor nucleus of the vagus nerve (Kovac, 2000). The vomiting center is activated by the chemoreceptor trigger zone (CTZ), which is located in the area postrema near the vomiting center on the floor of the fourth ventricle (Fetzer, 2010; Golembiewski & Tokumaru, 2006). The CTZ is abundant with serotonin type-3 (5-HT$_3$), histamine type-1 (H$_1$), muscarinic cholinergic type-1 (M$_1$), dopamine type-2 (D$_2$), neurokinin type-1 (NK$_1$), and *mu*-opioid receptors (Golembiewski & Tokumaru, 2006). Stimulation of these receptor sites results in activation of the vomiting center. Stimulation of receptors in the vestibular labyrinth can activate the vomiting center via the CTZ, and peripheral input via gastrointestinal vagal nerves can stimulate the vomiting center (Golembiewski & Tokumaru, 2006). Antiemetics are given to block stimuli to these neurochemical receptor sites (Kovac, 2000).

10. What medications are used for prophylaxis of PONV?

Stimulation of serotonin type-3 (5-HT$_3$), H$_1$, M$_1$, D$_2$, NK$_1$ and *mu*-opioid receptors in the CTZ in the brainstem activates the vomiting center. Also, stimulation of receptors in the vestibular labyrinth

and peripheral input can also stimulate the vomiting center (Golembiewski & Tokumaru, 2006).

- Medications that block serotonin receptors are ondansetron, granisetron, or dolasetron.
- Promethazine or diphenhydramine can be used to block histamine receptors, and glycopyrrolate or scopolamine patches can be used for the muscarinic receptors.
- Droperidol blocks the dopamine receptor site, but must be administered judiciously based on the FDA black box warning about QT prolongation and required EKG (electrocardiogram) monitoring. Metoclopramide and prochlorperazine also block the dopamine receptor sites.
- Dexamethasone is a glucocorticoid that is typically given in conjunction with a 5-HT$_3$ blocker. The exact method of action is unknown, but it appears to be more effective when administered before induction.
- Substance P belongs to the neurokinin family of neurotransmitters and is blocked by aprepitant. Aprepitant is available orally as a prophylactic agent (Fetzer, 2010; Golembiewski & Tokumaru, 2006; Odom-Forren, 2010). See Table 6-1.

11. What are other therapeutic modalities that may be used for prophylaxis of PONV?

Supplemental oxygen therapy has been proposed to attenuate the release of 5-HT$_3$ from vagal afferent nerves as a result of intestinal hypoperfusion and ischemia (Couture, Maye, O'Brien, & Smith, 2006). Most studies indicate that it is of

TABLE 6-1. Proposed Site(s) of Action, Usual Dose, and Adverse Effects of Select Antiemetic Drugs in Adults

Antiemetic drug	Proposed receptor site of action	Usual adult dose	Duration of action	Adverse effects	Comments
Droperidol	D_2	0.625–1.25 mg IV	Up to 12–24 hrs	Sedation, dizziness, anxiety, hypotension, EPS	Monitor ECG for QT prolongation/ torsades de pointes; more effective for nausea than vomiting
Metoclopramide	D_2	25 or 50 mg IV for prophylaxis	Up to 6 hrs	Sedation, hypotension, EPS	Doses <25 mg IV are not effective for prophylaxis in adults; consider 10 or 20 mg IV for rescue if N/V is thought to be the result of gastric stasis; give slow IV push
Prochlorperazine	D_2	5–10 mg IM or IV; 25 mg PR	4–6 hrs (12 hrs when given PR)	Sedation, hypotension, EPS	
Promethazine	D_2, H_1, M_1	12.5–25 mg IM or PR; 6.25–12.5 mg IV	4–6 hrs	Sedation, hypotension, EPS	For IV administration, dilute in 10 or 20 mL of normal saline or add to a minibag and give over 10–15 min
Dimenhydrinate	H_1, M_1	1–2 mg/kg or 50–100 mg IV, IM	6–8 hrs	Sedation, dry mouth, blurred vision, dizziness, urinary retention	
Diphenhydramine	H_1, M_1	12.5–50 mg IM or IV	4–6 hrs	Sedation, dry mouth, blurred vision, dizziness, urinary retention	
Scopolamine	M_1	1.5 mg transdermal patch[a]	72 hrs[b]	Sedation, dry mouth, visual disturbances; CNS effects in elderly patients, renal or hepatic impairment	Apply at least 4 hrs before the end of surgery for prophylaxis; wash hands after handling patch

Antiemetic drug	Proposed receptor site of action	Usual adult dose	Duration of action	Adverse effects	Comments
Dolasetron	5-HT$_3$	12.5 mg IV	Up to 24 hrs	Headache, lightheaded-ness, elevated liver enzymes	More effective for vomiting than nausea
Granisetron	5-HT$_3$	5 mcg/kg–1 mg IV	Up to 24 hrs	Headache, lightheaded-ness, elevated liver enzymes	More effective for vomiting than nausea
Ondansetron	5-HT$_3$	4 mg IV	Up to 24 hrs	Headache, lightheaded-ness, elevated liver enzymes	More effective for vomiting than nausea
Dexamethasone	None	4 mg IV	Up to 24 hrs	Vaginal itching or anal irritation with IV bolus	A single dose is well tolerated
Aprepitant	NK$_1$	40 mg PO	Up to 24 hrs	Headache, elevated liver enzymes	Give within 3 hrs before induction of anesthesia

Note: 5-HT$_3$, serotonin type 3 receptor; CNS, central nervous system; ECG, electrocardiogram; D$_2$, dopamine type 2 receptor; EPS, extrapyramidal symptoms (such as motor restlessness or acute dystonia [sustained muscle contraction causing twisting or abnormal positions]); H$_1$, histamine type 1 receptor; IM, intramuscular; IV, intravenous; M$_1$, muscarinic cholinergic type 1; N/V, nausea and/or vomiting; PO, per os (by mouth); PR, per rectum.
[a]Transdermal scopolamine has not been sufficiently studied in geriatric patients and cannot be recommended for those patients.
[b]Remove the patch 24 hours after surgery. Patient should be instructed to wash the site where the patch was located, as well as his or her hands thoroughly after removal of the patch.
Source: Used with permission. From Golembiewski and Tokumaru (2006).

limited or no benefit to the patient to use increased concentrations of intraoperative oxygen; the evidence is conflicting (Couture et al., 2006). More relaxed fasting guidelines were published by the ASA in 1999. The evidence supports allowing healthy adult patients to drink clear liquids as little as 2 hours before surgery, and that it can decrease the incidence of PONV (Couture et al., 2006). Fluid administration preoperatively may decrease the incidence of PONV, but liberal use of fluids is limited to adults who are not at risk of fluid volume overload (Couture et al., 2006).

12. What medications are used for rescue of patients who have PONV or PDNV after surgery?

Other causes of PONV should be ruled out as the cause, such as hypotension. Any medication used for prophylaxis should not be used

for rescue in the PACU. The rescue medication should have the ability to block a different receptor than the medication given for prophylaxis. For delayed PDNV, common medications used include ondansetron dissolving tablets, promethazine suppository or tablets, prochlorperazine oral tablet or suppository, or a scopolamine patch (Fetzer, 2010; Golembiewski & Tokumaru, 2006; Odom-Forren, Fetzer, & Moser, 2006).

13. How should PONV or PDNV be assessed?

The ASPAN guideline recommends that nausea be assessed with a numerical rating scale, usually verbal in the PACU (e.g., 0 as no nausea and 10 as the worst nausea one can imagine). Vomiting or retching can be assessed per episode and the amount of emesis described (ASPAN, 2006).

14. What nonpharmacologic methods of management are used for PONV?

Nonpharmacologic (or complementary therapy) methods of management for the symptoms of PONV can assist in the physical and emotional healing of a patient (Mamaril, Windle, & Burkard, 2006). Typically, nonpharmacologic interventions are used in addition to pharmacologic interventions. P6 stimulation, which includes acupressure, acupuncture, and transcutaneous electrical stimulation, has performed better than placebo to manage the symptoms of nausea and to reduce the incidence of PONV (ASPAN, 2006; Fetzer, 2010; Gan et al., 2007). Aromatherapy (e.g., oil of ginger, peppermint oil, and isopropyl alcohol) has also been used to treat PONV or PDNV. Limited studies have demonstrated some improvement in symptoms, and aromatherapy was identified by the ASPAN guideline as an option with limited evidence but with little risk to the patient (ASPAN, 2006; Odom-Forren, 2010).

15. What should be included in patient education?

- How to manage fluids and food (e.g., move slowly from fluid to soft to regular diet)

- How to take medications with food to decrease the chance of nausea

- Possible medications for PONV (prescription and over the counter)

- Nonpharmacologic methods of PONV management

- When to call healthcare provider (if unable to keep fluids down for over 24 hours or if PONV persists)

REFERENCES

American Society of PeriAnesthesia Nurses. (2006). ASPAN'S evidence-based clinical practice guideline for the prevention and/or management of PONV/PDNV. *Journal of Perianesthesia Nursing, 21*(4), 230–250.

Apfel, C. C., Laara, E., Koivuranta, M., Greim, C. A., & Roewer, N. (1999). A simplified risk score for predicting postoperative nausea and vomiting: Conclusions from cross-validations between two centers. *Anesthesiology, 91*(3), 693–700.

Apfel, C. C., Philip, B., Stader, A., Leslie, J., & Kovac, A. (2009). A prediction model for post-discharge nausea and vomiting after ambulatory surgery. Paper presented at the 2009 Annual Meeting of the American Society of Anesthesiologists, San Francisco, CA. Abstract retrieved from http://www.asa-abstracts.com/strands/asaabstracts/abstract.htm;jsessionid=CFDE470C93AA37A5D89BE9524AB3AAB6?year=2009&index=1&absnum=1896

Couture, D. J., Maye, J. P., O'Brien, D., & Smith, A. B. (2006). Therapeutic modalities for the prophylactic management of postoperative nausea and vomiting. *Journal of Perianesthesia Nursing, 21*(6), 398–403.

Fetzer, S. J. (2010). Postoperative nausea and vomiting. In L. Schick & P. Windle (Eds.), *PeriAnesthesia Nursing Core Curriculum: Preprocedure, Phase I and Phase II PACU Nursing* (2nd ed.). St. Louis: Saunders Elsevier.

Fetzer, S. J., Hand, M. A., Bouchard, P. A., Smith, H. B., & Jenkins, M. B. (2005). Self-care activities for postdischarge nausea and vomiting. *Journal of Perianesthesia Nursing, 20*(4), 249–254.

Gan, T., Meyer, T., Apfel, C., Chung, F., Davis, P., Habib, A. S., et al. (2007). Society for ambulatory anesthesia guidelines for the management of postoperative nausea and vomiting. *Anesthesia & Analgesia, 105*, 1615–1628.

Golembiewski, J., & Tokumaru, S. (2006). Pharmacological prophylaxis and management of adult postoperative/postdischarge nausea and vomiting. *Journal of Perianesthesia Nursing, 21*(6), 385–397.

Koivuranta, M., Laara, E., Snare, L., & Alahuhta, S. (1997). A survey of postoperative nausea and vomiting. *Anaesthesia, 52*(5), 443–449.

Kovac, A. L. (2000). Prevention and treatment of postoperative nausea and vomiting. *Drugs, 59*(2), 213–243.

Mamaril, M. E., Windle, P. E., & Burkard, J. F. (2006). Prevention and management of postoperative nausea and vomiting: A look at complementary techniques. *Journal of Perianesthesia Nursing, 21*(6), 404–410.

Murphy, M. J., Hooper, V. D., Sullivan, E., Clifford, T., & Apfel, C. C. (2006). Identification of risk factors for postoperative nausea and vomiting in the perianesthesia adult patient. *Journal of Perianesthesia Nursing, 21*(6), 377–384.

Odom-Forren, J. (2009). *Post discharge nausea and vomiting in ambulatory surgical patients: Incidence and management strategies.* Lexington, KY: University of Kentucky.

Odom-Forren, J. (Ed.). (2010). *Postanesthesia recovery* (2nd ed.). St. Louis, MO: Elsevier.

Odom-Forren, J., Fetzer, S. J., & Moser, D. K. (2006). Evidence-based interventions for post discharge nausea and vomiting: A review of the literature. *Journal of Perianesthesia Nursing, 21*(6), 411–430.

Ruiz, J. R., Kee, S. S., Frenzel, J. C., Ensor, J. E., Selvan, M., Riedel, B. J., & Apfel, C. (2010). The effect of an anatomically classified procedure on antiemetic administration in the postanesthesia care unit. *Anesthesia & Analgesia, 110*(2), 403–409.

Verheecke, G. (2003). Early postoperative vomiting and volatile anaesthetics or nitrous oxide. *British Journal of Anaesthesia, 90*, 109.

CHAPTER 7

Thermoregulation Issues

Vallire D. Hooper, PhD, MSN, RN, CPAN, FAAN

Patients in the perianesthesia setting are commonly susceptible to thermal imbalance issues, defined as a core body temperature outside of the normothermic range of 36° to 38°C (Hooper, 2009). This chapter reviews the most common thermoregulation issues seen in the perianesthesia setting: unplanned perioperative hypothermia (UPH) and malignant hyperthermia (MH). An overview of perioperative thermoregulation and temperature measurement is also provided.

PERIOPERATIVE THERMOREGULATION

1. What are the physiologic and behavioral mechanisms involved in normal thermoregulation?

Normal body temperature is maintained between a narrow range from 36° to 38°C through physiological regulation in the core and peripheral thermal compartments. The core thermal compartment comprises 50 to 60% of body mass and is comprised of the organs of the head and trunk area. This compartment maintains a uniform temperature that typically fluctuates no more than 0.2°C (Hooper, 2009, 2010; Sessler, 2000, 2001).

The peripheral thermal compartment, consisting of the arms and legs, is more sensitive to thermoregulatory responses and environmental changes in temperature. The temperature of the peripheral thermal compartment may be 2° to 4°C lower than that of the core thermal compartment (Hooper, 2009, 2010; Sessler, 2000).

Mechanisms of normal thermoregulation are coordinated by the hypothalamus and include behavioral, endocrine, and autonomic responses. Behavioral responses include adding or removing clothing, changing location, and/or adjusting the environmental temperature or the temperature of dietary intake. The endocrine response results in a hormonal release initiating organ and tissue responses in all systems, while the autonomic response triggers changes in the peripheral circulation (vasoconstriction or vasodilatation), that result in changes in the size of the peripheral shell or vascular space (Hooper, 2009, 2010; Sessler, 2000).

2. What are the primary mechanisms associated with normal heat production?

The primary mechanisms involve an increase in metabolic rate resulting in increased heat production. Metabolic rate can be increased through the normal generation of heat from body tissues, increased work or physical exercise, and thermogenesis, which is most commonly associated with shivering in the adult (Hooper, 2010; Sessler, 2000).

3. What are the primary mechanisms associated with heat loss in the perioperative/perianesthesia setting?

The primary mechanisms of heat loss in the perioperative/perianesthesia setting include radiation, convection, conduction, and evaporation (Hooper, 2009, 2010; Sessler, 2000; Welch, 2002).

- Radiation involves the loss of heat through radiant electromagnetic waves. Accounting for 40 to 60% of all heat loss in the operating room (OR) setting, heat loss via radiation occurs as heat radiates off of all exposed skin surfaces.

- Convection accounts for 25 to 50% of all heat loss in the OR and occurs as body heat is transferred to the surrounding cooler air. This transfer can occur passively, as warm air rises off of exposed skin. The transfer can also occur actively, as air is moved across the skin surface by wind or fans (a laminar flow system), resulting in heat transfer from the body to the cooler air.

- Conduction is the direct transfer of heat from the warmer body surface to a cooler object, such as the OR table, and accounts for up to 10% of heat loss in the OR.

- Evaporation accounts for up to 25% of heat loss in the OR and occurs when a liquid is changed into a gas, which most commonly occurs as a result of exposed viscera during surgery.

TEMPERATURE MEASUREMENT

4. What is a core temperature measurement?

A core temperature is the temperature of the core thermal compartment and is the most accurate indication of temperature during periods of rapid temperature fluctuation, such as in the OR environment. Core temperature can be directly measured via the pulmonary artery, distal esophagus, and nasopharynx (Hooper & Andrews, 2006; Hooper et al., 2009).

5. What is a near-core temperature measurement?

A near-core temperature measurement is a temperature obtained from a clinically available, noninvasive site that provides an accurate reflection of a core temperature measurement (Hooper & Andrews, 2006; Hooper et al., 2009; Langham et al., 2009).

- The most accurate near-core measurement is an oral temperature taken from the right or left sublingual pocket.

- Temporal artery measurements approximate the core temperature measurement at normothermic ranges; however, the evidence supporting their accuracy at temperature extremes is inconclusive.

- Infrared tympanic thermometry **does not** provide accurate temperature measurements in the perianesthesia period.

UNPLANNED PERIOPERATIVE HYPOTHERMIA

6. What is unplanned perioperative hypothermia?

Unplanned perioperative hypothermia (UPH) is defined as a core temperature of less than 36°C (Hooper et al., 2009; Mahoney & Odom, 1999; Sessler, 2001).

7. What are the adverse effects associated with UPH?

The adverse effects associated with UPH have been associated with increased hospital costs anywhere from $2500 to $7000 (Hooper et al., 2009; Mahoney & Odom, 1999; Sessler, 2001) and include the following:

- Patient discomfort
- Untoward cardiac events
- Coagulopathy
- Increased adrenergic stimulation
- Altered drug metabolism
- Prolonged postanesthesia care unit (PACU) stay
- Impaired wound healing/surgical site infection (SSI)

8. Who is at risk for developing UPH?

Risk factors most closely associated with the development of UPH include the following (Hooper et al., 2009):

- Extremes of ages
- Systolic blood pressure less than 140 mm/Hg
- Female gender
- Level of spinal blockade

Risk factors supported by insufficient evidence but worthy of consideration include the following (Hooper et al., 2009):

- Normal or below normal body mass index (BMI)
- Procedural duration
- Amount of body surface/wound area uncovered
- Anesthesia duration
- History of diabetes with autonomic dysfunction

9. What are passive thermal care measures?

Passive thermal care measures include the following (Hooper et al., 2009):

- Application of warmed cotton blankets
- Application of reflective blankets
- Application of socks and/or head coverings

- Limiting skin exposure to lower ambient room temperature

10. What are active warming measures?

Active warming measures include the following (Hooper et al., 2009):

- Forced-air warming
- Circulating-water mattresses
- Resistive heating blankets
- Radiant heat warmers
- Negative-pressure warming systems
- Warmed, humidified, inspired oxygen

11. What can be done preoperatively to promote perioperative normothermia?

Measures that can be taken to promote perioperative normothermia preoperatively include the following (Hooper et al., 2009):

- Passive thermal care measures for all patients
- Maintain ambient room temperature at or above 24°C
- Institute active warming measures for all hypothermic patients
- Prewarming the patient for a minimum of 30 minutes

12. How should the normothermic patient be managed in the PACU?

Normothermic patients should receive the following interventions (Hooper et al., 2009):

- Assessment of temperature on admission, at least hourly while in the PACU, at discharge, and as indicated by patient condition
- Assessment of thermal comfort level (e.g., asking the patient if he or she is cold) should occur on admission, discharge, and more frequently as indicated by patient condition
- Passive thermal care measures
- Maintain ambient room temperature at or above 24°C

13. How should the hypothermic patient be managed in the PACU?

Hypothermic patients should receive the following interventions (Hooper et al., 2009):

- Application of forced-air warming system
- Assessment of temperature and thermal comfort level every 15 minutes until normothermia is achieved

- Additional adjuvant measures such as warmed intravenous fluids and humidified warm oxygen may also be considered

MANAGEMENT OF THE FEBRILE PATIENT

14. How should the febrile patient be managed in the perioperative setting?

The primary treatment of the febrile patient in the perioperative setting should be focused on the underlying cause of the fever, most likely an underlying infection. While the cause of the fever is being evaluated, the underlying debate concerns whether the fever is harmful (and should be treated with an antipyretic or patient cooling) or part of a host-defense mechanism. There is evidence that fever is a beneficial part of a coordinated defense process. Additionally, antipyretic therapy is not without risk. However, an increase of 1°C may increase metabolic rate by 13%. It is recommended that the surgical team consult to weigh the benefits and risks of the elevated temperature and treat (or not treat) based on the risk/benefit analysis (Roth, 2009).

MALIGNANT HYPERTHERMIA

15. What is malignant hyperthermia?

Malignant hyperthermia (MH) is a hereditary abnormality of muscle metabolism initiated by certain triggering agents that results in a life-threatening hypermetabolic state most commonly associated with hypercarbia and hyperpyrexia (Hernandez, Secrest, Hill, & McClarty, 2009; Hooper, 2009).

16. What are preoperative assessment findings that may indicate a predisposition for MH?

The following assessment findings may indicate a risk for developing MH (Hernandez et al., 2009; Hooper 2009, 2010):

- A history of MH (Note that 50% of those susceptible will have had a previous anesthetic event without complications.)
- A family member with a history of MH
- A history of a family member with a death related to anesthesia and/or surgery
- A history of muscle weakness or abnormality
- A history of spontaneous muscle cramps, particularly associated with infectious illness or exercise
- A history of heat prostration during physical exertion associated with environmental heat stress

- The presence of myopathies associated with MH-like syndromes
  - Duchenne muscular dystrophy
  - Central core disease
  - Myotonia
  - Other unusual myopathies

17. What laboratory tests can be used to diagnose MH?

The gold standard for the diagnosis of MH is in vitro testing using one of the following diagnostic tests. These tests, however, are available only at limited centers throughout the United States (Hernandez et al., 2009; Rosenburg, 2006):

- Caffeine-Halothane Contracture Test (CHCT)
- In Vitro Contracture Test (IVCT)
- Ryanodine Contracture Test (RCT)
- 4-Chloro-M-cresol
- Molecular genetic testing
  - Still in development
  - Requires simple blood test

18. What are the primary triggering agents for MH?

The following are considered as unsafe agents for patients at risk for developing MH and can be thought of as triggering agents for the development of MH (Malignant Hyperthermia Association of the United States [MHAUS], 2009):

- Desflurane
- Enflurane
- Halothane
- Isoflurane
- Methoxyflurane
- Sevoflurane
- Succinylcholine

19. What are perioperative strategies for the management of the patient with MH susceptibility?

Patients with a suspected tendency for MH or a confirmed diagnosis should be managed using the following strategies (Hommertzheim & Steinke, 2006; Hooper, 2008; MHAUS, 2009; Naecsu, 2006):

- May pretreat with oral dantrolene for 1 to 3 days before anesthetic administration
  - Four divided doses of 4–7 mg/kg daily
- Avoid anticholinergics and phenothiazines preoperatively
- Avoid all triggering agents

20. What are signs and symptoms of MH?

The signs and symptoms of MH may appear immediately upon exposure to a triggering agent, or may be delayed for as long as 36 hours postexposure (Hernandez et al., 2009). These signs and symptoms include (Hernandez et al., 2009; Hooper, 2009, 2010; MHAUS, 2008):

- Elevated end-tidal carbon dioxide ($ETCO_2$)
- Muscle rigidity (particularly, masseter muscle rigidity upon administration of succinylcholine)
- Tachycardia
- Tachypnea
- Mixed respiratory and metabolic acidosis
- Myoglobinuria
- Hyperkalemia
- Fevers that may exceed 110°F (43°C) (may be a late sign)

21. What are the essential elements, medications, and equipment that any unit should have on hand in preparation for an MH crisis?

The following steps should be taken to maintain adequate preparation for a MH crisis (Hooper, 2010):

- Maintain an MH cart (may be shared with the OR) containing all drugs, fluid, and equipment needed to manage an MH crisis
- Keep clear instructions on the MH cart at all times
- Post-MH treatment protocols/posters in highly prominent places
- Develop a detailed MH crisis-response plan
  - Specify roles/functions for each staff member
- Monitor and update the education of all staff at least annually
- Conduct mock MH crisis drills involving all surgical team members using simulation technology when available on a regular basis
- Have dantrolene immediately available (minimum of 36 vials; never store in a locked cabinet or in the pharmacy)
- Have arterial blood gas laboratory immediately available

Information sources:

- Malignant Hyperthermia Association of the United States (MHAUS), P.O. Box 1069, 1139 East State St., Sherburne, NY 13460-1069

  Phone: 1-607-674-7901, 1-800-98-MHAUS, 1-800-MH-HYPER (MH hotline) www.mhaus.org

- North American Malignant
  Hyperthermia Registry
  1-888-274-7899
  http://naregistry.mhaus.org

22. What is the suggested treatment for MH?

The following steps should be taken in the treatment of an acute MH crisis (Hommertzheim & Steinke, 2006; Hooper, 2009; MHAUS, 2008; Naecsu, 2006):

- Discontinue use of any triggering agents and ask for additional assistance.
- Hyperventilate patient with large tidal volumes via a bag-valve-mask system and 100% oxygen at a flow rate greater than 10 L/min.
- Halt the surgical procedure as soon as possible.
- Intubate the patient if the airway is compromised.
- Insert arterial and central venous lines.
- Obtain blood specimens for arterial blood gas and electrolyte panel to include:
  - CK,
  - Myoglobin,
  - SMA-19,
  - PT/PTT,
  - Fibrinogen,
  - Fibrin split products,
  - CBC (complete blood count), and
  - Platelets.
- Reconstitute dantrolene for injection.
  - Dissolve 20 mg in each vial with at least 60 ml of sterile, preservative-free water.
- Administer 2.5 mg/kg of dantrolene rapidly through a large-bore IV if available.
  - Repeat until signs and symptoms of MH are reversed (may take more than 10 mg/kg total dose).
- Administer sodium bicarbonate to reverse the metabolic acidosis.
  - If blood gas results are unavailable, administer 1–2 mEq/kg.
  - Once blood gas results are available, administer sodium bicarbonate to correct the base deficit using the following formula:
    - Base deficit = $0.3 \times$ weight (kg) $\times$ base excess (mEq/L)
- If $PaCO_2$ is elevated:
  - Increase tidal ventilation of patient.
  - Do not correct respiratory acidosis with sodium bicarbonate.

- If core temperature is greater than 39°C, initiate cooling measures.
  - Cover all exposed areas with towels soaked in water.
  - Cover the wet towels with ice.
  - Use cooling blankets and fans if possible.
  - Use cold gastric lavage
  - Hydrate with iced intravenous fluids
- Discontinue cooling measures when temperature drops below 38°C.
- Treat hyperkalemia with bicarbonate, glucose/insulin, and calcium.
  - Bicarbonate: 1–2 mEq/kg IV
  - Glucose/insulin:
    - Pediatric: 0.1 units insulin/kg and 1 ml/kg 50% glucose
    - Adult: 10 units regular insulin IV and 50 ml 50% glucose
    - Check glucose levels hourly.
  - Administer calcium for life-threatening hyperkalemia.
    - 10 mg/kg calcium chloride, or
    - 10–50 mg/kg calcium gluconate
- Manage dysrhythmias.
  - Usually responds to the treatment of acidosis and hyperkalemia.
  - Can be treated with amiodarone, lidocaine, procainamide, adenosine, or other drugs per advanced cardiac life support (ACLS) protocol
  - Do not treat with calcium channel blockers
- Insert Foley catheter and monitor urinary output and appearance
  - Urinary output should be greater than 1 ml/kg/hr
  - If urinary output fall to less than 0.5 ml/kg/hr, induce diuresis using furosemide (1 mg/kg) or mannitol (1 g/kg)
- Continuously monitor:
  - $ETCO_2$
  - Core temperature
  - Vital signs
  - Electrolytes
  - Blood gases
  - CK
  - Coagulation studies
  - Neurological status
  - Urine output and color
  - Other parameters as indicated

23. What is the recommended follow-up treatment for MH following the acute management stage?

The recommended follow-up treatment for MH is as follows (Hooper, 2010; MHAUS, 2008):

- Supply IV or oral dantrolene (repeat every 4 to 6 hours for up to 48 hours).
- Monitor in ICU for MH recurrence for at least 24 to 48 hours.
- Monitor for development of disseminated intravascular coagulation (DIC).
- Follow serum creatine kinase levels until normalized.
- Counsel patient and family regarding MH and further precautions (refer to MHAUS, 2008).

24. What are complications that can be associated with MH?

Possible complications associated with MH include renal failure, consumption coagulopathies such as DIC, acute heart failure and pulmonary edema, and permanent brain damage, particularly for those patients who are not promptly diagnosed and/or who reach a core temperature of 41°C or greater (Hooper, 2009).

REFERENCES

Hernandez, J. F., Secrest, J. A., Hill, L., & McClarty, S. J. (2009). Scientific advances in the genetic understanding and diagnosis of malignant hyperthermia. *Journal of PeriAnesthesia Nursing, 24*(1), 19–31.

Hommertzheim, R., & Steinke, E. E. (2006). Malignant hyperthermia—The perioperative nurse's role [Review]. *AORN Journal, 83*(1), 151–156.

Hooper, V. D. (2008). *Unplanned perioperative hypothermia: The state of the science.* Paper presented at the 27th Annual ASPAN National Conference, Grapevine, TX.

Hooper, V. D. (2009). Care of the patient with thermal imbalance. In C. B. Drain & J. Odom-Forren (Eds.), *Perianesthesia nursing: A critical care approach* (5th ed., pp. 748–759). St. Louis, MO: Saunders Elsevier.

Hooper, V. D. (2010). Thermoregulation. In L. Schick & P. E. Windle (Eds.), *PeriAnesthesia nursing core curriculum: Preprocedure, phase I and phase II, PACU nursing* (2nd ed., pp. 484–505). St. Louis, MO: Saunders Elsevier.

Hooper, V. D., & Andrews, J. O. (2006). Accuracy of noninvasive core temperature measurement in acutely ill adults: The state of the science [Review]. *Biological Research for Nursing, 8*(1), 24–34.

Hooper, V. D., Chard, R., Clifford, T., Fetzer, S., Fossum, S., Godden, B., et al. (2009). ASPAN's evidence-based clinical practice guideline for the promotion of perioperative normothermia. *Journal of PeriAnesthesia Nursing, 24*(5), 271–287.

Langham, G. E., Maheshwari, A., Contrera, K., You, J., Mascha, E., & Sessler, D. I. (2009). Noninvasive temperature monitoring in postanesthesia care units. *Anesthesiology, 111*(1), 90–96.

Mahoney, C., & Odom, J. (1999). Maintaining intraoperative normothermia: A meta-analysis of outcomes with costs. *AANA Journal, 67,* 155–164.

Malignant Hyperthermia Association of the United States. (2008). Emergency treatment for MH. Retrieved from http://medical.mhaus.org/PubData/PDFs/treatmentposter.pdf

Malignant Hyperthermia Association of the United States. (2009). Anesthetic list for MH-susceptible patients. Retrieved from http://medical.mhaus.org/index.cfm/fuseaction/Content.Display/PagePK/AnestheticList.cfm

Naecsu, A. (2006). Malignant hyperthermia. *Nursing Standard, 20*(28), 51–57.

Rosenburg, H. (2006). Malignant hyperthermia syndrome: 2006. Retrieved March 15, 2007, from http://www.mhaus.org/NonFB/Slideshow_eng/SlideShow_ENG_files/frame.htm

Roth, J. V. (2009). Some unanswered questions about temperature management. *Analgesia & Anesthesia, 109*(5), 1695–1699.

Sessler, D. I. (2000). Perioperative heat balance. *Anesthesiology, 92,* 578–596.

Sessler, D. I. (2001). Complications and treatment of mild hypothermia. *Anesthesiology, 95,* 531–543.

Welch, T. C. (2002). AANA Journal Course. *AANA Journal, 70*(3), 227.

CHAPTER 8

Fluid, Electrolyte, and Acid-Base Imbalance

Kim A. Noble, PhD, RN, CPAN

For the surgical patient, fluid balance and acid-base homeostasis are difficult goals to achieve. This chapter will provide an overview of the physiologic principles of fluid, electrolyte, and acid-base balance with relevant questions incorporated for perianesthetic patient management priorities.

FLUID & ELECTROLYTE BALANCE

The Cell

It is estimated that based on body size, our bodies can be comprised of anywhere from 75 trillion (Shier, Butler, & Lewis, 1998) to more than 300 trillion cells (Porth & Matfin, 2009). This number is not static; approximately 10 million cells die and are replaced daily (Porth & Matfin, 2009). Cells contain a variety of structural elements based on the cell's function. All cells are encased by a cell membrane, which functions to regulate the movement of substances in and out of the cell. The biggest component inside a cell is water and the movement of water, termed osmosis, is determined by the solute concentration. The cell is able to concentrate ions on either side of the cell membrane based on the function of energy-dependent pumps.

1. How does hypotension affect a patient's cellular function?

Hypotension, or shock, affects the delivery of oxygen and nutrients to each individual body cell. Cells need a constant supply of oxygen and nutrients to fuel the active, energy-dependent pumps.

Without adequate tissue perfusion, the pumps cannot maintain the concentration of ions across the cell membrane, which are needed for normal cellular function. Hypotension and the reduction in the supply of nutrients to body tissues leads to global tissue dysfunction and to symptoms that are organ-specific, such as confusion due to a decrease in blood flow to neurologic tissue.

Hypotension and decreased tissue perfusion leads to the switch from an aerobic (oxygen-dependent) metabolism to an anaerobic (oxygen-deprived) metabolism. Anaerobic metabolism causes the production of lactic acid and metabolic acidosis.

Body Water Distribution

Total body water (TBW) accounts for approximately 60% of our weight, with approximately 42 liters of fluid found in a 70 kg person (Drain & Odom-Forren, 2009). Body water is divided into two major compartments: intracellular fluid and extracellular fluid. The extracellular fluid compartment is further divided into two compartments: the interstitial fluid and intravascular fluid. Approximately two thirds of TBW is found in the intracellular space, while only one third is found in the extracellular space (Berne & Levy, 1998).

Water is in constant flux, or movement, from one compartment to another as described by the Starling forces. The Starling forces are present on either side of the capillary and their sum determines the direction of movement across the capillary membrane. The forces found inside the capillary are the primary determinants of water

Arterial End   Venous End

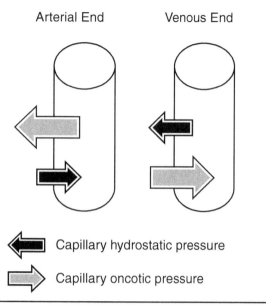

◀ Capillary hydrostatic pressure

▶ Capillary oncotic pressure

FIGURE 8-1. Starling forces

movement—the capillary hydrostatic pressure and capillary oncotic pressure. These two forces push and pull water across the capillary membrane, and the greater force determines the net direction of water movement. On the arterial end of the capillary, capillary hydrostatic, or "pump" pressure is greater and there is a net movement of water out of the capillary, called *filtration*. The fluid moves into the interstitial space and brings nutrients to the cells in that area. On the venous end of the capillary, the hydrostatic pressure declines and the greater force of capillary oncotic pressure (i.e., the pressure derived from the pull of albumin into the blood vessel), causes *reabsorption*. This leads to a net movement of fluid from the interstitial space back into the intravascular space (see Figure 1).

2. Why is my patient edematous?

There are several causes of edema in a patient:

- Increased hydrostatic pressure would be seen in the patient that has received a large volume of crystalloid replacement or when the cardiac pump begins to fail. In the example of over-hydration, the increased fluid in the vascular space moves into the interstitial space, termed "third spacing." In the case of left-sided heart failure, the failure of the left pump causes fluid to back up into the pulmonary capillary bed and fluid moves into the interstitial space surrounding the alveoli and eventually moves into the alveoli, termed pulmonary edema. The lymphatic system is responsible for collecting filtered water and returning it to the venous system. Any blockage of the lymphatic system (such as metastatic disease, venous obstruction, or the removal of lymph nodes) could lead to increased hydrostatic pressure and edema formation.

- Decreased oncotic pressure inside the vascular space can also lead to the development of edema. This would be seen in any patient with decreased serum albumin, which is the primary determinant of oncotic pressure. Decreased serum albumin is seen in patients who have either decreased production of albumin (such as nutritional deficiencies or liver disease) or protein losses (such as burns or nephrotic syndrome).

- The capillary endothelium provides a barrier to the movement of water and disease states (such as sepsis, inflammation, or allergic reactions) that could cause damage to the capillary endothelium and lead to the formation of edema.

3. How do I calculate my patient's fluid balance?

In most patients, intake should equal output; but in the perianesthetic patient, fluid balance goes beyond blood losses and intravenous fluids, as there are many factors that must be considered. Patient physical assessment should be of primary consideration, including vital signs, peripheral perfusion, and urine output. Assessment is complicated by the effects of endogenous endocrine mediators (such as catecholamines, cortisol, antidiuretic hormone [ADH], and aldosterone), sympathetic system activation with vasoconstriction and increased heart rate and blood pressure, and the impact of cool environmental temperatures and hypothermia (Drain & Odom-Forren, 2009).

Insensible fluid losses, or the losses of fluid that are not seen by the naked eye, should be considered in the calculation of fluid replacement. Exhaled air is saturated with water, and the water losses associated with breathing are increased in a cool environment. These losses are commonly prevented by the anesthesia care provider by adding humidification or heat-moisture exchangers to the ventilator circuit during the surgical procedure. Losses from vomiting and diarrhea (such as would accompany preoperative vomiting or bowel preparations) are obvious, but a significant amount of fluid can be lost through the abdominal cavity during bowel surgery. Again, this should be identified and addressed by the anesthesia care provider. Finally, insensible losses can also take place across the skin barrier and are worsened in an environment with decreased humidity.

Hormonal Regulation of Total Body Water (TBW): Antidiuretic Hormone

TBW is regulated by the hypothalamus through the monitoring of serum osmolarity within the range of 280–295 mOsm/kg (Porth & Matfin, 2009). An increase in serum osmolarity or a decrease in TBW by 1% is sufficient to cause the initiation of thirst mechanism (Berne & Levy, 1998). If thirst is ineffective, such as in the patient that is NPO for surgery, ADH is released from a stored supply in the posterior pituitary. Other triggers for the release of ADH include a decline in blood pressure and/or blood volume, nicotine, stress, anesthesia, or surgery. Alcohol inhibits the release of ADH (Porth & Matfin, 2009).

ADH, or vasopressin, travels to the distal tubule of the renal nephron and causes the insertion of water channels through plasma membranes of the distal tubular cells, literally "sucking" the water out of the tubular fluid (urine). Free water is rapidly reabsorbed, very effectively decreasing the urinary output. The corrected serum osmolarity has a negative feedback suppression on the release of ADH. Alterations in ADH secretion are relatively common in patients with neurologic injury or trauma and in patients having surgery or receiving anesthesia.

4. What is the syndrome of inappropriate ADH secretion (SIADH)?

SIADH follows the failure of the negative feedback mechanism control of the release of ADH and may result from an acute event, such as neurologic injury or surgery, or a chronic disorder like small cell or oat cell cancer of the lung or lymphatic, prostatic, or pancreatic tumors (Porth & Matfin, 2009). SIADH leads to an increase in water reabsorption from the distal tubule of the kidney, water intoxication, decreased serum osmolarity, and a very high urine osmolarity.

Symptoms of water intoxication or declines in serum osmolarity would include decreased urinary output and hyponatremia (decreased serum Na^+). Hyponatremia leads to the movement of water into cells as the dilute serum is pulled into the cells due to the higher intracellular solute concentration. Early symptoms commonly seen are neurologic, including complaints of headache or confusion, hostility, drowsiness, and seizures with the progression of cerebral edema. Patients with SIADH require ongoing monitoring of serum Na^+, sodium replacement with normal saline solution, fluid restriction, and diuresis with either mannitol or furosemide (Drain & Odom-Forren, 2009).

5. What is diabetes insipidus (DI)?

DI is caused by a decrease in the release of ADH from the posterior pituitary, causing a significant diuresis. Patients with DI have lost the ability to concentrate urine and may produce 3 to 20 liters of urine per day (Porth & Matfin, 2009). Patients with DI would present with copious urine output or a bulging urinary drainage bag. Their serum osmolarity would rapidly rise; they would have a very low urine osmolarity and an increased serum Na^+, indicating severe dehydration. Patients with DI require measurements of urine output every 30 minutes with fluid replacement geared to the replacement of water lost in the urine. ADH replacement may be used for neurogenic DI (Porth & Matfin, 2009).

Hormonal Regulation of TBW: Renin-Angiotensin-Aldosterone Secretion (RAA)

Renal function is dependent on adequate blood flow and pressure to filter and remove substances from the plasma portion of the blood. Each kidney contains 1.2 million nephrons and each is able to release the enzyme renin to autoregulate blood flow and blood pressure to maintain function. Renin has no direct effect on blood pressure, but it initiates a complex mechanism that increases both blood pressure and blood volume (see Figure 2).

Renin is released into the arteriole vessels in the distal nephron and causes the conversion of the plasma protein angiotensinogen to angiotensin I. Angiotensin I is an inactive substance that is converted to the active angiotensin II when it encounters the angiotensin-converting enzyme. This occurs almost entirely in the pulmonary capillary bed (Guyton, 1991). Angiotensin II has two effects: first, it causes

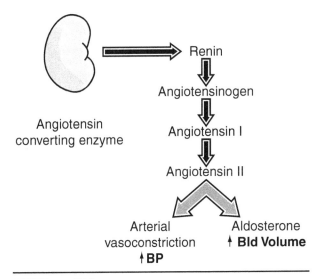

FIGURE 8-2. RAA

arterial vasoconstriction through a direct action in the smooth muscle of the arterial walls, leading to a significant increase in systemic blood pressure. Secondly, angiotensin II causes the release of aldosterone from the adrenal cortex, Na^+ (and H_2O) to be reabsorbed and K^+ excreted into the distal nephron, thus increasing blood volume. The resultant increase in blood pressure and blood volume would have a negative feedback effect and decrease the release of renin from the distal nephron.

The mechanism of aldosterone is different from ADH, but the end result is the same: Sodium and water are reabsorbed and blood volume increases. Although ACE inhibitors are primarily indicated for the treatment of hypertension, this class of drugs is also indicated to reduce the mortality associated with heart failure and as a prophylaxis for patients with significant risk for an adverse cardiovascular event. In addition to ACE inhibitors, the renin-angiotensin-aldosterone (RAA) system can be modulated with the following classes of drugs: angiotensin receptor blockers (ARBs), aldosterone antagonists, and renin inhibitors (Adams & Koch, 2010).

6. How do ACE inhibitors impact the patient after surgery or anesthesia?

There are currently 11 ACE inhibitors on the market, and they are a first line drug of choice for the treatment of hypertension (Adams & Koch, 2010). A patient taking ACE inhibitors has lost the ability to autoregulate blood pressure and blood volume. Patients receiving ACE inhibitors should have baseline vital signs and serum testing for renal function and electrolytes. These patients are at risk for orthostatic hypotension, but this risk is most commonly seen early in treatment. Patients receiving ACE inhibitors need to be well hydrated and may not tolerate mild blood losses as they have a pharmacologic inhibition of a hypotensive compensatory mechanism. Aldosterone is important for the excretion of K^+ in the distal nephron, and a decrease in aldosterone activity may predispose a patient to mild increases in serum potassium. ACE inhibitors are contraindicated in pregnancy and should be used with caution in patients with preexisting renal disease or hyperkalemia due to the risk of cardiac arrhythmias. A drug interaction may occur with the concurrent administration of ACE inhibitors and nonsteroidal anti-inflammatory drugs (NSAIDs) and lead to worsening of preexisting renal disease (Adams & Koch, 2010).

Electrolyte Balance: Sodium Regulation

Sodium (Na^+) is found in highest concentration in the extracellular space (135–145 mEq/L) and

in low concentration in the intracellular space (10–14 mEq/L) (Porth & Matfin, 2009). The concentration gradient of Na^+ across the cell membrane is maintained by the activity of the energy-dependent Na^+/K^+ ATPase pump. The ability to have differences in the ion concentrations between the extracellular fluid (ECF) and intracellular fluid (ICF) on either side of the cell membrane allows the cell membranes to be polarized or have a charge. This is the basis for most cellular activities in the human body.

Sodium and water are inversely proportional; that is, as one increases, the other decreases. Serum measurement of Na^+ can be used as an estimate of fluid balance as changes in the TBW will be seen in the serum Na^+ level. Na^+ is regulated by the secretion of aldosterone, leading to an increased reabsorption of Na^+ in the distal tubule in exchange for K^+, which would be excreted in the urine. A second mechanism for Na^+ regulation is atrial natriuretic peptide (ANP), which would be released from the atria of the heart in response to increased stretch from increased preload. ANP causes an increase in the excretion of Na^+ from the kidney, effectively decreasing preload and decreasing volume stretch on the atria.

Abnormalities in sodium balance are linked with changes in fluid balance. Overhydration, termed water intoxication, or sodium losses would lead to hyponatremia (or a serum Na^+ below 135 mEq/L) and a decline in serum osmolarity. This is one of the most common electrolyte abnormalities seen in both hospitalized and outpatients (Drain & Odom-Forren, 2009), and treatment should focus on reversal of the cause of the disorder. An increase in ADH release, termed the syndrome of inappropriate antidiuretic hormone (SIADH), would cause the reabsorption of free water from the distal kidney and hyponatremia. As mentioned previously, hyponatremia causes water to leave the extracellular space and move toward the higher solute concentration of the intracellular space. Early symptoms are related to cerebral edema and include confusion, agitation, and seizures. Patients with hyponatremia are treated with Na^+ replacement, reduced volume of intravenous fluids, diuretics, and careful recording of intake and output.

Hypernatremia, or a serum Na^+ greater than 145 mEq/L, is associated with dehydration from a reduction in oral intake (e.g., NPO status) or patients who have lost water (e.g., sweating or bowel preparations for colonic surgery). Hypernatremia from increased Na^+ intake is rare due to the rapid renal excretion of excess sodium. Hypernatremia is treated with fluid replacement.

7. What is the common presentation of hyponatremia in the PACU?

Patients who have had urologic surgery with bladder irrigation during the procedure are at risk for hyponatremia from the systemic absorption of irrigation fluid. Transurethral resection of the prostate (TURP) is the most common cause of surgical hyponatremia, as patients can absorb 10 to 30 ml/minute of irrigation fluid (Drain & Odom-Forren, 2009). Confusion is an early symptom of this disorder, and diagnosis is made by serum electrolyte analysis. Patients would be treated with the administration of diuretics and careful monitoring of intake and output.

8. What would happen if the Na^+/K^+ ATPase pump fails?

A common cause of the failure of the Na^+/K^+ ATPase pump would be present in hypotension (also known as shock) where there is not sufficient pressure to perfuse tissues and deliver oxygen and nutrients to each cell. As the single highest utilization of energy by the body is the Na^+/K^+ ATPase pump, this energy-dependent pump would no longer be able to maintain the concentration gradients of ions across the plasma membrane and cellular function would decline (Porth & Matfin, 2009). For example, with Na^+/K^+ ATPase pump failure, impulse passage (or the wave of change in polarization) would decline in neurologic tissue and patients would become confused. Other body systems would be affected as well, such as myocardial function would decline as a decrease in impulse passage would affect stroke volume, and renal function would decline as reabsorption is dependent on ion concentration gradients.

A second example of failure of the Na^+/K^+ ATPase pump can be seen with the administration of local anesthesia. Pain impulses cannot be passed by nerves that have been injected by local anesthetics because the drug inhibits the action of the Na^+/K^+ ATPase pump. Pain impulses do not arrive in the central nervous system (CNS) and are not perceived as painful with the pharmacologic interruption of the ion concentration gradients.

Electrolyte Balance: Potassium Regulation

Potassium balance is crucial for many body functions. Where Na^+ is the primary extracellular ion, potassium is the primary intracellular ion. The intracellular K^+ 140 to 160 mEq/L and extracellular K^+ 3.5 to 5.5 mEq/L is maintained by the Na^+/K^+ ATPase pump. Potassium is taken in by dietary sources and eliminated exclusively through the

action of the kidney: active excretion of potassium into the urine and the mechanism of action by aldosterone (Na^+ reabsorption in exchange for K^+ excretion in the urine).

Potassium has a large role in acid-base compensation, or the maintenance of the pH in the normal range of 7.35 to 7.45. As alterations occur in the pH in the blood, the positively charged K^+ is used as a shuttle and moves in and out of the cell in exchange for H^+ to normalize the pH.

Potassium has a large role in the contraction of nervous and muscular tissues. Alterations in the serum potassium can change impulse passage and negatively affect contraction. This is especially true in the heart as hypokalemia and hyperkalemia have very serious consequences on the ability of the heart to function as a pump.

Hyperkalemia, or a serum K^+ above 5.5 mEq/L, is rarely seen in an individual with normal renal function. Hyperkalemia is seen in three groups of patients: those with decreased renal function, patients who have received rapid K^+ replacement, and patients who have had a large scale disruption of cell membranes (e.g., crush injuries or burns) with the liberation of intracellular K^+. Hyperkalemia is most often seen in patients with a decline in renal function and the loss of excreting excess potassium. The symptoms associated with an accumulation of potassium would follow the inability to establish correct ion concentration gradients across cell membrane impacting skeletal and cardiac muscle contraction. Early in this disorder, characteristic elevations in the T waves would be seen on the electrocardiogram (ECG). These "peaked" T waves represent the inability of complete repolarization of the cardiac cycle. If the serum K^+ continues to rise, slow arrhythmias and cardiac standstill may occur.

Hypokalemia is also very dangerous for its effects on cardiac contraction. Hypokalemia is a serum potassium less than 3.5 mEq/L and may follow a reduced intake of K^+, a loss of potassium through the GI tract, kidney, or skin, or a movement of K^+ out of the extracellular fluids and into the intracellular space. A daily intake of potassium is needed to replace the daily losses of K^+ in the urine. Patients who do not have oral intake (e.g., surgical patients) need replacement of KCl. The most common cause of hypokalemia is from the increased losses of K^+ following the administration of diuretics and loss of K^+ in the urine (Porth & Matfin, 2009). Stress may also lead to the movement of K^+ from cells and the excretion of K^+ in the urine following stress hormone release. Patients with hypokalemia have abnormalities in the contraction of excitable tissue, including nausea and vomiting from the effect on GI smooth muscle; extracardiac contractions called ectopic beats; and muscle weakness, fatigue, and muscle cramping from the effect of decreased K^+ on skeletal muscle. Patients are treated with either oral or intravenous (IV) potassium replacement. IV replacement must be slow, as a rapid infusion of KCl can lead to cardiac arrest (Porth & Matfin, 2009).

9. What can be done for the acute treatment of hyperkalemia?

A temporary treatment for hyperkalemia is the IV administration of insulin, which drives the K^+ back into the intracellular space. The concurrent administration of dextrose is necessary to prevent hypoglycemia. The administration of sodium bicarbonate will also push K^+ into the cells due to an increase in the pH. Finally, the IV administration of calcium stabilizes the cell membrane and improves cardiac performance. These IV solutions are temporizing measures and are limited by time, lasting under 1 hour.

Electrolyte Balance: Calcium Regulation

The regulation and storage of calcium has a benefit not found in any other electrolyte regulation in the human body—the tremendous capacity of storage in the skeletal tissue. Approximately 99% of calcium is stored in bone, with the remaining 1% found in the intracellular compartment (Porth & Matfin, 2009). Extracellular calcium has vital regulatory functions. Calcium is derived from our dietary intake and is shuttled in and out of bone to ensure calcium homeostasis. Serum calcium is tightly regulated to be between 8.5 and 10.5 mg/dL (ionized, 1.0–1.2 mmol/L) through a negative feedback system of hormonal regulation (Porth & Matfin, 2009). When serum calcium increases from dietary intake, calcitonin is released from the thyroid gland, increasing the production of new bone until the serum calcium declines to a normal range. If serum Ca^{++} decreases, parathyroid hormone is released. Ca^{++} is maximally reabsorbed by the distal renal tubule and bone is demineralized to again normalize serum calcium. Calcium is found in the blood in three forms: bound to plasma proteins (40%); as a compound with citrate, phosphate, and sulfate (10%); and in an ionized form (50%). Ionized calcium is involved in cellular reactions, such as muscular contraction and the ability to polarize membranes by leaving the extracellular fluids. Calcium is also a very important cofactor in blood coagulation.

Hypocalcemia, or a serum calcium below 8.5 mg/dL, is associated with many forms of critical illness, estimated to be present in 70 to 90% of patients in intensive care settings (Porth & Matfin, 2009). It is considered to be a medical emergency and requires prompt IV replacement. Patients may have hypocalcemia for several reasons: they are unable to liberate Ca^{++} from boney storage; they have lost calcium from the renal tubule; or they have decreased protein binding from low serum albumin leading to an abnormal ratio between protein bound and ionized Ca^{++}. Citrate is used in banked blood as an anticoagulant, as it decreases ionized calcium and reduces clotting. Patients who have received banked blood are at risk for reduced ionized calcium due to circulating citrate. Hypocalcemia leads to twitching or tetany from a reduced neuromuscular threshold for muscular contraction. Patients may report tingling around the mouth or hands, and severe reduction of Ca^{++} is associated with laryngospasm and seizures (Porth & Matfin, 2009).

Hypercalcemia, or a serum calcium above 10.5 mg/dL, would be present if the body's ability to regulate Ca^{++} is overcome. High serum calcium is generally better tolerated than hypocalcemia, and is seen with boney malignancies or tumor of the parathyroid gland. Hypercalcemia places a patient at risk for renal calculi or pathologic fractures from bone destruction.

10. What symptoms would be present in a patient with hypocalcemia?

Severe hypocalcemia can impact myocardial contraction, leading to increased central venous pressure and hypotension. Skeletal muscle irritability may also be present with tremor and places the patient at increased risk for laryngospasm. Finally, patients with decreased serum Ca^{++} may have oozing and delayed clotting from a reduction in the activation of the clotting cascade. Hypocalcemia may be hidden in patients with renal failure due to abnormalities in fluid balance (Drain & Odom-Forren, 2009).

Fluid Replacement

Patients receiving surgery or anesthesia commonly have fluid balance abnormalities. Many factors can impact the regulation of fluid balance, including stress, NPO status, bowel preparations, blood and insensible fluid losses, or medications that lead to fluid abnormalities. Fluid losses can be replaced by either crystalloids or colloids, with research-based positive and negative aspects reported for each. Decisions for replacement should be based on the short-term treatment goals for the patient (Drain & Odom-Forren, 2009).

Crystalloid solutions contain electrolytes dissolved in fluid solutions that may or may not contain dextrose. They are freely permeable and rapidly leave the intravascular space. A variety of crystalloid solutions are available and they vary based on their electrolyte concentrations. They may reflect the normal serum osmolarity of 280 to 310 mOsm/L, called isotonic solutions; may contain more free water as compared to plasma, called hypotonic solutions; or have an increased electrolyte concentration as compared to plasma, called hypertonic solutions. Blood loss is commonly replaced using the formula: 1 ml of lost blood is replaced with 5 ml of isotonic solution, such as normal saline or lactated ringers. The replacement ratio is influenced by patient circumstances, increasing to 10 ml crystalloid for each 1 ml of lost blood volume with large traumatic injuries (Drain & Odom-Forren, 2009).

Colloid solutions contain human protein particles that are not able to cross the capillary membrane and exit the vascular space. Colloids contribute to fluid balance by influencing colloid oncotic pressure, which holds fluid within the vascular space. This class of replacement fluids tends to oppose the edema that accompanies replacement with crystalloid solutions. The volume for replacement needed for colloids is decreased because they remain in the vascular space, but they also tend to have a higher associated expense. Colloids can contribute to abnormalities in coagulation or anaphylaxis due to their protein basis. Examples of colloid solutions currently used in clinical practice include albumin (derived from human albumin), dextran 40%, and hetastarch 6% (Drain & Odom-Forren, 2009).

11. How is fluid replacement calculated for the surgical patient?

In order to accurately calculate fluid replacement, one must know the patient's weight in kilograms. The first fluid losses to be replaced are fluid losses from the patient's surgical preparation. These losses are replaced at a rate of 2 ml/kg/hour if the patient was NPO. If a bowel preparation was used, these replacement fluids would need to be increased. The second fluid to be replaced is the patient's surgical losses, based on the level of surgical trauma. The formula for replacement is as follows (Drain & Odom-Forren, 2009).

- Minimal trauma: 4 ml/kg/hr
- Moderate trauma: 6 ml/kg/hr
- Severe trauma: 8 ml/kg/hr

12. When would colloid replacement be indicated and how is colloid replacement calculated?

Colloid replacement is indicated when blood losses are above 20% of the total blood volume (e.g., 5000 ml total blood volume × 20% = losses > 1000 ml). Colloid replacement is generally milliliter for milliliter of blood loss (Drain & Odom-Forren, 2009).

Blood Replacement

Human blood contains formed elements and plasma. The formed elements include red blood cells (RBC), white blood cells (WBC), and platelets. RBCs function in the transportation of gasses from the lungs to the cells and back again. WBCs function in the prevention and treatment of infection: in the inflammatory and immune responses and in the surveillance of body cells for mutations or damage. The plasma portion of blood contains mostly water (approximately 90% by weight), plasma proteins, and other substances (such as hormones, electrolytes, gasses, or by-products of metabolism). Blood replacement may include whole blood, packed RBCs, fresh frozen plasma (FFP), platelets, or concentrated clotting factors. Additional individual blood products may be further processed (e.g., irradiated packed cells or washed or filtered cells to remove white blood cells) for sensitized individuals who are at risk for immune reactions to transfused blood products.

The human body is remarkably tolerant; up to 75% of circulating RBCs may be lost, and as long as the blood volume is supported with the administration of fluids, the patient may remain asymptomatic (Drain & Odom-Forren, 2009). The ability to pick up, transport, and release oxygen is the main function of the RBC, and when the number of RBCs declines and causes tissue hypoxia, the patient becomes symptomatic. Large volume blood replacement is not without complications and can lead to coagulopathies, fluid balance and electrolyte abnormalities, and acid-base derangements.

Red blood cells are classified in two ways. The first is based on surface antigens, which identify the blood as A, B, AB, or O (see Table 1).

The second means of classifying RBCs is by the presence of the D antigen, termed Rh factor. RBCs that contain the D antigen are called Rh-positive; individuals lacking the D antigen are Rh-negative. If persons lacking the D antigen (Rh-negative) are exposed to RBCs containing the D antigen (Rh-positive), their immune system is sensitized to the D antigen and subsequent blood exposures may lead to destruction of cells containing the D antigen (Porth & Matfin, 2009). A patient's blood

TABLE 8-1. Blood types

Blood type	RBC surface antigen	Serum antibodies	Rh factor
Type O	None (universal donor)	Anti-A & Anti-B	$+/-$ D-antigen
Type A	A	Anti-B	$+/-$ D-antigen
Type B	B	Anti-A	$+/-$ D-antigen
Type AB	AB	None (universal recipient)	$+/-$ D-antigen

type must be identified, and blood samples from the patient and the unit of blood to be used for replacement mixed to screen for incompatibilities, termed cross-matched. In the event of emergent blood replacement, blood type O is used, as it does not contain surface antigens. Blood plasma contains antibodies that identify RBCs not containing the correct antigen, and this can lead to an immune activation if a different RBC antigen is encountered.

Hemostasis (or the conversion of blood from a moving liquid to a solid stable clot) demonstrates the complex interaction of two separate components: platelets and the coagulation cascade. Platelets are a cellular fragment that is circulated in the plasma. Platelets adhere to irregular endothelial surfaces or, if exposed to underlying tissue, platelets activate, thereby releasing coagulation mediators causing a rapid clumping of platelets. The clumping and mediator release triggers the coagulation cascade and the production of a fibrin meshwork, which effectively contains and anchors the mass of platelets to the endothelial breech. An adequate number of circulating platelets and clotting factors are required to control surgical bleeding, and decreases in either component predispose the patient to have increased surgical blood loss.

A normal platelet count is 150,000 to 400,000 (Porth & Matfin, 2009). Platelet count can be depleted by abnormal bone marrow function or depletion due to clotting. Platelet replacement is recommended for platelet counts less than 100,000 (Drain & Odom-Forren, 2009), and platelet function is affected by a variety of antiplatelet agents that inhibit aggregation and clumping. Measurement of bleeding time is used to screen abnormalities for the time needed to establish a platelet clump. A normal bleeding time is 3 to 10 minutes and elevations of 1.5 times the normal place a patient at significant risk for bleeding (Drain & Odom-Forren, 2009).

The clotting cascade includes a variety of protein-based clotting factors that are produced by the liver. The clotting cascade can be activated in two ways: an extrinsic activation by the plasma coming into contact with body tissues and an intrinsic activation by damage to the capillary endothelium. Serum analysis of the coagulation cascade measures the time required for the formation of a clot and includes tests for each form of activation: prothrombin time (PT) for an extrinsic activation and partial thromboplastin time (PTT) for an intrinsic activation. Abnormalities in the clotting cascade are seen in patients with liver disease and depletion due to large-scale clotting. Deficiencies in clotting factors can be replaced with the administration of fresh frozen plasma or concentrated clotting factors.

13. What is an example of an Rh incompatibility?

An example of an Rh incompatibility is erythroblastosis fetalis, where an Rh-negative mother carries an Rh-positive infant to term, and the maternal immune system is exposed to the D antigen during birth. The mother's immune system becomes sensitized to the D antigen and with subsequent pregnancies with Rh-positive infants, the maternal Rh antibodies cross the placenta and destroy fetal Rh-positive RBCs. Rh incompatibility is prevented in an Rh-negative woman with the administration of RhoGAM, a passive immunization of banked anti-Rh antibodies to prevent the immune sensitization of the pregnant female (Adams & Koch, 2010).

14. How is blood administered?

The IV solution to use for blood administration is 0.9% normal saline. Lactated ringers contain calcium, which may cause banked blood to clot, and dextrose solutions may cause the lysis of red blood cells. An 18 gauge IV catheter is recommended, but a 20 gauge IV catheter may also be used, as well as blood filters based on hospital policy. Blood products may be warmed as indicated for the prevention of hypothermia. Blood removed from refrigeration should be hung within 30 minutes or returned to the refrigeration system. Blood products should have a maximum hang time of

4 hours, as there may be an increase in bacterial growth and RBC lysis after 4 hours. Follow hospital protocol for blood administration, but the initiation of transfusion with slow administration over the first 15 minutes with careful assessment for transfusion reaction is recommended (Miller, 2002). For adult men, the total blood volume is equal to 74 ml times their weight in kilograms. For adult females, the total blood volume is their weight in kilograms times 70 ml. Allowable blood loss (AL) can be calculated using the following formula (Drain & Odom-Forre, 2009):

$$AL = EBL \times \frac{Hb_{initial} - Hb_{target}}{Hb_{initial}}$$

15. How are platelets administered?

Platelets are obtained by plasmapheresis from a single or multiple donors in five to eight units per bag. Platelets are administered using blood tubing and may be infused rapidly as indicated. Platelets do not have a specific type or need to be cross-matched, as they do not contain surface antigens like the RBCs. Platelets need to be agitated every 10 to 15 minutes to prevent sticking to the plastic bag or tubing (Miller, 2002).

16. How is fresh frozen plasma (FFP) administered?

Fresh frozen plasma (FFP) is an excellent source of clotting factors and is indicated for a patient with prolongation of 1.5 times PT/PTT. FFP is separated from whole blood and is frozen within 6 hours. Each unit of FFP contains between 200 ml and 250 ml and has a very long shelf life (Miller, 2002). Similar to platelets, FFP should be A-, B-, or O-type specific when available, but as long as the FFP does not contain a large number of anti-A or anti-B antibodies, it does not need to be type-specific (O'Shaughnessy et al., 2004). Patients may receive FFP from donors with any Rh status (O'Shaughnessy et al., 2004). FFP is administered in a similar fashion as platelets, with straight blood tubing and it may be infused rapidly.

17. What would cause an abnormal PT?

A prothrombin time (PT) indicates extrinsic activation of the clotting cascade. The external activation of the clotting cascade is much faster than an intrinsic activation and would be seen in a traumatic injury such as a surgical incision. Calcium is required for the activation of clotting factors and the elimination of calcium in banked blood is used to prolong the shelf life of blood. A normal PT varies based on the laboratory analysis, but on average, is between 12 and 15 seconds. An international

normalized ration (INR) has been put into practice to give standardization for the PT analysis. A normal INR is 0.8 to 1.2 and is used to guide anticoagulation with Warfarin (Coumadin), vitamin K, and liver function. Patients with variation in PT/INR are first recommended to receive treatment with vitamin K and then FFP as clinically indicated (O'Shaughnessy et al., 2004).

18. What would cause an abnormal PTT?

An abnormal partial thromboplastin time (PTT) or activated thromboplastin time (aPTT) is a measure of the intrinsic or contact activation pathway activation. This side of the clotting cascade is much slower than the extrinsic arm; however, it also involves calcium and the activation of several factors in sequence. The administration of heparin would result in the prolongation of the PTT and can be reversed with the administration of protamine sulfate (Adams & Koch, 2010). Hemophilia also leads to an increased PTT. A normal PTT would be between 25 and 39 seconds, and increased PTT could be treated with the administration of FFP.

ACID-BASE BALANCE

Human physiology is maintained by the regulation of a very narrow range of pH in intracellular and extracellular fluids. pH is a measure of the amount of dissolved acid or H^+ in a solution and is normally between 7.35 and 7.45. The maintenance of pH takes place as a complex interaction between acid production and elimination and a series of buffer systems (Porth & Matfin, 2009). Normally, the levels of acid and buffer are maintained in a balance. Acid-base disease occurs when there is a loss on one side of the scale or a gain on the opposite side of the scale. When the body compensates for a disease, it will add or subtract on the opposite side of the abnormality so the scale again achieves balance.

Acids are derived from positively charged molecules and are classified into two groups based on the ease with which they give up acid (or a positive charge) in solution. Weak acids do not dissociate easily and tend to limit the release of a positive charge in a solution; strong acids readily give up their positive charge. Buffers serve to balance acids within the body as they accept the positive charge that is released from acids.

Acid Production

Carbonic acid (H_2CO_3) is a weak acid that is formed from the interaction of H_2O and the CO_2 produced as a by-product of cellular metabolism. A large amount of CO_2, approximately 15,000 mmol, is produced daily (Porth & Matfin, 2009), transported to the lungs, and is efficiently eliminated.

The second type of acid found in humans is termed a fixed acid. It is considered to be caustic due to its rapid dissociation or loss of the positive charge in a solution. Relatively small quantities of fixed acids are produced daily from the metabolism of ingested protein and are balanced by the production of buffers. Fixed acids are eliminated by the kidney.

Buffer Systems

There are three main buffer systems found in the body and they differ in their mechanism of action and timing of action. The goal for all buffer systems is to bind and prevent the release of additional acid into fluid or cells. The activity of the buffer system, called compensation, is the normalization of pH.

The first buffer system is active on a constant basis, becoming active in the neutralization of acid as soon as additional acid is produced. This system is found in three different sources: the extracellular fluids as bicarbonate (HCO_3^-), on the surface of bones, and as intracellular fixed proteins. HCO_3^- is present in all extracellular fluids and immediately binds and neutralizes weak acids. The surface of bone readily absorbs and neutralizes excess acid, releasing calcium carbonate or bicarbonate (HCO_3^-). Finally, intracellular proteins are able to accept acid by being amphoteric, meaning they can carry either a positive or negative charge. As acid accumulates in extracellular fluid, it immediately moves across the cell membrane in exchange for potassium (K^+). The H^+ that moves into the cell is rapidly buffered by the intracellular proteins so a physiologic intracellular pH is maintained. The end result in the activity of the immediate buffer system is a decline of serum bicarbonate (HCO_3^-) from binding with acid, a demineralization of bone and liberation of calcium, and an elevation in serum K^+ (Porth & Matfin, 2009).

The lungs are the second buffer system to become active in acute alterations in pH and changes in ventilatory rate and depth are seen within minutes. The accumulation of H^+ leads to an increase in elimination of CO_2 through Kussmaul respiration and hypoventilation, which would lead to a respiratory alkalosis. This very effective mechanism to compensate for acid-base abnormalities is short-lived, as it significantly can increase the work of breathing.

The final organ system involved in the long-term regulation of pH is the kidney. The kidney has a slower activation, but renal buffering can continue over the life of an individual. The kidney has several mechanisms to affect serum pH: HCO_3^- reabsorption, excretion of H^+ in the urine, and the production of new buffer. Bicarbonate is freely filtered in the nephron and, as acid accumulates, the nephron increases the amount of bicarbonate reabsorption. The excretion of H^+ in the urine and the production of new bicarbonate takes place in the distal nephron. In a single mechanism in the distal nephron, H^+ is pumped into the urine and the new HCO_3^- is reabsorbed.

Arterial Blood Gas Analysis

19. What is the normal range for an arterial blood gas?

pH:	7.35 to 7.45
PCO_2:	35 to 45
HCO_3^-:	22 to 26

The key to arterial blood gas (ABG) interpretation is to approach the analysis in a consistent, systematic fashion. As PO_2, CO_2, and saturation reflect airway and respiration—priority one for perianesthesia nurses—they are the first to be considered. To complete acid-base evaluation, PO_2 and saturation are eliminated from the analysis; what remains is pH, CO_2, and HCO_3^-, the three primary players in acid-base analysis. There are many different approaches that may be used for acid-base analysis; however, the three-step approach below is recommended to discover the cause of the acid-base abnormality:

The first step is to look at the pH and determine the "last name" of the acid-base disease. The normal range of the pH is between 7.35 and 7.45. If the pH is decreased (below 7.35) draw an arrow pointing downward ($\downarrow$) indicating acidosis; if the pH is increased (above 7.45) draw an arrow pointing upward ($\uparrow$) indicating alkalosis.

The second step is to look at the CO_2. Changes in CO_2 are controlled by respiratory function. If the acid-base abnormality is due to respiratory disease, the CO_2 will move in the opposite direction from the pH. For instance, if the acidosis is due to respiratory disease, the pH is $\downarrow$ and the CO_2 is $\uparrow$; the arrows move in different directions ($\downarrow\uparrow$), indicating respiratory disease. If the alkalosis is due to respiratory disease, the pH is $\uparrow$ and the CO_2 is $\downarrow$. The arrows move in different directions ($\uparrow\downarrow$), indicating a respiratory disease.

The third step is to look at the HCO_3^-. Metabolic disorders causing changes in HCO_3^- are due to the effect of the acid-base abnormality on HCO_3^-. Bicarbonate is controlled by renal function. If the acid-base abnormality is due to metabolic disorder, the HCO_3^- will move in the same direction as the pH. For instance, if the acidosis is due to metabolic disease, the pH is ↓ and the HCO_3^- is ↓; the arrows move in the same direction (↓↓), indicating metabolic disease. If the alkalosis is due to metabolic disease, the pH is ↑ and the HCO_3- is ↑; the arrows move in the same direction (↑↑), indicating a metabolic disease.

Advanced Arterial Blood Gas Analysis: Compensation

For those of you who are up to a challenge, look at what the body is doing to normalize the pH, termed compensation. When the body compensates for an acid-base disorder, the disease process is unimportant; the goal is to correct the pH through the manipulation of acid (CO_2) or buffer (HCO_3^-). There are only two compensations seen in the blood gas analysis: metabolic and respiratory.

In a metabolic disorder, the lungs will attempt to compensate; look to the CO_2. The use of arrows can also discriminate respiratory compensation from respiratory disease because in respiratory compensation, the arrows will move in the same direction as the pH (e.g., increasing ↑CO_2 to compensate for increased ↑pH [alkalosis] and decreasing ↓CO_2 to compensate for decreased ↓pH [acidosis]). As a reminder, if the disorder is due to respiratory disease, the arrows will be in opposite directions. Arrows in the same direction to pH indicates metabolic disease with respiratory compensation.

In a respiratory disorder, the kidney will attempt to compensate; look to the HCO_3^-. The use of arrows can also discriminate metabolic compensation from metabolic disease because in metabolic compensation, the arrows will move in the opposite direction as the pH (e.g., increasing ↑ HCO_3^- to compensate for decreased ↓pH [acidosis] or decreasing ↓HCO_3^- to compensate for increased ↑pH [acidosis]). As a reminder, if the disorder is due to metabolic disease, the arrows will be in same direction. Arrows in same direction to pH indicates respiratory disease with metabolic compensation.

Acid-Base Abnormalities: Metabolic Acidosis

Metabolic acidosis occurs when there is an increase in the production or intake of acid or a loss of base, tipping the scale to indicate an accumulation of acid. There are several causes of an increased production of acid and only one cause of a loss of bicarbonate. As acid accumulates, an increase in

serum K^+ is seen as the excess acid is buffered by intracellular proteins. The causes of metabolic acidosis are as follows:

- Increased production of lactic acid: This is a common cause of metabolic acidosis. Lactic acid is produced as a by-product of anaerobic metabolism, which would follow inadequate tissue perfusion, such as in a shock state. A reduction in the supply of oxygen to the cell decreases the efficiency of the production of ATP in the Krebs cycle. Instead of producing 36 to 38 molecules of ATP for each molecule of glucose in an oxygen-rich environment, anaerobic metabolism leads to the production of only two ATP and the by-product of lactic acid. The lactic acid must be returned to the Krebs cycle when oxygen is available and converted to ATP. This is a common finding in the perianesthetic environment. In lactic acidosis, the pH would be decreased and the bicarbonate would move in the same direction, indicating a metabolic disorder. If there is respiratory compensation for the acidosis, the CO_2 would also be decreased in an attempt to decrease acid and normalize the pH.

- Ketoacidosis: Ketoacidosis would be present in any situation when there is an inadequate intake of carbohydrate, and fatty acids are converted into ketones to be used as a fuel source. Ketoacidosis is present in diabetes mellitus when the cells are scavenging their own protein and fat as a fuel, termed diabetic ketoacidosis (DKA). Another source of ketoacidosis would be any disease process that would lead to malnutrition or starvation, such as severe dieting, anorexia or bulimia, or malignancy. Ketoacidosis is a normal finding associated with some types of diets where carbohydrates are eliminated from the diet and fat and protein are substituted. Compensation for ketoacidosis would result in a classic ventilatory pattern of deep, blowing breathing, termed Kussmaul respiration.

- Renal failure with a loss of the ability to excrete acid and produce bicarbonate: This is the most common cause of metabolic acidosis overall and impacts a large number of patients with diabetes. With chronic renal failure and a long-term acid-base disease, demineralization of bones and calcium losses are common as the bones serve as another short-term buffer. Hyperkalemia is common in any acidosis, but in chronic renal failure, the hyperkalemia is complicated by the loss of renal excretion of K^+.

- Salicylate toxicity, which occurs when an individual ingests a large amount of acetylsalicylic acid, causing an increased level of acid.
- Loss of HCO_3^- in the stool: This can be seen in diseases which cause severe diarrhea, such as small bowel obstruction, pancreatic or biliary fistulas, or ileostomy drainage (Porth & Matfin, 2009).

20. What is an example of an arterial blood gas that indicates metabolic acidosis?

     pH: 7.25   ↓

     PCO_2:   35   ↔

     HCO_3^-:   16   ↓

21. What is an example of an arterial blood gas that indicates metabolic acidosis with respiratory compensation?

     pH: 7.33   ↓

     PCO_2:   25   ↓

     HCO_3^-:   16   ↓

Acid-Base Abnormalities: Metabolic Alkalosis

Metabolic alkalosis occurs when there is an increase in buffer or a decrease in production or loss in acid, tipping the scale to indicate an accumulation of buffer. Metabolic acidosis has two common causes:

- Increased buffer: An increased intake of antacids can lead to the accumulation of buffer and the development of metabolic alkalosis. The resultant hypokalemia from the outward movement of acid from the intracellular space to the extracellular space may be the first symptom.
- Loss of acid, which can be seen with prolonged gastric suction, chronic vomiting , bulimia, or chemotherapy-associated vomiting. From bulimia or chemotherapy-associated vomiting: Gastric acid contains a high concentration of hydrochloric acid (HCl), and each secretion of acid into the lumen of the stomach generates a newly secreted bicarbonate molecule in the portal circulation.

22. What is an example of an arterial blood gas that indicates metabolic alkalosis?

     pH: 7.55   ↑

     PCO_2:   45   ↔

     HCO_3^-:   38   ↑

23. What is an example of an arterial blood gas that indicates metabolic alkalosis with respiratory compensation?

     pH: 7.48   ↑

     PCO_2:   55   ↑

     HCO_3^-:   30   ↑

Acid-Base Abnormalities: Respiratory Acidosis

Respiratory acidosis is caused by a disorder that impairs ventilation or the exchange of gases in and out of the alveoli. The impairment of gas exchange would lead to the retention of CO_2, increased weak acid, and respiratory acidosis. The difference between acute and chronic respiratory acidosis is time and the ability of the kidney to become involved and excrete acid and increase the level of buffer in the body. There are many possible causes of respiratory acidosis. For the sake of clarification, it has been divided into three broad classifications: acute respiratory acidosis, chronic respiratory acidosis, and respiratory alkalosis.

Acute Respiratory Acidosis

Acute respiratory acidosis would occur in a time frame where the kidney does not have the opportunity to compensate. There are three large classifications of acute respiratory disorders:

- Respiratory control: In this classification, there is a loss in the control of ventilation. This form of acute respiratory failure would be seen in neuromuscular disorders that would impact the muscle contraction required for ventilation, such as multiple sclerosis, paralytic agent administration, or a high spinal. A second example of this classification of respiratory disorder is impaired activity or depression of the respiratory center in the brain stem, which could be present in drug overdose or head injury. Either of these examples would result in the acute onset of decreased ventilation and would not allow for renal compensation.
- Chest wall activity: In this classification, there would be a loss in the ability of the chest wall to change shape to allow for ventilation. An example of this type of disorder would be flail chest, pneumothorax, or hemothorax, where there would be impaired ventilation due to decreased ability for lung expansion. Another example of this form of disorder would be the acute impact of scoliosis or surgical insult and incisional pain, which may accompany thoracic procedures.

- Any type of disorder that would impact the ability of respiration or the exchange of gasses across the alveolocapillary membrane: There are a large number of diseases that would lead to this type of disorder, such as pneumonia, asthma, aspiration, pulmonary embolus, acute pulmonary edema, or airway obstruction. All of these disorders would acutely decrease gas exchange and lead to increased CO_2 levels

24. What is an example of an arterial blood gas that indicates acute respiratory acidosis?

pH:	7.25	↓
PCO_2:	55	↑
HCO_3^-:	25	↔

Chronic Respiratory Acidosis

Any situation that impairs gas exchange and would lead to CO_2 retention over a period of time where the kidney could compensate would lead to the development of chronic respiratory acidosis. Examples of this type of acid-base abnormality would be emphysema or chronic bronchitis, long-standing pneumonia, pulmonary fibrosis, or long-standing neuromuscular disorder. The difference between chronic and acute respiratory acidosis would be an increased bicarbonate level on arterial blood gas analysis.

25. What is an example of an arterial blood gas that indicates chronic respiratory acidosis?

pH:	7.28	↓
PCO_2:	55	↑
HCO_3^-:	38	↑

Respiratory Alkalosis

Respiratory alkalosis is seen primarily in panic attacks or hyperventilation. Respiratory alkalosis may be present in pregnancy, but would be compensated over time.

26. What is an example of an arterial blood gas that indicates chronic respiratory acidosis?

pH:	7.55	↑
PCO_2:	25	↓
HCO_3^-:	24	↔

REFERENCES

Adams, M. P., & Koch, R. W. (2010). *Pharmacology: Connections to nursing practice.* Upper Saddle River, NJ: Pearson.

Berne, M. B., & Levy, M. N. (1998). *Physiology* (4th ed.). St. Louis, MO: Mosby.

Drain, C. B., & Odom-Forren, J. (2009). *Perianesthesia nursing: A critical care approach* (5th ed.). St. Louis, MO: Saunders Elsevier.

Guyton, A.C. (1991). Textbook of Medical Physiology, 8th ed., Philadelphia: W.B. Saunders Company.

Miller, R. L. S. (2002). Blood component therapy. *Urologic Nursing, 22*(5), 331–339.

O'Shaughnessy, D. F., Atterbury, C., Bolton Maggs, P., Murphy, M., Thomas, D., Yates, S., et al. (2004). Guidelines for the use of fresh frozen plasma, cryoprecipitate and cryosupernatant. *British Journal of Haematology, 126,* 11–28.

Porth, C. M., & Matfin, G. (2009). *Pathophysiology: Concepts of altered health states* (8th ed.). Philadelphia: Lippincott Williams & Wilkins.

Shier, D., Butler, J., & Lewis, R. (1998). *Hole's human anatomy & physiology* (7th ed.). Boston: McGraw Hill.

SECTION I

SECTION II

SECTION III

CHAPTER 9

Integumentary Issues

Maureen F. McLaughlin, MS, RN, CPAN, CAPA

The integumentary system is comprised of skin, hair, glands, and nails. Of those, the skin is the largest and, in fact, is considered the largest organ in the body. The skin receives one third of the body's circulating blood volume. The primary function of the skin is protection, serving as a barrier against ultraviolet radiation, loss of body fluids, invasion of microorganisms, and stress of mechanical factors. The skin also aids in maintaining a constant body temperature (Huether, 2002). Disruptions in skin integrity can adversely affect outcomes following surgery. In addition, many disease states (such as diabetes and peripheral vascular disease) significantly increase the risk of skin breakdown and pressure ulcer formation in the perianesthesia setting.

STRUCTURE AND FUNCTION OF THE SKIN

1. What are the three layers of skin?

The skin consists of three layers: the epidermis, dermis, and hypodermis. The epidermis is the outer layer and is approximately 0.12 mm in depth. Despite its relatively small size, the dermis is considered the most important layer of the skin, serving as an immunity barrier. The dermis prevents dehydration of the deeper skin layers through the process of cornification. Melanocytes are specialized cells located in the dermis and are responsible for synthesizing and secreting melanin, which provides a barrier against ultraviolet radiation. Langerhans cells migrate to the dermis from the bone marrow and initiate an immune response as needed.

The dermis ranges from 1 to 4 mm in thickness and contains nerves, lymphatic and blood vessels, hair follicles, sebaceous glands, and sweat glands. Cells within the dermis participate in immune response and hypersensitivity skin reactions. In addition, muscles at the base of hair follicles, arrector pili muscles, are responsible for the appearance of "goose bumps," tiny bumps on skin that involuntarily develop in response to cold or strong emotions.

The hypodermis is the third layer of skin and is considered the subcutaneous layer. In addition to a layer of fat, the hypodermis contains appendages of elements of the dermal layer, including hair follicles, sebaceous glands, nails, and the supplying blood vessels for the dermis (Huether, 2002).

2. How is heat loss regulated by the skin?

One critical role of the skin is to regulate body temperature. Heat loss is prevented or facilitated by regulating blood flow to the skin. Thermoregulatory processes are largely autonomic responses. The primary autonomic defenses against heat loss are arteriovenous shunt vasoconstriction and shivering.

Located in the dermis, thermoregulatory arteriovenous shunts are anastomoses linking arterioles with venules. They are largely restricted to fingers and toes. Regulated by the sympathetic nervous system, these arteriovenous shunts prevent or reduce heat loss by diminishing blood flow to the skin. By closing the shunt, blood flow is reduced to the body's periphery, and the arms and legs gradually cool. In turn, metabolic heat, generated by the deep organs, is restricted to the body's central core and not allowed to escape into the peripheral tissues. Thus, the core body temperature is maintained under normal conditions.

In addition to regulating blood flow, the skin serves to regulate heat loss through insulation. The subcutaneous layer consists of adipose tissue and provides insulation for temperature control (Jarvis, 2004; Sessler, 2009).

3. What is shivering?

Shivering is defined as involuntary oscillatory skeletal muscle activity, often in response to hypothermia. Shivering is initiated by the hypothalamus in response to a decrease in the core body temperature. The temperature threshold for shivering is less than that of vasoconstriction; vasoconstriction is the body's first autonomic response to a decrease in temperature.

The intent of shivering is to raise the core body temperature by generating heat from the increased metabolic rate from the act of shivering. The metabolic rate can double as a result of shivering, thus increasing oxygen consumption, often a harmful side effect of shivering. Overall, shivering is less effective than vasoconstriction in preventing heat loss and preserving core body temperature.

Of note, postoperative patients report that shivering and the feeling of being cold were the most unpleasant experience following surgery (Paulikas, 2008; Sessler, 2009).

4. How does the skin cool the body?

The eccrine sweat glands are distributed throughout the body, with the greatest concentration in the soles of the feet, the palms of the hands, and the forehead. The apocrine sweat glands are located in the groin, axilla, scalp, genital area, face, and abdomen. Combined, secretions from these glands are important in the body's thermoregulation; the secretions cool the body through evaporation. Evaporation accounts for about 20% of heat loss. Insensible fluid loss, in the absence of active sweating, can amount to 600 ml per day (Drain, 2003; Huether, 2002).

5. What role does the skin's flora have on postoperative wound infection?

The source of many surgical site infections is actually the patient's own skin flora. Many studies have determined a correlation between postoperative wound infection and the presence of

Staphylococcus aureus in nasal passages. The Centers for Disease Control (CDC) recommend an antiseptic shower at least the night before surgery; repeating the shower in the morning of surgery may have an additional benefit in reducing the microbial colony counts (Centers for Disease Control [CDC], n. d.; Strelczyk, 2008).

AGE-SPECIFIC PATIENT CONSIDERATIONS

6. What are some developmental considerations related to skin in the pediatric patient population?

A newborn's skin is similar to that of an adult; however, several of the skin's functions are not fully developed at birth. The newborn's skin is more permeable than that of an adult, placing the infant at greater risk for fluid loss through the process of evaporation.

Temperature regulation is immature and ineffective. The eccrine sweat glands do not secrete in response to heat until the infant is older. In addition, the infant's skin provides minimal protection against the cold because the shivering response in inactive and the subcutaneous layer of adipose tissue is ineffective at this age. Heat loss can be reduced by covering the largest part of the infant's body, the head (Jarvis, 2004).

7. Is the presence of jaundice in a newborn a matter of concern?

Physiologic jaundice occurs frequently during the first week of life in otherwise healthy infants. This type of jaundice is caused by mild unconjugated hyperbilirubinemia. Physiologic jaundice presents as a yellowing of the skin, sclera, and mucous membranes, and often develops after the third or fourth day after birth. It is attributed to the increased number of red blood cells that hemolyze after birth (Evers, 2002; Jarvis, 2004).

8. What are some special considerations related to skin in the elderly patient population?

The aging process involves a slow atrophy of the skin's structures; as we age, the skin loses its elasticity. The outer layer, the epidermis, thins, thereby reducing the protective function of the skin. Chemicals and other elements have easier access to the body. There is also a reduction in adipose fat, reducing the insulating properties of the skin and thus placing the elderly patient at increased risk of heat loss. Aging results in a loss of collagen, so the elderly are at increased risk of skin tears. Decreased sweat production and reduced sebaceous gland secretions will result in comparatively drier skin in the elderly (Jarvis, 2004).

PREOPERATIVE ASSESSMENT OF THE SKIN

9. What elements of a skin assessment should be part of the preoperative patient interview?

During the preoperative interview, the patient should be asked if they have a previous history of a skin disease; if yes, the patient should be asked how that disease was treated. The patient should be asked if he or she has currently or has had in the past any rashes or lesions. If any are present, these should be examined prior to surgery.

Patients should be asked if they have any tattoos. Use of nonsterile equipment during the tattooing process increases the patient's risk of acquiring hepatitis C.

Patients should also be assessed for the presence of any pressure ulcers, defined as localized injury to the skin and/or underlying tissue, usually over a bony prominence (Jarvis, 2004).

10. What special considerations regarding the pediatric patient should be included in the pre-operative interview?

The presence of any birthmarks, rashes (including diaper rash), or sores should be noted. A history of jaundice and its duration should also be recorded. Information regarding exposure to any contagious skin disorders, such as lice or scabies, should also be elicited (Jarvis, 2004).

11. What special considerations regarding the elderly patient should be included in the preoperative interview?

Additional information should include history of peripheral vascular disease and/or diabetes, recent history of falls, and any recent changes in the appearance or the integrity of the skin (Jarvis, 2004).

12. What is the correlation between allergies and skin assessment?

Very often, the skin presents the first indication of an allergic reaction, either in the form of hives or erythematous changes in the skin. During the patient interview, it is important to inquire about any allergies to medications, foods, and other allergens. Document the type of allergy; a history of hives following administration of a medication is also important information for the prescriber (Jarvis, 2004).

13. What are hives?

Hives, or urticaria, are described as wheals or fluid-filled blisters that coalesce to cover a large surface area of the skin. They are intensely pruritic or itchy. The underlying mechanism is the localized release of histamine in response to an antigen (Jarvis, 2004; Rote, 2002).

14. What type of risk assessment regarding pressure ulcers should be performed?

Patients should be assessed for the following risk factors related to pressure ulcers:

- Inability to respond to or perceive pressure-related discomfort
- Incontinence or the degree to which skin is exposed to moisture
- Decreased activity level (e.g., confined to chair or bed)
- Inability to reposition
- Poor nutritional intake
- History of friction or tearing injuries
- Requiring assistance when moving

These factors may predispose a patient to the development of a pressure ulcer during hospitalization (Ayello & Braden, 2002).

DAY-OF-SURGERY SKIN ASSESSMENT

15. What are elements of the skin assessment for the day of surgery?

All data collected during the preadmission interview should be reviewed; any documented skin lesions or disruptions in skin integrity should be reassessed. Patients should be assessed for the presence of any pressure sores; if present, carefully and clearly document the size, location, and the stage. The presence of any pressure sores the morning of surgery would classify them as present on admission. In addition, the presence of any bruises should be noted and carefully documented. Patient populations at risk for abuse include both the very young as well as the elderly. Be attentive to the potential for abuse in a patient, such as bruising, marks associated with cigarette burns, and/or linear whip marks (Jarvis, 2004). Any deviation from normal skin should be passed on in a hand-off report from the preoperative area to the operating room (OR) staff.

16. What is the best method to identify patients at high risk for pressure ulcers?

On the day of surgery, patients should be assessed for the presence of any pressure ulcers. The risk factors previously listed should also be reassessed. In addition, any surgical procedure expected to last longer than 4 hours increases the risk of a pressure ulcer.

Depending on intuitional protocols and practices, additional position aids or padding can be utilized during surgery to reduce the risk of pressure ulcer formation for patients identified to be at increased risk (Courtney, Ruppman, & Cooper, 2006).

POSTOPERATIVE SKIN ASSESSMENT

17. What are the elements of a postoperative skin assessment?

All patients must have their skin assessed upon arrival to the postanesthesia care unit (PACU). Elements of this assessment include condition and color of skin. It is essential to turn patients and to perform both an anterior as well as posterior skin assessment.

Normally, skin color is consistent with the patient's genetic background. Pallor may indicate hypothermia, anxiety or stress, and/or the loss of oxygenated hemoglobin in the blood stream. Mucous membranes, lips, and nail beds are specific locations to assess for generalized pallor. Cyanosis is a bluish mottled color that signifies decreased perfusion or hypoxemia. It may occur in shock states, heart failure, or vasoconstriction. Correlation of the patient's skin color with other objective signs, such as oxygen saturation, heart rate, blood pressure, and temperature must be made to measure the significance of the skin's appearance. The skin must be assessed for any bruising, redness, or ulceration. Any disruption in skin integrity must be compared to the preoperative skin assessment. Any new alteration in skin integrity must be carefully documented. Most surgical patients have some type of dressing or covering of the surgical site. The integrity of the surgical dressing must be assessed and documented (Jarvis, 2004).

18. What special considerations related to skin should be included in assessing and caring for the elderly patient?

The elderly patient is at increased risk of disruption in skin integrity, infection, and delayed wound healing due to the loss of elasticity, collagen, muscle, and adipose tissue as part of the aging process. The elderly patient is at increased risk for skin tears, even during simple turning. Take care to avoid shearing forces when repositioning the elderly patient. Provide additional padding and/or protective surfaces, reduce the use of tape on fragile skin, and ensure that limbs and joints are in neutral positions to minimize stress. Encourage early ambulation or reposition the elderly patient frequently to reduce the risk of postoperative complications (Allen, 2010).

DISORDERS OF THE SKIN: PRESSURE ULCERS

19. What is a pressure ulcer?

A pressure ulcer (PU) is defined as a localized injury to the skin and/or underlying tissue that often forms over a bony prominence and is the result of pressure or pressure in combination with shear and/or friction (Walton-Geer, 2009).

20. How are PUs staged?

The National Pressure Ulcer Advisory Panel (NPUAP) has developed a pressure ulcer staging system that is one of the most widely used in the country. According to the NPUAP, stages of PUs may be categorized as Stages I through IV, deep tissue injury, and unstageable (National Pressure Ulcer Advisory Panel [NPUAP], n. d.):

- Stage I is intact skin with nonblanchable redness of a localized area, usually over a bony prominence. The area may be painful, firm or soft, and warmer or cooler as compared to the surrounding tissue. Patients should be considered to be at increased risk for further pressure ulcer formation if a Stage I PU is identified.

- Stage II is partial thickness loss of dermis presenting as a shiny or dry, shallow, open ulcer with a red-pink wound bed, without slough. A Stage II PU may also present as an intact or open/ruptured serum-filled blister.

- Stage III is a full-thickness tissue loss; subcutaneous fat may be visible, but bone, tendons, or muscle are not exposed. Slough may be present in these ulcers.

- Stage IV ulcers have full thickness loss with exposed bone, tendon, or muscle. Slough may be present and this ulcer often includes tunneling.

- An unstageable ulcer has full-thickness tissue loss in which the base of the ulcer is covered by slough (yellow, tan, gray, green, or brown) and/or eschar in the wound bed.

- Suspected deep tissue injury is described as a purple or maroon localized area of discolored intact skin or blood-filled blister due to damage of underlying soft tissue from pressure and/or shear.

21. What tools should be used for the assessment of PUs and associated risk factors?

There are several standardized risk assessment tools that are widely used. These include, but are not limited to, the Norton Scale, the Waterlow

Scale, and, perhaps the most common, the Braden Scale. The Institute for Healthcare Improvement (IHI) recommends that all patients be assessed for risk and presence of a PU using a standardized assessment tool. Such standardization across an institution will facilitate standardized assessments and interventions (Balzer, Pohl, Dassen, & Halferns, 2007; Institute for Healthcare Improvement [IHI], 2008).

22. Why are surgical patients at increased risk for developing PUs?

All surgical patients should be considered to be at risk for the development of a PU due to the effects of anesthesia and the length of time in surgery. The incidence of PUs in surgical patients can be as high as 45%. One of the risk factors for the development of a PU is pressure. PUs are formed by compression of soft tissue between a bony prominence and an external surface, such as an OR table. When the external pressure exceeds the normal capillary filling pressure, local blood flow is occluded. This can result in tissue ischemia and subsequent necrosis of both the skin and underlying tissue. Sometimes the underlying tissue becomes necrotic before a lesion even presents on the skin.

A patient's body must be positioned in the OR to facilitate the surgical procedure. As an example, surgeries of the spine require that the patient be positioned to ensure that the surgeon has the best visualization of the surgical site. Even with careful positioning and maximum padding and protection, there is often pressure of bony prominences against the firm surface of the OR table and support structures.

In addition, anesthesia increases the patient's risk of developing PUs. Anesthesia blocks the patient's sensitivity to pain and prevents the patient's ability to reposition himself or herself in response to increasing pain and pressure. Anesthetic agents are also potent vasodilators, which may result in a decrease in blood pressure and concomitant decrease in tissue perfusion.

The length of time that the patient is in one position may increase the risk of developing a PU, as most tissue can only withstand excessive pressure for brief periods of time. Any lengthy surgical procedure increases the risk of PU formation (Walton-Geer, 2009).

Additional risk factors for PU formation include, but are not limited to, bariatric patients, patients with altered immune function secondary to disease or chemotherapy, and the very old and the very young patients.

23. What are some important postoperative nursing interventions that can reduce the risk of developing a PU?

Nursing care should be directed at reducing all of the identified risks for PU formation to the greatest extent possible. Assessment and reassessment practices should be implemented. Patients who are unable to turn or reposition themselves should be turned frequently, and additional padding should be provided over bony prominences. Patients should be kept dry. If the patient is incontinent, ensure the frequent changing of diapers or pads, and consider the benefits and risks of inserting an indwelling urinary catheter to prevent incontinence and possible skin maceration. Encourage early mobility and/or ambulation whenever possible. Resume diet as soon as the patient is able; be mindful of the risk of diminished nutritional intake. Prevent friction and shearing injuries during turning and repositioning. Implement institution-specific skin care regimes for patients in whom a PU has been identified (IHI, 2008).

DISORDERS OF THE SKIN: DIABETES

24. Why are diabetic patients at increased risk for impaired wound healing?

Diabetes is a disease characterized by chronic hyperglycemia and resultant alterations in carbohydrate, fat, and protein metabolism. Patients with diabetes have impaired wound healing and are at increased risk for developing wound infections. Elevated glucose contents in body fluids provide an ideal medium for bacterial proliferation, thereby increasing the risk for infection. Surgical patients often have a blunted immune response to pathogens. Vascular changes associated with diabetes may result in the impaired migration of neutrophils to the surgical site, which can delay wound healing and adversely affect the patient's ability to mount an immune response (Patel, 2008).

25. What postoperative strategies can be implemented to reduce complications in the diabetic patient?

Surgical patients with diabetes should be identified as such preoperatively. These patients should have physician orders for blood glucose monitoring postoperatively with the goal of maintaining blood glucose levels within normal ranges. Scheduled prandial insulin doses should be given in relation to meals as applicable; surgical patients who remain NPO should have appropriate coverage of their blood glucose levels. Insulin infusions could be considered for the patient who is unlikely to resume a diet by postoperative day one. A plan for treating hypoglycemia should be established. Postoperative diabetic patients should be observed closely for wound infections, delayed wound healing, and disruptions in skin integrity (Patel, 2008).

REFERENCES

Allen, J. (2010). The geriatric patient. In L. Schick & P. E. Windle (Eds.), *Perianesthesia nursing core curriculum* (pp. 221–242). St. Louis: Saunders.

Ayello, E. A., & Braden, B. (2002). How and why to do pressure ulcer risk assessment. *Advances in Skin and Wound Care, 15*(3), 125–131.

Balzer, K., Pohl, C., Dassen, T., & Halferns, R. (2007). The norton, waterlow, braden, and care dependency scales. *Journal of Wound Ostomy Continence Nursing, 34*(4), 389–398.

Centers for Disease Control. (n. d.). *Guide for prevention of surgical site infection.* Retrieved from http://www.cdc.gov/NCIDOD/DHQP/pdf/guidelines/SSI.pdf

Courtney, B. A., Ruppman, J. B., & Cooper, H. M. (2006). Save our skin: Initiative cuts pressure ulcer incidence in half. *Nursing Management, 37*(4), 36–45.

Drain, C. (2003). *Perianesthesia nursing: A critical care approach.* St. Louis, MO: Saunders.

Evers, D. B. (2002). Alteration of digestive function in children. In K. L. McCance & S. E. Huether (Eds.), *Pathophysiology: The biologic basis for disease in adults and children* (pp. 1314–1337). St. Louis, MO: Mosby.

Huether, S. E. (2002). Structure, function, and disorders of the integument. In K. L. McCance & S. E. Huether (Eds.), *Pathophysiology: The biologic basis for disease in adults and children* (pp. 1434–1468). St. Louis, MO: Mosby.

Institute for Healthcare Improvement. (2008). *Prevent pressure ulcers.* Retrieved from http://www.ihi.org/NR/rdonlyres/74373FC5-4615-48AB-ADA4-CCAAE801C0E0/0/IntrotoPUP.ppt

Jarvis, C. (2004). *Physical examination and health assessment.* St. Louis, MO: Saunders.

National Pressure Ulcer Advisory Panel (n. d.) Retrieved from http://npuap.org/pr2.htm

Patel, K. (2008). Impact of tight glycemic control on postoperative infection rates and wound healing in cardiac surgery patients. *Journal Wound Ostomy Continence Nursing, 35*(4), 397–404.

Paulikas, C. A. (2008). Prevention of unplanned perioperative hypothermia. *AORN, 88*(3), 358–364.

Rote, N. S. (2002). Infection and alteration in immunity and inflammation. In K. L. McCance & S. E. Huether (Eds.), *Pathophysiology: The biologic basis for disease in adults and children* (pp. 227–271). St Louis, MO: Mosby.

Sessler, D. I. (2009). Thermoregulatory defense mechanisms. *Critical Care Medicine, 37*(7), S203–S210.

Strelczyk, K. (2008). SSIs: What are the host factors? *AORN, 2*(8), 10–13.

Walton-Geer, P. S. (2009). Prevention of pressure ulcers in the surgical patient. *AORN, 89*(3), 538–548.

CHAPTER 10

Infection Prevention Strategies

Amy D. Nichols, RN, MBA, CIC

*"Certainly infections cannot be attributed to the interven-
tion of the devil but must be laid at the surgeon's door."*
(Cushing, 1915)

Infection prevention strategies are documented in
the Qur'an, Old Testament, and the Torah, and
forward throughout history (Cule, 1987; Forder,
2007; Miller, Rahimi, & Lee, 2005). Holmes (infection transmission), Semmelweis (hand hygiene),
Pasteur (germ theory), Nightingale, Lister, and Keen
(surgical sterility), Bergmann (steam sterilization),
Neuber, Mikulicz, and Halstead (personal protective
equipment), Fleming (penicillin), and Haley (infection prevention discipline) have built on previous
knowledge culminating in a compendium of infection prevention strategies, which, if applied, can
reduce the risk of infection in hospitalized patients
to nearly zero. Unfortunately, infection continues
to plague the hospitalized patient (Brennan et al.,
1991), though not as widespread as with the historic
50% mortality potential for a soldier undergoing
surgical intervention during the mid-19th century
Crimean or Civil Wars.

In 1995, Hecht estimated that by 2000, approximately 75% of all surgical procedures in the
United States would be performed in an out-of-
hospital environment, such as in an ambulatory
or same-day setting (Hecht, 1995). National
statistics for 2006 demonstrate that this prediction
was optimistic (Cullen, Hall, & Golosinskiy, 2009;
DeFrances, Lucas, Buie, & Golosinskiy, 2006),
with more than 50% of all surgical procedures
performed as ambulatory procedures (Maki &

Crnich, 2005). The significance of this phenomenon is the potential to miss an untoward event,
such as the development of surgical site infection,
as patients may be lost to follow-up in the ambulatory setting (see Table 10-1).

In 1999, the Institute of Medicine (IOM) released its report, *To Err is Human: Building a Safer
Health System,* which reported that up to 98,000
people die each year because of medical errors, and
wound infections were the second most common
adverse event to occur to hospitalized patients after
drug complications (John & Donaldson, 1999). The
Institute for Healthcare Improvement (IHI) estimates that 2.6% of surgical procedures are complicated by surgical site infections (SSIs) each year
(IHI, 2008), with rates up to 11% for some procedures (Cruse, 1994). Each infection is estimated to
increase a hospital stay by an average of 7 days and
add over $3000 in charges (CDC, 1992).

Legislative mandates and reimbursement limits
designed to accelerate healthcare facilities' implementation of infection risk-reduction strategies are
now in effect for many states in the United States.
In California, for example, the requirement to
report deep and organ space infections as the result
of select surgical procedures was effected in 2009.
The state department of health is required to
publicly report statewide data for surgical site
infections in January 2012. In response to the
federal Deficit Reduction Act of 2005, the Centers
for Medicare and Medicaid Services (CMS) (2007)
instituted their Value-Based Purchasing initiative,
intended to link "payment more directly to the

TABLE 10-1. Surgical procedure volume, United States, 2006

Inpatient surgical procedures (in millions)	Overall ambulatory surgical procedures (in millions)	
46	54.6	
	Ambulatory surgical procedures performed in hospitals (percent of overall ambulatory surgical procedures)	Ambulatory surgical procedures performed in free-standing centers (percent of overall ambulatory surgical procedures)
	34.7 (64%)	19.9 (36%)

quality of care provided, [as] a strategy that can help to transform the current payment system by rewarding providers for delivering high quality, efficient clinical care." Legislative and reimbursement decisions have spurred healthcare facilities to implement strategies with demonstrated positive outcome effects, as well as unproven risk-reduction strategies (Mangram, Horan, Pearson, Silver, & Jarvis, 1999; Chavez et al., 2005). This chapter will provide the reader with strategies for demonstrated positive outcome effects.

INFECTION PREVENTION STRATEGIES

Infection prevention in the Post Anesthesia Care Unit (PACU) begins long before the patient arrives, and encompasses the entire environment. The four basic critical elements of infection and prevention are:

- Hand hygiene
- Surface disinfection
- Appropriate use of personal protective equipment
- Proper patient placement

However, every aspect of planning the physical space, purchasing equipment, developing and implementing policy, and monitoring workflow are critical elements in the systematic effort to reduce infection risk. This section begins with the planning phases of PACU development and concludes with infection risk reduction strategies that can be used during direct patient care. Each section describes the key considerations for each element from the viewpoint of infection risk reduction.

1. What is a written functional program?

A written functional program is critical to ensure that infection prevention strategies are considered in all aspects of PACU functioning. Designers, planners, and administrators are required by The Joint Commission (TJC) to involve specialists in infection prevention in planning new or renovated spaces. Some areas of planning from an infection prevention perspective include:

- Adequate space for storage and safe movement for current and anticipated equipment and personnel
- Adequate storage for linens and supplies to discourage cross-contamination
- Purchased equipment able to withstand routine cleaning products
- Procedures in place or consideration made for alternate products if routine cleaning products cannot be used
- Adequate volume of equipment purchased to allow appropriate handling, cleaning, storage, and maintenance ("turn-around" time)

2. What are important aspects to the physical layout of a PACU that should be considered to reduce infection risks?

- Great potential exists when a PACU space is being planned to create an efficient, safe environment for both patients and personnel. Along with state-mandated construction and spacing requirements, the American Institute of Architects (AIA) *Guideline for Design and Construction for Healthcare* (2006) provides excellent, practical guidance for designing a new space. If a PACU already exists, the AIA Guideline provides information to safely and efficiently use existing space.
- Each patient care "station" must be a "minimum of 80 square feet (7.43 square meters) for each patient bed, exclusive of general circulation space within the PACU, with a space for additional equipment described in the functional program and for clearance of at least 5 feet (1.52 meters) between patient

beds and 4 feet (1.22 meters) between patient bedsides and adjacent walls" (AIA, 2006, 5.3.3.2.1).

- Phase II recovery areas (where patients receive class B or class C sedation) requires 50 square feet of space for every lounge chair "and for clearance of 4 feet (1.22 meters) on the sides of the lounge chairs and the foot of the lounge chairs" and 100 square feet of clear space for single bed areas (AIA, 2006, 5.3.3.3.2).

- A medication station, hand washing sink, staff toilet, and patient toilet (in phase II recovery areas) are required by AIA guidelines for a PACU.

- At least one hand washing station with hands-free or wrist blade-operable controls shall be available for very four beds or lounge chairs, uniformly distributed to provide equal access from each bed (AIA, 2006).

- An airborne isolation room is not required in a PACU. However, policies and procedures must be developed to protect healthcare personnel from exposure.

3. What air handling (airflow and air exchange) is necessary to protect both patients and personnel in the PACU?

- At least six air changes per hour (ACH) are required in most states for the PACU.

- Fresh air intakes must be located at least 25 feet from an exhaust output and at least 6 feet from ground level. Prevailing winds should be taken into consideration when locating both air intakes and the exhaust output.

- Semiannual monitoring is usually adequate to ensure appropriate ACH in a stable facility. In a facility undergoing construction or demolition, more frequent monitoring of ACH must be accomplished and should be undertaken on a schedule determined by personnel knowledgeable in air handling in a healthcare facility.

- High-efficiency particulate air (HEPA) filters are not required for a PACU.

4. What workflow elements in the PACU should be considered to reduce infection risks?

Workflow can often be greatly aided by building a full-sized mock-up of a planned space or observing in an existing (working) space. The use of a disinterested third-party observer trained in infection prevention and human factors analysis is valuable to identify workflow patterns that minimize or

eliminate infection risks. Elements to consider include:

- Adequate space is provided for people and equipment to move and pass without cross-contamination.

- Adequate space is provided in a patient space for personnel to move without cross contamination.

- Adequate hand cleaning opportunities, such as hand washing sinks or alcohol-based hand rub (ABHR) dispensers, should be appropriately placed.

- In order to gain the most efficiency in a PACU, all supplies and equipment, including waste and soiled linen disposal, should be located within 10 paces of the patient space.

- Only supplies intended for the current patient should be located in the patient's space. ("Leftover" disposable supplies should be discarded when a patient is moved out of the bay or room, as unrecognized contaminating events are likely to have occurred, causing cross-contamination of packaging, supplies, and equipment for subsequent patients).

- If PACU staff feel the urge to "stockpile" supplies in the patient areas, it is critical to determine and correct the root causes for that urge through a systematic review of workflow.

5. How can storage in the PACU support workflow and reduce infection risks?

Storage of appropriate size, location, and appointments (such as electrical wiring, cabling, plumbing, air) are critical to supporting workflow.

- Spatially separating clean items from used or visibly soiled items is critical to minimizing cross-contamination risks. Clean and used/soiled areas should be completely separated by impervious barriers, such as walls, rather than a counter separated by a strip of electrical tape.

- Space for pillows, linens, and clean and sterile supplies should be configured to allow easy and efficient access, removal, and disposal, as well as for appropriate documentation for patient charges.

- Space and sufficient/appropriate wiring/cabling for current and strategically planned computerized equipment is critical for supporting workflow and documentation.

- Cleaning supplies must be clearly identifiable, easily available, and appropriate for the surfaces to be cleaned.

6. What hospital finishes are appropriate for a PACU?

There is movement to make hospital environments less "sterile" and more "homelike." Even so, hospitals must be built with finishes that are designed to withstand rigorous cleaning agents and processes, and that will encourage appropriate and frequent attention. Critically evaluate every surface in the PACU for its ease of and availability to cleaning and compatibility with cleaning products. For example:

- Internal corners should be coved so matter does not accumulate in 90° crevices.

- All furnishings and cabinetry should be solid, rather than veneer (which can lift and trap matter).

- Determine the chemical components of the facility's cleaning products used or planned for use in the PACU and choose furnishings, wall treatments, floor coverings, and cabinetry built to withstand the active components. Caution: Read the warranties of items considered for purchase and determine if a warranty will be voided due to use of the facility's routine cleaning products.

- Current and developing technologies often contain viewing screens and lenses with special cleaning requirements. See the following for a discussion on cleaning products appropriate for hospital environments, and ensure compatibility between equipment and cleaning products.

- Avoid unnecessary horizontal ledges and shelving.

- Equipment suspended from ceiling-hung booms can be remarkably efficient. Ensure cleaning policies include specific instructions to clean the horizontal surfaces of the mounts/booms.

- Floor-mounted equipment and cabinetry must be either moveable or mounted such that the equipment and the floor beneath it can be easily and completely cleaned. Be wary of enclosed spaces that can hide accumulated matter, such as under a cabinet, around floor-embedded shelving, or under low shelving. Allow 10 inches between the floor and the solid bottom shelf to allow for floor cleaning.

- Ensure the bottom shelf (10 inches from the floor) is constructed of solid material rather than wire to prevent contamination from floor cleaning activities.

- Ensure that all finishes are able to be wiped, smooth, and nonporous.

- Semigloss paint is preferable to vinyl wall covering. Mold growth under vinyl wall covering has been reported, leading to poor patient outcomes (A. Streifel, personal communication, March 2007)

- Avoid carpeting. Floor coverings should be monolithic, such as welded seams or poured epoxy. Many current and developing flooring options provide a pleasant environment, are easy to clean, can withstand industrial cleaners, are noise-reducing, and can be ergonomically superior for healthcare personnel.

- Walls and cabinetry should be constructed using simple lines, without reveals or recesses.

- Upholstered furniture must be able to be wiped and to withstand fluid contaminants without soaking into the fabric or cushion material. There is no technology at present capable of adequately cleaning woven fabric upholstery contaminated with blood, urine, or liquid stool.

7. What are important elements to include in a cleaning policy and who should be involved in developing and revising the policy?

All policies referring to cleaning should be developed with consideration of evidence-based guidelines (Sehulster & Chinn, 2003) and created in conjunction with the leadership from the department with cleaning responsibility. In many facilities, cleaning is a shared responsibility between direct patient care personnel, those who perform environmental sanitation activities, and those who reprocess equipment. Capturing assigned responsibilities in policy, training, and monitoring is key to standardizing efficient and thorough cleaning of the patient care environment.

- Involve facility leaders for environmental cleaning and equipment reprocessing in PACU cleaning policy development.

- All surfaces that touch multiple patients must be cleaned after each patient contact. Examples of these items include blood pressure cuffs, bed/lounge chairs, stretchers and side rails, call bells, pillows, pulse oximeter probes, monitor cables, patient transfer devices, glucometers, and over-the-bed table/bedside cabinets.

- Surfaces in the individual patient care area should be cleaned daily or more frequently, if soiled. Examples of these items include IV pumps, patient warming machines, cardiac monitor touch pads, and thermometers.

- Disposable wipes impregnated with hospital-approved detergent or disinfectant should be placed in key locations in the PACU. This has been a successful strategy to encourage appropriate cleaning of frequently used surfaces and multiple-patient items.

- Responsibility for approving cleaning products for a healthcare facility is usually accorded to the infection prevention and control committee. Usual routine hospital-approved detergents and disinfectants contain an EPA-registered disinfectant (EPA: 7 United States Code [USC] § 136 et seq.). Do not use alcohol, high-level disinfectants, or sterilants to disinfect environmental surfaces larger than a few square centimeters.

- Quality control monitoring of surface cleaning should be incorporated into cleaning policies, and reports of monitoring results should be reported to the organization.

8. What information is important to include in a hand hygiene policy?

The facility's hand hygiene policy should reflect recommendations made by the Centers for Disease Control and Prevention (CDC) (Boyce & Pittet, 2002) or the World Health Organization (WHO, 2009), if a facility desires to be accredited by TJC (National Patient Safety Goal #7a). Alcohol-based hand rub (ABHR) use has been shown to be superior for decontaminating hands without visible soiling and for preserving the integrity of the skin on the hands. Healthcare personnel who have demonstrated sensitivity to hand hygiene products selected for routine use in the facility should be evaluated by occupational health specialists, and accommodation with alternate products should be considered. Some extreme cases may need to transition out of the patient care environment. Certain recommendations for hand cleaning, however, cannot be abridged. Monitoring hand hygiene compliance has become recognized as an effective means of feedback to healthcare personnel. Monitoring should be accomplished by personnel internal and external to the PACU and should include peer feedback. Results of hand hygiene compliance audits should be reported to the organization.

- Use ABHR for routine hand cleaning when hands are not visibly soiled. Use sufficient quantity to remain wet on all aspects of the hands and fingers for a minimum of 15 seconds.

- Use ABHR or antimicrobial soap for hand washing before an invasive procedure such as IV insertion, bronchoscopy, or urinary catheter insertion.

- Use soap and water hand washing for visibly soiled hands.

- Use soap and water hand washing after contact with patients or their environments with *Clostridium difficile.*

- Use a surgical hand preparation before performing surgery.

- Clean hands at the following times:
  - At the beginning of work
  - Upon entering and exiting the patient environment
  - Before and after patient contact, including dry skin contact
  - After removing gloves
  - Before performing invasive procedures
  - Before and after contact with wounds
  - After contact with patients' bodily substances
  - After handling equipment, supplies, or linen contaminated with bodily substances
  - Before handling sterile or clean supplies
  - After using the restroom
  - After touching or blowing your nose
  - Before leaving the unit

- Use hand lotion to prevent skin dryness and damage. However, limitations include:
  - Lotion may promote the growth of bacteria. Do not refill containers.
  - Petroleum and mineral oil-based lotions degrade latex (including latex-containing gloves).
  - Petroleum-based lotions negate the persistent antimicrobial effect of chlorhexidine gluconate (CHG).

9. What personal protective equipment (PPE) should be used in the PACU?

PPE is used to prevent the transmission of infectious matter to the healthcare worker. Critical assessment of the patient's condition is necessary to anticipate appropriate garb when caring for the PACU patient. For example:

- Wear a mask with eye protection when suctioning or extubating a patient, or encouraging the patient to breathe deeply, cough, or when administering therapies that may cause coughing.

- Wear a fit-tested respirator and eye protection when engaging in aerosol-generating procedures, such as intubation or bronchoscopy (Siegel, Rhinehart, Jackson, & Chiarello, 2007).

- Wear examination gloves when touching mucous membranes, broken skin, or when anticipating a hand-contaminating event, such as emptying a drain or urinary catheter.

- Wear a fluid-resistant gown when anticipating a splash of blood or bodily fluid, such as uncontrolled bleeding or placement of an arterial line.

Monitoring compliance with the appropriate PPE should be accomplished by personnel both internal and external to the PACU, with peer feedback. Results of compliance audits should be reported to the organization. All PPE should be discarded and hands cleaned when the healthcare worker leaves the individual patient's care area (bay, cubicle, etc.). For example, pulling a mask under the chin and replacing it affords two separate hand-contaminating events and, therefore, is not recommended.

10. Many PACUs are designed with open bays. What isolation precautions can be used in the PACU?

Patient placement decisions must be made for patients with confirmed or suspected communicable diseases that present a risk to other patients. The Guideline for Isolation Precautions provides an isolation scheme for patients (Siegel et al., 2007).

- Standard precautions are used for all patient interactions and consist of three cardinal rules:

  ○ Clean hands at all the appropriate times, for the appropriate length of time, using the appropriate agent (see previous).

  ○ Disinfect surfaces at all appropriate times, for the appropriate length of time, using the appropriate agent (see previous).

  ○ Appropriate use of PPE based upon assessed risk.

- Transmission-based precautions consist of three types of precautions, which are used in addition to standard precautions. Any combination or all of the precautions types may be applied to a patient:

  ○ Airborne precautions are applied to patients with diseases transmitted by the airborne route. Airborne transmission occurs when droplet nuclei (<0.5 micron) are released via cough, sneeze, spit, or speech, then desiccate and travel on air currents to locations away from the infected patient. Patients with confirmed or suspected pulmonary tuberculosis, measles, or varicella zoster virus (chicken pox or disseminated [shingles]) should be placed in airborne precautions.

These patients must be housed in an airborne isolation (negative pressure) private room. When caring for a patient with confirmed or suspected tuberculosis, the healthcare worker must wear a fit-tested respirator. When caring for a patient with measles or varicella (vaccine-preventable diseases), the nonimmune healthcare worker should not care for the patient until vaccinated. The reader will recall that an airborne isolation room is not required in a PACU. However, facility-specific policies must be developed to recover a patient with confirmed or suspected airborne-transmitted disease. Some facilities will recover such a patient in the operating room (OR) or in an airborne isolation room in another area of the facility.

○ Contact precautions are applied to patients with diseases transmitted by direct or indirect touch. Patients diagnosed with multiple drug-resistant organisms (MDRO) should be placed according to the facility's policy, which may include placing patients with MDRO in contact precautions. Patients with confirmed or suspected *C. difficile* associated disease (CDAD), patients with draining wounds not contained by dressings, and patients with skin lesions are nearly universally placed in contact precautions. The appropriate application of standard and contact precautions precludes the necessity for special placement consideration (e.g., cohorts, specific spatial separation). However, workflow stresses should be taken into consideration when placing patients requiring the healthcare worker to wear PPE. For example, if two patients in contact precautions are adjacent, the healthcare worker may be tempted to wear the same gown and gloves for both patients, thereby increasing the potential for pathogen transmission between the patients.

○ Droplet precautions are applied to patients with diseases spread by the droplet route of transmission. Droplet transmission occurs when large, macroscopic droplets are released via cough, sneeze, shout, or spit. The droplets travel only a few feet, then drop. Therefore, when the healthcare worker is in the "cough zone," or within about 3 feet of the patient who is infected with a droplet-transmitted disease (such as influenza, pertussis, bacterial meningitis), he or she should wear a surgical mask and eye protection. Because infectious droplets contaminate the area around the patient, gloves may be worn to decrease the risk of insensate touch contamination. Even if gloves are worn, hand hygiene must be performed as previously outlined. The use of gloves does not preclude hand hygiene.

11. What considerations should be given to occupational health?

- Immunization status for vaccine-preventable diseases: Healthcare personnel should know their immunization status for the vaccine-preventable diseases they are likely to encounter in the course of their work. Health-care facilities often provide no-cost vaccines to nonimmune healthcare personnel. Vaccine-preventable diseases to which healthcare personnel should be immunized or against which healthcare personnel should demonstrate immunity include hepatitis B, measles, mumps, rubella, varicella, and influenza. Healthcare personnel caring for pediatric patients should also be vaccinated against pertussis, as adults represent the reservoir for disease for the undervaccinated pediatric population.

- Work restrictions for those with a communicable disease: Healthcare organizations should enforce work restrictions to healthcare personnel demonstrating a communicable disease. The risk to the remainder of the workforce and to patients recovering from surgery has been demonstrated. For example, a healthcare worker with upper respiratory symptoms should not be allowed to work until the fever has abated for more than 24 hours and respiratory symptoms improve. Facility policies should be developed to provide guidance for symptomatic healthcare personnel management.

12. What attire should PACU nurses wear and what personal appearance practices should PACU nurses keep?

- Scrub wear: There is no evidence that hospital-laundered scrub wear present less risk to patients than home-laundered scrub wear. However, some facilities opt to provide location-specific scrub wear to assist in identifying healthcare worker groups, to control traffic, to satisfy employees, or to satisfy labor union agreements. If scrub wear is considered personal protective equipment by the facility, the facility is obligated to provide and launder the scrub wear.

- Shoes: Close-toed shoes should be worn to prevent exposure of blood and bodily fluids to the healthcare worker.

- Fingernails: Incontrovertible evidence of infection caused by long, natural fingernails and fingernails with enhancements (e.g., tips, extensions, overlays, artificial nails, embedded jewels) has been published for over 15 years. Facility policy should clearly require short, natural fingernails. "Short" means that the tip of the nail is not visible over the tip of the finger when viewed from the palmar surface of the hand, with tips of the finger at eye level.

REFERENCES

American Institute of Architects. (2006). *Guidelines for design and construction of health care facilities*. Retrieved from http://www.filterair.info/library_files/1-2009aj.pdf

Boyce, J. M., & Pittet, D. (2002). Guideline for hand hygiene in health-care settings: Recommendations of the healthcare infection control practices advisory committee and the HICPAC/SHEA/APIC/IDSA hand hygiene task force. *Morbidity and Mortality Weekly Report, 51*(RR-16), 1–45.

Brennan, T. A., Leape, L. L., Laird, N. M., Hebert, L., Localio, A. R., Lawthers, A. G., et al. (1991). Incidence of adverse events and negligence in hospitalized patients: Results of the Harvard medical practice study I. *New England Journal of Medicine, 324*, 370–376.

CDC. (1992). Public health focus surveillance, prevention, and control of nosocomial infections. *MMWR, 41*, 783-787.

Centers for Medicare and Medicaid Services. (2007). *U.S. Department of Health and Human Services Medicare hospital value-based purchasing plan development*. Retrieved from www.cms.gov/AcuteInpatientPPS/downloads/hospital_VBP_plan_issues_paper.pdf

Chavez, G. F., Delahanty, K. M., Cahill, C., Eck, E., Graham, J., LaBouyer, B., et al. (2005). *Recommendations for reducing morbidity and mortality related to healthcare-associated infections in California*. Retrieved from www.cdph.ca.gov/HealthInfo/discond/Documents/RecforReducingMorbandMortRelatedtoHAIinCaRpttoDHS.pdf

Cruse, P. J. E. (1994). History of surgical infection. In D. E. Fry (Ed.), *Surgical infections* (pp. 3–10). Boston: Little, Brown.

Cule, J. (1987). Biblical ills and remedies. *Journal of Religion & Sociology in Medicine, 80*, 534–535.

Cullen, K. A., Hall, M. J., & Golosinskiy, A. (2009). Ambulatory surgery in the United States: 2006. *National Health Statistics Reports, 11*, 1–25.

Cushing, H. (1915). Concerning the results of operations for brain tumor. *Journal of the American Medical Association, 64*, 189–195.

DeFrances, C. J., Lucas, C. A., Buie, V. C., & Golosinskiy, A. (2008). 2006 National hospital discharge survey. *National Health Statistics Reports, 5*, 1–20.

Forder, A. (2007). A brief history of infection control: Past and present. *South African Medical Journal, 97*(3), 1161–1164.

Hecht, A. D. (1995). Creating greater efficiency in ambulatory surgery. *Journal of Clinical Anesthesia, 7*(7), 581-584.

Institute for Healthcare Improvement. (2008). *Getting started kit: Prevent surgical site infections how-to guide.* Retrieved from www.ihi.org

John, L. T., & Donaldson, M. S. (ed.). (1999). *To err is human: Building a safer health system.* Washington, DC: National Academy Press.

Maki, D., & Crnich, C. J. (2005). History forgotten is history relived: Nosocomial infection control is also essential in the outpatient setting. *Archives of Internal Medicine, 165*, 2565–2567.

Mangram A. J., Horan, T. C., Pearson, M. L., Silver, L. C., & Jarvis, W. R. (1999). Guideline for the prevention of surgical site infection. *Infection Control & Hospital Epidemiology, 20*, 247–280.

Miller, J. T., Rahimi, S. Y., & Lee, M. (2005). History of infection control and its contributions to the development and success of brain tumor operations. *Neurosurgical Focus, 18*(4), e4.

Sehulster, L., & Chinn, R. Y. W. (2003). Guidelines for environmental infection control in health-care facilities: Recommendations of CDC and the Health-care Infection Control Practices Advisory Committee (HICPAC). *Morbidity and Mortality Weekly Report, 52*(RR10), 1–42.

Siegel J. D., Rhinehart E., Jackson M., & Chiarello L. (2007). *Guideline for isolation precautions: Preventing transmission of infectious agents in healthcare settings.* Retrieved from www.cdc.gov/hicpac/pdf/isolation/Isolation2007.pdf

World Health Organization. (2009). *WHO guidelines on hand hygiene in health care.* Retrieved from http://whqlibdoc.who.int/publications/2009/9789241597906_eng.pdf

CHAPTER 11

Principles of Anesthesia

John M. Taylor, MD

The term "anesthesia" was coined in 1846 by Oliver Wendell Holmes, Sr. to describe the state produced following the administration of ether. Today, anesthesia care refers to perioperative patient care. The anesthesia provider draws upon knowledge of anatomy, physiology, and pharmacology to care for neonatal, pediatric, adult, and geriatric patients in environments ranging from preoperative evaluation to outpatient procedures to operating rooms involving cardiopulmonary bypass to postoperative care units. This chapter will focus on the general principles of anesthesia as applied to adult patients in the perioperative environment.

1. What is anesthesia?

Anesthesia is a continuum of care or perioperative care. Surgical anesthesia is comprised of three components: amnesia, analgesia, and immobilization or muscle relaxation. These three components provide favorable conditions for surgical procedures.

2. What is the American Society of Anesthesiologists (ASA) classification system?

The ASA classification system, formally called the ASA Physical Status Classification System, was developed in 1941 and last modified in 1963 by the ASA (American Society of Anesthesiologists [ASA], 2008). Today it contains six categories and is intended to describe the physical status of a patient prior to undergoing surgery. It is not intended to estimate perioperative risk (see Table 11-1).

3. What are the major categories of anesthesia?

- Moderate sedation
- Monitored anesthesia care (MAC)
- General anesthesia
- Local anesthesia
- Regional anesthesia
- Balanced anesthesia

4. What is moderate sedation?

Formerly referred to as conscious sedation, moderate sedation involves the administration of sedatives and/or analgesics to control anxiety and pain during diagnostic or therapeutic procedures.

5. What is MAC?

MAC is an anesthetic technique that combines local anesthetic (for the surgical procedure) with sedatives and analgesics designed to produce minimum reduction in patient consciousness to allow for the procedure, while still allowing the patient to protect his or her airway. As stated in the ASA (2009) publication *Distinguishing Monitored Anesthesia Care ("MAC") From Moderate Sedation/Analgesia*, an essential component of monitored anesthesia care is the anesthesia assessment and management of a patient's actual or anticipated physiological derangements or medical problems that may occur during a diagnostic or therapeutic procedure. While MAC may include the administration of sedatives and/or analgesics often used for moderate sedation, the provider of MAC must be prepared and qualified to convert to general

TABLE 11-1. ASA Classification System

ASA category	Description and examples
ASA 1	A normal healthy patient (this excludes the very young and the very old)
ASA 2	A patient with mild systemic disease (no significant physiologic limitations; well-controlled disease involving one organ system; examples include hypertension, diabetes mellitus, obesity, cigarette smoking, and pregnancy)
ASA 3	A patient with severe systemic disease (some physiologic limitations; controlled disease involving more than one organ system; no immediate threat of death; examples include previous myocardial infarction, congestive heart failure, chronic renal failure, morbid obesity, and poorly controlled COPD)
ASA 4	A patient with severe systemic disease with a constant threat to life (symptomatic organ failure with the possibility of death; examples include unstable angina, controlled COPD, acute renal failure, and recent stroke)
ASA 5	A moribund patient not expected to survive more than 24 hours without the operation (possibility of immediate death exists; examples include severe sepsis, multiple organ system failure, ongoing myocardial infarction, and intracranial hemorrhage)
ASA 6	A declared brain-dead patient whose organs are being removed for donation
ASA #E	E is a modifier that designates a patient as an emergency or having an unplanned surgery; the ASA number (1 through 6) is followed by the letter E (e.g., ASA 6E)

anesthesia when necessary. Additionally, a provider's ability to intervene to rescue a patient's airway from any sedation-induced compromise is a prerequisite to the qualifications to provide MAC. By contrast, moderate sedation is not expected to induce depths of sedation that would impair the patient's own ability to maintain the integrity of his or her airway. These components of MAC are unique aspects of an anesthesia service that are not part of moderate sedation (ASA, 2009).

Monitored anesthesia care should not be confused with minimum alveolar concentration (also abbreviated as MAC). Minimum alveolar concentration describes the relative potency of different anesthetic gases. It is for this reason that the acronym for monitored anesthesia care (MAC) has fallen out of favor.

6. How does monitored anesthesia care differ from general anesthesia?

The major difference is the ability of the patient with monitored anesthesia care to protect or maintain a patent airway. A patient receiving general anesthesia cannot maintain a patent airway on his or her own and, thus, cannot provide verbal response to the experience of pain or discomfort. Patients receiving MAC anesthesia are intended to maintain a patent airway and to breathe independently, although airway management must be

provided by the anesthesia provider in the event of oversedation or unexpected loss of airway control.

7. What are the indications and contraindications for monitored anesthesia care?

The indications for moderate anesthesia care include an environment of safe sedation, control of patient anxiety, and pain control that allows for rapid discharge of the patient following the procedure. Full stomach, patient refusal, or a patient's inability to follow directions are absolute contraindications for MAC. Other relative contraindications include language barriers, young age, and altered mental status.

8. What are common medications used during monitored anesthesia care?

Common medications used during monitored anesthesia care are short acting benzodiazepines, short acting narcotics, propofol, dexmedetomidine, and ketamine. Monitored anesthesia care is not defined by the individual medications; it is defined by the patient's level of consciousness and the ability to protect his or her airway.

9. What are postprocedure concerns for patients receiving monitored anesthesia care?

Concerns for patients who received monitored anesthesia care are the same as those who receive general anesthesia (e.g., level of consciousness, cardiopulmonary stability, pain control, nausea control, ability to void). Discharge criteria are the same for all patients in the postanesthesia care unit (PACU) setting, regardless of the type of anesthesia used.

10. How does regional anesthesia differ from local anesthesia?

Local anesthesia provides pain relief to nerve endings in an area infiltrated with local anesthetic medication. Local anesthesia is used for suturing lacerations (i.e., getting stitches) in a conscious person to ensure comfort during the procedure. Regional anesthesia provides sensory and motor blockade to a much larger area as a result of local anesthetic effects on the nerves supplying innervation to a region of the body.

11. What are the major types of regional anesthesia?

Regional anesthesia can be divided into three broad categories:

- Peripheral nerve blocks
- Spinal anesthesia (also called subarachnoid block)
- Epidural anesthesia

12. What is a peripheral nerve block?

A peripheral nerve block provides sensory and motor blockade in the distribution of selected peripheral nerves. This is achieved by depositing local anesthetic near a peripheral nerve with the aid of a nerve stimulator and/or ultrasound guidance. Examples of peripheral nerve blocks are axillary block, interscalene block, femoral nerve block, and sciatic nerve block.

Peripheral nerve blocks can be given either as a single shot or a continuous infusion of local anesthetic depending on the duration of the surgery and the proposed postoperative pain management strategy.

A single shot peripheral nerve block involves locating the desired nerve and administering local anesthetic with a duration profile congruent with the procedure in question.

A continuous infusion of local anesthetic can be delivered to selected peripheral nerves. This allows for targeted analgesia to persist independent of the agent's pharmacokinetic and pharmacodynamic profile. Risks of continuous infusion include possible intravenous administration and systemic toxicity.

13. What is spinal anesthesia?

Spinal anesthesia is achieved by depositing local anesthetic, with or without additives like narcotics,

in the subarachnoid space. To do this, a lumbar puncture is performed with a 25 to 18 gauge needle. Then the anesthetic mixture is administered, typically 2 to 5 ml. Depending on the volume of anesthetic used, the result is a dense sensory and motor blockade of the lower extremities and abdomen. Most often, this is a single dose of medication, although a catheter can be introduced into the subarachnoid space under special circumstances.

14. What is an epidural?

Epidural anesthesia is most often provided after a catheter is introduced into the epidural space. Through this catheter, bolus doses or continuous infusion of local anesthetics can be given. Local anesthetics with or without additives can be administered. Typical bolus volumes are 2 to 10 ml and continuous infusion rates may be in the range of 4 to 14 ml/h.

15. How do the different anesthetic agents differ when used for a peripheral block, spinal anesthesia, and epidural anesthesia?

The duration of local anesthetic action is due to the agent's lipid solubility, diffusion characteristics, protein binding, ionization at physiologic pH, ability to produce vasodilation, and blood flow to the area receiving the local anesthetic. Those medications that are more lipid soluble and able to diffuse into the nerve fiber will have a longer duration of action. Those medications that are closer to physiologic pH have a more rapid onset of action. It is important to remember that the nonionized fraction of the local anesthesia produces anesthetic properties by binding to sodium channels.

All local anesthetics (except cocaine) are vasodilators; vasodilation leads to increased blood flow, a more rapid rate of absorption, and shorter duration of action. Due to relatively high blood flow rates, local infiltration has the shortest duration of action. Peripheral nerve blocks and epidural administration tend to have a more similar duration of action due, in part, to similar blood flow characteristics.

Subarachnoid, or spinal, administration of local anesthetic provides dense and lasting anesthesia to the area of the body below the level of administration. Spinal anesthetics are typically administered at or below the L3–L4 vertebral interspace. This is below the terminus of the spinal cord and is meant to avoid a complication of direct spinal cord injury due to needle trauma. The volume of local anesthetic administered in the subarachnoid space is far less than volumes used for peripheral or epidural anesthesia (Cousins & Bridenbaugh, 1998; New

TABLE 11-2. Anesthetic Agents and Duration of Action in Minutes (Duration of Action Influenced by Concentration and Volume Administered)

Medication	Infiltration	Peripheral	Epidural	Spinal
Lidocaine	60–90	90–120	70–120	60–90
Lidocaine + Epinephrine	90–180	120–180	100–180	90–120
Bupivacaine	180–360	240–600	120–180	90–180
Bupivacaine + Epinephrine	200–480	480–900	180–300	120–300
Ropivacaine		120–480	150–210	
Ropivacaine + Epinephrine		240–540	180–240	

York School of Regional Anesthesia, 2009a, 2009b, 2009c; PDR Staff, 2010) (see Table 11-2).

16. What are the side effects of local anesthetics?

- Nerve damage from administration
- Seizures
- Coma
- Respiratory arrest
- Cardiac conduction abnormalities
  ○ Intravenous administration of bupivacaine has been associated with cardiac toxicity and cardiac arrest
- Allergic reactions
  ○ Allergic reactions are extremely rare and should be treated as any other allergic or anaphylactic reaction would be treated

17. How does local anesthetic toxicity present and how is it treated?

Local anesthetic toxicity can affect multiple organ systems. The most commonly affected are the central nervous, cardiovascular, and hematologic systems. Effects on the central nervous system include dizziness, disorientation, auditory changes (tinnitus), muscle twitching, seizures, and coma. Seizures can be treated with benzodiazepines or propofol, but avoid phenytoin because it acts through sodium channels (as do local anesthetics).

Cardiovascular system manifestations include vasodilation, hypotension, palpitations, chest pain, dysrhythmias, and direct myocardial depression. Symptomatic intravenous bupivacaine administration can cause cardiac arrest and must be treated immediately. A 20% lipid emulsion bolus of 1 ml/kg should be administered as soon as possible.

Overdose of topical benzocaine, most often applied to the oral mucosa for pain relief or procedural comfort, can cause methemoglobinemia. Manifestations include fatigue, dyspnea, cyanosis, and metabolic acidosis. Methemoglobinemia is treated with methylene blue.

18. What are common categories and examples of anesthetic agents?

Anesthetic agents can be classified into the following categories:

- Sedatives/hypnotics
- Analgesics
- Muscle relaxants
- Inhaled agents (see Table 11-3)

19. What is the mechanism of action of benzodiazepines?

Benzodiazepines increase the gamma-aminobutyric acid (GABA) receptor affinity for GABA in the brain. This increased affinity results in increased GABA activity. The result is sedation, amnesia, anxiolysis, and hypnotic and anticonvulsant properties.

20. How are benzodiazepines metabolized in the body?

Benzodiazepines are principally metabolized by the liver and excreted by the kidneys (PDR Staff, 2010) (see Table 11-4).

21. What affects the rate of metabolism and clearance of benzodiazepines?

- Liver disease
- Age
- Synergistic effects of narcotics and other sedatives

TABLE 11-3. Common Anesthetic Agents and Examples

Medication type	Examples
Sedative/ hypnotic	Benzodiazepines (midazolam, lorazepam, valium)
	Propofol
	Central nervous system alpha-2 receptor agonist (dexmedeto- midine)
Analgesics	Narcotics (fentanyl, hydromor- phone, morphine, remifentanil)
	Nonsteroidal anti-inflammatory agents (ketorolac, ibuprofen, acetaminophen)
Muscle relaxants	Depolarizing (succinylcholine)
	Nondepolarizing (rocuronium, vecuronium, pancuronium)
Inhaled agents	Nitrous oxide (N_2O), desflurane, sevoflurane, isoflurane

22. What is the mechanism of action of common narcotics?

Narcotics such as fentanyl, morphine, hydromor-phone, codeine, and remifentanil are *mu*-receptor agonists. These receptors are primarily located presynaptically in the periaqueductal gray region of the brain and in the dorsal horn of the spinal cord. Activation of *mu* receptors produces analgesia. *Mu* receptors are also found in the intestinal tract. Activation of these intestinal receptors results in constipation due to decreased peristalsis.

Remifentanil is an ultrashort-acting synthetic narcotic. It exerts analgesic properties by binding to *mu* receptors like other narcotics. Unlike other narcotics that undergo clearance by hepatic metabolism, remifentanil undergoes rapid hydrolysis by nonspecific tissue and plasma esterases. The result is a high potency narcotic infusion that maintains a constant elimination half-life of approximately 4 minutes. This ultra-short duration of action can leave patients in a great deal of discomfort due to acute withdrawal symptoms.

23. What is the mechanism of action for nonnar-cotic analgesics like ketorolac and acetaminophen? What are some considerations with administration of these medications?

Ketorolac is a parenteral nonsteroidal anti-inflammatory (NSAID) medication used to treat pain and inflammation. Ketorolac acts by decreasing prostaglandin production, which directly decreases pain and inflammation. Patients with an allergy to aspirin or other NSAIDs should not receive ketorolac. Patients with thrombocytopenia, platelet dysfunction,

TABLE 11-4. Benzodiazepine Metabolism and Excretion

Generic drug name (Trade name)	Typical dose	Onset of action	Elimination half-life	Metabolism
Midazolam (Versed)	1–2 mg IV	1–2 minutes	2–3 hours	Hepatic with renal excretion
Lorazepam (Ativan)	0.5–1 mg IV	1–2 minutes	8–18 hours	Hepatic with renal excretion
Diazepam (Valium)	2–10 mg IV	1–4 minutes	15–40 hours (100 hours in elderly patients)	Hepatic (active metabolites) with renal excretion
Alprazolam (Xanax)	0.5–5 mg/day PO	1–2 hours	8–20 hours	Hepatic with renal excretion
Temazepam (Restoril)	7.5–30 mg PO	30–60 minutes	8–9 hours	Hepatic with renal excretion

bleeding tendencies, intracranial bleeding, or renal insufficiency should be carefully evaluated before receiving NSAIDs.

Acetaminophen is a centrally acting analgesic and antipyretic. The mechanism of analgesia is not known, though it appears to act by increasing the pain threshold. Metabolism of acetaminophen is a three-step process that occurs in the liver. Acetaminophen should be administered to patients with liver dysfunction only after very careful consideration.

24. What are the differences between selected narcotics in relation to dose and duration?

Lipid solubility defines opiate action; a more lipid-soluble compound will have a more rapid onset of action and a shorter duration of action. Increased lipid solubility allows the medication to cross cell membranes and affect change. This increased solubility also causes a more rapid metabolism and decreased duration of action. For example, morphine is less lipid soluble than fentanyl. If both agents were to be administered intravenously, the fentanyl would have a more rapid onset of action and shorter duration of action due to increased lipid solubility (Miller, 2005; PDR Staff, 2010) (see Table 11-5).

25. What are the manifestations of and treatments for narcotic overdose?

Narcotics have numerous side effects, including dizziness, somnolence, altered mental status, pruritus, urticaria, difficulty urinating, abdominal pain, constipation, and, most importantly, respiratory depression. Hypoventilation and resultant respiratory acidosis may lead to cardiac dysrhythmias and, possibly, death. A patient suspected of receiving an overdose of narcotics resulting in altered mental status and respiratory depression should be treated with a narcotic antagonist like naloxone, supplemental oxygen, continuous pulse oximetry, and hemodynamic monitoring in a closely monitored environment. Patients who receive a narcotic overdose may require advanced airway support and cardiopulmonary resuscitation.

26. What are the criteria for endotracheal extubation?

- Return to baseline mental status
- Patent airway
- Ability to protect airway
- Intact cough and/or gag

TABLE 11-5. Narcotic Dose, Onset, and Duration of Action

Name	Usual dose	Onset of action	Duration	Metabolism
Fentanyl	25–50 mcg IV	1–3 minutes	10–30 minutes	Hepatic with renal and fecal excretion
Morphine	2–10 mg IV	2–5 minutes	1–2 hours	Hepatic with renal and fecal excretion
Hydromorphone	0.2–0.6 mg IV	1–3 minutes	20–40 minutes	Hepatic with renal excretion
Remifentanil	0.05–2 mcg/kg/min (1–2 mcg/kg bolus)	1–2 minutes	3–9 minutes	Hydrolysis, plasma esterases
Methadone	2.5–40 mg IV/PO daily	30–60 minutes	8–20 hours	Hepatic with renal and fecal excretion
Hydrocodone	7.5–15 mg PO	20–40 minutes	4–6 hours	Hepatic with renal excretion
Oxycodone	5–15 mg PO	20–40 minutes	4–6 hours	Hepatic with renal excretion

Adapted from Miller, 2005.

TABLE 11-6. Indications for Intubation

Reason	Examples
Airway protection	Poor mental status, head injury
Increased work of breathing (respiratory rate >35)	Sepsis, pulmonary injury, increased dead space, pulmonary shunt
Ventilatory failure	$PaCO_2$ >55 mmHg, hypopnea, apnea
Oxygenation failure	ARDS with PaO_2 to FiO_2 ratio <200, acute hypoxemia
Severe metabolic derangement	Severe acidosis, carbon monoxide poisoning
Procedures	Surgery, other diagnostic or therapeutic procedure

- Ability to maintain appropriate minute ventilation
- Ability to handle secretions

27. What are the indications for emergent intubation or reintubation? What are signs and symptoms of respiratory insufficiency?

Respiratory insufficiency, also referred to as respiratory failure, is the inadequate exchange of respiratory gases. The result is hypoxemia and/or hypercapnia. Hypoxemia leads to end organ dysfunction and, if severe, eventual death. Hypercapnia is the result of inadequate minute ventilation (the product of depressed respiratory rate and/or tidal volume). The indications for intubation are presented in Table 11-6.

28. What is emergence?

Emergence is defined as the transition from sleep or anesthetized state to a wakeful state. This is a typically smooth and uneventful transition from stage III to stage I anesthesia (Miller, 2005) (see Table 11-7).

29. What is delirium?

Delirium is a reversible syndrome characterized by an acute onset of perceptual disturbance, altered sleep–wake cycle, physiologic lability, disturbance of consciousness, and cognitive dysfunction. Patients most at risk for postoperative delirium are elderly patients with prior history of psychiatric disorders undergoing long surgical procedures requiring general anesthesia

TABLE 11-7. Stages of Anesthesia

Stage of anesthesia	Description
Stage I	Induction phase; medications given to cause loss of consciousness. Patients experience amnesia in this phase.
Stage II	Excitation phase; a period between induction and adequate surgical anesthesia. This period includes marked irregularity in heart rate, blood pressure, and respirations. Airway compromise due to laryngospasm is a risk in this stage.
Stage III	Surgical anesthesia phase; respirations and other vital signs return to baseline. The patient is able to tolerate surgery.
Stage IV	Overdose; too much medication resulting in brainstem depression and potential cardiovascular collapse. This stage is lethal without cardiovascular support.

with volatile anesthetics. Elderly patients who receive benzodiazepines are also more likely to experience delirium.

30. What are possible causes of hypotension in the PACU?

The most common cause of hypotension in the PACU is hypovolemia resulting from NPO (nothing by mouth) status, insensible operating room (OR) fluid losses, or blood loss. The most acute and serious cause of hypotension is acute hemorrhage.

Insensible losses in the OR are greatest for open abdominal cases, open thoracic cases, and cases involving large débridements or burns. Peripheral vasodilation due to anesthetic agents or generalized inflammatory response can contribute to hypotension. Urine output causing a net negative fluid status may also contribute to hypotension. Of course, any type of shock (e.g., septic, cardiogenic, neurogenic) can cause hypotension. Treatment of hypotension should be based on the cause of volume loss or the type of shock.

31. What are the most common causes of hypoxemia in the PACU?

Hypoxemia is a commonly encountered problem in the PACU. Unless absolutely contraindicated, all postoperative patients should receive supplemental oxygen until they have met discharge criteria (see Table 11-8).

32. What are common problems caused by hypothermia?

Hypothermia results in impaired wound healing, slowed metabolism of medications, coagulopathy, and generalized patient discomfort.

33. What are the risk factors for postoperative nausea and vomiting (PONV)?

Demographic risk factors for PONV are younger patients, female gender, history of motion sickness, and history of PONV. Surgical procedures with a high incidence of PONV are those involving strabismus surgery, middle ear surgery, urologic surgery, gynecologic surgery, and any surgery resulting in blood being swallowed. Patients who receive volatile anesthetic agents have a greater risk of PONV as compared to patients who receive total intravenous anesthesia (TIVA). Administration of nitrous oxide (N_2O) and/or narcotics may increase the incidence of nausea and vomiting. A history of smoking decreases the likelihood of PONV.

34. What are PACU discharge criteria?

The ASA 2002 *Practice Guidelines for Postanesthetic Care* identify nine areas for evaluation of the postanesthetic patient. The nine areas for evaluation are as follows (ASA, 2002):

- Respiratory status
- Cardiovascular status
- Neuromuscular function
- Mental status
- Temperature
- Pain assessment
- Fluid management
- Urine output
- Drainage and bleeding

35. What is the modified Aldrete score?

The modified Aldrete score is an evaluation tool used to determine the readiness for patient discharge from phase I recovery to phase II recovery or another inpatient care setting. The score ranges from 1 to 10. Patients scoring greater than 8 (and/or who are determined to be at preoperative baseline) are considered to be fit for transition to phase II recovery.

The categories and scoring for the modified Aldrete score are as follows:

Respiration
2 = Able to take deep breaths and cough
1 = Dyspnea/shallow breathing
0 = Apnea

O_2 saturation
2 = Maintains more than 92% on room air
1 = Needs O_2 inhalation to maintain O_2 saturation greater than 90%
0 = Saturation less than 90% even with supplemental oxygen

Consciousness
2 = Fully awake
1 = Able to be aroused on calling
0 = Not responding

Circulation
2 = BP+ 20 mmHg preop
1 = BP+ 20–50 mmHg preop
0 = BP+ 50 mmHg preop

Activity
2 = Able to move four extremities
1 = Able to move two extremities
0 = Not able to move any extremities

TABLE 11-8. Common Causes of Hypoxemia

Problem	Corrective actions
Airway obstruction	Jaw thrust, head tilt, nasal or oral airway, hand ventilation, endotracheal intubation, cricothyrotomy
Residual sedation	Stimulation and verbal cues, pharmacologic reversal of narcotics or benzodiazepines
Hypoventilation	Stimulate the patient, assist respirations, consider airway adjuncts, and consider calling for help. Administer narcotic or benzodiazepine antagonist, if appropriate. Consider neurology consultation.
Atelectasis causing V/Q (ventilation/perfusion) mismatch	Deep breathing, incentive spirometry, lung segment recruitment maneuvers, hand ventilation, high flow oxygen, endotracheal intubation
Residual neuromuscular blockade	Pharmacologic reversal (if possible), hand ventilation, endotracheal intubation with mechanical ventilation
Primary cardiac dysfunction	Treat specific underlying cause (hypovolemia, myocardial dysfunction, etc.), initiate ACLS (advanced cardiac life support)

REFERENCES

American Society of Anesthesiologists. (2008). ASA physical status classification system. Retrieved from http://www.asahq.org/clinical/physical status.htm

American Society of Anesthesiologists. (2009). Distinguishing monitored anesthesia care ("MAC") from moderate sedation/analgesia (conscious sedation). Retrieved from http://www.asahq.org/publications AndServices/standards/35.pdf

American Society of Anesthesiologists, Task Force on Postanesthetic Care. (2002). Practice guidelines for postanesthetic care: A report by the American Society of Anesthesiologists. *Anesthesiology, 96,* 742–752.

Cousins, M. J., & Bridenbaugh, P. O. (Eds.). (1998). *Neural blockade in clinical anesthesia and management of pain* (3rd ed.). Philadelphia: Lippincott-Raven.

Miller, R. D. (Ed.). (2005). *Miller's anesthesia* (6th ed.). Philadelphia: Elsevier.

New York School of Regional Anesthesia. (2009a). *Local anesthetics.* Retrieved from http://www.nysora .com/regional_anesthesia/equipment/3116-local_ anesthetics.html

New York School of Regional Anesthesia. (2009b). *Spinal anesthesia.* Retrieved from http://www.nysora.com/ regional_anesthesia/neuraxial_techniques/3119-spinal_ anesthesia.html

New York School of Regional Anesthesia. (2009c), *Epidural blockade.* Retrieved from http://www.nysora .com/regional_anesthesia/neuraxial_techniques/ 3026-Epidural-Blockade.html

PDR Staff. (2010). *Physicians' desk reference* (64th ed.). Montvale, NJ: PDR Network, LLC.

Population-Specific Principles

CHAPTER 12

Bariatric Patients

Janet Laughlin, RN, BSN, CPAN

The prevalence of obesity is increasing throughout the world and is estimated to affect more than 250 million people worldwide, based on statistics from 2000 (Owens, 2006). An estimated 65% of Americans over the age of 20 are overweight. The significance of the problem becomes even more staggering as it is estimated that this number will increase as obesity increases in children (Owens, 2006). A 1999–2000 survey of children between the ages of 2 and 19 showed that more than 25% were overweight or obese. The morbidly obese are at an increased risk of developing chronic diseases such as type II diabetes, obstructive sleep apnea (OSA), gastroesophageal reflux disease (GERD), and osteoarthritis of the weight-bearing joints. While obesity predisposes this population to chronic diseases, it also puts caregivers at risk for injury when mobilizing bariatric patients. An often over-looked problem is the prejudice and discrimination that this population experiences (Camden, 2006).

1. What is the definition of a bariatric patient?

Bariatrics is concerned with the prevention and treatment of obesity. Bariatric patients include those who are obese or morbidly obese. Morbid obesity, or clinically severe obesity, is a term used by the American Society of Bariatric Surgery. Morbid obesity is further defined by a body mass index (BMI; BMW = weight[kg]/height[m]^2) greater than 40 or a weight twice as much as predicted for age, gender, body build, and height (Owens, 2006).

2. What are the major effects of obesity on the respiratory system?

There are marked decreases in expiratory reserve volume due to the inability to effectively expand the chest. Diaphragmatic movement is limited due to anatomic changes such as excess abdominal fat. Functional residual capacity may be decreased when sitting and in a supine position, thus closing off the dependent lung zones that can lead to mismatching of ventilation and perfusion.

3. What are the other effects of obesity on the respiratory system?

One major effect of obesity on the respiratory system includes obstructive sleep apnea (OSA). OSA, which reportedly occurs in 5% of the morbidly obese population, results in multiple episodes of significant apnea (>10 seconds) during sleep. When partial or complete airway obstruction occurs, the cause is usually the redundant excess tissue in the posterior aspect of the throat, which closes the airway and results in the cessation of breathing. OSA is frequently undiagnosed.

When the airflow is decreased by 50%, it is significant enough to lead to a 4% decrease in oxygen saturation. The result of these interruptions in airflow can lead to hypoxia, hypercapnia, systemic and pulmonary hypertension, and cardiac arrhythmias.

4. What are the major effects of obesity on the cardiovascular system?

- An increase in oxygen consumption and cardiac output
- Prolonged Q/T interval, which may contribute to an increased risk of ventricular arrhythmias
- Elevated systemic blood pressure due to the stress of excess body weight on the cardiovascular system

5. What other disorders are more common in the obese population?

- Diabetes is a common chronic condition among the bariatric population and inconsistencies in postoperative glucose management further complicate a bariatric patient's postoperative course. Increased adipose tissue can lead to insulin resistance.
- Gastroesophageal reflux disease (GERD) results from the excess abdominal weight pushing gastric acid from the stomach into the esophagus.
  - There is also a correlation with aspiration of gastric acid and asthma.
- Osteoarthritis of the weight-bearing joints is also common, resulting from wear and tear due to the excess weight on the joints and the breakdown of cartilage, which further leads to painful inflammation (Owens, 2006).
  - In addition to the hip and knee joints, this population often has back pain and disc degeneration.

6. What are the preoperative concerns for the bariatric patient?

As a result of excessive weight, patients may suffer from multiple respiratory, cardiovascular, endocrine, and musculoskeletal system issues that make them a greater anesthetic risk. If possible, a bariatric bed should be ordered ahead of time so that the bariatric patient can be as comfortable as possible in the preoperative area.

7. What special considerations are necessary when caring for a patient with OSA?

OSA is common in morbidly obese patients. This condition may be diagnosed and treated, undiagnosed and untreated, or diagnosed with compliance issues with the prescribed treatment. If the patient uses home CPAP (continuous positive airway pressure) or Bi-PAP (bilevel positive airway pressure), it is ideal for the patient to be on their own machine, which has been fitted and adjusted for the individual patient. If a patient comes into your facility with a home CPAP/Bi-PAP machine, follow institutional protocols in dealing with the equipment.

8. What other special considerations should be addressed in the preoperative area?

- Skin assessment must be thorough because there may be hidden skin breakdown in the skin folds. This may be challenging especially for those patients who have mobility issues.
- IV access may also present a challenge because veins are buried in the subcutaneous tissue.

9. What intraoperative concerns need to be addressed?

- A bariatric patient is at higher risk for aspiration. As such, the anesthesia provider may elect to perform an awake intubation or rapid sequence induction with cricoid pressure.
- A bariatric patient is at higher risk for skin breakdown due to maceration, skin folds, and positioning.
- The procedure may be attempted laparoscopically and then switched to an open procedure due to necessity for greater visualization on the part of the surgeon.
- A bariatric patient often needs a special operating room table and extra padding, along with an adequate lift device and/or personnel to transfer the patient from the bed to the operating room (OR) table and back.

10. What are some considerations for weight-loss surgery?

- There may be a medical need due to the patient's weight-related health conditions, or this may be the patient's best option for sustained weight loss.
- Nonsurgical attempts often involve diets that do not provide a sustainable weight loss and often put the person at risk for health problems related to severe nutritional restriction.
- The loss of muscle mass leads to a reduction in metabolic rate, which further exacerbates the problem.
- Bariatric patients who do not undergo weight-loss surgery are often at greater risk for death than from the possible complications commonly associated with the surgery itself.

11. What is the history of bariatric surgery?

The first bariatric procedure, a jejuno-ileal bypass, was performed in 1954. It has evolved from this initial anatomic procedure to variations from small intestine bypass to gastric bypass in the late 1980s (e.g., Roux-en-Y duodenojejunostomy with stomach volume reduction). The gastric banding device, an inflatable band with a balloon as its lining, was developed by Dr. Kuzmak in 1990. Gastric bypasses are now most often performed laparoscopically, reducing the risk for infection, hernias, and decreasing the length of stay in a hospital.

12. What are the current procedures for bariatric surgery?

- The most commonly performed procedures are divided into three categories: restrictive, malabsorptive (see Question 13), and combination procedures. (see Question 14)
- An example of a restrictive procedure is adjustable gastric banding, which involves the placement of a silastic band around the uppermost portion of the stomach. The result is a restriction in the amount of food that can be ingested. There can be band adjustments via the port, which is accessed by a Huber needle (Owens, 2006).

Advantages include:

- Reduction in stomach size, leading to decreased caloric consumption
- No effect on the digestive process or absorption of nutrients
- Adjustable and removable band

Disadvantages include:

- May not make the person feel satisfied, which could lead to increase in snacking
- Reports of less weight loss when compared with other weight-loss surgeries

Risks include:

- Gastric perforation or tearing of the stomach wall, leading to additional surgery
- Access port twisting or leaking
- Nausea and vomiting
- Outlet obstruction
- Pouch dilatation
- Band migration/slippage
- Gastric wall erosion or ulceration

13. What are the malabsorptive procedures for bariatric surgery?

Biliopancreatic diversion and biliopancreatic diversion/duodenal switch are the two most commonly performed malabsorptive procedures.

In a biliopancreatic diversion (BPD), a small gastric pouch is created with an anastomosis of the proximal ileum, creating a gastroileostomy. The proximal limb is then anastomosed to the side of the distal ileum, proximal to the ileocecal valve. In this procedure, the distal stomach, duodenum, and entire jejunum are bypassed.

A biliopancreatic diversion/duodenal switch (BPD/DS) preserves the first portion of the duodenum and pylorus. There is a vertical subtotal gastrectomy to create the pouch, then a division of the duodenum is performed with the closure of one end of the duodenum and an anastomosis of the other end to the distal small bowel (Owens, 2006).

Advantages include:

- The possibility of producing greater weight loss because of the greatest malabsorption (mean weight loss is 70% of excess body weight) (Buchwald et al., 2004)
- A somewhat larger pouch that allows patients to consume more food, which some patients prefer

Disadvantages include:

- A potential for gastrointestinal leak at the anastomotic site
- An increased risk for developing gall bladder disease due to changes in the intestinal absorption
- A frequent liquid stool can be caused by the malabsorptive component of the procedure
- Abdominal bloating and gas. (Patients should be monitored for protein malnutrition, anemia, and bone disease. It is recommended that the patient take vitamin supplements.)

Risks include:

- Fat-soluble vitamin deficiencies (A, D, E, and K)
- Intestinal irritation and ulceration due to rerouting of bile and digestive juices
- Malabsorption of vitamin B12 and iron resulting in menstruating women being more prone to anemia
- Osteoporosis and metabolic bone disease resulting from the decreased absorption of calcium

SECTION I

SECTION II

SECTION III

- "Dumping syndrome," where stomach contents rapidly move to the small intestines. (This syndrome is characterized by nausea, weakness, sweating, faintness, and sometimes diarrhea after eating.)

14. What is the combination or hybrid gastric bypass procedure?

Roux-en-Y gastric bypass is considered the most common procedure for weight-loss surgery and involves the creation of a reduced-sized stomach by stapling or surgically separating the stomach across the fundus—the restrictive portion of the surgery. The distal stomach, duodenum, and proximal jejunum are bypassed with the creation of a gastrojejunostomy and biliopancreatic conduit connection.
 Advantages include:

- A higher percentage of excess weight loss for the compliant patient (as compared with restrictive procedures)
- Weight loss averaging 77% of excess body weight after just 1 year (Wittgrove & Clark, 2000)
- Maintaining 60% of excess weight loss over a period of 10 to 14 years
- Improvement or resolution of certain associated health conditions such as diabetes, hypertension, sleep apnea, back pain, and depression (Wittgrove & Clark, 2000)

Disadvantages include poorer demonstrated results if the created stomach pouch volume exceeds 15–30 ml or if the stomach pouch expands due to overeating.
 Risks include:

- Potential for anastomotic leaks at the sites of gastrojejunostomy and/or enteroenterostomy
- Vitamin deficiencies (similar to malabsorptive procedures)
- Anemia due to malabsorption of iron
- Early onset of osteoporosis due to calcium malabsorption
- Chronic anemias and neurologic deficiencies related to vitamin B12 deficiency

15. What are the benefits of bariatric surgery other than weight loss?

- Reduction or elimination of comorbidities, which provides an improvement in quality of life and eliminates the need for medications to manage conditions such as hypertension, diabetes, and hyperlipidemia

- Gastric banding and Roux-en-Y bypass prevent proximal stomach acid from reaching the esophagus, thus eliminating GERD
- Elimination or "curing" of OSA

16. What compromises postoperative respiratory status?

- Excess abdominal fat interferes with the diaphragm's movement, as well as excess adipose tissue in the thorax affects the diaphragm's ability to expand. This can lead to atelectasis, which may compound other respiratory issues in the postoperative period.
- The effects of general anesthesia and administration of opioids lead to hypoventilation, which leads to hypercarbia and lowered oxygen saturation and a decrease in arousability.
- Arterial hypoxemia should be avoided, because the patient may not be able to compensate for an increased cardiac output demand with pulmonary vasoconstriction caused by reduced arterial oxygen tension.

17. What interventions are implemented to prevent respiratory complications?

- The head of bed should be elevated at all times while the patient is in bed unless they have cardiovascular compromise.
  - Positioning the patient with the head of bed elevated at least 30° allows for increased lung expansion.
  - Positioning the patient with the use of pillows to elevate the head and upper body can assist in relieving the pressure on the diaphragm.
  - The supine position should be avoided because of further compromising alveolar ventilation, which can lead to hypoxemia.
- Early intervention with incentive spirometry will assist the patient in decreasing their risk for atelectasis and pneumonia.
- If the patient has orders for patient controlled analgesia (PCA) for postoperative pain management, careful monitoring is necessary. The patient may require continuous oximetry monitoring as well as supplemental oxygen (Drain, 2003).
- The use of CPAP or Bi-PAP may be indicated to improve ventilation and oxygenation.

18. What interventions must be implemented for the patient who remains intubated postoperatively?

- The patient should be placed on the ventilator with settings that reflect the management plan.
- The effectiveness of the ventilatory plan should be evaluated by periodic arterial blood gas tests.
- Auscultation for bilateral breath sounds is essential in determining proper tube placement.
- A portable chest x-ray should also be obtained to determine proper tube placement.
- If the tube becomes dislodged, the patient should be ventilated with a bag-valve-mask system and the anesthesia provider should be immediately notified.

19. Obese patients have an increased risk for cardiovascular compromise. What are the necessary postoperative interventions?

- All bariatric surgery patients should have cardiac monitoring because of their risk for developing arrhythmias.
- Elevated heart rate may require treatment with beta-blockers.
- When patients complain of chest pain, an electrocardiogram (ECG) should be obtained to rule out myocardial ischemia.
- Selecting the proper size and location of the blood pressure cuff is essential in determining the patient's systemic blood pressure. The blood pressure cuff must cover one third to one half the length of the upper arm. If the patient was monitored using a forearm cuff, that practice should continue in the postanesthesia care unit (PACU) for comparison of values.

20. What are the signs and symptoms of an anastomotic leak?

- Whether the procedure is performed laparoscopically or as an open procedure, a leak can occur and can be fatal if not detected early.
- Anastomotic sites are checked with methylene blue intraoperatively, but that does not guarantee that a leak will not develop postoperatively.
- Symptoms of a leak may be subtle and can include abdominal tenderness, left shoulder pain, tachycardia, decrease in urine output, elevated temperature, elevated white blood cell count (WBC), and a decrease in oxygen saturation.

21. How are anastomotic leaks managed?

- Depending on the hemodynamic stability of the patient, the patient may be surgically reexplored. If the patient has symptoms of peritonitis but is stable, surgical reexploration may be indicated.
- If the patient has a controlled or contained leak or abscess, he or she may be taken to interventional radiology for placement of an abdominal drain (Owens, 2006).

22. Obese patients have an increased risk for developing deep vein thrombosis (DVT). What interventions can be implemented to prevent this complication?

- Placement of compression stockings during surgery and while the patient is in bed can help prevent DVT (Owens, 2006).
- Patients who have had a history of DVT or pulmonary embolism may have a vena caval filter placed prior to surgery.
- Patients need to be educated on the importance of early ambulation.

23. What preventative measures should be taken to ensure skin integrity?

- Thorough skin assessments through all phases of the perioperative experience are imperative in the prevention of skin breakdown.
- Correct the misconception commonly held by healthcare professionals that bariatric patients are not at risk for skin breakdown because they have plenty of padding. The bariatric patient is actually at an increased risk for skin breakdown because of the decreased blood supply to distal subcutaneous tissue and the excess weight on bony prominences.
- Skin folds are an area that must have vigilant care to ensure that moisture does not have an opportunity to cause skin breakdown.
- The OR nurse is responsible for ensuring that prep solution does not remain in skin folds. Proper padding placement and monitoring of skin over pressure points is essential in the prevention of skin breakdown.

24. Fluid dynamics is a factor in the care of the postoperative patient. What is the cause of differences in fluid requirements?

Adipose tissue is 6–10% water as compared to lean tissue (which is 70–80% water). As a result, the bariatric patient may experience alteration in their fluid volume status. In the healthy patient, body water is 65%, as compared to the obese patient whose body water is approximately 40% of body weight. Without adjustments in the fluid volume to compensate for this difference, the bariatric patient may experience hypovolemia.

25. What are some of the barriers that healthcare professionals must overcome to provide optimal care to bariatric patients?

- Healthcare professionals need to respond to bariatric patients with an expression of sincere empathy, showing an understanding of the disease and the discrimination that these patients have to endure in their everyday life.
- Prejudice, described as prejudgment, and discrimination based on this judgment, stem from an ill-conceived notion that obesity is related to lack of self-discipline.
- There is a strong genetic predisposition associated with morbid obesity; healthcare professionals must overcome their belief that these patients could lose weight if they just reduce their intake and increase their exercise.

- Healthcare professionals should be aware that bariatric patients may overcompensate by trying to do too much and may actually injure themselves in the process of trying to "help" the nurse by doing activities of daily living themselves (e.g., repositioning in bed) (Camden, 2006).

REFERENCES

Buchwald, H., Avidor, Y., Braunwald, E., Jensen, M. D., Pories, W., Fahrbach, K., et al. (2004). Bariatric surgery: A systematic review and meta-analysis. *Journal of the American Medical Association, 292*(14), 1724–1737.

Camden, S. G. (2006). Nursing care of the bariatric patient. *Bariatric Nursing and Surgical Patient Care, 1*(1), 21–30.

Drain, C. B. (2003). *Perianesthesia nursing: A critical care approach* (4th ed.). St. Louis, MO: Saunders.

Owens, T. M. (2006). Bariatric surgery risks, benefits, and care of the morbidly obese. *Nursing Clinics of North America, 41*(2), 249–263.

Wittgrove, A. C., & Clark, G. W. (2000). Laparoscopic gastric bypass, Roux-en-Y 500 patients techniques and results, with 3–60 month follow-up. *Obesity Surgery, 10*(3), 233–239.

CHAPTER 13

Patients with Chronic Diseases

Kathy Daley, RN, MSN, CNS, CCRN-CMC-CSC, CPAN

A chronic disease, as defined by the US National Center for Health Statistics, is one lasting 3 months or more. More than 133 million Americans, or 45% of the population, have at least one chronic condition (The Partnership to Fight Chronic Disease [PFCD], 2008). There is an immense likelihood that the perianesthesia nurse will care for a patient with a chronic comorbidity in a typical workday. This chapter will briefly explore 11 chronic diseases: hypertension, stroke, coronary artery disease, chronic obstructive pulmonary disease, asthma, sleep apnea, diabetes, arthritis, cancer, chronic renal insufficiency, and morbid obesity. Each disease state will have a definition and overview followed by preoperative considerations and postoperative implications.

1. What is hypertension?

It is estimated that approximately 33% of Americans (or 1 in 3) have hypertension (HTN) and more than 30% of those cases are undiagnosed. This is especially true for those who do not seek regular medical care. It is not surprising that the initial diagnosis is often found when the patient presents for surgery.

HTN is an abbreviation for high pressure (tension) in the arteries. High blood pressure increases one's chance for developing heart disease, stroke, and other chronic diseases. Normal blood pressure is below 120/80; blood pressure between 120/80 and 139/89 is called prehypertension, and a blood pressure of 140/90 or above is considered high. HTN directly raises the myocardial oxygen demand. In the presence of coronary artery disease, this demand may not be able to be met. These patients have a risk of increased blood pressure instability during anesthesia and ischemic complications postoperatively. Chronic HTN results in an enlarged heart, myocardial damage, and lung and renal abnormalities (Chummun, 2009). HTN is the leading risk factor for developing a stroke.

2. What are the preoperative considerations for patients with chronic HTN?

Antihypertensive medications should be continued until immediately before the surgery or procedure, with a small sip of water during the preoperative period when patients are allowed nothing by mouth (NPO). Withdrawal of some antihypertensive agents such as beta-blockers (β-blockers) can cause rebound HTN or can unmask myocardial ischemia that may not have been previously recognized. Therefore, patient education concerning the importance of continuing antihypertensive treatment is essential. Reducing the risk of cardiac events by 30 to 90% may be achieved by perioperative use of β-blockers. β-blockers are started in the preoperative phase to reduce the stress and demands of surgery by slowing down the heart rate. The stress of surgery increases the myocardial oxygen demand, which can lead to cardiac events such as myocardial infarction (MI), angina, and congestive heart failure (Mathias, 2007).

3. What are the postoperative implications for patients with chronic HTN?

Postoperative HTN may also cause a ventricle with systolic dysfunction to fail, resulting in pulmonary edema. Diastolic dysfunction may lead to intolerance of tachycardia, often seen postoperatively because of inadequate ventricular filling time. Antihypertensive therapy should be resumed as soon as possible postoperatively. β-blocker protocols have been instituted in patients with chronic HTN and in those with coronary artery disease (CAD) as a risk factor. This helps not only with blood pressure control, but also with controlling tachycardia and protecting the heart from ischemia in the perioperative period.

4. What is a stroke?

A stroke or brain attack occurs when a blood clot blocks an artery or a blood vessel breaks, interrupting blood flow to an area of the brain. When either of these events occurs, brain cells begin to die and brain damage results. When brain cells die during a stroke, abilities controlled by that area of the brain are lost. These abilities include speech, movement, and memory. How a stroke patient is affected depends on where the stroke occurs in the brain and how much of the brain is damaged. Strokes affect roughly 780,000 people per year, and 5.8 million people live with the consequences of stroke.

A transient ischemic attack (TIA) is a warning stroke or ministroke that produces strokelike symptoms lasting for less than 24 hours, with no lasting damage. Recognizing and treating TIAs can reduce the risk of a major stroke. In people who have had one or more TIAs, more than one-third will later have a stroke. Unlike TIAs, a RIND, or reversible ischemic neurological deficit, lasts for more than 24 hours, but for less than 3 weeks.

5. What are the preoperative considerations with the patient who has had a previous stroke?

The preoperative nurse should focus on the neurologic status from the prior stroke with clear documentation of any deficits. Again, if the patient has chronic HTN, it is imperative that antihypertensive therapy continues. Another consideration is the etiology of the original stroke. Atrial fibrillation and atherosclerosis are often precursors to embolic or ischemic strokes. Therefore, anticoagulant or antiplatelet therapy is usually in the treatment regime and must be reversed prior to surgery. In patients who have had multiple strokes, the benefit of continuing the antiplatelet therapy up to the time of surgery may outweigh the risk of increased surgical bleeding.

6. What are the postoperative implications for patients who have had a previous stroke?

One postoperative implication for patients who have had a previous stroke includes keeping the blood pressure normotensive. Profound hypotension or HTN in the immediate postoperative period

can cause decreased cerebral perfusion, resulting in the risk for an additional stroke. Careful neurological assessment compared with preoperative neurologic status in the postoperative period is crucial to determine if an insult has occurred.

Postoperatively, antiplatelet therapy can safely be resumed if surgical hemostasis is satisfactory and there is no evidence of bleeding. In patients who have been chronically anticoagulated with warfarin, the perceived risk of perioperative stroke determines whether a patient needs a heparin drip or low-dose heparin postoperatively. If the risk factor is considered low, warfarin should resume when the patient can take pills postoperatively. If the risk factor is moderate to high, interim anticoagulation with heparin drip or low-molecular heparin once surgical bleeding risk has subsided is often implemented and continued until the protime is therapeutic on warfarin.

Any patient with a history of nonhemorrhagic stroke should be considered for prophylactic β-blocker therapy, given the very high incidence of coexisting coronary artery disease and the proven increased perioperative cardiac risk among patients who have had a prior stroke.

7. What is coronary artery disease?

According to the 2006 publication by the American Heart Association (AHA) and the American Stroke Association (ASA) on heart disease and stroke statistics, cardiovascular disease remains the leading cause of mortality in the United States in men and women of every major ethnic group. Approximately 13 million individuals have a history of coronary artery disease (CAD) and 7.2 million have suffered a myocardial infarction (MI).

CAD is a type of heart disease. The heart gets oxygen and nutrients from the blood that flows through the coronary arteries. In CAD, plaque sticks to the walls of the coronary arteries. As the plaque thickens, artery openings get narrow and blood flow slows. This causes the heart to receive less blood and oxygen, resulting in myocardial ischemia. Over time, the heart must work harder and the ventricle can be hypertrophic causing dysfunction and end-organ damage.

8. What are preoperative considerations for patients with CAD?

Current studies suggest that β-blockers reduce perioperative ischemia and may reduce the risk of MI and death in patients with known CAD. Evidence suggests that therapy should be started days to weeks before surgery, if possible, and should continue throughout the perioperative period. The basic clinical evaluation obtained by history, physical examination, and review of the electrocardiogram (ECG) usually provides the clinician with sufficient data to estimate cardiac risk (American College of Cardiology [ACC] & AHA, 2007). Additional tests may be indicated with increased risk. Anemia can exacerbate myocardial ischemia and aggravate heart failure; therefore, a preoperative hematocrit may be indicated for high-risk blood loss surgeries.

9. What are the postoperative implications for patients with CAD?

Continuation of β-blocker therapy is crucial for optimum myocardial protection. Perioperative MIs can be documented by assessing clinical symptoms, serial ECGs (compared to the preoperative ECG), cardiac-specific biomarkers, and comparative ventriculographic studies before and after surgery. Perioperative surveillance for acute coronary syndromes with routine ECG and cardiac serum biomarkers is unnecessary in clinically low-risk patients undergoing low-risk operative procedures (ACC & AHA, 2007).

Pain management is vital in the perioperative care of the cardiac patient. Tachycardia can ensue as a result of catecholamine release with acute pain. This, in turn, can increase myocardial oxygen consumption, resulting in MI. Therefore, an effective analgesic regimen must be included in the perioperative plan.

10. What is chronic obstructive pulmonary disease (COPD)?

COPD is a lung disease characterized by chronic obstruction of lung airflow that interferes with normal breathing. It is not fully reversible. The more familiar terms chronic bronchitis and emphysema are no longer used, but are now included within the COPD diagnosis. COPD is not simply a "smoker's cough" but an underdiagnosed, life-threatening lung disease (World Health Organization [WHO], 2010).

Over 16 million people suffer from this disease in the United States. According to the American Lung Association, approximately 14 million people suffer with chronic bronchitis, and there are an estimated 1.9 million people suffering with emphysema. According to the WHO, 75% of deaths from COPD that occur in developed countries are directly related to smoking tobacco.

In a healthy person, increasing CO_2 levels in the blood drives respiration. In patients who are diagnosed with COPD, because of their increased level of CO_2, a deficiency of oxygen is necessary to stimulate respiration (hypoxic drive). In these patients, high-dose oxygen can reduce respiration and can cause respiratory depression.

The phenomena of "air-trapping" is one of the primary insults of COPD. Expiratory times are prolonged due to a loss of integrity of the airways, causing hyperinflated lungs. Hypotension may occur from the decreasing venous return to the heart because of an increase in intrathoracic pressure.

11. What are preoperative considerations for the patient with COPD?

Preoperative incentive spirometry can be utilized to establish baseline volumes. Pulmonary function testing may be useful as a predictor of postoperative success. Many of these patients are on home oxygen (O_2) and liter flow and oxygen saturation (SPO_2) must be established. These patients may have a baseline SPO_2 of less than 90%.

Use of metered dose inhalers (MDIs) containing bronchodilators and corticosteroids, as well as handheld nebulizers, should be given per the daily routine. Physical assessment of the pulmonary status is an important preoperative consideration for patients with COPD. This includes auscultation and documentation of breath sounds to establish the patient's baseline.

12. What are the postoperative implications for patients with COPD?

Fast-acting bronchodilators (albuterol) should be given postoperatively for audible wheezing. Incentive spirometry should begin as soon as feasible. If mechanical ventilation is required, attention must be given to air trapping. Time must be given to exhale by adjusting the inspiration to expiration ratio. Arterial blood gases (ABGs) may be ordered. With the ABG results, the acid-base balance (pH) is the key element in deciding treatment, not the $PaCO_2$. Capnography, or end-tidal CO_2 monitoring, can be used to trend values in COPD patients.

13. What is asthma?

Asthma is a chronic respiratory illness characterized by bronchial inflammation and hyperresponsiveness, resulting in recurrent episodes of bronchoconstriction, airway edema, mucus plugs, coughing, and wheezing. In the United States, there are 16.4 million, or 7.3% adults, and 7 million, or 9.4% children, that have been diagnosed with asthma.

14. What are preoperative considerations for patients with asthma?

Bronchodilators and corticosteroids should be continued per the routine and care must be given to avoid triggers. Preoperative physical assessment—giving detail to auscultation—is imperative to establish a baseline.

15. What are the postoperative implications for patients with asthma?

Due to patients' reactive airways, bronchodilators should be continued in the postoperative period. Care should be given to avoid known triggers and additional corticosteroid therapy may be indicated.

16. What is obstructive sleep apnea?

Approximately 31.2% of adults aged 20 years or older have been diagnosed with obstructive sleep apnea (OSA) (Centers for Disease Control [CDC], 2010). OSA syndrome is the most common form of breathing-related sleep disorder. It is characterized by repeated episodes of upper airway obstruction (apneas and hypopneas) during sleep. The central drive for respiration and respiratory movements in the chest and abdomen are preserved. OSA usually occurs in overweight individuals and leads to a complaint of excessive sleepiness. OSA syndrome is characterized by loud snores or brief gasps that alternate with episodes of silence, usually lasting 20 to 30 seconds. Snoring is caused by breathing through a partially obstructed airway. Silent periods are caused by obstructive apneas, and the cessation of breathing is caused by complete airway obstruction. OSA has been shown to have a negative impact on certain aspects of cognitive function, which can be evident during the waking hours. Sequelae include excessive daytime sleepiness, depression, and attention and concentration problems.

17. What are preoperative considerations for patients with OSA?

Patients that require continuous positive airway pressure (CPAP) should be instructed to bring their own machines and nasal or oral masks with them to the hospital. The use of sedatives in these patients must be carefully weighed, as they suppress upper airway muscle activity. Each facility that cares for these patients should have a process and policy in place to check the home machine for safety prior to patient use.

18. What are the postoperative implications for patients with OSA?

Many patients with OSA require postoperative intubation and mechanical ventilation until fully awake. Patients who already use a prescribed CPAP machine should utilize it during this time, but the pressure should be monitored to ascertain that it is adequate. CPAP can also be employed postoperatively in other patients that do not utilize this technology at home to support their breathing in the immediate postoperative period. There may also be some upper airway swelling secondary to intubation and extubation. The lingering sedative and respiratory depressant effects of the anesthetic can pose difficulty with breathing (American Sleep Apnea Association, 2008).

19. What is diabetes?

Diabetes mellitus (DM) results when the body cannot use blood glucose as energy because too little insulin is produced by the body or the body is unable to use the insulin. Type I diabetes is a condition in which the pancreas makes so little insulin that the body cannot use blood glucose as energy. People with type 1 diabetes need to take insulin every day. Type 2 diabetes is a condition in which the body either makes too little insulin or cannot use the insulin it has in order to use blood glucose as energy. Type 2 diabetes is the most common form of diabetes (CDC, 2010).

It is estimated that DM affects 10% of the US population of adults aged 20 years and older (7.5% are diagnosed and 2.5% go undiagnosed). DM accounts for 8% of all legal blindness, is the leading cause of end-stage renal disease, and patients with diabetes are twice as likely to develop cardiovascular disease. Elevated blood glucose adversely affects every tissue of the body, with the possible exception of hair. Long-term effects of DM can also lead to such conditions as peripheral neuropathies, gastroparesis, foot ulcers, and infections due to delayed wound healing.

20. What are the preoperative considerations for patients with DM?

The type of DM and the patient's individual treatment regime should be documented. Accurate glucose monitoring is a vital step in promoting wound healing and in preventing infection. Hyperglycemic protocols should be in place, starting with the day of surgery and including a fasting preoperative blood sugar.

Surgery and anesthesia invoke a stress response, which causes an increase in peripheral insulin resistance, increased glucose production, impaired insulin secretion, and the breakdown of protein and fat. This leads to a potential for hyperglycemia and, in more severe cases, ketosis. The degree of this response depends on the complexity of the surgery and any postsurgical complications (Marks, 2003). In addition, a serum creatinine and possibly BUN (blood urea nitrogen) may be ordered preoperatively for all diabetic patients because of the possibility of coexisting renal dysfunction.

21. What are the postoperative implications for patients with DM?

Patients with DM have a muted immune response to invading organisms; therefore, even a small bacterial load can result in an infection (Nortcliffe & Buggy, 2003). Preexisting vascular changes, impaired immunity, and delayed healing also can contribute to increased risk for postoperative infection in the diabetic patient. The stress of surgery and anesthesia can exacerbate hyperglycemia by increasing insulin resistance. This is a result of an increase of counterregulatory hormones (glucagon, epinephrine, cortisol, and growth hormone). This stress response also prevents the hepatic glucose to undergo gluconeogenesis and glycogenolysis. During the perioperative period, adequate insulin must be present to prevent metabolic breakdown (Marks, 2003). For these reasons, strict glycemic control is imperative in the perioperative period.

22. What is arthritis?

Arthritis is inflammation of one or more joints. Approximately 46 million (or nearly one out of five adults) have been diagnosed with arthritis in the United States. Arthritis is one of the most prevalent chronic health problems and the nation's leading cause of disability among Americans over the age of 15. It is estimated that 67 million adults older than the age of 18 will be diagnosed with arthritis by 2030 (CDC, n.d.). There are many different types of arthritis. Two common types are rheumatoid arthritis (RA) and osteoarthritis (OA). RA is an autoimmune disease; the synovial fluid lining the joints is chronically inflamed. This transforms the synovium from a smooth membrane to one that is thickened and protrudes into the joint cavity. The resultant erosions cause pain and limited motion and function. When the lining of the joint becomes inflamed, it gives off more fluid and the joint becomes swollen and painful. This inflammation can spread to surrounding tissues and can affect other organs. OA is also called degenerative arthritis and is the most common form of arthritis. OA is characterized by a loss of cartilage and destruction of musculoskeletal tissue in the affected joint. It is neither not an inflammatory process nor the result of wear and tear of the joints due to the aging process. Cartilage absorbs shock of movement and when it is lost, bones rub together causing pain, swelling, and decreased mobility of the affected joint.

23. What are the preoperative considerations for patients with arthritis?

Patients with arthritis may be at an increased risk for perioperative complications because of systemic manifestations of the disease, medication effects, or specific joint-related problems. Patients who have received long-term corticosteroid therapy are at highest risk of having cervical spine instability, which influences tactics for airway management. Home pain medications and adjuncts, such as aspirin (ASA) or nonsteroidal anti-inflammatory agents (NSAIDs) should be documented. These medications may increase the risk for developing perioperative bleeding complications. Mobility limitations must be identified in the preoperative period to provide a baseline.

24. What are the postoperative implications for patients with arthritis?

Many medications used to treat arthritis are immunosuppressive, so there is a concern for postoperative infection and delayed wound healing. Ketorolac (intravenous NSAID) may be used as an adjunct for analgesic management in those patients with chronic pain. NSAIDs must be used with caution in patients with impaired renal function. The need for careful positioning and stabilization of the neck should be considered in patients with advanced arthritis of the cervical spine.

25. What is cancer?

Cancer accounts for nearly one fourth of deaths in the United States, exceeded only by heart disease. Presently, the risk for an American man developing cancer over his lifetime is one in two. The leading cancer sites are prostate, lung, colon, and rectum (American Cancer Society, n.d.). Approximately one in three women in the United States will develop cancer over her lifetime. Cancer begins when cells in a part of the body start to grow out of control and can invade other tissues. There are many kinds of cancer, but they all start because of out-of-control growth and metastasis of abnormal cells. A tumor is an abnormal mass of tissue that results when cells divide more than they should or do not die when they should. Tumors may be benign (not cancer) or malignant (cancer). When patients are diagnosed with cancer, staging is usually the first step in determining treatment. Staging describes the extent or severity of an individual's cancer based on the extent of the original (primary) tumor and the extent of spread in the body. The common elements considered in most staging systems are: location of where the tumor started, the size and number of tumors, if the cancer has spread into the lymph nodes, the cell type and how closely the cancer resembles normal tissue, and if metastasis has occurred. Treatment of cancer can include chemotherapy, radiation, surgery, or a combination of all of these treatment regimens.

26. What are the preoperative considerations for patients undergoing cancer treatment?

Many of the considerations for the patient with cancer are due to the treatment of cancer. Chronic pain, malnourishment, electrolyte imbalance, immunosuppression, and skin fragility are all side effects of chemotherapy treatment. A complete physical assessment, including chemistry and hematology labs, and the patient's current pain management regime is indicated to determine the baseline. It is also good practice to create and implement a pain management plan for the patient's anticipated postoperative pain needs.

27. What are the postoperative implications for patients with cancer?

Pain management in the cancer patient is often a challenge due to the presence of chronic pain. The preoperative regime should begin as appropriate with additional analgesic therapies for the acute-on-chronic pain during the postoperative period. Careful positioning and attention to skin in the postoperative period is important to prevent skin breakdown and tears. Because of the immunosuppressive side effects of many chemotherapeutic agents, skin is often fragile and delayed wound healing is a concern.

28. What is renal insufficiency?

The Third National Health and Nutrition Examination Survey (NHANES III) estimates that the prevalence of chronic renal disease in adults in the United States is 11% of the population (19.2 million). The two leading causes of chronic renal insufficiency are HTN and DM (Coresh et al, 2003).

Chronic renal insufficiency (CRI) is defined as when the filtering capacity of the kidneys is slowly and gradually destroyed. It is sometimes referred to as progressive renal insufficiency, chronic kidney disease, or chronic renal failure (CRF). This kind of damage cannot currently be repaired, and, as such, it is irreversible. A person may have CRF for many years, even decades, before dialysis or a kidney transplant becomes necessary. CRI does not, by itself, mean complete shutdown of the kidneys, and a person with CRI may still pass urine normally and may have more than enough kidney function left for normal functioning of the body. One cannot judge kidney function by the amount of urine one produces. Patients with quite advanced renal insufficiency and even patients on dialysis may still produce a fair amount of urine. But this does not mean that the kidneys are filtering waste or regulating serum electrolyte levels efficiently. As CRI

progresses, the condition may eventually reach the point where it is considered to be end-stage renal disease (ESRD). One important aspect of kidney disease is that, once a kidney is damaged to a certain degree, it continues to deteriorate even if the underlying kidney disease can or could be cured. This is commonly referred to as the point of no return. As the CRI continues to progress on its own, scarring of the glomeruli continues, and kidney function continues to gradually decline. The point of no return is generally considered to be when serum creatinine reaches 2.0 mg/dl (Chronic Renal Insufficiency, n. d.). Long-term sequelae of renal insufficiency include anemia, osteodystrophy due to hyperphosphatemia and hypocalcemia, electrolyte and acid-base disturbance, alterations in nutrition and protein metabolism, and end-stage renal disease. Infants and children with CRI may be malnourished, have growth retardation, and neurologic disorders.

29. What are the preoperative considerations for patients with renal insufficiency?

Certain procedures increase the risk of acute renal failure in nondialysis chronic renal patients such as those procedures involving radiographic contrast material. N-acetylcysteine and sodium bicarbonate can be given intravenously in the preoperative or postoperative setting to prevent and protect kidney function.

30. What are the postoperative implications for patients with renal insufficiency or chronic renal failure?

Chronic kidney disease is associated with impaired hemostasis; therefore, there is a higher risk for bleeding and patients should be closely monitored. Many drugs are metabolized and cleared by the kidney, such as metoclopramide and cefazolin. Drug profiles should be reviewed by a pharmacist for dose adjustments in the postoperative arena. Additionally, care should be given to not volume overload these patients.

31. What is morbid obesity?

It is estimated that 33% of US adults age 20 years and older are overweight, 34% are obese, and 6% are extremely obese. Morbidly obese individuals generally exceed ideal body weight (IBW) by 100 pounds or more, are 100% over IBW, or have a body mass index (BMI) greater than 40 kg/m². Morbid obesity is a risk factor for HTN, CAD, stroke, COPD, DM, asthma, OSA, renal disease, and arthritis. In addition, these patients are predisposed to hiatal hernia and reflux and are at greater risk for aspiration at the time of intubation and extubation.

32. What are the preoperative considerations for patients with morbid obesity?

Thought must be given to all of the possible comorbidities with which the morbidly obese patient presents. A thorough preoperative assessment with appropriate diagnostic labs should be conducted. Deep vein thrombus (DVT) prophylaxis is also warranted in these patients.

33. What are the postoperative implications for patients with morbid obesity?

Obesity can significantly change the anatomy of the airway and can lead to a difficult intubation (Noble, 2009). Respiratory complications following anesthesia are increased because of lung volume constriction due to intra-abdominal fat. Skin breakdown and the risk of developing pressure ulcers is a concern for prolonged supine positioning and requires diligent skin care and special equipment, such as a larger bed or gurney.

Many analgesic agents that are used perioperatively are stored in the adipose tissue of the morbidly obese, which increases the risk for medication-related respiratory depression. However, the morbidly obese patient may have difficulty breathing without pain control; therefore, careful assessment, ongoing monitoring, and careful titration of analgesics is required.

REFERENCES

American Cancer Society (n. d.) Retrieved from http://www.cancer.org

American College of Cardiology & American Heart Association. (2008, March). 2007 guidelines on perioperative cardiovascular evaluation and care for noncardiac surgery: executive summary: a report of the American College of Cardiology/American Heart Association Task Force on Practice Guidelines. *Anesthesia & Analgesia, 106*(3), 685–712.

American Sleep Apnea Association. (2008). Sleep apnea and same-day surgery. Retrieved from http://www.sleepapnea.org/resources/pubs/sameday.html

Centers for Disease Control. (2010) Retrieved from http://www.cdc.gov/

Chronic renal insufficiency. (n. d.) Retrieved from http://www.mcw.edu/FileLibrary/Groups/Medicine Nephrology/ChronicRenalInsufficiency.pdf

Chummun, H. (2009, July). Hypertension—a contemporary approach to nursing care. *British Journal of Nursing, 18*(13), 784–789.

Coresh, J., Astor, B. C., Greene, T., Eknoyan, G., Levey, A.S. (2003, January) Prevalence of chronic kidney disease and decreased kidney function in the adult US population: Third National Health and Nutrition Examination Survey. *American Journal of Kidney Disease, 41*(1),1–12.

Marks, J. B. (2003, January). Perioperative management of diabetes. *American Family Physician, 67*(1), 93–100.

Mathias, J. M. (2007, March). Setting up a beta blocker protocol. *OR Manager Supplement, 23*(3), 20–22.

Noble, K. A. (2009, December). The obesity epidemic: The impact of obesity on the perianesthesia patient. *Journal of PeriAnesthesia Nursing, 23*(6), 418–425.

Nortcliffe, S. A., & Buggy, D. J. (2003). Implications of anesthesia for infection and wound healing. *International Anesthesiology Clinics, 41*(1), 31–64.

The Partnership to Fight Chronic Disease. (2008). Almanac of chronic disease (2008 ed.). Retrieved from www.fightchronicdisease.org/pdfs/PFCD_FINAL_PRINT.pdf

World Health Organization. (2010). Chronic respiratory diseases, COPD-definition. Retrieved from http://www.who.int/respiratory/copd/definition/en/index.html

CHAPTER 14

Critically Ill Patients

Hildy Schell-Chaple, RN, MS, CCNS, CCRN

This chapter will provide an evidence-based review of general critical care topics that cross the span of diagnosis and surgical procedure and that are essential knowledge for nurses caring for this patient population regardless of care location.

1. What is critical care?

Florence Nightingale was an advocate of separate care areas for specific patient populations, in particular, postsurgical patients. Due to the historic events of the early 1900s, invention of healthcare technologies (e.g., mechanical ventilators), and thoughtful clinicians, intensive care units (ICUs) began to open in the United States. The first multidisciplinary ICU with 24-hour physician coverage was opened in 1958 at Baltimore City Hospital, now known as The Johns Hopkins Hospital. By 2004, there were over 87,000 critical care beds in the United States. The specialty practice of critical care has evolved over the years to meet the needs of patients with severe life-threatening illness or injury and/or for those who require specialty monitoring or complex interventions requiring specialty training of clinicians.

2. When does a postanesthesia recovery patient become a critical care patient?

The location where a patient receives care (e.g., ICU or postanesthesia care unit [PACU]) and/or specific clinical criteria cannot define or differentiate critical care. In the PACU, the patient in phase I recovery with an unstable airway or hemodynamic compromise is a critically ill patient. In another scenario, the postsurgical patient becomes a critically ill

patient when their clinical course plan changes due to delayed anesthesia recovery and/or changes in their clinical status that require ongoing monitoring and/or critical care interventions. In still another scenario, in some hospitals, it is routine for critically ill patients that already have a reserved ICU bed to go first to the PACU for initial stabilization. Finally, some PACUs across the country routinely care for and hold the critical care patient until an ICU bed becomes available. For these reasons, critical care will be used throughout this chapter to describe the constellation of vigilant monitoring and aggressive practices that can occur in PACUs that provide this care or in ICUs.

Common reasons postanesthesia patients require critical care include monitoring for potential complications due to the high risk nature of their operative procedure and/or the risks related to their comorbid conditions. For example, the postoperative renal transplant patient who also has severe coronary artery disease may require ischemia monitoring beyond the anesthesia recovery time period.

3. What infections are common to critical care patients?

A recent epidemiologic study of 1265 ICUs in 75 countries revealed a 51% prevalence rate of infections in ICU patients (Vincent et al., 2009). The most common location of infection is the lungs (pneumonia) with gram negative organisms as the most common pathogen. Common sources and locations of infections in critical care patients are central venous catheters, surgical sites, the sinuses, and intra-abdominal locations. ICU patients with infections have a clinically significant higher ICU and hospital mortality rate than patients without infection. The prevention of hospital-associated infections for patients is important nursing work. Nurses can prevent infections through diligent hand hygiene practice, use of aseptic principles for specified care, and following evidence-based procedures for routine and complex nursing care such as oral care, suctioning, central venous catheter care, Foley catheter care, and access of tubing and invasive devices. The priority of infection prevention that nurses have traditionally paid attention to now has the public and federal government's attention as a patient safety concern. The US Health and Human Services requires all states to have a 5-year goal and action plan to reduce hospital-associated infections such as ventilator associated pneumonia, surgical site infections, and central venous catheter-related blood stream infections by 2010.

4. What are important assessment tips for early detection of infection in critical care patients?

Early detection of infection through thorough physical exam and assessment of patient risk factors, signs, and symptoms can positively impact outcomes through early appropriate interventions.
Risk factors include the following:

- Immunosuppressive medications (corticosteroids, chemotherapy, transplant antirejection medications, and immunotherapy for autoimmune disorders)

- Immunosuppressive therapies (plasmapheresis, radiation therapy)

- Chronic diseases (diabetes, end-stage renal disease, end-stage liver disease)

- Invasive devices, wounds, and surgical sites

- Extreme ages

- Malnutrition

- Antibiotic therapy (increases risk of secondary infections by *Clostridium difficile* and *Candida albicans*)

Signs and symptoms include the following:

- Fever (>38.3°C) or hypothermia (<36°C)

- Elevated white blood cell (WBC) count (>12,000 cells/mm³) or leucopenia (<4,000 cells/mm³)

- New onset diarrhea and recent or current antibiotic use (increases risk of secondary infection by *C. difficile*)

- Red rash with small pustules along edges in perineum, axilla, skin folds, and around incisions, wounds or device dressing sites (e.g., cutaneous fungal infection)

- Persistent nasal drainage and presence of a nasal tube (e.g., sinusitis)

- Increased pulmonary secretions, increased oxygen requirements, and infiltrates on chest x-ray (e.g., ventilator-associated pneumonia)

- Redness, induration, tenderness near incisions or wounds, device insertion sites, or over joints (e.g., cellulitis or abscess)

- Lip and/or perineal lesions, which may be recurrent viral infections (e.g., *Herpes simplex*) and are often mistaken for pressure injury from an endotracheal tube or from being bed bound

- Persistent purulent eye drainage and redness (i.e., conjunctivitis)

5. How should fever be managed in critically ill patients?

Fever is defined as a regulated increase in temperature to at least 38.3°C in critically ill patients. The method of temperature monitoring should be based on the most accurate and reliable method that is the least invasive to patients. Intravascular (pulmonary artery catheter), esophageal, rectal, bladder, and oral thermometry are accurate methods for most patients. Axillary, temporal artery, and chemical dot thermometry are not recommended in adult ICU patients. Differentiating "postoperative fever" from fever of infectious or noninfectious etiology can be challenging and, therefore, requires a comprehensive assessment. Physical examination and review of the patient's history and laboratory values is warranted to evaluate risk and other potential etiologies of fever before initiating diagnostic tests in the first 72 hours of the postoperative period. There is no evidence to support routine suppression of fever in critical care patients (O'Grady et al., 2008). Assessment of the patient's respiratory, hemodynamic, neurologic, and metabolic response to the fever should be considered when deciding on the administration of antipyretic agents or physical cooling measures.

6. What practices prevent central venous catheter-related blood stream infections (CRBSI)?

It is estimated that there are 250,000 hospital-acquired CRBSIs each year in the United States. CRBSI is associated with increased morbidity, mortality, and economic burden. Attributed mortality estimates range from 4 to 20%. Hand hygiene prior to contact with any part of the central venous catheter (CVC) or attached circuit is always the first step of prevention.

Infection prevention strategies can be bundled into four areas for CVC care:

1. CVC insertion technique: full barrier precautions including drapes, masks, and hats; skin disinfection with chlorhexadine friction scrub

2. Daily assessment of CVC criteria: nursing review of need for the CVC by established criteria such as pressure monitoring, rapid fluid administration, medications or therapies requiring central access, and inability to obtain alternate IV access

3. CVC site assessment and care: assess site for signs of infection and that the dressing is dry and intact; care of site with a chlorhexidine friction scrub and application of chlorhexadine impregnated patch at insertion site under occlusive dressing

4. Circuit maintenance: scrub injection hubs with alcohol or chlorhexidine prior to access, ensure blood and debris are cleared from injection hubs and stopcock lumens, ensure a closed circuit is maintained, minimize entry into circuit for medication administration or blood draws as much as possible, and change circuit tubing at least every 96 hours

7. What is sepsis, and how does it differ from severe sepsis and septic shock?

Sepsis terminology and diagnostic criteria have been standardized by an international expert consensus group as part of the Surviving Sepsis Campaign (Dellinger et al., 2008). This global campaign strives to reduce death from sepsis by providing research-based guidelines that focus on improving early identification, diagnosis, and management of sepsis. Sepsis is the body's systemic inflammatory response to an infection. The infection may be anything from a urinary tract infection to an infected wound site. The diagnostic criteria for sepsis are a suspected or known infection with systemic signs of infection by two or more of the criteria found in Table 1. Severe

TABLE 14-1. Signs and Symptoms of Sepsis

General variables & vital signs
• Core temperature greater than 38.3°C or less than 36°C • Heart rate greater than 90 beats per minute • Respiratory rate greater than 20 per minute • Altered mental status (lethargy or confusion) • Significant edema formation or positive fluid balance (>20 mL/kg over 24 hours) • Hyperglycemia (blood glucose greater than 140 mg/dL [nondiabetic])
Inflammatory variables
• White blood cell (WBC) count greater than 12,000 or less than 4,000 • Normal WBC count with differential of greater than 10% bands (immature neutrophils) • Plasma C-reactive protein level greater than two standard deviations of normal lab • Plasma procalcitonin level greater than two standard deviations of normal lab
Hemodynamic variables
• Hypotension (SBP less than 90 mmHg, MAP less than 70 mmHg or a SBP decrease greater than 40 mmHg from baseline)
Organ dysfunction variables
• Hypoxemia (PaO_2 less than 60 mmHg, SpO_2 less than 90%) • Low urine output less than 0.5 mL/kg/hour despite adequate fluid resuscitation • Increased plasma creatinine level by >150% • Coagulation abnormalities (INR greater than 1.5 and/or PTT greater than 60 seconds) • Thrombocytopenia (platelet count less than 100,000) • Hyperbilirubinemia (total bilirubin greater than 4 mg/dL)
Tissue perfusion variables
• Elevated serum lactate level greater than the upper limit of normal lab • Decreased capillary refill or presence of mottling (in extremities, knee caps, abdomen, trunk)

sepsis is sepsis plus related organ dysfunction and/or tissue hypoperfusion. Septic shock is sepsis plus hypotension that persists despite adequate fluid resuscitation.

8. What are resuscitation priorities for severe sepsis?

The Surviving Sepsis Campaign (Dellinger et al., 2008) endorses a sepsis resuscitation bundle of care interventions that should be completed as soon as possible and within 6 hours of suspecting sepsis along with interventions to identify the source of infection.

1. Measure serum lactate levels to monitor severity of anaerobic metabolism as proxy monitor of tissue oxygenation adequacy.

2. Obtain blood cultures prior to antibiotic administration.

3. Administer broad spectrum antibiotics within 1 hour of suspected sepsis for hospital inpatients.

4. Ensure patient has adequate IV access for resuscitation fluids and medications.

5. If serum lactate is greater than 4 mmol/L or the patient has hypotension, optimize oxygen delivery to tissues and organs with the following interventions:

   a. Administer 20 mL/kg bolus of crystalloid IV fluids over 30 minutes to target goals of a CVP of 8 to 12 mmHg and/or a central venous blood oxygen saturation ($ScvO_2$) of greater than 70%.

   b. Initiate vasopressor therapy if mean arterial pressure (MAP) is less than 65 mm Hg after initial fluid bolus. Target MAP is greater than 65 mmHg.

   c. If $ScvO_2$ is less than 70% or hypotension persists after fluids and vasopressors, initiate dobutamine infusion and consider blood transfusion if hemoglobin level is less than 7 gm/dL.

9. What are the management priorities for severe sepsis after resuscitation?

The sepsis management bundle of care interventions are evidence-based supportive therapies.

1. Consider the administration of drotrecogin alfa activated (human recombinant activated protein C) at 24 mcg/kg/hr for 96 hours to patients with severe sepsis who are at a high risk of dying (e.g., APACHE II score of greater than or equal to 25) and present with multiple organ dysfunction. Mortality was reduced by 13% in randomized controlled trials using drotrecogin alfa activated to treat severe sepsis in patients at a high risk of death (Bernard et al., 2001). This intravenous medication has anticoagulant and anti-inflammatory properties. Since bleeding is the potential major adverse effect, evaluating the patient for identified contraindications and monitoring for bleeding is essential. The infusion should be held 2 hours prior to the start of any invasive procedures (e.g., CVC insertion or removal). It is recommended that the infusion be restarted 12 hours after a major invasive procedure (e.g., surgical procedure and continued until total dose is administered). Contraindications and cautions are primarily related to the risk of bleeding, and essential monitoring during administration includes laboratory monitoring (e.g., platelet count, partial thromboplastin time [PTT], partial thrombin time/international normalized ratio [PT/INR] values), and assessment for signs of bleeding.

2. Monitor blood glucose levels and initiate insulin therapy when levels are greater than 180 mg/dL. Maintain insulin therapy with a target around 150 mg/dL. Monitor patients closely for signs and symptoms of hypoglycemia and treat with a dextrose source when indicated.

3. Treat patients with acute lung injury or acute respiratory distress syndrome related to their sepsis with low tidal volume ventilation to maintain inspiratory plateau pressures less than 30 cmH_2O.

10. What is propofol infusion syndrome?

Propofol infusion syndrome is a potentially lethal adverse effect of the anesthetic/sedative infusion commonly used in critical care and perioperative settings. The clinical syndrome that presents is cardiac failure (arrhythmias and/or hypotension), severe metabolic acidosis (low pH, low bicarbonate, and a base deficit), acute kidney injury (decreased urine output and elevated creatinine level), and rhabdomyolysis (elevated creatine kinase, troponin, and myoglobin levels due to muscle lysis). The associated risk factor for this syndrome is the stress response of critical illness, which increases glucocorticoid secretion and catecholamine release. Critically ill patients receiving vasoactive infusions (e.g., norepinephrine and other vasopressors), glucocorticoid therapy, and propofol at higher doses (>65 mcg/kg/min and infusions greater than 48 hours) are at risk of this potentially lethal adverse effect of propofol. The combination of propofol and risk factors leads to cardiac and skeletal muscle dysfunction as utilization of fuel sources for cellular and metabolic activity are impaired. The cellular dysfunction results in impaired utilization of free fatty acids for energy production and excess levels in the blood that manifests as hypertriglyceridemia. The lack of fuel to meet the body's metabolic demands leads to catabolism (ischemic breakdown of cardiac and skeletal muscle) and presents with increased lactate, creatine kinase, myoglobin, and troponin I levels (Zaccheo & Bucher, 2008).

The clinical signs of propofol infusion syndrome include:

- Metabolic acidosis
- Elevated serum lactate levels
- Hypotension
- Elevated serum triglyceride levels
- Arrhythmias (sudden onset bradycardia)
- Acute kidney injury
- Rhabdomyolysis (elevated serum myoglobin and creatine kinase)
- Hepatomegaly

11. How is propofol infusion syndrome prevented and treated?

Nurses caring for patients receiving propofol infusions can contribute to early detection through awareness of the associated risk factors and clinical signs of this syndrome. Propofol infusion syndrome can be prevented through assessment of risk factors, use of doses within manufacturer recommendations, and consideration of an alternate sedative agent if the patient is at risk. Nurses are key to the early detection by considering their patient's signs of a lower heart rate, trend to a mild metabolic acidosis, and increase in vasopressor dose titration by responding to the hypotension as potential propofol infusion syndrome and discussing their assessment with their care team.

Treatment for suspected or diagnosed propofol infusion syndrome includes discontinuation of the propofol and support care for organ dysfunction and related tissue injury. Cardiac pacing may be considered if the bradycardia is refractory to medical interventions. Fluids, vasopressors, and positive inotropic medications can be used to support oxygen delivery through increased cardiac output. Continuous renal replacement therapy (CRRT) may be initiated to prevent rhabdomyolysis-induced kidney injury

through clearance of myoglobin and/or to treat the metabolic acidosis and the sequelae of acute kidney injury.

12. What are some clinical concerns about bariatric critically ill patients?

Bariatric patients are at risk for complications related to their obesity-associated comorbid conditions (e.g., pulmonary hypertension, diabetes, obstructive sleep apnea [OSA], venous stasis) in conjunction with the different impact of routine medications and care interventions they may experience. They are at risk for airway obstruction and/or hypoxemia with body positioning requirements during diagnostic or therapeutic procedures (e.g., CT scan or central line insertion) and routine care (e.g., shifting up in bed). Bariatric patients that receive sedatives or neuromuscular blocking agents are at extreme risk for reduced compliance of their respiratory system related to the effects on the musculature of the upper airway and due to the ventilation-perfusion mismatch caused by low lung volumes from increased intra-abdominal pressure. Positioning bariatric patients with the head of bed elevated to at least 30° or use of reverse Trendelenberg position and application of continuous positive airway pressure (CPAP) may prevent these complications in bariatric patients with or without the diagnosis of OSA. Cautious use of benzodiazepine and opioid medications and close monitoring during their use is recommended due to the respiratory risks. Pulmonary embolus is a risk for most critically ill patients, including bariatric patients. Venous stasis, OSA, and a BMI greater than 60 is associated with high risk for pulmonary embolism, and the insertion of an inferior vena cava filter is recommended in this population (Kaw et al., 2008).

13. What is pressure-induced rhabdomyolysis in bariatric patients?

A rare postoperative complication of bariatric patients is pressure-induced rhabdomyolysis. Muscle injury and necrosis occurs from pressure-induced ischemia from unrelieved, prolonged immobility on the operating room (OR) table. The risk factors associated with this injury include morbid obesity, prolonged OR time, and diabetes. The muscle areas affected are the lower limbs, buttocks, and lumbar area. Clinical signs to monitor in at risk, postoperative patients are dark or brown-tinged urine from muscle breakdown products (myoglobin), positive urine dipstick for hemoglobin, negative red blood cells on urinalysis, increased serum creatine phosphokinase (CPK) levels, complaints of muscle pain or numbness over affected muscle areas, and/or presence of bullae or purpura on the skin near the affected muscle areas due to ischemia. Early interventions can prevent the extent of acute kidney injury from the toxic myoglobin released during rhabdomyolysis. Treatment includes administration of IV fluids, bicarbonate therapy to alkalize the urine, diuretics, and removal of myoglobin with CRRT (Pieracci, Barie, & Pomp, 2006).

14. What is acute lung injury (ALI) and acute respiratory distress syndrome (ARDS)?

ALI and ARDS are the most severe types of acute respiratory failure. Severe inflammation in the lungs occurs after indirect or direct lung injury or infection. Diagnostic criteria for ALI and ARDS are acute onset of respiratory distress, bilateral infiltrates on chest x-ray, no clinical evidence of elevated left atrial pressures or a pulmonary capillary wedge pressure (PCWP) of less than 18 mmHg, and a PaO_2/F_IO_2 ratio (P/F ratio) of less than or equal to 300 for ALI and a P/F ratio of less than or equal to 200 for ARDS. The P/F ratio is an oxygen tension-based index that reflects the severity of hypoxemia related to an intrapulmonary shunt (venous blood flows by collapsed or fluid-filled alveoli to arterial circulation). Lower P/F ratio values reflect more severe hypoxemia and higher intrapulmonary shunt values. The estimated incidence of ALI and ARDS is 190,000 patients per year in the United States with an attributed mortality of over 74,000 patients per year (Matthay, 2008).

15. What causes ALI and ARDS?

The lung may be directly injured as with aspiration or chest trauma or indirectly injured as with sepsis or transfusion reaction in ALI and ARDS. There are many clinical conditions associated with ALI and ARDS, such as sepsis or systemic inflammatory response syndrome (SIRS), multiple or single blood transfusions, acute pancreatitis, aspiration of gastric contents, trauma, and toxic gas inhalation.

16. What are priority nursing care interventions for patients with ALI and ARDS?

Assessment includes the following:

- Patient's general appearance (assess for difficulty breathing and use of accessory muscles for inhalation and exhalation, assess synchrony with mechanical ventilation, color, and presence of diaphoresis)
- Airway: assess artificial airway type, patency and securement, and presence of secretions

- Oxygenation: assess PaO_2 and SpO_2 in relation to F_IO_2 and positive end-expiratory pressure (PEEP) levels, PaO_2/F_IO_2 ratio
- Ventilation: assess respiratory rate, tidal volume, minute ventilation, and $PaCO_2$ in relation to minute ventilation
- Barotrauma risk and detection: palpate the neck and chest to assess for subcutaneous air (early sign of barotrauma), and assess inspiratory plateau pressure (goal of <30 cmH$_2$0), breath sounds, new onset of higher peak inspiratory pressures
- Chest tube assessment (when present): assess the insertion site examination for signs of subcutaneous air, bleeding and infection; assess the chest tube system to ensure intact, secure connections, and suction settings as prescribed; assess the chest drainage system for the presence of tidaling and for an air leak (bubbling) in the water seal chamber; and assess the amount and characteristics of drainage when present

Interventions include the following:

- Achieve appropriate sedation level to facilitate synchrony with mechanical ventilation
- Assess pulmonary positioning to optimize ventilation-perfusion (VQ) matching and enhance pulmonary gas exchange
- Suction per procedure to minimize loss of end-expiratory lung pressure by use of inline device and/or a PEEP valve on the Ambu bag (aseptic procedure to prevent infection)

Anticipatory planning includes the following:

- Ensure supplies are available for emergent pneumothorax treatment: chest tube insertion tray and chest drainage system or large bore angio catheter with stopcock and 60 mL syringe
- Anticipate chest x-ray procedures to confirm diagnosis and to evaluate reexpansion of the lung postintervention

17. What management strategies can reduce ventilator days and reduce mortality in ARDS patients?

Mortality rates for patients with ARDS were as high as 60% in the 1990s and have decreased by 20% since the implementation of low tidal volume ventilation and advances in supportive care in ICUs over the past decade. The ARDS Network is a multicenter research collaborative in the

United States supported by the National Heart, Lung, and Blood Institute that has contributed to the science and practice changes that have improved care of patients with ARDS. The first intervention study that found significant impact on reducing mortality in ALI and ARDS was the use of low tidal volume (tidal volume of 6 mL/kg of predicted body weight) with a plateau pressure limit of 30 cmH$_2$0. The patients that received low tidal volume also had less ventilator days and less nonpulmonary organ dysfunction. Interventions that are not recommended since there is evidence that they do not improve survival or reduce ventilator days are high PEEP levels and the use of steroids for persistent ARDS. Conservative fluid management goals ("keeping them normovolemic") for patients with ALI and ARDS compared to liberal fluid management ("fluid overload") has been shown to reduce ventilator days (Matthay, 2008).

18. Why is ventilator-associated pneumonia (VAP) a priority concern in ICUs?

VAP is the most common ICU-associated infection. Prevalence of VAP ranges from 6 to 52 cases per 100 ICU patients. Patients intubated longer than 24 hours are up to 21 times more likely to develop ventilator-associated pneumonia. The risk for VAP increases with each additional day of mechanical ventilation and the attributed mortality from VAP ranges from 20 to 41%. ICUs that have implemented VAP prevention care bundles have reduced morbidity, mortality, and costs associated with VAP. Reduction in VAP rates is a national critical care priority.

19. Who is at risk for VAP?

Patients on a mechanical ventilator or who have a tracheal tube have an increased risk of VAP. Because the tube is a direct path to the lower airways, it interferes with the cough reflex, stimulates mucus production, and promotes dry mouth. Plaque is a prime reservoir for bacterial growth. Saliva contains immune factors and facilitates plaque breakdown. The other risk factors for VAP include a depressed level of consciousness, head of bed (HOB) flat position, gastric distention, presence of an enteral tube, enteral feeds, and having a COPD or trauma diagnosis. The mechanisms that contribute to VAP development are (a) colonization and/or contamination of the tracheal tube and ventilator circuit and (b) aspiration of gastric and/or oral secretions (Munro, Grap, Jones, McClish, & Sessler, 2009).

20. How is VAP prevented?

- By preventing colonization and contamination
  - Wash hands before and after glove use when performing any procedures related to suctioning, oral care, and/or manipulation of the ventilator circuit.
  - Rinse mouth with an antiseptic solution (e.g., 0.12% chlorhexidine at least every 12 hours). Oral care with tooth brushing or swab cleaning is acceptable for VAP prevention. Moisturizing the oral mucosa and lips after cleansing facilitates saliva production, prevents fissure formation, and promotes comfort.
  - Maintain clean technique principles and a closed system when handling suction and ventilator tubing or circuit supplies; routine ventilator circuit changes based on hours in use is not recommended.
  - Use appropriate antibiotics and isolate patients with colonization and/or infections from multidrug resistant pathogens to reduce cross contamination
- By preventing aspiration
  - Keep the patient's HOB elevation greater than 30° unless contraindicated. Use the gauge on the bed or a measurement device to assess HOB degrees as simultaneous comparisons of nurse perceptions based on "eyeballing" the patient's position do not agree with actual HOB degrees.
  - Monitor to ensure adequate volumes on tracheal tube cuff pressures without excessive pressure, especially after repositioning tubes and/or transporting patients.
  - Review indications for nasotracheal or nasogastric tubes and remove or relocate to oral tubes when possible. Higher rates of respiratory and sinus infections are associated with nasal tubes.
  - Use continuous subglottic suction endotracheal tube systems when possible to facilitate the removal of organism-laden secretions from above the tracheal tube cuff.
  - Avoid gastric overdistention through continuous or intermittent gastric suction and avoidance of procedures that result in gastric insufflation.

- By ventilator weaning and extubation

  - Provide respiratory therapy and nurse-driven ventilator weaning protocols to ensure appropriate and timely weaning.

  - Assess the patient's readiness to extubate on a regular basis (e.g., daily spontaneous breathing trial).

  - Use a sedation holiday to assess appropriate sedative needs on a regular basis (e.g., daily sedation wake up protocol).

21. What are the goals of hemodynamic monitoring?

The ultimate goal of the critical analysis of hemodynamic data, along with the patient's history, diagnosis and physical exam, and interventions implemented to optimize these parameters, is to optimize oxygen delivery and function of organ systems. Hemodynamic monitoring includes the measurement or calculation of physiologic indices of pressure, resistance, and flow in the cardiovascular system: heart rate (HR) and rhythm, blood pressure (BP), central venous pressure (CVP), pulmonary artery occlusion pressure (PAOP), pulmonary artery pressure (PAP), cardiac output/ cardiac index (CO/CI), stroke volume (SV), and systemic and pulmonary vascular resistance (SVR and PVR). The goals of monitoring hemodynamic variables are to obtain data for differential diagnosis (e.g., cardiogenic versus septic shock), to monitor for changes in clinical conditions that may lead to early intervention, and to evaluate response to therapies (e.g., vasoactive medications, fluid resuscitation, cardiopulmonary support devices).

22. What steps ensure accurate hemodynamic monitoring?

- Ensure patients are positioned correctly prior to obtaining measurements

  - CVP: supine (not lying on side) & HOB 0–60°

  - PAP: supine & HOB 0–60°

  - CO: supine & HOB 0–45°

- Level transducer (air-fluid interface) to the phlebostatic axis and verify accuracy of transducer monitoring system by performing the square wave test (dynamic response test).

- Use graphic print of ECG rhythm and CVP/ PAOP waveform to identify the mean of the wave and end expiration phase of respiration.

- Ensure CO system components are verified and procedures are followed.

  - Verify PAC tip in PA position

- Verify that the computation constant entered is appropriate based on:

  - PAC model number (length & diameter of catheter is important)

  - Injectate solution temperature range (iced or room temperature ranges)

  - Injectate solution volume (5 mL or 10 mL)

- Inject CO injectate rapidly without interruption (over less than 4 seconds) and evaluate CO curves for smooth form

- Perform at least three CO measurements and ensure they are within 10% of median value. Repeat measurements to obtain 3 to meet this target

- Determine cardiac index (CI) based on patient's body surface area

23. What tools can be used to assess the level of sedation in ICU patients?

There are a few commonly used sedation assessment tools used for ICU patients. The newer tools have more specific assessment procedures, which enhance reliability between nurses. The recommended sedation assessment scale is the Richmond Agitation Sedation Scale (RASS) due to the increased reliability and ease of use in a clinical practice. The Motor Activity Assessment Scale (MAAS), Sedation Agitation Scale (SAS), and the Ramsay Scale are other valid and reliable tools that can be used. The use of these sedation assessment tools can improve appropriate sedation use to meet the goals of sedation while minimizing the negative sequelae associated with excessive sedation. They can also provide a more consistent measure of a patient's level of sedation that can lead to early detection of neurologic changes.

24. How are risks associated with sedation use in ICU patients minimized?

ICU patients that receive continuous infusions of sedation have associated risks of prolonged mechanical ventilation, prolonged ICU length of stay, delirium, and other adverse effects of critical illness (O'Connor, Bucknall, & Manias, 2009). It makes sense that administering the right amount of sedation to achieve the desired effect while avoiding excessive dosing that could lead to adverse outcomes is the desired goal. Interventions that have been shown to help achieve this goal include: (a) the use of sedation orders that target a sedation level as measured by a valid and reliable sedation assessment tool, (b) the use of a sedation interruption protocol with specific indication criteria that includes at least daily assessment of patients after stopping sedation infusions, and (c) the use of nurse driven sedation protocols. Changing practice to include use of sedation interruption has been slow to happen in ICUs due to concerns about potential risks of tube dislodgement, negative physiological and psychological stress and discomfort for the patient when sedation is held, and nurse concern about the inability to safely manage potential severe agitation. Although further research in this area is warranted, identification of the goal of sedation for each patient and the reevaluation of sedation effects in relation to the goal is a best practice.

25. What is delirium?

Delirium is an acute syndrome of fluctuating levels of consciousness and cognition that can be classified as hyperactive, hypoactive, or mixed (mixed hyperactive and hypoactive signs) depending on the patient's clinical presentation. Delirium is common in the ICU and can go unrecognized when valid screening tools are not used or if there is limited awareness of diagnostic criteria. Delirium is associated with a prolonged ICU and hospital length of stay, as well as increased risk of death and lower quality of life reports after ICU discharge as compared to patients without delirium (Van Rompaey et al., 2009). Delirium has many precipitating and predisposing risk factors including medications (benzodiazepines, opioids, and psychoactive agents), infection or sepsis, metabolic disturbances, cerebral hypoperfusion, dehydration, and alcohol withdrawal.

Clinical signs and symptoms of delirium include the following:

- In hyperactive delirium:
  - Agitation
  - Combativeness
  - Lack of awareness about environment
  - Confusion
  - Memory deficits
  - Disorientation
- In hypoactive delirium:
  - Flat affect
  - Confusion
  - Periods of inattention or lack of focus (inconsistent follow of commands)
  - Memory deficits
  - Disorientation

26. How is delirium screened for in ICU patients?

There are a handful of validated tools used for delirium screening in the ICU. The Confusion Assessment Method for the ICU (CAM-ICU) has high inter-rater reliability and is commonly used in research studies and practice settings. It assesses four key criteria: mental status changes, inattention, disorganized thinking, and altered level of consciousness. Other screening tools used in ICUs include the ICU Delirium Screening Checklist, the Nursing Delirium Screening Scale, and the Delirium Detection Score. Patients receiving sedating medications and their inability to self-report are limitations with all delirium screening tools used in the ICU.

27. What interventions can help prevent and treat delirium in ICU patients?

Prevention strategies for delirium include minimizing risk factors through a review of the patient's history, diagnosis, and treatments (especially medication review). Nonpharmacologic interventions include frequently reorientating, providing activities that stimulate cognitive function, enhancing sleep and quiet time to minimize overstimulation, providing exercise and early mobilization in the ICU, and ensuring patients have their eyeglasses and hearing aids. The recommended pharmacologic intervention for delirium is haloperidol. Other antipsychotic and neuroleptic medications (e.g., risperidone, olanzapine, ziprasidone) may also be used.

28. What is the target blood glucose (BG) level for ICU patients?

Hyperglycemia is common in patients with critical illness regardless of whether they have a diabetes diagnosis. The movement toward tight glycemic control (BG target of 81–110 mg/dL) with insulin therapy in ICU patients was popular over the past decade based on evidence of improved outcomes. Recent studies have evaluated a broadened BG target range of up to 180 mg/dL and found the same benefits and a lower incidence of hypoglycemia (Fahy, Sheehy, & Coursin, 2009). Current recommendations are to monitor BG levels and to treat with insulin therapy to a target of less than 150 and up to 180 mg/dL with adequate monitoring for hypoglycemia. The conflicting evidence is not surprising as the study methods and insulin protocols used varied significantly. Changes in future BG target recommendations are likely with ongoing research of glycemic control benefits in ICU patients. It is important to ensure that the insulin therapy protocol used at your institution has safe monitoring and treatment procedures for hypoglycemia (BG target of <40 mg/dL).

29. What are risks and signs of acute kidney injury (AKI)?

Acute kidney injury (AKI) is an abrupt and sustained cessation of renal function. It is common in critically ill patients and has an attributed mortality of up to 80%. AKI risk factors in ICU patients are associated with comorbid diseases, altered perfusion and increased metabolic demand states associated with critical illness, and toxic side effects of diagnostic and therapeutic interventions. AKI is diagnosed using consensus derived diagnostic criteria (RIFLE criteria outlines three degrees of kidney injury severity based on risk, injury, failure, loss, and end-stage disease), which includes serum creatinine level change, urine output change, and creatinine clearance rates (Dennen, Douglas, & Anderson, 2010).

Risk factors for AKI include the following:

- Hypoperfused states (hypovolemia, obstructed renal flow, low cardiac output)
- Sepsis (inflammation, intrarenal cellular ischemia, hypoperfusion)
- Rhabdomyolysis (intrarenal cellular damage)
- Intra-abdominal compartment syndrome (perfusion and edema-related ischemia)
- Toxicities (IV contrast media, medications [antimicrobials])

Assessment and prevention for AKI includes the following:

- Reviewing patient's history and diagnosis for risk
- Reviewing baseline creatinine, blood pressure, and urine output
- Reviewing medications and therapies for toxicity risk
- Monitoring urine output and intake: output ratio
- Monitoring serum creatinine levels
- Assessing urine and serum analysis for fraction of excreted sodium (FeNa) to aid classification of AKI (prerenal versus intrarenal injury)
- Consider 24-hour urine for creatinine clearance data
- Considering hydration and bicarbonate administration plan before and during the procedure when IV contrast media is essential if chronic renal insufficiency or high risk of AKI present

AKI management includes the following:

- Identifying and treating the cause of AKI (volume repletion, cardiac support, stenosis, or obstruction relief procedure; alter medication selection or dose if appropriate)
- Renal replacement therapy (intermittent hemodialysis [IHD] or continuous renal replacement therapy [CRRT] based on assessment of symptomatic uremia, electrolyte imbalance, symptomatic fluid overload, acid-base status, and hemodynamic and neurologic tolerance of IHD)

REFERENCES

Bernard, G. R., Vincent, J. L., Laterre, P. F., LaRosa, S. P., Dhainaut, J. F., Lopez-Rodriguez, A., et al. (2001). Efficacy and safety of recombinant human activated protein C for severe sepsis. *New England Journal of Medicine, 344*(10), 699–709.

Dellinger, R. P., Levy, M. M., Carlet, J. M., Bion, J., Parker, M. M., Jaeschke, R., et al. (2008). Surviving sepsis campaign: International guidelines for management of severe sepsis and septic shock: 2008. *Critical Care Medicine, 36*(1), 296–327.

Dennen, P., Douglas, I. S., & Anderson, R. (2010). Acute kidney injury in the intensive care unit: An update and primer for the intensivist. *Critical Care Medicine, 38*(1), 261–275.

Fahy, B. G., Sheehy, A. M., & Coursin, D. B. (2009). Glucose control in the intensive care unit. *Critical Care Medicine, 37*(5), 1769–1776.

Kaw, R., Aboussouan, L., Auckley, D., Bae, C., Gugliotti, D., Grant, P., et al. (2008). Challenges in pulmonary risk assessment and perioperative management in bariatric surgery patients. *Obesity Surgery, 18*(1), 134–138.

Levy, M. M., Dellinger, P., Townsend, S. R., & Linde-Zwirble, W. T. (2010). The surviving sepsis campaign: Results of an international guideline-based performance improvement program targeting severe sepsis. *Critical Care Medicine, 38*(2), 367–374.

Matthay, M. A. (2008). Treatment of acute lung injury: Clinical and experimental studies. *Proceedings of the American Thoracic Society, 5*(3), 297–299.

Munro, C. L., Grap, M. J., Jones, D. J., McClish, D. K., & Sessler, C. N. (2009). Chlorhexidine, toothbrushing, and preventing ventilator-associated pneumonia in critically ill adults. *American Journal of Critical Care, 18*(5), 428–437.

O'Connor, M., Bucknall, T., & Manias, E. (2009). A critical review of daily sedation interruption in the intensive care unit. *Journal of Clinical Nursing, 18*(9), 1239–1249.

O'Grady, N. P., Barie, P. S., Bartlett, J. G., Bleck, T., Carroll, K., Kalil, A. C., et al. (2008). Guidelines for evaluation of new fever in critically ill adult patients: 2008 update from the American College of Critical

Care Medicine and the Infectious Diseases Society of America. *Critical Care Medicine, 36*(4), 1330–1349.

Pulmonary Artery Catheter Education Project (PACEP). Retrieved from www.pacep.org

Pieracci, F. M., Barie, P. S., & Pomp, A. (2006). Critical care of the bariatric patient. *Critical Care Medicine, 34*(6), 1796–1804.

Surviving Sepsis Campaign: http://www.survivingsepsis .org/Pages/default.aspx

Van Rompaey, B., Schuurmans, M. J., Shortridge-Baggett, L. M., Truijen, S., Elseviers, M., & Bossaert, L.

(2009). Long term outcome after delirium in the intensive care unit. *Journal of Clinical Nursing, 18*(23), 3349–3357.

Vincent, J. L., Rello, J. Marshall, J. Silva, E., Anzueto, A., Martin, C. D., et al. (2009). International study of the prevalence and outcomes of infection in the intensive care unit. *Journal of the American Medical Association, 302*(21), 2323–2329.

Zaccheo, M. M., & Bucher, D. H. (2008). Propofol infusion syndrome: A rare complication with potentially fatal results. *Critical Care Nurse, 28*(3), 18–26.

CHAPTER 15

Extended Care/ Observation Care Patients

Lois Schick, MN, MBA, RN, CPAN, CAPA

Extended care is the period when care and interventions are required following discharge from Phase I and Phase II recovery. Many patients require further observation and extra time prior to being transported to an inpatient care bed or leaving the healthcare facility. They may be awaiting transportation, have no care provider at home, require further observation for potential complications, or are waiting for the availability of an inpatient bed. This chapter describes some of the regulations and practice considerations as they relate to extended care patients. The terms *extended care* and *observation care* will be used interchangeably throughout this chapter.

1. What is observation care?

The Centers for Medicare and Medicaid Services (CMS) defines outpatient observation services as

> a well-defined set of specifically appropriate services, which include ongoing short-term treatment, assessment, and reassessment before a decision can be made regarding whether patients will require further treatment as hospital inpatients or if they are able to be discharged from the hospital. (Sturgeon, 2009)

A person receiving observation services may improve and be released or be admitted as an inpatient.

Observation level of care is, by definition, the use of appropriate monitoring, diagnostic testing, therapy, and assessment of patient symptoms, signs, laboratory tests, and response to therapy for the

purpose of determining whether a patient will require further treatments as an inpatient or can be discharged home. According to the Medicare Outpatient Observation Physician Guidelines (2007), observation is an outpatient diagnostic treatment category and is a billing status and not a place. Observation allows the physician time to make a decision and then rapidly move the patient to the most appropriate setting. Observation is not a holding zone. When the American College of Emergency Physicians (ACEP) recognized the need for observation units, they described the keys to a successful observation unit as having clearly defined admission criteria, well-planned policies and procedures, a clear chain of command, proper staffing, adequate location, appropriate equipment, and a carefully developed quality assurance and utilization program (Brillman et al., 1994).

2. What criteria are used to utilize the post anesthesia care unit (PACU) for observation care?

Patients cannot be preadmitted into an observation status. If the patient develops a complication during the normal PACU time (typically 4–6 hours), observation status is warranted. Observation is an unplanned stay of some hours because the patient needs to be observed more closely. If the patient is already an inpatient, he or she cannot typically be converted to observation status. Some postoperative complications that warrant outpatient observation status include persistent postoperative nausea and vomiting (PONV), uncontrolled pain, excessive or uncontrolled bleeding, an unstable level of consciousness, fluid or electrolyte imbalance, dysrhythmias, and a deficit in mobility or coordination (Flagler Hospital and Status Health, 2007).

3. Is short stay, 23-hour observation equivalent to extended care?

Short stay units hold patients up to 72 hours and, in some facilities, are known as clinical decision units. The three main functions identified in short stay units are to provide observation, to involve specialists to make assessments and diagnoses, and to provide short-term, high-level management of the patient. Some facilities identify a perioperative unit as a short-stay unit, but most are affiliated with emergency departments (Runy, 2006). Patients in short-stay units must have the ability to meet basic self-care needs, and there must be a likelihood of reasonable pain control. A surgical observation unit is considered a specialized unit designed to receive postoperative and postprocedural patients with stays ranging from 1 to 24 hours.

4. Should there be a limit on the length of time a patient can be classified as an extended care patient?

According to the CMS, if reimbursement is to be received, the time a patient can be considered in observation status is 24 hours, and all costs beyond 24 hours will be included in the composite ambulatory payment group (APG) payments. Patients may be in an observation category for up to 48 hours (American College of Emergency Physicians, 2010; Brillman et al., 1994; Runy, 2006).

5. What CMS rules and regulations will be imposed in creating an observation category?

According to the Medicare Outpatient Observation Physician Guidelines (2007), observation is an active treatment to determine if a patient's condition is going to require hospitalization or if the patient may be discharged home due to problem resolution. CMS has updated the outpatient prospective payment system (OPPS) such that general orders for observation services following outpatient surgery are not recognized. This refers to the services that are part of another Part B service, such as postoperative monitoring during the standard recovery period (4–6 hours) that are billed with PACU services. Observation services should not be billed for diagnostic or therapeutic services that are included as part of the procedure (such as a colonoscopy). CMS identifies that the end time for observation is when all medically necessary services related to the observation are completed. If a patient is waiting for transportation home, this time is not part of the observation time—even though the patient is still under a nurse's care.

Medicare and private insurers establish stricter criteria for hospital admissions each year. Patients may be placed in observation status and Medicare may not cover their expenses longer than 24 hours. A hospital cannot bill Medicare, as the facility risks being charged with fraud when it bills for an inpatient stay that is not covered or for an observation stay that is greater than 24 hours. Patients are then charged the difference. It is important that the patient be alerted to the fact that expenses may be incurred in the event that he or she is placed in an observation category.

6. What does not qualify for outpatient observation?

The Medicare Outpatient Observation Physician Guidelines (Flagler Hospital and Status Health, 2007) identifies the following services that are not covered as outpatient observation.

- Services that are not reasonable or necessary for the diagnosis or treatment of the patient
- Services that are provided for the convenience of the patient, patient's family, or a physician
- Services that are covered under Part A (e.g., medically appropriate inpatient admission)
- General standing orders for observation following outpatient surgery
- Patients undergoing diagnostic testing in a hospital outpatient department

Observation should not be billed concurrently with therapeutic services for which active monitoring is a part of the procedure such as chemotherapy or colonoscopy procedures.

Furthermore, CMS states that outpatient observation is *not* indicated for the following situations (Flagler Hospital and Status Health, 2007):

- As a substitute for inpatient admission
- For continuous monitoring
- For medically stable patients needing diagnostic testing
- For patients needing therapeutic procedures such as blood transfusion, chemotherapy, or dialysis that is routinely provided in outpatient settings
- For patients waiting for long-term care facility placement
- For the convenience of the patient, his or her family, or the physician

- For routine preparation or recovery prior to or following diagnostic or surgical services
- A routine stop between the emergency department and an inpatient admission

7. What standards of care are utilized for extended care patients?

Each of the American Society of PeriAnesthesia Nurses (ASPAN) Standards of Perianesthesia Nursing Practice (2010) must be considered when caring for patients placed in an observation category. Patient rights must be honored, and autonomy, confidentiality, privacy, dignity, and self-worth must be maintained. The environment where the observation care is provided must be safe, comfortable, and therapeutic. Appropriate staffing must be available. Performance improvement activities (including monitoring and evaluating care utilizing a multidisciplinary approach) should be implemented. The nursing process of assessment, planning, implementation, and evaluation are essential and should be individualized for each patient admitted to extended observation status (ASPAN, 2010).

8. Are there specific admission criteria for a patient to be considered an extended care patient?

Patients should not be scheduled as extended care patients. However, patients should be evaluated for the need for possible admission. Patients who are treated should be expected to be stabilized with release within 24 hours. Those patients who should be considered an extended care patient are those following a complication of an outpatient procedure; however, these patients are placed in observation only if a complication develops during or after the procedure that requires further care beyond the usual recovery period of 4–6 hours.

There are no standing orders for observation. After 4–6 hours of a routine recovery, the physician should be called to notify that the patient is not safe to go home so that updated orders for extended recovery or observation can be completed. A physician's order is needed to place the patient in the most appropriate setting.

9. What staffing requirements are needed to cover extended care patients?

The intensity of service needs should be limited and consistent with the staffing pattern for the unit. For unmonitored beds, a nurse-to-patient ratio similar to the hospital ward would dictate a ratio of one nurse to five patients based on the acuity of the patients. For monitored beds, a nurse–patient ratio

similar to hospital monitored beds would be one nurse to four patients, depending on patient acuity (California Nurses Association, 2004). Some states have mandated staffing ratios in place. One must follow institutional protocols.

10. Is there a specific nurse–patient ratio requirement for extended care?

The nurse–patient ratio should be no different than that proposed in the ASPAN Standards. Observation care could consist of one nurse for three to five patients, depending on the acuity and type of patients. Critical care patient ratios should be no different than the ratio used in the intensive care unit (ICU), namely, one nurse to two patients, unless the patient's acuity dictates otherwise. The standards reflect that there needs to be two competent personnel, one of whom is an RN possessing competence appropriate to the patient population and in the same unit where the patient is receiving extended observation level of care. The need for additional nurses and support staff is dependent on the patient acuity, patient census, and the physical facility (ASPAN, 2010; Brillman et al., 1994).

11. What types of nursing personnel are needed?

According to the ASPAN standards (2010, p. 14), "An appropriate number of registered nursing staff with demonstrated competence is available to meet the individual needs of patients and families in each level of perianesthesia care based on patient acuity, census, and physical facility." Resource 2 of the ASPAN standards (2010, p. 61) recommends that the extended observation level of care include "two competent personnel, one of whom is a RN possessing competence appropriate to the patient population, are in the same unit where the patient is receiving extended observation level of care. The need for additional RNs and support staff is dependent on the patient acuity, patient census, and the physical facility." The recommendation is to have a ratio of no more than one nurse for every three to five patients (ASPAN, 2010). The number of patients assigned should be based on patient acuity and the number of patients in the unit. If the observation patient is in an unmonitored bed, the staffing ratio could be the same as that on a hospital ward or unit where patients are in unmonitored beds. If the observation patient is on a monitored bed, the staffing ratio should match that of a monitored bed. Consideration must also be given to the actual physical makeup of the unit utilized for observation.

If ICU patients are housed in this observation unit, the staffing ratio will need to be one nurse to two patients, based on staffing literature and ASPAN standards. This represents one nurse to two patients based on the patient's acuity (ASPAN, 2010; California Nurses Association, 2004). Nurses caring for patients as observation patients in the PACU should have limited responsibility for other patients in the unit, and every attempt to separate the PACU patient from the observation patient should be made.

Support personnel and those assisting in the unit should have had an orientation to the policies and procedures and setup of the unit. Asking just anyone to assist and be the second person is inappropriate and can impact the quality of care provided. Use of float personnel, unless adequately trained, is discouraged.

12. What monitoring requirements for observation care are needed?

If monitoring equipment is available in the unit, it can be used for monitoring the observation patient. Most PACUs have the appropriate equipment available in the unit if the PACU is used as the observation, boarder, or extended care area. Essential PACU equipment that can be used for the observation patient includes airway management supplies, suction, oxygen delivery equipment, means to monitor blood pressure and temperature, ECG monitor, pulse oximetry, glucose monitoring equipment, lab drawing supplies, emergency equipment, thermoregulation equipment, respiratory therapy assistance (including ventilator availability), plus all the stock supplies that are needed for routine patient care (ASPAN, 2010).

If a special unit is set up to house the observation patients, essential equipment should include airway management supplies, suction, oxygen delivery equipment, and the means to monitor blood pressure, temperature, and oximetry. Emergency equipment and supplies should always be readily available in any unit where patients are housed.

13. Can ICU patients be managed in this category while awaiting bed placement in the ICU?

ICU patients can be monitored in the PACU with appropriate staffing, but the CMS does not reimburse the facility in this scenario as an observation patient. Patients who are kept as overflow patients in the PACU are often referred to as "boarders," "extended stay," or "ICU overflow" (Drain & Odom-Forren, 2009).

Staffing the ICU overflow patient in the PACU presents a challenge. If the patient is stable, the nurse may have another patient assigned to his or her care. As recommended by the ASPAN standards 2010 and ICU staffing ratios (utilizing the California ratios), the PACU nurse should have no more than two patients at any time (ASPAN, 2010; California Nurses Association, 2004).

14. What documentation requirements are needed?

Vital signs, including pulse, blood pressure, respirations, pulse oximetry, and temperature, should be measured. The fifth vital sign of pain assessment should also be considered. Patient education, including self-care measures after discharge, should be included in patient teaching. Follow-up care, including when to contact the physician and what to do in the case of an emergency, should be reinforced in the discharge instructions.

15. How frequently are vital signs required?

Frequency of vital signs is dependent on the patient's condition and unit policies. Most patients placed in the observation category have received phase I level of care, so they have stabilized to advance their vital signs from a range of 1 to 4 hours to every 4 to 6 hours, depending on their acuity and current condition. Minimum vital signs include temperature, blood pressure, pulse, respirations, pulse oximetry, and pain assessment.

16. Who is responsible for the ultimate management of the patient?

Hospital and ambulatory surgery center policies and procedures should identify the team ultimately responsible for the management of the patient. Each facility should have a designated position as the physician resource and one as the nurse resource for patients and others to contact if questions, issues, or concerns arise. The anesthesia department works collaboratively with surgeons related to the management of patients in the observation unit. If it is a teaching facility, an intern or resident may be assigned to manage problems. If hospitalists are available in the hospital, they may be assigned to be responsible to manage the department. A physician is ultimately responsible for managing the observation of a patient.

17. Is there a time limit attached to the category of extended observation?

According to the CMS, the time for an observation patient is usually 23 hours, but this may extend to 48 hours. By that time, the patient's response to the therapy instituted can be evaluated and a decision can be made as to whether the patient will be admitted as an inpatient or be discharged.

18. Is extended observation an extension of phase II PACU care?

Phase II level of care and extended observation are two separate and distinct entities. Phase II level of care is characterized by the nurse focusing on preparing the patient for care in the home, extended observation, or an extended care environment. Observation or extended care is defined as the time when it is anticipated that the patient's condition will rapidly improve or require treatment or further evaluation, which can only be provided within a 24–48 hours period. If it is not anticipated that the patient's condition will rapidly improve, the patient is admitted as an inpatient. Observation allows time to determine if the inpatient admission is necessary.

19. What criteria are required for discharge?

Discharge criteria should be developed in consultation with the physicians using the following assessment parameters: vital signs (e.g., blood pressure, pulse, respirations, oxygen saturation, temperature, level of consciousness); comfort level (e.g., assessment of pain, nausea, and oral analgesia); surgical site care and maintenance; hydration and nourishment; activity level (i.e., ability to ambulate); postoperative instructions; support of a responsible adult; and the need to urinate if appropriate (Burden, O'Brien, Quinn, & Dawes, 2000; Schick & Windle, 2010).

20. Where will the patient be discharged or transported to following observation care?

The patient may be discharged from observation care to inpatient care, a skilled nursing facility, or to the patient's home depending on if he or she meets the extended observation criteria. If sent to the ICU or acute care ward, an inpatient order will be needed. If the patient is going to a skilled nursing facility, a discharge order and an admit order for the skilled facility will be required. If the patient is being discharged home, a discharge order will suffice.

21. Are transport policies and procedures necessary for sending patients to a higher level of care from a freestanding facility?

Most freestanding facilities have written transfer arrangements with hospitals or extended care facilities that enable the freestanding facility to admit patients if they do not meet discharge criteria from observation status. It is not a transfer of care, but rather an admission to the hospital or extended care facility from the freestanding facility. Reasons for moving patients from a freestanding facility to a hospital or extended care facility can include unplanned medical emergencies (such as cardiac or respiratory problems); more extensive surgery is required; and/or a surgical complication has occurred (e.g., hemorrhage or dehiscence) (Burden et al., 2000; Schick & Windle, 2010).

22. When are discharge instructions given?

Discharge instructions are reviewed with the patient and the responsible adult or family throughout the period of time that the patient is being cared for in the extended observation level of care setting.

23. Should patients be discharged with a "responsible adult" or is this not necessary because they have recovered from extended care?

It behooves patients to be transported with a responsible adult when being discharged from extended observation. Being discharged to the care of a "responsible adult" provides the patient and family with the reinforcement of self-care instructions, including who to contact in case of an emergency (Schick & Windle, 2010; Ziser, Alkovi, Mardovits, & Rozenberg, 2002)

24. Are post procedure/post discharge phone calls necessary?

Postprocedure or postdischarge telephone calls reinforce the caring concept of the staff toward the patient and family. Follow-up phone calls also give the patient the opportunity to vent both positive and negative feelings as well as to offer suggestions for unit improvement or for improving the process of observation. The postprocedure or postdischarge phone call is an excellent tool to identify if the patient has had delayed responses to any medications or any other adverse reaction. Patients are always referred to their primary care giver for any questions or concerns that may arise (Schick & Windle, 2010; Ziser et al., 2002).

25. Will family members have the opportunity to visit and assist with patient care in the observation unit?

It would be optimal for family members to be intimately involved in the patient's postprocedure care during observation. The concern becomes the location of where this care is being provided. Some open units, such as the PACU, do not offer much privacy due to the layout of the typical environment. PACUs are usually open rooms with curtains around the bedside that are not conducive to privacy. Whenever possible, cohorting the observation patient away from other patients provides the privacy that allows for more meaningful family involvement in the extended observation patient's care and recovery (Ziser et al., 2002).

26. What level of care is provided to patients who are categorized as extended care?

It is an ideal situation when patients are placed in an observation level of care to provide them with the best quality of safe care, which may include a comfortable bed or gurney that will allow them the comfort of recovery. Routine postoperative orders are instituted. If the patient is scheduled for more definitive testing (e.g., initiating PT or OT), the CMS does not reimburse the facility for the time the patient is off the unit during this testing period.

27. Is there a limit to the types of orders implemented during the patient's stay as an extended care or observation care patient?

The goal for the extended observation period is to stabilize and treat the patient. Observation care is an active treatment to determine if the patient's condition is going to require that he or she be admitted as an inpatient or if the condition resolves itself so that the patient may be discharged. Types of orders include appropriate monitoring (including vital sign measurement), intravenous fluids, medications, activity, diagnostic testing (including lab and radiology), and teaching for preparation of discharging the patient. If diagnostic procedures are performed (such as colonoscopy or chemotherapy), the charges and reimbursement will not be reflected within the observation charges, but as part of the procedure. Physician orders must be specific for the period of time that the patient is in the observation category.

REFERENCES

American College of Emergency Physicians. (2010). Observation care payments to hospitals FAQ. Retrieved from www.acep.org/practres.aspx?id=30486

American Society of Perianesthesia Nurses. (2010). Perianesthesia nursing standards and practice recommendations: 2010–2012. Cherry Hill, NJ: Author.

Brillman, J., Mathers-Dunbar, L., Graff, L., Joseph, T., Leikin, J. B., Schultz, C., et al. (1994). *Management of observation units*. Retrieved from www.acep.org/practres.aspx?LinkIdentifier=ifier=id&id=29872#&fid=2630&Mo=No

Burden, N., Quinn, D., O'Brien, D., & Dawes, B. (2000). *Ambulatory surgical nursing* (2nd ed.). Philadelphia: W. B. Saunders.

California Nurses Association. (2004). *RN ratio alert*. Retrieved from www.calnurse.org/assets/pdf/ratios/ratios_basics_unit_0704.pdf

Drain, C., & Odom-Forren, J. (2009). *Perianesthesia nursing: A critical care approach* (5th ed.). Saint Louis, MO: Saunders.

Flagler Hospital and Status Health. (2007). Medicare outpatient observation physician guidelines. Retrieved from www.pepperresources.org/LinkClick.aspx?fileticket=0sm78M7X;A4%3D&tabid=748mid=395

Runy, L. A. (2006). Clinical observation units. *Hopitals & Health Networks, 80*(3): 59–65. Retrieved from http://www.hhnmag.com/hhnmag_app/jsp/articledisplay.jsp?dcrpath=HHNMAG/PubsNewsArticle/data/2006March/0603HHN_FEA_gatefold&domain=HHNMAG

Schick, L., & Windle, P. (2010). *PeriAnesthesia nursing core curriculum: Preprocedure, phase I and phase II PACU nursing* (2nd ed.). Saint Louis, MO: Saunders.

Sturgeon, J. (2009). *Observations on "observation" for the record*. Retrieved from www.forthrecordmag.com/archives/01709p8.shtml

Ziser, A., Alkovi, M., Markovits, R., & Rozenberg, B. (2002). The postanesthesia care unit as a temporary admission location due to intensive care and ward overflow. *British Journal of Anaesthesia, 88*(4), 577–579.

CHAPTER 16

Geriatric Patients

Melissa Lee, MS, RN, CNS-BC & Carla Graf, MS, RN, CNS-BC

The care of the older adult undergoing surgery is often more complex than for younger patients. Healthcare providers must understand and consider both the normal changes in body systems that occur with aging as well as other factors (such as the presence of common chronic illnesses, smoking, alcohol overuse, polypharmacy, obesity, sedentary lifestyles, and malnutrition) that may contribute to morbidity and mortality postoperatively. Aging can be viewed not only as one's chronologic age, but also one's physiologic or biologic age. Because older adults are an extremely heterogeneous group, systemic changes that occur across this population may not be consistent. Persons who maintain an active and healthy lifestyle, for example, may have less postoperative complications than a younger person who is sedentary.

1. What are the implications of aging demographics?

There will continue to be significant growth of the older adult population as the "baby boom" generation reaches age 65. The term "older adult" generally refers to persons aged 65 and older, a definition originally established by the Social Security Administration. Today, gerontologists view older adults as young–old (ages 65 to 74), middle–old (ages 75 to 84), and old–old (ages 85 and older) (Mauk, 2006). We are also becoming more ethnically diverse; minority populations are predicted to increase to approximately 24% of all older adults by 2020. The average life expectancy of those persons reaching age 65 today is an additional 19.0 years (females, 20.3 years; males, 17.4 years).

Currently, 12.6% of the population is aged 65 and older (1 in every 8). By 2030, it is anticipated that there will be 72.1 million older adults in the United States (19.3% of the total US population). In addition, the old–old population, those persons age 85 and older, is projected to increase to 6.6 million by 2020 (Administration on Aging [AOA], 2008).

Hospitalization rates for those aged 64 and younger have decreased in the last several decades; however, rates for those aged 65 and older, and specifically aged 75 and older have continued to increase (DeFrances, Lucas, Buie, & Golosinskiy, 2008). Lengths of stay are also highest for persons aged 65 and older (DeFrances et al., 2008).

2. What are the most common surgical interventions in older adults?

Current advances in care have decreased surgical risks, thereby, altering the risk–benefit ratio to favor surgery in older patients with more complex conditions (Christmas & Pompei, 2010). Older adults account for more than half of all surgical procedures performed. In addition, they experience disproportionately higher rates of postoperative morbidity and mortality due, in part, because of the decrease in physiologic reserve that occurs with aging.

Common surgical procedures include the following (Schick, 2004):

- Ophthalmic (cataract and vitrectomy)
- Orthopedic (open reduction and internal fixation, joint replacements)

- Cardiovascular (pacemaker placement, carotid endarterectomy)
- Genitourinary (cystoscopy, transurethral resection of the prostate)
- General (herniorrhaphy)

3. What are surgical intervention outcomes of older adults?

Standard surgical measurement of outcomes includes morbidity and mortality within a usual defined period, often 30 days. Mortality rates at 30 days vary by surgery, but are higher in patients over 80 years of age. Hamel, Henderson, Khuri, and Daley (2005) reported on data from the Veterans Administration National Surgical Quality Improvement Program (NSQIP) ($n = 26,648$ patients aged 80 or over with the median age of 82 years and 568,263 patients were over 80 median, with a median age of 62 years). Hernia repair, vertebral disc surgery, knee replacements, transurethral prostatectomy, carotid endarterectomy, and laryngectomy were associated with mortality rates as low as 2% or less. However, rates of complications and the impact of these complications, especially on recovery of function, increased with aging. One fifth of patients over 80 years of age had at least one complication; the presence of complications increased mortality from 4 to 26%. Usual complications were respiratory and urinary tract related.

PHYSIOLOGIC CHANGES WITH AGING AND SURGICAL IMPLICATIONS: CARDIOVASCULAR

4. What are the age-related changes?

Cardiovascular disease is the most common cause of mortality in adults aged 65 and older. Commonly, pathology rather than normal aging changes is evident in this body system.

Structural changes with aging include (Plahuta & Hamrick-King, 2006; Schick, 2004; Sloane, 2002):

- Overall decrease in myocardial cells, decreased aortic distensibility, and decreased vascular tone, which may cause pooling of blood in the periphery, thus, increasing the risk for deep vein thrombosis (DVT)
- Increases in myocardial weight, size of the left atrium, left ventricular wall thickness, and arterial stiffness
- Increases in elastin and collagen levels
- Loss of pacemaker cells in the sinoatrial node, predisposing the older adult to bradyarrhythmias and atrial fibrillation

Functional changes with aging include (Plahuta & Hamrick-King, 2006; Schick, 2004; Sloane, 2002):

- Increased systolic blood pressure
- Decreased diastolic filling and decreased reaction to β-adrenergic stimulus; decreased tolerance to changes in volume status, leading to orthostatic hypotension
- Small decrease in cardiac output, and slowed circulation time leading to prolonged onset of action and clearing of drugs
- Cardiac reserve declines

There are no changes in ejection fraction, stroke volume, or overall systolic function as a normal course of aging.

Peripheral changes include (Schick, 2004):

- Impaired circulation, causing difficulty with venipuncture due to aging collagen (rolling veins)
- Increased bleeding and bruising at venipuncture sites, occurring because of decreased elasticity of blood vessels

5. What are the perioperative implications in older adults?

Older adults are more reliant on ventricular filling and stroke volume to maintain sufficient cardiac output and have a decreased ability to tolerate hypovolemia; close hemodynamic monitoring is warranted. Extreme changes in blood pressure should be prevented. Because older adults have slowed circulation times, such patients may require lower ranges of medication doses, as well as adequate time for full effect before repeating. Tachyarrhythmias, atrial fibrillation, and dysthymias are common with aging and necessitate monitoring and management. Orthostatic hypotension is common and requires slow changes in positioning, especially when moving to a sitting or standing position (Schick, 2004).

From a vascular perspective, use gentle venipuncture techniques, avoiding tourniquets if possible. Ensure adequate pressure on puncture sites or removal of catheters (Schick, 2004). Encourage early ambulation for DVT prophylaxis. Perioperative β-blockade, statins, antiplatelets (aspirin, clopidogrel), anticoagulants, amiodarone, and hydrocortisone are recommended to reduce cardiovascular complications from surgery in certain high-risk patients. Antibiotics may be used to prevent infective endocarditis in patients with specific cardiac conditions who are undergoing dental, respiratory tract, infected skin, or musculo-skeletal tissue procedures (Rueben et al., 2009).

PHYSIOLOGIC CHANGES WITH AGING AND SURGICAL IMPLICATIONS: PULMONARY

6. What are the age-related changes?

Aging of the respiratory system includes the following (Plahuta & Hamrick-King, 2006; Schick, 2004; Sloane, 2002):

- Alveolar surface area decreases
- Alveoli become flatter and shallower
- Lung elasticity decreases, leading to a reduced inspiratory capacity; however, total lung capacity remains relatively normal
- Oxygen delivery may be negatively impacted by this decrease in lung elasticity, ultimately leading to lower air flow through lung bases, resulting in less efficient oxygen delivery to the body tissues
- As a compensatory mechanism to maintain normal gas exchange, older adults need to breathe in more air
- Lung vital capacity decreases by 17% between the ages of 30 and 70
- Older adults rely on the diaphragm for chest cavity expansion and contraction because of age-related calcification of the cartilage that attaches the ribs to breastbone; respiration may be somewhat limited due to these changes as well as overall loss of muscle mass
- Ciliary activity decreases and diminished responses to hypoxia and hypercarbia
- Cough and swallowing can be less efficient, leading to increased aspiration risk

Intubation may be more difficult when the older adult is edentulous (toothless) and/or has cervical arthritis, which limits flexion and extension of the neck (Silverstein, 2007; Stoelting & Miller, 2000). Two major respiratory pathologies, chronic obstructive pulmonary disease (COPD) and pneumonia, occur more commonly in older adults and may have more significant consequences (Plahuta & Hamrick-King, 2006). In addition, risk factors such as smoking, obesity, and abdominal and thoracic surgery contribute to postoperative complications.

7. What are the perioperative implications?

The older adult needs close monitoring and head-elevated positioning, if possible, to prevent aspiration. Postoperative use of incentive spirometry, coughing and deep breathing, suctioning, and ambulation are all interventions that can prevent pulmonary complications. Some patients may need chest physiotherapy, intermittent positive-pressure breathing, and/or continuous positive-airway pressure, as well as aggressive drug management of COPD. Smoking cessation is recommended 6 to 8 weeks preoperatively (Rueben et al., 2009). Older adults need to be observed for hypoxemia and be supported with oxygen, if necessary. Effective pain management and frequent assessment for fluid overload while maintaining adequate hydration is imperative.

PHYSIOLOGIC CHANGES WITH AGING AND SURGICAL IMPLICATIONS: NEUROPSYCHIATRIC

8. What are the age-related changes?

Common nervous system changes with aging include an overall decrease in central nervous system (CNS) activity related to a decline in neuronal density, decreased cerebral oxygen metabolism, decreased cerebral blood flow, and a reduction in numbers and functioning of neurotransmitters. Reaction times may be slower because of neuronal loss. Dementias and depression occur commonly with aging and contribute to poor surgical outcomes. Patients with dementia are at increased risk for developing delirium; patients with delirium are at higher risk for iatrogenic events such as aspiration, falls, and functional decline (Plahuta & Hamrick-King, 2006; Schick, 2004; Sloane, 2002):

9. What is postoperative delirium?

Delirium is an acute change in mental status with alterations in attention and level of consciousness, usually occurring within 48 hours after surgery in 10 to 50% of patients. If patients require ICU postoperatively, delirium rates may be higher. In the postoperative patient, the common contributing factors to development of delirium are medications with CNS effects, the stress of surgery, and an unfamiliar environment; additional risk factors are older age, having baseline cognitive impairment such as dementia, functional decline, alcohol abuse, metabolic abnormalities, infection, and having a postoperative hematocrit less than 30% (Marcantonio, Flacker, Wright, & Resnick, 2001; Marcantonio, Goldman, Orav, Cook, & Lee, 1998).

Complications of postoperative delirium include pressure ulcers, aspiration, falls, pulmonary embolism, dehydration, psychologic stress, death, functional decline, and long-term cognitive impairment.

10. What are the perioperative implications?

Delirium leads to poor patient outcomes such as death, long-term cognitive impairment and nursing home placement, increased nursing care costs, increased lengths of stay, and increased health system costs. Since dementia represents a significant risk factor for delirium, preoperative cognitive screening is indicated. The Mini-Cog (Borson, Scanlon, Brush, Vitaliano & Dokmak, 2000) is a simple screening instrument that takes about 3 minutes to complete. The results of this assessment should be part of the medical record and communicated to the PACU nurse as well as to the receiving patient care unit.

Because delirium can be difficult to detect, use of a reliable and valid screening instrument is recommended. There are several screening instruments available for use in the postoperative patient. One widely used instrument is the Confusion Assessment Method (CAM) (Wei, Fearing, Sternberg, & Inouye, 2008). Once identified, communication with the team is imperative, as delirium represents a medical emergency.

Patients and families should be educated about delirium. Delirium symptoms, including delusions and hallucinations, may persist for days to months and can cause psychologic distress.

11. Can delirium be prevented?

A randomized study by Inouye (2006), utilizing multicomponent interventions, reduced the incidence of delirium by one third in medically ill older adults. These same interventions can be utilized in surgical patients. The interventions include the following:

- Minimizing deliriogenic medications
- Promoting sleep using a nonpharmacologic approach
- Mobilization
- Dehydration prevention protocols
- Orientation protocols
- Adequate pain management
- Providing sensory aides such as hearing amplifiers and magnifying lenses or glasses

Additional interventions to prevent or minimize the duration and severity of delirium include family presence, the removal of tethering devices such as IVs and Foley catheters as soon as medically feasible, restraint reduction, and assessment for and treatment of metabolic abnormalities. Treatment of delirium is focused on the management of underlying causes such as infection or hypoxia.

PHYSIOLOGIC CHANGES WITH AGING AND SURGICAL IMPLICATIONS: SKIN

12. What are the age-related changes?

There are many skin changes associated with aging, such as loss of skin thickness, elasticity, and strength that can delay the healing process and increase the risk of skin injury. The loss of subcutaneous fat can affect temperature control. The decrease in sebaceous and sweat gland activity also affects thermoregulation and decreases sweating. These changes lead the skin to become more fragile, unable to respond to heat or cold quickly, and prone to pressure injury (Clayton, 2008; Doerflinger, 2009; Monarch & Wren, 2004; Walton-Geer, 2009).

13. What are the perioperative implications?

Patients who are 65 years of age or older experience the highest incidence of pressure ulcer development (Walton-Geer, 2009). Skin needs to be handled gently because normal age-related changes place the older adult at increased risk of pressure injury, bruising, skin tears, infection, and impaired thermoregulation. Pressure ulcer prevention with positioning and padding and thorough skin assessment during all perioperative phases can identify skin changes early to reduce injury severity. Temperature regulation monitoring is important given the older adults reduced efficiency to compensate for temperatures changes (Schick, 2004).

PHYSIOLOGIC CHANGES WITH AGING AND SURGICAL IMPLICATIONS: GASTROINTESTINAL (GI) TRACT

14. What are the age-related changes?

In the mouth and oral cavity, there is a decrease in saliva production in older adults. The decrease in saliva leads to decreased protection of teeth and possible decay or loss of teeth. Loss of teeth can lead to diet changes and an increase in the risk of malnutrition. The decrease in gag-reflex sensitivity increases the risk of choking and aspiration. In the stomach, there is a decrease in gastric acid production. Also seen is a decrease in iron and folic acid absorption, which can lead to anemia. Digestion slows because acid production decreases. Motility in the stomach also slows, delaying gastric emptying. There are several age-related changes in the colon—the most troublesome is the atrophy and decreased strength of the muscle wall which slows peristalsis and may cause constipation (Amella, 2006; Saufl, 2004). Bleeding of the upper GI tract is also more common in older adults. Two common causes of GI bleeding are due to nonsteroidal anti-inflammatory drug (NSAID) use and ulcers and erosions (Doerflinger, 2009).

In the liver, the size of the liver and blood flow are both reduced with aging. These changes lead to an impaired ability to meet the increased demands of metabolism, biotransformation, and protein synthesis after surgery. Hepatic blood flow is responsible for drug delivery to the liver. Drugs that rely on hepatic metabolism have a prolonged impact in older adults.

Liver metabolism can be divided into two general categories: oxidative (phase I) and conjugative (phase II). Phase I metabolism is impaired the most in the older adult (Doerflinger, 2009; Rivera & Antognini, 2009). Long-acting benzodiazepines are one group of drugs that undergo significant phase I metabolism. The elimination half-life of long-acting benzodiazepines is prolonged in the older adult versus in younger persons. Additionally, older adults can have a paradoxical response to benzodiazepines (Beliveau & Multach, 2003; Fick et al., 2003).

15. What are the perioperative implications?

Older adults may have decreased absorption of medications because of decreased blood flow to the GI tract and alterations with gastric motility. Monitoring for adverse effects of medications is important. If an older adult has a GI bleed, they are at an increased risk of becoming hemodynamically unstable because of their lack of reserve to changes in blood volume. Slowed gastric motility puts the older adult at increased risk of developing paralytic ileus postoperatively. Prevention measures to prevent aspiration events need to be in place (HOB >30 degrees and frequent oral care). Oxygen masks may be difficult to fit because of lost teeth or decreased bony mass in the jaw (Clayton, 2008; Doerflinger, 2009; Saufl, 2004).

PHYSIOLOGIC CHANGES WITH AGING AND SURGICAL IMPLICATIONS: MUSCULOSKELETAL SYSTEM

16. What are the age-related changes?

Older adults are at risk for osteoporosis, a condition characterized by low bone mass and bone density, resulting in skeletal support compromise. Osteoporosis is most common in postmenopausal women; however, it can be seen in older men. Degenerative changes in vertebrae can cause difficulty with intubation and spinal anesthesia. Kyphosis may limit the ability of the chest to expand normally, thus decreasing lung capacity.

Osteoarthritis (OA), the most common form of arthritis, increases with age and wear and tear on the joints. OA causes decreased joint mobility, pain, difficulty with ambulation, and decreased flexibility. Weight-bearing joints are commonly affected.

With aging, lean muscles mass is replaced by fat, and there is decreased size and number of muscle fibers (Plahuta & Hamrick-King, 2006; Schick, 2004; Sloane, 2002).

17. What are the perioperative implications?

Perioperative positioning may be compromised due to decreased flexibility. The back should be supported and proper body alignment maintained with bony prominences protected. Patient movement should be gentle (Schick, 2004). Presence of chronic pain from OA or other types of arthritis will need to be managed along with treating the acute postoperative pain. Patients may need to be assisted or use assistive devices such as walkers in the immediate postoperative period. A fall prevention program is imperative for all perioperative and ambulatory surgery areas because changes in the musculoskeletal system, coupled with anesthesia, anxiolytics, and pain medication, lead to gait and balance problems. Close monitoring of medication effects and changes in electrolytes is important, as older adults have decreased lean body mass and decreased total body water, leading to an impaired ability to compensate for fluid changes. Functional decline, meaning an older adult may lose ability to independently perform an activity of daily living, can occur early during the hospital admission; therefore, it is imperative that an ambulation or mobility regimen be established.

PHYSIOLOGIC CHANGES WITH AGING AND SURGICAL IMPLICATIONS: ENDOCRINE SYSTEM

18. What are the age-related changes?

Pancreatic function declines with age, and the incidence of diabetes mellitus becomes more common as the ability to metabolize glucose becomes impaired. Diabetes places the older adult at risk for cardiovascular and infectious complications. Cardiovascular complications are common because diabetes is a risk factor for atherosclerosis, and cardiac reserve is diminished. In all diabetic patients undergoing surgery, it is important to monitor blood glucose levels frequently before, during, and after surgery.

Thyroid disease, if undetected, can result in complications perioperatively. Hypothyroidism causes patients to metabolize medications more slowly, and their increased sensitivity to CNS depressants can result in respiratory insufficiency. Perioperative risks associated with hyperthyroidism include hyperpyrexia, dysrhythmias, and heart failure (Amella, 2006; Saufl, 2004).

19. What are the perioperative implications?

Diabetic preoperative evaluation should include the type of diabetes, current therapy and management, trends of glucose control, and prior surgical complications. The perioperative goal is to avoid ketosis and to maintain glucose levels. In addition to monitoring blood glucose levels, it is important to monitor diabetic surgical patients for infections and impaired wound healing. Myocardial ischemia in the older adult can be silent and may be detected unexpectedly on a postoperative electrocardiogram (ECG). Review of current thyroid lab results can reveal abnormalities in function, which can lead to perioperative complications.

PHYSIOLOGIC CHANGES WITH AGING AND SURGICAL IMPLICATIONS: IMMUNE SYSTEM

20. What are the age-related changes?

It is believed that immunity deteriorates with age as a result of decreasing T lymphocyte function. There is also a decrease in thymus mass and production. As a result, the antibody response to stimuli is depressed, and this places the older adult at increased risk of infection because of the decreased efficiency of the immune system (Amella, 2006).

21. What are the perioperative implications?

Immunosuppression causes a decreased ability to recognize and fight infection. Because of the delayed response, infections can go undetected in older adults until the infection has reached an acute stage. In addition, older adults may have atypical symptoms of infection. For example, confusion may be the first symptom of a urinary tract infection (UTI). Vigilant assessment and monitoring is needed to pick up on small changes from the older adult's baseline.

PHYSIOLOGIC CHANGES WITH AGING AND SURGICAL IMPLICATIONS: SENSORY SYSTEM

22. What are the age-related changes?

Both vision and auditory changes occur commonly with aging. Pupils are less refractive to light and the cornea flattens causing scattering of light rays and sensitivity to glare. Overall, there is decreased visual acuity, peripheral vision, and accommodation. There is increased incidence of cataracts and glaucoma. Impaired color discrimination occurs due to increased yellow pigmentation in the lens. Less aqueous humor is produced, leading to increased eye dryness and risk of eye infection. Field cuts, or hemianopsia, may be present after

a stroke (Plahuta & Hamrick-King, 2006; Schick, 2004; Sloane, 2002).

The tympanic membrane becomes thinner and less resilient, causing impairment in auditory function. The ossicular chain can calcify, causing decreased sensitivity to high-pitched tones and difficulty localizing sound, as well as balance problems.

Tactile changes include decreased sensation and decreased response to pain. Taste is diminished due to tongue atrophy, decreased salivary production, or use of upper dentures (Plahuta & Hamrick-King, 2006; Schick, 2004; Sloane, 2002).

23. What are the perioperative implications?

Sensory impairment is a contributing factor to delirium; allow sensory devices such as glasses and hearing aides for as long as possible preoperatively, and replace them as soon as possible in the PACU. Any written educational materials should be designed to accommodate older eyes such as utilizing size 14 font on nonglare paper. If providing information about medications, do not identify them by color. Also, having hearing amplifiers and magnifiers in all perioperative areas can be very helpful for the older patient. Finally, be aware that many medications taken by older adults for chronic conditions may affect the senses, such as furosemide resulting in tinnitus, decreased hearing, and dry mouth (Schick, 2004).

PHYSIOLOGIC CHANGES WITH AGING AND SURGICAL IMPLICATIONS: RENAL SYSTEM

24. What are the age-related changes?

Renal function declines with age. There is a loss of renal mass, primarily in the cortex, which results in less glomeruli. The loss of filtering surface is associated with a fall in renal blood flow. These factors lead to a decreased glomerular filtration rate (GFR), which contributes to a diminished ability to concentrate urine. The loss of nephrons and impaired drug clearance place older adults at risk for volume and electrolyte abnormalities. Renal and glomerular blood flow decreases with age but does so without a correlating increase in serum creatinine. This occurs because as renal function declines, muscle mass also declines, and creatinine is a by-product of muscle metabolism. Changes in GFR are variable; some older adults have little change over time and others having a marked decrease. Therefore, serum creatinine levels may not be an accurate indicator of GFR. Creatinine clearance, which depends on the GRF, may be a more accurate indicator and can be estimated using the Cockroft-Gault formula

(Beliveau & Multach, 2003; Doerflinger, 2009; Rivera & Antognini, 2009):

$$\frac{(140-age) \times wt\ (kg) \times (0.85\ if\ female)}{72 \times serum\ creatinine\ (mg/mL)}$$

25. What are the perioperative implications?

The kidneys play a crucial role in fluid and electrolyte balance. The altered thirst response and decreased ability to concentrate urine are likely to facilitate sodium and volume depletion. Urine output is less reliable as a surrogate for renal perfusion in older adults. The kidneys may still excrete urine in the face of hypovolemia or in a dehydrated state. Maintenance of appropriate fluid balance is difficult in the older adult population. Fluctuations in blood pressure (especially during position changes) and new cognitive changes may be indicative of intravascular volume depletion.

Creatinine clearance provides a way to estimate renal function. IV fluids and intake/output must be closely monitored because of the impaired ability of the kidney to maintain sodium and hydration equilibrium. The older adult has a decreased ability to respond to these volume changes. Postoperative renal failure increases in frequency because of impaired preoperative function coupled with the impaired renal reserve of the older adult.

PHYSIOLOGIC CHANGES WITH AGING AND SURGICAL IMPLICATIONS: LAB CHANGES WITH AGING

26. What are the age-related changes?

Accurate interpretation of lab values is a challenge because normal ranges may change with age. Nurses aware of the effects of aging are better equipped to make appropriate decisions about what is normal and abnormal. There are multiple confounding factors making interpretation challenging, including: varying degrees of age-related changes, the presence of chronic conditions, changes in fluid and nutrition status, and medications. Some lab values considered abnormal for younger adults are within reference ranges for older adults. There is no trend to how age effects normal lab ranges; values can be less than, more than, or the same as the accepted ranges in younger adults.

Examples of select lab values affected by age include:

- Serum glucose levels may be higher or lower. Decreased sensitivity of muscles to insulin and/or insulin resistance may account for the increased serum glucose levels. Poor nutritional status or losses in body mass may lead to lower glucose levels

- Creatinine clearance decreases with age but serum creatinine may not change due to the decrease in muscle mass. Therefore, serum creatinine tends to overestimate renal function. Creatinine clearance should be used to assess renal function and can be calculated by the Cockcroft-Gault formula.

- The serum albumin value in healthy older adults may be low, usually due to diet. However, low values, especially when accompanied by malnutrition, may also indicate disease.

- Arterial blood gas (ABG) ranges in older adults may differ from younger adults. What would be considered hypoxemia may be normal in older adults. Age-related changes in lung function like stiffening of the lungs, decrease in alveoli, and decrease in diaphragm and intercostal muscle strength, result in diminished partial pressure of arterial oxygen tension (PaO_2) (Edwards & Baird, 2005; Hoot-Martin, Larsen, & Hazen, 1997; Merck Sharp & Dohme Corp., 2009–2010).

27. What are the perioperative implications?

Interpretation of lab values in older adults is a complex task. Small changes outside of expected ranges may lead to adverse outcomes due to the loss of reserve in the older adult to respond to acute illness. Having a baseline value for comparison can assist the nurse in responding to changes that place the older adult at risk for complications.

PHYSIOLOGIC CHANGES WITH AGING AND SURGICAL IMPLICATIONS: PSYCHOSOCIAL CONSIDERATIONS

28. What elements are required to ensure that a patient's choice is ethically and legally binding?

In order for a patient's choice to be ethically and legally binding, the following three elements are required (Goldstein, 2002):

- Is there a capable decision maker? Capacity is decision specific; for example, a patient with dementia may be capable of consenting to a blood transfusion, but not a heart transplant. If there is sufficient impairment, a surrogate decision maker is necessary.

- The person voluntarily participates in the decision-making process.

- The person must be sufficiently informed of the following aspects diagnosis; costs, risks, benefits of intervention; alternative treatments including risk, benefit, costs; the likely outcome of no treatment; and the likelihood of success.

29. How is decisional capacity determined?

Decisional capacity (Rueben et al., 2009) can be explored using the following questions:

- Can the patient make and express personal preferences at all?
- Can the patient comprehend the risks and benefits?
- Does the patient comprehend the implications?
- Can the patient give reasons for the alternative selected?
- Are supporting reasons rational?

30. What is competency?

Competency is a legal term that refers to a court judge's determination of an individual's ability to make decisions and his or her ability to understand the meaning and importance of a legal document. Competency may also be situation specific; for example, a person may be competent to make a will, but not to run a business. If a person is deemed not to be competent, then, someone else must assume the decision-making role. This can be a family member who becomes the guardian or an unrelated person appointed as a conservator (Goldstein, 2002).

31. What are effective communication strategies?

Communication can be more difficult with older adults due to sensory losses as well as with diagnoses such as dementia, depression, stroke, or delirium. Taking a history or doing an admission assessment may take more time, and may need to be done over more than one session, especially if the patient is in pain or becomes fatigued. Older adults are an extremely heterogeneous group; it is important to not stereotype or patronize. Examples of patronizing communication include using simple vocabulary with a loud or slow voice, using childish terms, using terms of endearment such as "honey" or "dear," or childlike terms such as "good girl" or "cute little man" (Ryan, Hummert, & Boich, 1995).

For patients with vision and hearing loss, it is important to find out the preferred method of communication rather than speaking loudly or by using short sentences. For hearing loss, communication may be written, videotaped, computerized, or presented with the use of aides. When speaking with the patient, stand or sit face-to-face and use lower pitched tones rather than shouting. For vision loss, let the patient know who you are,

where you are, and what you are doing. Also let them know when you are stepping away.

In general, being respectful, listening to the patient's historic narrative as time permits, and recognizing intergenerational differences leads to a trusting and meaningful relationship.

32. Why assess for elder abuse or mistreatment?

In the United States, it is estimated that 2.16 million older Americans are victims of elder abuse or mistreatment each year. Although the actual incidence and prevalence of elder abuse in the United States is not known, the 1998 National Elder Abuse Incidence Study estimated that for every one reported case of elder abuse, approximately five more cases go unreported. The abused older adult is likely to be female, 80 years of age or older, frail, chronically ill, and dependent on someone else with assistance with activities of daily living (ADLs). Most cases of elder abuse occur when the older adult is living at home; however, abuse also occurs in care facilities (such as nursing homes or assistive living residences). The abusers most likely are family members, commonly the spouse or adult child, who serves as a caregiver. Elder abuse occurs across all cultural and socioeconomic classes.

33. Why is elder mistreatment hidden?

Elder mistreatment remains hidden for several reasons. One problem is the lack of uniform definitions. States differ on the types of abuse included in the law (some exclude abandonment and self-neglect) and the definition of older adults varies. Ageism also contributes to underreporting. Healthcare providers may assume behavior is due to a dementia, confusion, or paranoia and may minimize the elder's report of mistreatment. Cognitive impairment may distort the ability to recollect events, adding to the challenge of reporting and data collection. Older adults may be ashamed or embarrassed to talk about abuse they experience. Social isolation can obstruct the detection of mistreatment. And when the older adult presents with injuries from abuse, they may be attributed to chronic disease sequelae (e.g., hip fracture attributed to osteoporosis instead of investigating the possibility of being injured from being pushed). Finally, the older adult may be reluctant to report abuse for fear of repercussions from the abuser.

34. What are elements of elder mistreatment assessment?

When screening an older adult for elder mistreatment, ask direct and simple questions in a nonjudgmental and nonthreatening manner. For example, if the older adult has a physical injury requiring additional assessment, one potential question could be, "Injuries like this usually do not happen by accident. Was anybody else involved?" Start with general questions and become progressively more specific if the older adult's responses indicate elder mistreatment may be occurring. Arrange time to interview the patient and caregiver together and separately; this not only can detect abusive behavior, but can also allow one to detect disparities in stories and/or to assess for caregiver stress. Caregivers may be reluctant to discuss personal problems in the presence of the person who depends on their care.

35. What are some signs and symptoms that demand further investigation?

Although there is not one set marker of abuse, there are several clinical situations suggestive of abuse that warrants further assessment. Clues to the possibility of elder abuse include the following:

- Observations that either the caregiver is reluctant to leave the client alone with healthcare providers, or the older adult defers excessively to the caregiver to answer questions.

- There are delays between injuries and when treatment is sought.

- There are inconsistencies between an observed injury and explanation.

- There is a lack of appropriate clothing or hygiene.

- There is a history of "doctor shopping".

A positive finding does not necessarily mean abuse has occurred. Instead, treat such findings as signs that further assessment is needed.

36. What if elder mistreatment is suspected?

If elder mistreatment is suspected, follow the facility's policy or procedure for reporting abuse. Laws in all 50 states protect elderly victims of mistreatment and most states require healthcare professionals to report incidents of actual or suspected mistreatment to Adult Protective Services. However, specific requirements and penalties vary considerably among states. Proper documentation is important in recording suspected cases of elder mistreatment. Precise recording of findings is crucial since medical records may become part of the legal record. If possible, document verbatim descriptions of events, and draw or photograph physical findings (Bonnie & Wallace, 2003; Fulmer, 2008; Kruger & Moon, 1999; Lachs & Pillemer, 1995; Plitnick, 2008; Tatara & Kuzmeskus, 1999; Tatara et al., 1998).

AGE-ASSOCIATED CHANGES IN PHARMACOKINETICS AND PHARMACODYNAMICS

Physiological, age-related changes will affect the pharmacokinetics and pharmacodynamics of many drugs used before, during, and after surgery.

37. What are pharmacokinetic changes that occur with age?

Pharmacokinetics refer to the concentration of the drug at the sites of action or what the body does to the drug. Pharmacokinetic responses includes drug absorption, distribution, metabolism, and elimination. Absorption is generally complete but may occur more slowly in older adults. For a given drug dose, the plasma concentration and the volume of distribution of a drug are inversely related. Changes in body composition (loss of lean body mass and total body water with an increase in adipose tissue) may influence the distribution of drugs in the older adult. With a decrease in kidney and liver functioning, clearance and excretion of drugs takes longer. Monitoring serum protein levels and albumin levels, as well as renal and liver functions, may help the older adult avoid toxicity or undertreatment (Amella, 2006; Monarch & Wren, 2004; Rivera & Antognini, 2009).

38. What are the effects of water-soluble drugs?

Total body water decreases with age (the use of diuretics exacerbates this change). Because there is less fluid available, water-soluble medications (such as aspirin or lithium) have a smaller volume of distribution and will attain a higher plasma concentration. This will generate a greater pharmacologic effect and can lead to toxic levels more quickly (Rivera & Antognini, 2009).

39. What are the effects of lipid-soluble drugs?

With the increase of body fat, the volume of distribution of lipid-soluble drugs increases and may prolong medication action. Lipid-soluble drugs (such as diazepam, midazolam, and verapamil) will attain a lower concentration because of increased uptake by adipose tissue. It takes longer for the drug to reach a therapeutic level and prolongs elimination because the volume of drug that must be cleared is increased (Rivera & Antognini, 2009).

40. What role does protein have in drug availability?

Added to this are changes in protein binding that alter free-drug availability. Protein malnutrition is common in both underweight and obese older adults. This means that there are fewer binding sites for protein-binding drugs, thereby increasing the amount of the available (free, unbound) drug to circulate. The free drug is active, increasing the pharmacologic effect. High protein-bound drugs (e.g., lidocaine, propanolol, etomidate, thiopental, propofol, alfentanil) may have an exaggerated clinical effect because of a higher level of unbound or free drug (Monarch & Wren, 2004; Rivera & Antognini, 2009).

41. What are pharmacodynamic changes with age?

Pharmacodynamics is defined as what the drug does to the body or the response by the body to the drug. It is the set of pharmacologic actions produced by the drug—both desired and undesired. Pharmacodynamic changes with aging (i.e., end-organ effects) have been more difficult to define than pharmacokinetic changes. In general, older adults will be sensitive to drugs because of changes in pharmacokinetics that lead to a higher concentration for a given dose, because of pharmacodynamic changes (i.e., increased sensitivity for a given drug concentration), or because of both. As a result of marked heterogeneity of drug responses in the older adult, no age-based rules can be applied across the older population. Doses of medications should be modified based on pharmacokinetic predictions, but actual pharmacodynamic responses to the medications should be used to adjust the dose as needed (Amella, 2006; Monarch & Wren, 2004; Rivera & Antognini, 2009).

PREOPERATIVE ASSESSMENT

Because of organ system changes with aging, often accompanied by concomitant disease conditions, the older adult is at higher risk for morbidity and mortality in the perioperative period. For that reason, a thorough preoperative patient assessment should be completed on an older adult. The preoperative assessment should include medical, cognitive, functional, and social and environmental domains. Additional assessments not already covered in this chapter include nutritional status, smoking status, alcohol and drug history, weight, dentition, risk for delirium, balance and gait, falls history and risk, living and financial status, and advanced directives (Silverstein, 2007).

The American Society of Anesthesiologists (ASA) has identified risk factors for screening older adults in the preoperative period for postoperative cardiovascular and pulmonary complications. These include emergency surgery, renal failure, mild to severe systemic disease, unstable angina, recent myocardial infarction or heart failure, COPD,

malnutrition, anemia, ADL dependence, delirium, and prolonged surgery time (Rueben et al., 2009).

INTRAOPERATIVE ASSESSMENT

Changes in organ function manifest as decreased margins of reserve. Older adults may be able to maintain homeostasis, but become increasingly less able to restore it when they are subjected to trauma, disease, or drugs.

42. What are anesthetic considerations in the older adult?

Age-related changes in body composition may have a significant effect on anesthetic management and monitoring. Overall, the loss of muscle and lean body mass and a reduction in blood volume is seen. The contracted state of the vasculature may produce a higher initial plasma concentration when anesthetic medications are administered. An increase in the amount of adipose tissue also occurs, with an increased availability of lipid-soluble anesthetic medications. There is prolonged elimination because of the volume of drug that must be cleared from storage sites, and hypotension may be seen.

The older adult has a decrease in pulmonary and cardiac reserve and a decreased response to catecholamine stimulation. Therefore, the half-lives and an increased sensitivity to medications are important considerations when caring for an older adult who has received an anesthetic. With decreased liver and kidney function, medication metabolism and clearance often decreases in older adults. The minimum anesthetic concentration required declines with age (Clayton, 2008; Rivera & Antognini, 2009).

43. What are thermoregulation changes in the older adult?

All patients are at risk of hypothermia because of the cool temperature of the operating room (OR) and the effect of anesthetic agents. Older adults are at increased risk because of age-related changes (e.g., the loss of subcutaneous tissue in the skin and lower basal metabolic rates). Shivering increases oxygen consumption and may lead to hypoxia and acidosis, and can deprive the heart and brain of necessary oxygen. The circulating nurse and anesthesia provider together can help to prevent hypothermia by increasing the room temperature until the patient is completely draped, by using warm IV and irrigating solutions, by warming the patient interoperatively (i.e., using forced-air warming, circulating-water garments), and by humidifying and warming the airway.

44. What are interoperative skin considerations?

Positioning and padding of the older adult requires extra care and attention because of fragile skin and decrease in subcutaneous fat. The overall goal of positioning is to reduce stress and pressure on the older adult patient's pressure points. Patients with arthritis or other limitations in range of motion (ROM), to the extent possible, should be positioned on the OR table in a position comfortable for them prior to the induction of anesthesia. Comfortable positioning avoids strain on ligaments and joints that can be painful in the postoperative period. Older adults may have kyphotic spines that benefit from additional support padding. If not contraindicated, a pillow placed under the patient's knees can prevent postoperative stiffness that may limit early mobility.

45. What are the risks to fluid and electrolyte balance?

In older adults, the ability to maintain homeostatic levels of fluid and electrolytes is reduced, resulting in a narrow window between too little and too much fluid. Decreases in renal function caused by aging affect fluid, electrolyte, and acid-base balance. The stress of the surgical procedure, pain, anesthetics, and some medications given preoperatively increase the patient's serum levels of sodium and fluid-retaining hormones. An excess of these electrolytes and hormones and a decrease ability of the cardiovascular system to expand make the older patient prone to hypovolemia. Electrolyte imbalances occur because the kidneys are no longer able to reabsorb or adequately secrete electrolytes well. Acid-base imbalances may occur as the kidneys lose their ability to secrete ammonia. Hypovolemia, electrolyte, and acid-base imbalances can be minimized by monitoring and responding to intake and output.

POSTOPERATIVE ASSESSMENT

46. What are the top complications to be prevented in the older adult?

The goal of providing care to all patients in the postoperative period is to reduce morbidity and mortality associated with surgery and anesthesia. For the older adult, restoration of functional capacity to at least the preoperative level and quality of life may be more important than survival alone. When a complication occurs, older adults have less reserve to overcome the complication without overall decline. For example, the response to hypoxemia and hypercarbia is blunted by aging and by residual anesthesia and narcotics.

Postoperatively, older adults may lack the reserve required to meet the added demands residual anesthetics place on ventilatory capability. As a result, the older adult may be predisposed to hypoxemia and respiratory failure. The most common postoperative medical complications in older adults include respiratory problems, congestive heart failure (CHF), delirium, and thromboembolism. Therefore, postoperative interventions for the older adult should focus on maintaining adequate cardiopulmonary function, fluid management, pain management, comfort, and mobility.

47. What are thermoregulation changes in the older adult in the postoperative period?

Age is considered a predisposing factor for perioperative hypothermia, which may impose increased demands on the cardiovascular system. Older patients are at increased risk for hypothermia because of lower basal metabolic ranges, which results in lower body temperature and the loss of subcutaneous tissue. In the early postoperative period, mild hypothermia can elevate norepinephrine concentrations and increase peripheral vasoconstriction and arterial blood pressure. This may lead to cardiovascular ischemia and dysrhythmias (Cheng, Yang, Jeng, Lee, Liu, & Liu, 2007). Other hypothermia-adverse effects include prolonged drug action, oxygen imbalance, immune dysfunction, and subsequent increased incidence of wound infection. There is up to a four-fold increase in oxygen consumption associated with shivering. Special care to maintain normothermia can minimize the risk of postoperative hypothermia in older adults. Being able to refer to the patient's baseline temperature allows the PACU nurse to compare any change in temperature to help prevent hypothermia and assess for infection.

48. What are the airway management concerns with the older adult?

Monitoring with a pulse oximeter may indicate the need for supplemental oxygen or ventilation during the postoperative period. Clearance of anesthetic and pain medications may be slower in the older adult due to age-related physiologic changes. The older adult is susceptible to aspiration from a reduction in airway reflexes. The head of bed (HOB) should be kept higher than 30° when possible.

49. What reorientation measures assist the older adult?

Assistive devices that increase sensory perception (i.e., hearing aids, glasses) should be returned to the older adult as soon as possible, and family members should be allowed to be with the patient as soon as feasible. As the patient wakes up from anesthesia, reintroduce staff members and reorient the patient to the surroundings.

50. What are infection risks for older adults?

Postoperative infections are an important source of morbidity and mortality in older adults. The risk of iatrogenesis (i.e., health care acquired, inadvertent, preventable disease or complications) is increased by the loss of homeostatic reserves that occur with aging. They develop more easily in older adults because of immune system changes. The most common sites of postoperative infection are the urinary tract, the surgical site, and the lungs (e.g., pneumonia). Symptoms of an infectious process in the older adult can be atypical and easily missed. Symptoms include confusion, lethargy, and anorexia, in addition to the typical signs associated with any age group. The same preventative measures with all patients should be used in the older adult population, including the following:

- Promote good nutrition and hydration
- Monitor vital signs and mental status
- Ensure coughing and deep breathing and use of an incentive spirometer
- Maintain intact skin and avoid immobility

Early mobilization, removal of lines and tubes (e.g., indwelling urinary catheter and movement limiting equipment) can help decrease the risk of infection and the sequelae of immobility. Preservation of mobility will assist in reducing the risk of skin breakdown, muscle atrophy, stiffening of joints, and DVT. Early and adequate mobilization improves the possibility that the older adult may return to his or her previous living situation.

51. How are older adults at risk for dehydration?

Dehydration is common in older adults because decreased muscle mass leads to less free water, the extracellular water in muscle tissue. Additionally, the thirst response is blunted with age, and this can result in inadequate fluid intake. The kidneys also have an impaired ability to concentrate urine, which can lead to further dehydration.

PAIN MANAGEMENT

52. What are the barriers to effective pain management in older adults?

Common factors affecting pain control in the older adult patient include misconceptions regarding use

and effects of analgesics, cognitive impairment, impaired communication, and physiologic age-related changes that affect how drugs are metabolized.

Misconceptions about pain management in the older adult population may lead to inadequate pain control. One misconception is that older adults have a higher pain threshold than younger patients and that pain perception decreases with age. The majority of older adults describe moderate to severe pain at some point after major surgery. Even though older adults report pain similar to younger adults, older adults continue to be undertreated for postoperative pain. Another potential barrier is the fear of becoming addicted. Perioperative nurses can help minimize the concern by educating patients that the incidence of opioid addiction (<1%) is very rare when taken for pain relief (McCaffery & Pasero, 1999). Preoperative education about pain management can decrease postoperative pain. Pain management should take into account concurrent treatments for preexisting chronic pain problems using an approach that incorporates opioids, nonopioids, and nonpharmacologic interventions. One example is an older adult with osteoarthritis. Arthritis is a common source of pain in older adults. Nonpharmacologic preventative measures, such as positioning during and after surgery, can help to reduce the pain experienced from arthritis.

53. What are some complications of ineffective pain management in older adults?

Untreated or undertreated postoperative pain can have significant negative impact on the recovery of the older adult following surgery. Pain causes tachycardia, increases myocardial oxygen consumption, and may lead to myocardia ischemia. Older adults often decrease their activity to decrease pain, which can lead to the negative sequelae of immobility, including the potential for skin breakdown, thromboembolic disorders, and declines associated with deconditioning and functional decline. The anticipation of pain may lead to splinting and poor inspiratory effort with subsequent atelectasis and increased risk of pneumonia.

54. What are the basics of pain assessment in the older adult?

Pain assessment should be based on the patient's perception of pain. The patient's report is the most reliable indicator of pain. In cognitively intact older adults, the same assessment instruments used in the younger population may be used to quantify the patient's pain. Some older adults use different words to describe pain such as hurting, aching, sore, and/or discomfort. During the initial pain assessment, ask the older adult to describe the pain using their own words and description. On subsequent pain assessments and reassessments, use the patient's preferred pain terminology. In addition to using consistent words during the assessment, pain intensity should be measured using a consistent scale. The pain thermometer, verbal description scale, and faces pain scale have been used in the older adult population. Postoperative pain assessment during movement provides a more accurate pain measure than pain described at rest.

Older adults with cognitive impairment can often report their pain and report pain intensity similar to cognitively intact individuals. Those who cannot accurately communicate their pain should be assessed using behavioral indicators like facial expressions (i.e., grimacing), verbal cues (i.e., groaning, crying out), or body language (i.e., guarding the injured areas or resisting care). Several tools are available to aid in the assessment of nonverbal pain assessment. Family members and caregivers can assist in identifying behaviors that may be indicative of pain. Asking family and caregivers preoperatively to identify behaviors associated with pain can assist the perioperative nurse in providing pain management in the cognitively impaired older adult. When pain cannot be adequately assessed, assume that pain is present in a patient who has undergone a painful procedure and treat pain preemptively.

55. What are opioid dosing guidelines in older adults?

In general, to adjust for the potential for age related changes, opioid doses should be started at a dose 25% to 50% lower than the recommended dosage for adults and increased slowly by 25% to 50% increments until pain relief is achieved. Older adults experience side effects from opioids more frequently than younger adults. Common side effects include constipation, urinary retention, pruritus, delirium, nausea and vomiting, sedation, bradypnea, and hypotension. Constipation may not be identified as a problem in the perianesthesia period, but may occur later. Prophylaxis to prevent constipation should be initiated postoperatively, and bowel function should be monitored. If nausea and vomiting occur, metoclopramide use avoids the anticholinergic side effects of many antiemetics. The goal for treating all patients, including older adults, with opioid analgesics is to provide the dose that will relieve their pain to an acceptable level with manageable and tolerable side effects.

56. Can patient-controlled analgesia or patient-controlled epidural analgesia therapy be used in the older adult population?

Cognitively intact older adults may be treated with patient-controlled analgesia (PCA) or patient-controlled epidural analgesia (PCEA) to enhance pain management while reducing narcotic use. Pain medication dosages should be adjusted to compensate for an older person's decreased hepatic function and reduced glomerular filtration rate. PCA and PCEA allows for a more constant level of analgesia, minimizing the peaks and troughs associated with PRN analgesia. PCA and PCEA can also give older adults better pain control with fewer complications, less sedation, and better patient satisfaction. The older adult must be able to understand the instructions and use the button before the pain becomes too intense to maintain an effective level of pain control. If an older adult is on PCA or PCEA therapy but is unable to understand instructions and/or push the button appropriately, he or she is at risk for pain to be undertreated.

57. What is the role of nonpharmacologic pain interventions?

When pharmacologic and nonpharmacologic interventions are used together, the dose requirement of analgesics may be decreased, which can lead to a lower incidence of side effects. Examples of nonpharmacologic interventions include cold, heat, relaxation, guided imagery, distraction, and massage therapy (American Pain Society, 2003; Cheng et al., 2007; Herr, Bjoro, Steffensmeier & Rakel, 2006; Leung et al., 2006; Paynter & Mamaril, 2004).

SAFETY AND CHALLENGES IN THE PACU

58. What is emergence delirium?

Emergence delirium (ED) is the transition from the sleep state to becoming fully conscious. ED is uncommon (<10% of surgical cases), but there are specific patient populations who are at high risk (Burns, 2003). Older adults are considered a high-risk population, and risk may be associated with certain medications or presence of baseline cognitive impairment. Medications used during surgery or procedures that can contribute to ED include:

- Ketamine
- Droperidol
- Benzodiazepines
- Metoclopramide
- Atropine
- Scopolamine

Contributing physiologic factors for the development of ED may include hypoxemia, hypercapnia, hypoglycemia, hyponatremia, sepsis, hypothermia, full bladder, and alcohol withdrawal.

Signs and symptoms in the PACU include excitement, alternating periods of lethargy and excitement, and disorientation. Patient behavior may be quite violent and can include kicking, thrashing, screaming, and removal of tubes and catheters. There is risk for injury to the patient and staff (Burns, 2003).

DISCHARGE PREPARATION FROM AMBULATORY SURGERY CENTERS

59. What are the common issues with discharging older adults from ambulatory surgery centers?

Older adults comprise more than one third of all ambulatory surgeries and may take up to 48 hours longer to regain independence than younger adults. A study in Ireland found that almost 12% of older adults scheduled for ambulatory surgery were noncompliant with fasting, 37% took medications despite instructions not to, 13% planned to drive themselves home after surgery, and 7% had no one to stay with them the night after surgery (Lafferty, Carroll, Donnelly & Boylan, 1998).

60. What are recommendations to improve care for older adults undergoing ambulatory surgery?

Ambulatory surgery nursing staff need to provide evidence-based care to older adults. This encompasses developing systems to assess and plan for their special needs. A survey study was conducted to determine what types of preoperative assessments, patient teaching, and discharge planning were performed for older adults undergoing ambulatory surgery.

Recommendations from this study include (Tappen, Muzic, & Kennedy, 2001):

- Developing a separate process for preoperative assessment and evaluation,
- Using multiple screens for adult patients,
- Improving communication among providers,
- Improving collaboration of laboratory and x-ray results,
- Avoiding discharge from the facility with unfilled prescriptions, and
- Educating staff members about the unique needs of older adults undergoing surgery.

Additional recommendations include follow-up phone calls to assess for pain, tolerance of food and fluids, ambulation status, mental status, and the ability to understand discharge instructions and medications (McGory et al., 2009).

REFERENCES

Administration on Aging. (2009). *A profile of older Americans*. Retrieved from http://www.aoa.gov?AoARoot/Aging_Statistics/index.aspx

Amella, E. T. (2006). Presentation of illness in older adults: If you think you know what you're looking for, think again. *AORN Journal, 83*(2), 372–389.

American Pain Society. (2003). *Principles of analgesic use in the treatment of acute pain and cancer pain*. Glenview, IL: Author.

Beliveau, M. M., & Multach, M. (2003). Perioperative care for the elderly patient. *Medical Clinics of North America, 87*, 273–289.

Bonnie, R. J., & Wallace, R. B. (2003). *Elder mistreatment: Abuse, neglect, and exploitation in an aging America*. Washington, DC: National Academy of Sciences.

Borson, S., Scanlon, J., Brush, M., Vitaliano, P., & Dokmak, A. (2000). The mini-cog: A cognitive "vital signs" measure for dementia screening in multilingual elderly. *International Journal of Geriatric Psychiatry, 15*(11), 1021–1027.

Burns, S. M. (2003). Delirium during emergence from anesthesia: A case study. *Critical Care Nurse, 23*(1), 66–69.

Cheng, S. P., Yang, T. L., Jeng, K. S., Lee, J. J., Liu, T. P., & Liu, C. L. (2007). Perioperative care of the elderly. *International Journal of Gerontology, 1*(2), 89–97.

Christmas, C., & Pompei, P. (2010). *AGS geriatric review syllabus: A core curriculum in geriatric medicine-perioperative care*. Retrieved from http://www.frycomm.com/ags/teachingslides

Clayton, J. L. (2008). Special needs of older adults undergoing surgery. *AORN Journal, 87*(3), 557–570.

DeFrances, C. J., Lucas, C. A., Buie, V. C., & Golosinskiy, A. (2008). 2006 National hospital discharge survey. *National Health Statistic Report, 30*(5), 1–20.

Doerflinger, D. C. (2009). Older adult surgical patients: Presentation and challenges. *AORN Journal, 90*(2), 223–240.

Edwards, N. & Baird, C. (2005). Interpreting laboratory values in older adults. *Medsurg Nursing, 14*(4), 220–229.

Fick, D. M., Cooper, J. W., Wade, W. E., Waller, J. L., Maclean, J. R., & Beers, M. H. (2003). Updating the beers criteria for potentially inappropriate medication use in older adults: Results of a US consensus panel of experts. *Archives of Internal Medicine, 163*, 2716–2724.

Fulmer, T. (2008). How to try this: Screening for mistreatment of older adults. *American Journal of Nursing, 108*(12), 52–59.

Goldstein, M. K. (2002). Ethics (pp. 165–182). In R. J. Ham, P. D. Sloane, & G. A. Warshaw (Eds.), *Primary care geriatrics: A case based approach* (4th ed.). St. Louis, MO: Mosby.

Hamel, M. B., Henderson, W. G., Khuri, S. F., & Daley, J. (2005). Surgical outcomes for patients aged 80 and older: Morbidity and mortality from major noncardiac surgery. *Journal of the American Geriatrics Society, 53,* 424–429.

Herr K., Bjoro, K., Steffensmeier, J., & Rakel, B. (2006). Acute pain management in older adults. Retrieved from http://www.guideline.gov/summary/summary. aspx?ss=15&doc_id=10198&string

Hoot-Martin, J., Larsen, P., & Hazen, S. (1997). Interpreting laboratory values in elderly surgical patients. *AORN Journal, 65*(3), 621–626.

Inouye, S. K. (2006). Delirium in older persons. *New England Journal of Medicine, 354*(11), 1157–1165.

Kruger, R. M., & Moon, C. H. (1999). Can you spot the signs of elder mistreatment? *Postgraduate Medicine, 106*(2), 169–173, 177–178, 183.

Lachs, M., & Pillemer, K. (1995). Abuse and neglect of elderly persons. *New England Journal of Medicine, 332*(7), 437–443.

Lafferty, J., Carroll, M., Donnelly, N., & Boylan, J. F. (1998). Instructions for ambulatory surgery-patient comprehension and compliance. *Irish Journal of Medical Science, 167*(3), 160–163.

Leung, J. M., Sands, L. P., Paul, S., Joseph, T., Kinjo, S., & Tsai, T. (2009). Does postoperative delirium limit the use of patient-controlled analgesia in older surgical patients? *Anesthesiology, 111*(3), 625–631.

Marcantonio, E. R., Goldman, L., Orav, E. J., Cook, E. F., & Lee, T. H. (1998). The association of intraoperative factors with the development of postoperative delirium. *American Journal of Medicine, 105*(5): 380–384.

Marcantonio, E. R., Flacker, J. M., Wright, R. J., & Resnick, N. M. (2001). Reducing delirium after hip fracture: A randomized trial. *Journal of the American Geriatrics Society, 49*(5), 516–522.

Mauk, K. L. (2006). Introduction to gerontological nursing (p. 7). In K. L. Mauk (Ed.), *Gerontological nursing competencies for care.* Boston: Jones and Bartlett.

McCaffery, M., & Pasero, C. (1999). *Pain: Clinical Manual.* St. Louis, MO: Mosby.

McDonald, D. D. (2006). Postoperative pain management for the aging patient. *Geriatrics & Aging, 9*(6), 395–398.

McGory, M. L., Kao, K. K., Shekelle, P. G., Rubenstein, L. Z., Leonardi M. J., Parikh, J. A., et al. (2009). Developing quality indicators for elderly surgical patients. *Annals of Surgery, 250*(2), 338–347.

Merck Sharp & Dohme Corp. (2009–2010). *Manual of geriatrics manual. Appendix I: Laboratory values.* Retrieved from http://www.merck.com/mkgr/mmg/appndxs/app1.jsp

Monarch, S., & Wren, K. (2004). Geriatric anesthesia implications. *Journal of PeriAnesthesia Nursing, 19*(6), 379–384.

Paynter, D., & Mamaril, M. E. (2004). Perianesthesia challenges in geriatric pain management. *Journal of PeriAnesthesia Nursing, 19*(6), 385–391.

Plahuta, J. M., & Hamrick-King, J. (2006). Review of the aging of physiological systems (pp. 143–264). In K. L. Mauk (Ed.), *Gerontological nursing competencies for care.* Boston: Jones and Bartlett.

Plitnick, K. R. (2008). Elder abuse. *AORN Journal, 87*(2), 422–427.

Rivera, R., & Antognini, J. F. (2009). Perioperative drug therapy in elderly patients. *Anesthesiology, 100*(5), 1176–1181.

Rueben, D. B., Herr, K. H., Pacala, J. T., Pollock, B. G., Potter, J. E., & Semla, T. P. (2009). *Geriatrics at your fingertips* (11th ed.). New York: American Geriatrics Society.

Ryan, E. B., Hummert, M. L., & Boich, L. H. (1995). Communication predicaments of aging patronizing behavior toward older adults. *Journal of Language and Social Psychology, 14*(1–2), 144–166.

Saufl, N. M. (2004). Preparing the older adult for surgery and anesthesia. *Journal of PeriAnesthesia Nursing, 19*(6), 372–378.

Schick, L. (2004). The elderly patient (pp. 209–225). In D. M. DeFazio Quinn & L. Schick (Eds.), *PeriAnesthesia nursing core curriculum: Preoperative, phase I and phase II PACU nursing.* St. Louis, MO: Saunders.

Silverstein, J. H. (2007). The practice of geriatric anesthesia. In J. H. Silverstein, G. A. Rooke, J. G. Reeves, & C. H. McLeskey (Eds.), *Geriatric anesthesiology* (2nd ed.). New York: Springer.

Sloane, P. D. (2002). Normal aging (pp. 15–28). In R. J. Ham, P. D. Sloane, & G. A. Warshaw (Eds.), *Primary care geriatrics: A case based approach* (4th ed.). St. Louis, MO: Mosby.

Stoelting, R. N., & Miller, R. D. (2000). *Basics of anesthesia* (4th ed.). New York: Churchill Livingstone.

Tappen, R. M., Muzic, J. & Kennedy, P. (2001). Preoperative assessment and discharge planning for older adults undergoing ambulatory surgery. *AORN Journal, 73*(2), 464–474.

Tatara, T. & Kuzmeskus, L.M. (1999). *Elder abuse information series No. 1–3.* National Center on Elder Abuse Grant No. 90-am-0600. Washington, D. C.

Tatara, T., Kuzmeskus, L. B., Duckhorn, E., Bivens, L., Thomas, C., Gertig, J., Jay, K., Hartley, A., Rust, K., & Croos, J. (1998). *National elder abuse incidence study.* Retrieved from http://www.aoa.gov/AoARoot/AoA_Programs/Elder_Rights/Elder_Abuse/docs/ABuseReport_Full.pdf

Walton-Geer, P. S. (2009). Prevention of pressure ulcers in the surgical patient. *AORN Journal, 89*(3), 539–552.

Wei, L., Fearing, M., Sternberg, E., & Inouye, S. (2008). The confusion assessment method: A systematic review of current usage. *Journal of the American Geriatrics Society, 56*(5), 823–830.

SECTION I

SECTION II

SECTION III

CHAPTER 17

Patients with Mental Health Considerations

Joni M. Brady, MSN, RN, CAPA, CLC

According to the National Institute of Mental Health (NIMH), approximately 25% of persons aged 18 years and older has a diagnosable mental condition (2010). Such conditions represent the leading cause of disability in the United States in the 15- to 44-year-old demographic annually. Around 6% of those affected experience a serious type of mental illness. Mental health ailments typically encountered in the perianesthesia population comprise anxiety disorders, mood disorders, schizophrenia, autism spectrum disorder, attention deficit hyperactivity disorder, and dementia associated with Alzheimer's disease. Some of these diagnoses may have accompanying complex communication needs. This chapter briefly explores nursing considerations for the more frequently encountered mental health impaired patients treated in the perianesthesia setting and offers strategies to help promote patient- and family-centered care. These considerations are intended for incorporation into routine perianesthesia nursing care practices.

Medication reconciliation and diagnosis specific perianesthesia medication management is paramount to patient safety. Although patients treated with psychotropic medications may be at increased risk for complications associated with administration of procedural sedation or surgical anesthesia, the available literature on this topic is quite limited; therefore, practice recommendations are largely presented from the expert opinion or consensus level of evidence. Preoperatively, all patients or legal guardians should compile a current medication list that includes the dose, frequency, and times administered. Preanesthetic consultation with a mental health provider should occur when indicated to determine maintenance of routine medication schedules and/or appropriate discontinuation of any psychotropic agents contraindicated in the anesthetic period. Postoperatively, the timely resumption of psychotropic medications supports good continuity of care.

For the patient entering a healthcare facility to have surgery or an invasive procedure, the feeling of loss of control is very powerful and disturbing. For those with a mental health diagnosis, this anxiety and fear can be amplified. The perianesthesia nurse is more likely to circumvent aggressive behavior and achieve success in meeting the emotional needs of a mentally impaired patient when demonstrating knowledge and understanding of the presenting condition. By employing engaging and supportive interpersonal communications throughout the perianesthesia care continuum, the nurse can alleviate a patient's stress and foster feelings of control. Permitting the patient to make choices and involving significant others at the point of care helps to minimize patient and family anxiety. In addition, the use of complementary therapies, distraction techniques, and fostering a quiet, calm environment has proven to be beneficial. The importance of identification and implementation of the most effective means of communication in the patient with complex communication needs cannot be overstated.

Safe care practices in perianesthesia units have been a nursing focus for some time, with evidence-based practice recommendations continually evolving. Due to the small number of studies involving care of the mentally ill patient in the perianesthesia practice setting, much more research is needed to guide care delivery and establish best practices for this population.

1. When is a patient diagnosed with mental illness not legally capable of giving informed consent for a procedure?

Informed consent is a communication process involving patient respect, understanding, and self-rule. The signing of this legal document should follow facility-based protocol and involve an actual discussion between the clinician who will perform the procedure and the patient and his or her legal guardian. Special considerations apply in the case of a minor or compromised patient with a legal health-care proxy. In every case, the nurse has a responsibility to speak out if any question of the patient's competence to consent is identified (Sullivan, 2004). For elective procedures, the consent process should take place in advance to promote a frank discussion regarding clinical options and to permit the patient to ask questions and obtain any clarification needed (Tartaglia, Faulkner, & Roberson, 2009). A patient with a diagnosed mental illness may not give legal consent when the disorder prevents that person from understanding exactly what he or she is consenting to, communicating his or her consent, possessing the ability to act decisively, and/or recognizing the need for therapeutic intervention. The competence to grant informed consent should be based on these criteria and assessed at the specific time when informed consent must be provided or confirmed (Van Staden & Krüger, 2003).

2. What is anxiety disorder?

Every person experiences some anxiety as an innate physiologic response to stress. With anxiety disorder, the individual cannot cope with daily stressors and his or her anxiety progresses to a disabling disorder characterized by an irrational fright of typical life situations. Annually, around 40 million Americans age 18 years and older, representing roughly 18% of men and women in this age group, experience an anxiety disorder. The onset generally occurs at the early end of the age spectrum because almost 75% of those diagnosed have an initial anxiety related event by age 21. Most people that have one anxiety disorder have a coexisting second type of the disorder, and the diagnosis often coincides with substance abuse or

a depressive disorder (NIMH, 2010). The five major forms of anxiety disorders are:

- Panic disorder
- Obsessive-compulsive disorder
- Generalized anxiety disorder
- Social phobia
- Posttraumatic stress disorder

3. What is panic disorder?

Panic disorder (PD) affects approximately 6 million American adults, and women are twice as likely to experience PD as men. Although many people encounter one panic attack, they will not go on to develop PD. Panic attacks often begin during the early adult or late adolescent years and have a genetic correlation. Recurring full-scale panic attacks may occur at any time, can be debilitating, and may cause the individual to avoid the situations or locations in which they occur. A panic attack generally lasts about 10 minutes and its symptoms include chills, numbness or tingling of extremities, weakness, dizziness, faintness, nausea, chest pain or pounding, and a sense of being smothered. The event is accompanied by feelings of loss of control and impending doom (NIMH, 2010). PD, often undiagnosed by primary and secondary care providers, is responsive to combination therapy and medication treatment. Early treatment is needed to prevent the development of social agoraphobia (Baldwin et al., 2005).

4. What is obsessive-compulsive disorder?

Obsessive-compulsive disorder (OCD) impacts over 2 million American adults and is manifested by unrelenting troubling thoughts (i.e., obsession) and a ritual performed to control anxiety related to those thoughts (i.e., compulsion). Ultimately, the individual becomes controlled by a continual performance of rituals, which produce only temporary relief from the anxiety. OCD most frequently begins during childhood, adolescence, or early adulthood, and has a chronic impact with intermittent severity and significant comorbidity with major depression and eating disorders. While psychotherapy promoting desensitization and/or medication treatment has been effective (Baldwin et al., 2005; NIMH, 2010), new research on neurosurgical procedures and brain stimulation is underway to help those not responsive to therapies currently available (Greenberg et al., 2010; NIMH, 2010).

5. What is generalized anxiety disorder?

Generalized anxiety disorder (GAD), which is one of the most common mental health disorders found in the primary care setting (Baldwin et al., 2005), evolves gradually and may occur at any time during the life span. It impacts almost 7 million American adults. The usual onset, most often originating in childhood through middle adulthood, is marked by exaggerated worry and tension associated with everyday life experiences. Females are affected twice as often as males, and some genetic link appears to be involved. Persons affected by GAD have undue anxiety and experience difficulty relaxing, sleeping, resting, concentrating, and may startle easily. Physical symptoms include muscle tension and aching, irritability, sweating, hot flashes, trembling, breathlessness, lightheadedness, and dysphagia. GAD regularly occurs in combination with depression, substance abuse, and another form of anxiety disorder. Treatment includes cognitive behavioral therapy, medication to alleviate symptoms, and targeted therapy aimed at dealing with the accompanying condition(s) identified (NIMH, 2010).

6. What is social phobia?

Social phobia (SP), also called social anxiety disorder, affects around 15 million American adults. It has no gender predominance and may be associated with genetic predisposition. The condition is frequently overlooked in primary care settings and may be labeled as shyness (Baldwin et al., 2005). The typical onset occurs in childhood or early adolescence. SP sufferers dread certain situations and may worry about a potential encounter far in advance. They experience a chronic, powerful fear of self-embarrassment and the unfounded perception that others are judging or watching them. The fear and personal distress associated with SP and a tendency toward situational avoidance impedes friendships, ordinary life activities, school, and work. The disorder is often accompanied by depression. Use of alcohol and/or drugs to alleviate anxiety-related symptoms predisposes the individual to substance abuse (Baldwin et al., 2005; NIMH, 2010).

7. What is posttraumatic stress disorder?

Posttraumatic stress disorder (PTSD) results from some horrifying event involving the threat of harm or actual physical harm. The sufferer may have sustained a direct injury or closely witnessed a terrifying situation involving another person or persons. PTSD currently affects approximately 7.7 million American adults, may be genetically linked, and is more prevalent in women. It can occur at any time during the life span. PTSD is characterized by hyperarousal, reexperiencing the traumatic event, avoidance of stimuli associated with the event, and emotional numbing. The individual

often feels scared or stressed when no danger or threat is present, and relives the event in their in thoughts while awake and in nightmares when asleep. It is frequently accompanied by comorbidities related to chronic stress, other anxiety disorders, depression, and substance abuse. Treatment involves a combination of psychotherapy and medication to control symptoms (NIMH, 2010).

8. What therapeutic medical interventions are indicated for the treatment of anxiety disorders?

Upon completion of a comprehensive medical exam and symptom-based diagnostic determination, principal treatment for an anxiety disorder typically includes some type of psychotherapy combined with medication for symptom management and implementation of self-help strategies (Baldwin et al., 2005). Cognitive behavioral therapy promotes a change in fearful thought patterns and uses applied techniques to desensitize the patient's anxiety triggers (NIMH, 2010). Selective serotonin reuptake inhibitors (SSRIs) have broad-spectrum anxiolytic effects and are most often the first-line medication used. Tricyclic antidepressants and monoamine oxidase inhibitors (MAOIs) are used when SSRIs prove ineffective and are associated with more side effects. Benzodiazepines have proven effective but can produce troublesome sedation and dependence. A beta-blocker, such as propranolol, may be prescribed to treat physical symptoms associated with the disorder. See Table 17-1 for a summary of frequently prescribed antianxiety medications (Baldwin et al., 2005; NIMH, 2010).

9. What perianesthesia nursing strategies are helpful when caring for the patient with an anxiety disorder?

Fear of anesthesia and fear of not waking up after becoming anesthetized are among the greatest fears that a patient (and family) experience. Preoperative anxiety is commonly associated with unpleasant memories of a prior experience, apprehension about the unknown, the anticipation of nausea, and the patient's baseline personality. Anxiety can alter vital signs and the way a person behaves, thinks, and feels. High levels of preoperative anxiety are associated with greater intraoperative anesthetic requirements and increased postoperative pain and analgesic requirements (Rosén, Svensson, & Nilsson, 2008; Sveinsdóttir, 2010). Sveinsdóttir reported a 13–33% range of undiagnosed anxiety and depression found in surgical inpatients. Hospitalization for surgery and interventional procedures is associated with the patient feeling a loss of control. Because anxiety disorders involve underlying fear and intense feelings of loss

TABLE 17-1. Common Medications Used to Treat Anxiety Disorders

Condition	Frequently prescribed medications	Comments
Panic disorder	Alprazolam Imipramine Isocarboxazid Lorazepam Phenelzine Tranylcypromine	• Benzodiazepines may be prescribed for up to 1 year. • Dose tapering should occur for benzodiazepine discontinuation to prevent exacerbation of disorder and onset of withdrawal symptoms.
Obsessive-compulsive disorder (OCD)	Escitalopram Clomipramine Fluoxetine Sertraline	• With the exception of clomipramine, tricyclic antidepressants are less effective in the treatment of OCD.
Generalized anxiety disorder (GAD)	Alprazolam Azapirone Buspirone Clonazepam Imipramine Venlafaxine	• Benzodiazepines are usually prescribed for a brief time due to dependency potential. • Buspirone requires 2 week dosing to attain desired effect. • Venlafaxine use requires baseline blood pressure (BP) and electrocardiogram (ECG) assessment and is contraindicated in patients with hypertension, cardiac disease, or electrolyte imbalance.
Social phobia	Clonazepam Escitalopram Fluoxetine Isocarboxazid Phenelzine Propranolol Sertraline Tranylcypromine	• Treatment with buspirone, imipramine, and atenolol was found to be nonefficacious.
Posttraumatic stress disorder (PTSD)	Escitalopram Fluoxetine Paroxetine Sertraline	• Evidence for an optimal treatment pathway is under investigation.

Source: Baldwin et al., 2005; NIMH, 2010

of control, it is extremely important for the preanesthesia nurse to ascertain the type of anxiety disorder affecting the patient and to assess and document factors that trigger the patient's anxiety. This information should be included in hand-off reporting throughout the perianesthesia continuum. An explanation of the sequencing of events and the time involved in those events should be regularly integrated into care delivery. The nurse can foster a sense of control for the patient through active listening and by offering encouragement to articulate his or her needs. By acknowledging the patient's feelings when control must be relinquished to members of the surgical or procedural team, the nurse can assuage feelings of helplessness or fear. The simple act of being heard and having personal feelings validated can increase the patient's sense of control (Susleck et al., 2007). The patient should always be given an opportunity to assist in the development of a plan of care (Schick, 2009), while permitting the patient to incorporate significant others into the perianesthesia experience (including PACU visitation). The involvement of a trusted person in the preanesthetic and postanesthetic period helps the patient establish a comfort connection throughout the unfamiliar experience (Susleck et al., 2007). Other useful anxiety reduction strategies include adjuvant complementary approaches such as relaxation breathing, music therapy, and use of lavandin essential oil (Braden, Reichow, & Halm, 2009).

10. What additional considerations should the nurse be cognizant of when caring for the perianesthesia patient with PTSD?

An increased risk for emergence delirium exists in the PTSD patient. Upon emergence from anesthesia, the postanesthesia nurse should give frequent orientation to person, place, and time, and employ a soft, calming voice while observing the patient for agitation, sudden hysterical outbursts, or a blank stare. Because individuals with PTSD may startle easily, a calm and quiet environment should be maintained. In extreme PTSD cases, collaboration with the anesthesia provider regarding resedation may be indicated. Family presence in the early postanesthesia period can be beneficial for comforting and reassuring the patient (Mamaril, 2009). PTSD has long been associated with uniformed military service members. Poorly treated pain in the early posttrauma period has recently been associated with increased rates of PTSD in soldiers; therefore, it is important that operative or procedural pain be treated aggressively. Although it has been suggested that use of midazolam in patients with PTSD can enhance the memory of the traumatic event, a study involving soldiers with PTSD did not find any differences with the intensity of memories between those getting midazolam and those who did not (McGhee et al., 2009). Interestingly, a recent study conducted by Brzezinski and his team, found that US military veterans with a history of PTSD had a significant and independent risk for increased mortality during the year following a surgical procedure as compared to their non-PTSD counterparts (Fossum, 2009). Based on the high number of veterans returning from often repetitive combat tours in the Iraq and Afghanistan wars, this study finding may present future challenges in the perioperative setting.

11. Does a history of anesthesia awareness cause PTSD?

Anesthesia awareness, associated with explicit recall, causes patient discomfort, dissatisfaction, and long-term psychological symptoms (Samuelsson, Brudin, & Sandin, 2007). While unintentional awareness under anesthesia occurs in less than 1% of the population receiving anesthesia, this equates to approximately 20,000–40,000 persons annually.

Patients who experience this phenomenon can develop varying degrees of anxiety disorders, including PTSD. While those identified most at risk include cardiac patients, pregnant women undergoing emergency cesarean section, and trauma patients in unstable hemodynamic condition (Geisz-Everson & Wren, 2007; Saufl, 2007), Samuelsson and colleagues (2007) found that anesthesia awareness is not limited to high-risk patients or dangerous surgical procedures. Leslie, Chan, Myles, Forbes, and McCulloch (2010) found that PTSD was frequent and unyielding in confirmed awareness patients and produced varying degrees of lasting consequences. Some of the patients studied experienced delayed psychological problems or PTSD, while others did not encounter sustained emotional difficulties. The preoperative surgical patient should be interviewed to find out if he or she experienced unintentional awareness during a prior procedure. A positive response must be documented and reported to other members of the surgical and anesthetic care teams (Geisz-Everson & Wren, 2007) and included throughout hand-off reporting. The team should make every possible effort to alleviate the patient's anxiety by using therapeutic anxiety related strategies previously discussed.

12. What is a mood disorder?

Mood disorder includes major depressive disorder, dysthymic disorder (also known as chronic mild depression), and bipolar disorder. Annually, nearly 21 million Americans older than the age of 18, representing approximately 10% of the population, experience a mood disorder. The median age for onset of mood disorders is 30. Persons with depressive disorders frequently have concomitant anxiety disorder and substance abuse. The optimal treatment for mild-to-moderate depression is psychotherapy. Generally speaking, clinical depression requires a combination therapy of medication and psychotherapy; this is especially effective in decreasing the probability of recurrence in the adolescent population. Bipolar disorder involves alternating periods of depression and mania. The disorder often begins with an episode of depression that evolves into a mania in which the person displays unusually high energy levels, irritability, and/or pomposity. Evidence has shown that a manic phase can occur when a person is receiving antidepressant therapy in the case of unrecognized bipolar disorder (NIMH, 2010). Catatonia, a condition marked by posturing, mutism, mannerisms, and cataplexy (sudden, transient loss of muscle tone) is associated with bipolar disorder. Catatonia can be effectively treated with electroconvulsive therapy (ECT) (Zisselman & Jaffe, 2010).

13. What are perianesthesia nursing implications for the patient with a mood disorder?

Comprehensive preanesthesia assessment of the mood disorder patient is important due to potential medication interactions, especially in the MAOI class of drugs. Consultation with the patient's psychiatric provider and coordination of a psychotropic medication regimen during the perianesthetic period is frequently indicated (see Table 17-2).

Clarification on when to restart psychotropic medications postoperatively should be identified and documented during the preoperative assessment period. Substance use and abuse may be a factor in this patient population and should be assessed. Many mood disorder patients self-medicate with St. John's Wort, which has been studied and found ineffective in the treatment of major and minor depression. St. John's Wort may cause adverse drug interactions, which prompted a 2010 US Food and Drug Administration advisory regarding simultaneous ingestion with medications used to treat depression, particular cancers, seizures, heart disease, and organ transplantation rejection (NIMH, 2010). Involvement of significant persons and/or family is important, and education regarding possible withdrawal symptoms and exacerbation of depression should be performed. In some facilities, ECTs are performed in the PACU. The nurse should ensure that the consent process for such patients meets ethical, legal, and regulatory standards, and that proper emergency treatment equipment is readily available.

14. What is schizophrenia?

Each year, roughly 2.4 million adult Americans age 18 years and over will be diagnosed with schizophrenia. While there is no gender predominance, schizophrenia often appears in women during the early 20-to-30 year range, while the onset in men occurs in the late teens to early 20s. Schizophrenics suffer from auditory hallucinations and paranoia, which causes fear and social withdrawal. Other symptoms include movement disorders, cognitive deficits, flat affect, delusions, and disordered thinking. The cause for this disease remains unidentified and research in this area is ongoing. Treatment currently focuses on medication for symptom management (NIMH, 2010). First generation antipsychotics have effectively decreased symptoms but cause extrapyramidal symptoms

such as tremors, slow movements, and muscle stiffening. Today, second generation antipsychotics (e.g., clozapine, olanzapine, ziprasidone, risperdone, apriprazole) are often prescribed because they produce significantly fewer extrapyramidal symptoms than does haloperidol; comparable symptoms are noted when compared to low dose first generation antipsychotics. The newer class of antipsychotics, however, has been found to induce more weight gain than the former (Leucht et al., 2008).

15. What perianesthesia nursing actions best support the patient with schizophrenia?

A review of the literature revealed very few inpatient studies in this topic area, and none performed specifically in the perianesthesia patient population. Kudoh (2005) reported on management of the schizophrenic patient noting that a heightened risk for perioperative complications exists due to an altered biologic stress response. These patients have an increased risk for diabetes and respiratory and cardiovascular disease. They can also exhibit endocrine, immune, and cardiovascular system abnormalities. Further, patients on a chronic antipsychotic medication regimen have higher postoperative mortality rates and lack pain sensitivity. Adverse responses encountered during anesthesia include hypotension, arrhythmias, hyperpyrexia, prolonged narcosis or coma, postoperative confusion, and postoperative ileus. Similar to the other mental disorders discussed in this chapter, a thorough preanesthesia assessment, psychiatric evaluation, and coordination of perianesthetic care is essential. Communication difficulties may be encountered throughout the course of care, so strategies to accommodate communication deficits must be explored. The nurse should ensure that the consent process meets ethical, legal, and regulatory standards.

Because these patients are known to have difficulty maintaining social relationships, social service consults should be initiated when indicated. Second generation antipsychotic medications used to treat schizophrenia are relatively new and require a psychiatric provider's determination for management during the perioperative period. This type of medication should be tapered and not abruptly discontinued. Dosing directions should be established and documented preoperatively. For example, clozapine, used to treat hallucinations and psychotic symptoms, can cause agranulocytosis (see Table 17-2). The patient's white blood cell count should be monitored weekly or biweekly (Kudoh, 2005). In the PACU,

TABLE 17-2. Anesthetic Considerations for Psychotropic Medications

Medication	Discontinue preoperatively?	Risk of relapse	Interactions/ side effects	Direct effects	Withdrawal symptoms	Psychiatric consult	Integrated case management
Clozapine	Yes	Yes	Hypotension; possible sedation	Seizures; agranulocytosis	Yes	Yes, done as early as possible due to high rate of relapse	Yes
First-generation antipsychotics	No; perform baseline ECG evaluation for prolonged QT interval, and assess comorbidities.	Yes	Potentiate sedation; Possible: antacids, ACE-inhibitors	Possible: extrapyramidal symptoms, decreased cardiac conduction, agranulocytosis, anticholinergic effect	Possible cholinergic rebound	Yes	As clinically indicated
Lithium	Yes	Yes	NSAIDS, ACE-inhibitors, diuretics	GI symptoms, cardiac conduction, CNS	None	Yes	Yes
Monoamine oxidase inhibitors (MAOI)	Discontinue irreversible MAOI 2 weeks in advance; recommend rotating to a reversible MAOI to shorten the discontinuation period.	Rapid discontinuation can cause serious withdrawal syndromes such as severe depression, suicidal behavior, paranoid delusions, and hallucinations.	Epinephrine: blood pressure elevation; seratogenic symptoms	None	Nonselective class: hypertension	Yes	Yes

Selective serotonin reuptake inhibitors (SSRI)	Not necessary in ASA class I and II patients, except when administered in combination with NSAID or aspirin.	Requires further investigation	Midazolam: cognitive impairment; sodium channel blocker antiarrhythmics; Possible cytochrome P450 inhibition; serotonergics	Possible: GI bleeding, serotonergic symptoms	Agitation, anxiety, dizziness, lethargy, sleep disturbances, palpitations, GI disturbances, general malaise	As clinically indicated	As clinically indicated
Tricyclic antidepressants	Yes; gradually discontinue during the 2 weeks prior to surgery and obtain baseline ECG. Restart as soon as possible in postoperative period.	Relapse rate in persons on maintenance therapy is two to four times greater than those who continue medication management.	Enflurane: seizures; sympathomimetics: arrhythmias, hypertension, tachycardia; changes in cytochrome P450	Anticholinergic symptoms; cardiac arrhythmias	GI; vivid dreams/ sleep disturbances; general malaise	Yes	As clinically indicated

Source: Adapted from Huyse, Touw, Van Schijndel, De Lange, & Slaets, 2006.

frequent orientation should be provided to the patient. Due to altered pain sensitivity and the possible lack of self-reporting, the nurse can assume pain is present in the early postoperative period and should provide appropriate starting doses of pain medication per anesthesia orders (Pasero, 2009). Agitation and delirium are possible, so protective safety measures must be taken to prevent injury to the patient and staff. Early involvement of significant others can help promote communication and calm for the patient.

16. What evidence is available regarding psychotropic medications and anesthetic interactions, and related patient management recommendations?

While the available evidence surrounding specific psychotropic medication groups is somewhat limited at this time, nonsystematic reviews and case reports point to an increased risk for complications during the perioperative period (Huyse et al., 2006). MAOIs are known to have a serious interaction with amphetamines, reserpine, methylphenidate, and ephedrine or pseudoephedrine that can cause a hypertensive crisis. Meperidine administered in addition to a MAOI causes restlessness, agitation, hypertension, convulsions, rigidity, and hyperpyrexia. Rapid MAOI discontinuation can cause severe withdrawal symptoms and exacerbation of depression to include suicidal ideation and/or attempts and paranoid delusions. The administration of fentanyl, morphine, and direct-acting sympathomimetics is considered acceptable for patients taking MAOIs (Golembiewski, 2006). Huyse et al. (2006) performed a review of psychotropic medication characteristics and existing management recommendations for patients undergoing anesthesia and concluded that the preanesthesia unit provides an excellent opportunity to perform a risk assessment and develop an integrated, patient-centered approach to care. The preanesthesia assessment should focus on risk management for perioperative complications, the potential for physiologic withdrawal symptoms, acute/long-term mental condition relapse, and prevention of late cancellation of surgery.

17. What is attention deficit hyperactivity disorder (ADHD)?

This disorder typically appears in children during the preschool or early elementary school years with onset at the median age of 7 years. ADHD is among the most common mental disorders found in children and adolescents affecting approximately 4% of adults age 18 to 44 years old each year. Causes of ADHD include prenatal exposure to alcohol and nicotine, traumatic brain injury, and genetic predisposition. Symptom clusters include hyperactivity, impulsiveness, and inattention (NIMH, 2010).

- Hyperactivity symptoms
  - Difficulty sitting still/in constant motion
  - Talking incessantly
  - Struggling with quiet activities and tasks
  - Squirming or fidgeting
  - Touching everything within sight or reach
- Impulsivity symptoms
  - Difficulty waiting for things
  - Very impatient
  - Frequently interrupting others
  - Making inappropriate comments
  - Unrestrained emotions
  - Taking action without thinking about consequences
- Inattention symptoms
  - Difficulty focusing or completing a task, processing information, or following instructions
  - Easily bored
  - Frequently switching activities
  - Easily distracted
  - Daydreaming, appearing as if not listening
  - Losing objects often

Current ADHD treatment includes a combination of education and behavior modification techniques, medication for functional improvement and symptom reduction, and psychotherapy. Stimulants, the medication of choice, are believed to work by increasing the brain's dopamine levels. Stimulants appear to decrease hyperactivity and impulsivity, and increase impulse control, concentration levels, planning, and follow through (NIMH, 2010).

18. How can the perianesthesia nurse best support an ADHD patient?

The limited amount of literature on ADHD in the perianesthesia setting centers on the study of children. Approximately 65% of children have intense fear and anxiety during the preoperative period and, particularly, during anesthesia induction. Parental anxiety is positively linked to children's preoperative anxiety. This is important to note because children experiencing preoperative distress, anxiety, and fear exhibit more difficult postoperative behaviors and emergence delirium (Sadhasivam et al., 2009). Another research team compared children with and without ADHD to assess behaviors during anesthesia induction, emergence, and in the postoperative period (Tait, Voepel-Lewis, Burke, & Doherty, 2010). The researchers concluded that ADHD children were considerably more uncooperative at induction and had more maladaptive behaviors in the postoperative period (e.g., impulsive, restless, disobedient, has temper tantrums, difficulty communicating, problem making decisions, has poor appetite, and poor concentration following surgery). Clearly, all perianesthesia nursing actions that serve to minimize anxiety in both the parent and child are indicated. Comfort strategies and family education should be employed early during the preanesthesia assessment and throughout the continuum of care. Nursing care planning should be based on the symptoms encountered with the type of ADHD diagnosed. Premedication to reduce anxiety and hyperactivity could be beneficial. Anesthetic emergence safety measures should be observed due to the high potential for delirium. Pain assessment and adequate treatment is important. Parents should be informed that maladaptive behaviors are frequently encountered in the postoperative period after the ADHD child returns home (Tait et al., 2010) and that these behaviors are most effectively handled with positive discipline techniques. The patient on chronic amphetamine therapy will have a lower anesthetic requirement, possibly resulting from catecholamine depletion in the central nervous system (CNS), and a reduced pressor response to ephedrine. Phenylephrine and epinephrine should be immediately available to treat potential bradycardia or hypotension. Perioperative discontinuation of the medication has not been proven necessary, but continuation in the perianesthesia period warrants caution (Fischer, Healzer, Brook, & Brock-Utne, 2000). Medication dosing instructions must be determined by the mental health provider in collaboration with the anesthesia team, documented in the preanesthesia assessment period, and then communicated to the patient and/or family.

19. What is autism spectrum disorder?

Autism spectrum disorder (ASD) includes pervasive developmental disorder and Asperger syndrome, and comprises a range of neurodevelopmental conditions characterized by behavioral, social, and communication impairments. The incidence of ASD is rising although the reason for its increase is not clear (Dell et al., 2008). A recent study estimated that autism occurs in 3.4 of every 1000 children age 3 to 10 years. While ASD disproportionately affects males, females are inclined to experience more pronounced cognitive impairment and more severe symptoms (NIMH, 2010). Typical ASD behavior patterns can involve repetitive physical actions, continued fixation with a particular interest or object, and a rigid observance of nonproductive routines. Social connections are hampered by the deficient use of nonverbal communication and a lack of peer relationships. Impaired communication manifests in speech development delays or absence or the inability of the ASD patient to conduct a conversation. Combination treatment for ASD includes varied therapies (behavioral speech/language, physical, occupational) and school-based interventions. Medications are prescribed for symptom control and may include tricyclic antidepressants, antianxiety agents, SSRIs, antipsychotics, and stimulants (Dell et al., 2008).

20. What perianesthesia nursing actions support optimal care of an ASD patient?

An individual with ASD presents challenges to healthcare workers who are unfamiliar with that person's communication patterns for personal needs and his or her usual behaviors. The inclusion of parents, close family members, or significant others in all aspects of care can be extremely beneficial to the ASD patient and the nurse. Burke et al. (2009) reported on several studies that assessed the impact of family presence in procedural or specialty care areas. The study findings showed that family presence had no increased risks, but did provide high levels of parent satisfaction. Additionally, this study found that parents want to be given the choice whether or not to be present during care. Allaying anxiety in both the parent and ASD patient is important. The care team should always assess parental coping levels because it has been found that allowing a very anxious parent to accompany a child into the OR can increase anxiety in a calm or somewhat nervous child (Kain, Mayes, Caldwell-Andrews, Karas, & McClain, 2006). Preanesthesia assessment should include a discussion with the parents about the child's usual and most effective communication method; sensory, behavioral, and social skills; and behavioral strengths and limitations. Care planning should be based on the type of ASD diagnosed and the respective symptoms encountered (Souders, DePau, Freeman, & Levy, 2002). Medication reconciliation, withholding or the continuation of medication, and proper dosing instructions must be identified and documented preoperatively. Persons with Asperger syndrome and those possessing a normal intelligence level may be competent to give informed consent (Dell et al., 2008). Souders et al. (2002) offer these strategies to promote the successful care of the ASD patient:

- Prepare parents for their role in care delivery.
- Allow the patient to make choices.
- Use distraction techniques to decrease anxiety.
- Model desired behaviors for the child.
- Present information visually instead of verbally.
- Encourage family to bring a familiar, favorite toy.
- Sing songs while performing procedures to distract the patient's focus from the task.
- Avoid the use of restraints and use gentle holding when necessary.

Postoperatively, a potential exists for delayed agitation after premedication with midazolam. In cases where delayed agitation occurs, a review of medications administered may reveal a possible need for flumazenil to reverse midazolam (Voepel-Lewis, Mitchell, & Malviya, 2007). Early reunification with parents is advised. Assessing for anxiety and pain in a nonverbal and/or cognitively impaired ASD patient presents a challenge. Parental feedback on the patient's physical cues and behavioral or observation-based assessment by the nurse, and the use of picture communication offer a best practice approach in the PACU (Dell et al., 2008; Mesko, 2010). Discharge education should include the possibility of delayed agitation.

21. What is Alzheimer's disease?

Approximately 5.3 million Americans have Alzheimer's disease (AD), which is the most common cause of dementia and the seventh leading cause of death in the United States. African Americans and Hispanics are at higher risk for developing AD. The cause for the disease is presently unknown, and research is underway to identify the root cause. In AD, information transfer at the synapses begins to fail, the amount of synapses decline, and the cells ultimately die. The advanced AD brain reveals a dramatic reduction in size due to cell losses and dying neurons.

Advancing age is the greatest risk factor for AD, and the primary symptom involves a gradual decline in the recall of new information. There is currently no treatment to stop the brain cell deterioration found in AD and many experimental therapies are under investigation (Alzheimer's Association, 2010).

22. Are there special perianesthesia considerations for the AD patient?

The AD affected patient requires perianesthesia care management that addresses possible challenges with informed consent, preoperative disease progression, and postoperative support. As the volume of older surgical patients rises, it is likely that comorbidities will have an impact on a patient's physical ability and autonomy level; therefore, the elderly patient requires a thorough mental status and physical evaluation. It is important to assess and determine if the patient has the ability to make medical decisions or whether a legal guardian or healthcare proxy must be involved. Equally important is the identification of who will participate in preoperative care and be present on the day of the surgery or procedure. Anesthetic drugs are known to interfere with cholinergic function in the brain and several anesthetic agents yield a neurotoxic effect. AD patients frequently encounter CNS complications after anesthesia and may need a higher level of care due to postoperative declines in cognitive function. Anesthetic drug interactions are also an important consideration in AD patients. For example, galantamine, used to manage senile dementia symptoms, has been used to reverse tubocurarine-like neuromuscular blockade agents. Chronic use of tacrine, an anticholinesterase used to manage Alzheimer's dementia, could affect the response to nondepolarizing neuromuscular blocking agents. The cholinesterase inhibitor, donepezil, antagonizes the effects of atracurium (Fodale, Quattrone, Trecrocia, Caminiti, & Santamaria, 2006). Communication is a key factor in care delivery to this patient population. When questioned, AD patients will frequently give the same answer to incongruous questions. In order to obtain the most accurate information from the patient, it is advisable to ask open-ended questions. Involvement of family members or usual caregivers will aid in the collection of pertinent information and the development of a complete plan of care (Williams, 2009). As always, documentation of patient information and inclusion of that information in the hand-off report is essential to patient safety. In order for the nurse to plan and

TABLE 17-3. Stages and Symptoms of Alzheimer's Disease

Early stage (mild)
• Difficulty learning new information and recalling familiar words • Recent memory loss that is not readily apparent to others • Shortened attention span, problem organizing thoughts and thinking logically • Remains quiet to circumvent verbal errors • Asks repetitive questions • Becomes irritable or angry when tired or frustrated, unusually insensitive to the feelings of others • Reluctant to make decisions
Middle stage (moderate)
• Cannot follow logical explanations or organize thoughts • Obvious hygiene, appearance, behavioral, and sleep changes noted • Confuses peoples' identities, difficulty recognizing familiar objects • Safety issues related to poor judgment encountered • Demonstrates repetitive words, statements, stories • Experiences restless, repetitive movements in late afternoon or evening • Can yell, curse, accuse, threaten, squirm, and/or become physically aggressive • Difficulty finishing tasks and following written instructions • May smell, see, taste, or hear things that are not present • Encounters more difficulty when positioning body in a chair or onto the toilet • Displays improper sexual behavior, such as masturbating or disrobing in public
Late stage (severe)
• Requires full assistance to accomplish activities of daily living • No longer recognizes self or significant others • May call out loudly or appear uncomfortable or when touched • Communication is impaired, is difficult to understand, or remains silent • May refuse food, forget to swallow, or choke • Loss of weight and bladder or bowel control • Skin becomes fragile and easily tears • Possible seizures and frequent falls • Frequent infections encountered • Difficulty or absence of ambulation

Source: Williams, 2009

deliver comprehensive care across the perianesthesia care continuum, he or she must become familiar with the Alzheimer's patient's stage of disease progression and the general characteristics found in that stage (See Table 17-3).

23. What postoperative nursing implications are indicated when the patient has Alzheimer's disease?

Assessing the patient's level of orientation to time, situation, and place should occur frequently, and the nurse should provide orientation as indicated. Involvement of family or usual caregivers can enhance communication and interpretation of the patient's needs. Agitation and delirium may occur due to anesthetic medications administered, along with hypoxia or hypercapnia. Safety measures should be in place to protect the patient and staff members from harm. Offering reassurance in a soft voice and maintaining a calm, quiet PACU environment is helpful. Pain assessment and the related need for pain medication will depend on the patient's communication ability. Frequently, the AD patient may have a lower pain tolerance than before the onset of the disease and will have increased sensitivity to the effects of an opioid. For those who cannot communicate at all, the nurse should assume pain is present when the procedure is known to be painful (Pasero, 2009) and medicate beginning with low doses based on regular patient observations and family member consultation regarding verbal cues (Williams, 2009). Generally speaking, the nurse can expect a delayed response to anesthesia recovery and a prolonged postanesthesia recovery period.

24. How can the perianesthesia nurse communicate more effectively with patients having complex communication needs?

The mentally impaired patient with complex communication needs requires creative nursing strategies to facilitate information exchange. Both patients and nurses have reported deep frustration and concern over inadequate communication. The use of augmentative and alternative communication helps communicate more effectively when speech is not possible. Finke, Light, and Kitko (2008) share the following strategies to improve communication.

- Partner preoperatively with a speech or language pathologist.
- Establish a calm environment to support communication efforts.
- Wait patiently for the person to convey thoughts.
- Look directly at the person to pick up verbal cues.
- Establish a yes/no response system with the patient.

Pictures that tell a story or convey a thought are very useful when speech is lacking. Ono, Oikawa, Hirabayashi, and Manabe (2008) performed postoperative interviews and found that the use of a picture book allowed parents to preoperatively familiarize a child with hospitalization and enhanced the child's autonomy on the day of surgery. Similar use of a picture communication board and integrated social stories has proven successful with nonverbal perianesthesia autism patients (Mesko, 2010). Ultimately, when innovative strategies are needed to bridge a communication gap, the preanesthesia nurse should encourage early multidisciplinary collaboration during the preanesthesia unit assessment and on the day anesthesia is administered to ensure optimal care delivery for the patient with complex communication needs.

REFERENCES

Alzheimer's Association. (2010). Alzheimer's facts and figures. Retrieved from http://www.alz.org/alzheimers_disease_facts_figures.asp?type=homepage#aa

Baldwin, D. S., Anderson, I. M., Nutt, D. J., Bandelow, B., Bond, A., Davidson, J. R., et al. (2005). Evidence-based guidelines for the pharmacological treatment of anxiety disorders: Recommendations from the British Association for Psychopharmacology. *Journal of Psychopharmacology, 19*(6), 567–596.

Braden, R., Reichow, S., & Halm, M. A. (2009). The use of the essential oil lavandin to reduce preoperative anxiety in surgical patients. *Journal of PeriAnesthesia Nursing, 24*(6), 348–355.

Burke, C. N., Voepel-Lewis, T., Hadden, S., DeGrandis, M., Skotcher, S., D'Agostino, R., et al. (2009). Parental presence on emergence: Effect on postanesthesia agitation and parent satisfaction. *Journal of PeriAnesthesia Nursing, 24*(4), 216–221.

Dell, D., Feleccia, M., Hicks, L., Longstreth-Papsun, E., Politsky, S., & Trommer, C. (2008). Care of patients with autism spectrum disorder undergoing surgery for cancer. *Oncology Nursing Forum, 35*(2), 177–183.

Finke, E. H., Light, J., & Kitko, L. (2008). A systematic review of the effectiveness of nurse communication with patients with complex communication needs with a focus on the use of augmentative and alternative communication. *Journal of Clinical Nursing, 17*(16), 2102–2115.

Fischer, S. P., Healzer, J. M., Brook, M. W., & Brock-Utne, J. G. (2000). General anesthesia in a patient on long-term amphetamine therapy: Is there cause for concern? *Anesthesia & Analgesia, 91*(3), 758–759.

Fodale, V., Quattrone, D., Trecroci, C., Caminiti, V., & Santamaria, L. B. (2006). Alzheimer's disease and anaesthesia: Implications for the central cholinergic system. *British Journal of Anaesthesia, 97*(4), 445–452.

Fossum, S. (2010). Notes from the 2009 American Society of Anesthesiologists' annual meeting. *Journal of PeriAnesthesia Nursing, 25*(2), 128–132.

Geisz-Everson, M., & Wren, K. R. (2007). Awareness under anesthesia. *Journal of PeriAnesthesia Nursing, 22*(2), 85–90.

Golembiewski, J. (2006). Antidepressants: Pharmacology and implications in the perioperative period. *Journal of PeriAnesthesia Nursing, 21*(4), 285–287.

Greenberg, B. D., Gabriels, L. A., Malone, D. A., Rezai, A. R., Friehs, G. M., & Okun, M. S. (2010). Deep brain stimulation of the ventral internal capsule/ventral striatum for obsessive-compulsive disorder: Worldwide experience. *Molecular Psychiatry, 15*(1), 64–79.

Huyse, F. J., Touw, D. J., Van Schijndel, R. S., De Lange, J. J., & Slaets, J. P. (2006). Psychotropic drugs and the perioperative period: A proposal for a guideline in elective surgery. *Psychosomatics, 47*(1), 8–22.

Kain, Z. N., Mayes, L. C., Caldwell-Andrews, A. A., Karas, D. E., & McClain, B. C. (2006). Preoperative anxiety, postoperative pain, and behavioral recovery in young children undergoing surgery. *Pediatrics, 118*(2), 651–658.

Kudoh, A. (2005). Perioperative management for chronic schizophrenic patients. *Anesthesia & Analgesia, 101*(6), 1867–1872.

Leslie, K., Chan, M. T., Myles, P. S., Forbes, A., & McCulloch, T. J. (2010). Posttraumatic stress disorder in aware patients from the B-aware trial. *Anesthesia & Analgesia, 110*(3), 823–828.

Leucht, S., Corves, C., Arbter, D., Engel, R. R., Li, C., & Davis, J. M. (2008). Second-generation versus first-generation antipsychotic drugs for schizophrenia: A meta-analysis. *Lancet, 373*(9657), 31–41.

Mamaril, M. E. (2009). Care of the shock trauma patient (pp. 760–780). In C. B. Drain & J. Odom-Forren (Eds.), *Perianesthesia nursing: A critical care approach.* St. Louis, MO: Saunders.

McGhee, L. L., Maani, C. V., Garza, T. H., DeSocio, P. A., Gaylord, K. M., & Black, I. H. (2009). The relationship of intravenous midazolam and posttraumatic stress disorder development in burned soldiers. *The Journal of Trauma, 66*(Suppl. 4), 186–190.

Mesko, P. J. (2010). Use of picture communication tools in the perianesthesia care unit. *Breathline, 30*(1), 12–15.

National Institute of Mental Health. (2010). *The numbers count: Mental disorders in America.* Retrieved from http://www.nimh.nih.gov/health/publications/the-numbers-count-mental-disorders-in-america/index.shtml

Ono, S., Oikawa, I., Hirabayashi, Y., & Manabe, Y. (2008). Preparation of a picture book to support parents and autonomy in preschool children facing day surgery. *Pediatric Nursing, 34*(1), 82–88.

Pasero, C. (2009). Challenges in pain assessment. *Journal of PeriAnesthesia Nursing, 24*(1), 50–54.

Rosén, S., Svensson, M., & Nilsson, U. (2008). Calm or not calm: The question of anxiety in the perianesthesia patient. *Journal of PeriAnesthesia Nursing, 23*(4), 237–246.

Sadhasivam, S., Cohen, L. L., Szabova, A., Varughese, A., Kurth, C.D., Willging, P., et al. (2009). Real-time assessment of perioperative behaviors and prediction of perioperative outcomes. *Anesthesia & Analgesia, 108*(3), 822–826.

Samuelsson, P., Brudin, L., & Sandin, R. H. (2007). Late psychological symptoms after awareness among consecutively included surgical patients. *Anesthesiology, 106*(1), 26–32.

Saufl, N. M. (2007). Prevention of anesthesia awareness. *Journal of PeriAnesthesia Nursing, 20*(2), 130–131.

Schick, L. (2009). Assessment and monitoring of the perianesthesia patient (pp. 360–389). In C. B. Drain & J. Odom-Forren (Eds.), *Perianesthesia nursing: A critical care approach.* St. Louis, MO: Saunders.

Souders, M. C., DePaul, D., Freeman, K. G., & Levy, S.J. (2002). Caring for children and adolescents with autism who require challenging procedures. *Pediatric Nursing, 28*(6), 555–562.

Sullivan, E. E. (2004). Issues of informed consent in the geriatric population. *Journal of PeriAnesthesia Nursing, 19*(6), 430–432.

Susleck, D., Willocks, A., Secrest, J., Norwood, B. K., Holweger, J., Davis, M., et al. (2007). The perianesthesia experience from the patient's perspective. *Journal of PeriAnesthesia Nursing, 22*(1), 10–20.

Sveinsdóttir, J. (2010). Factors associated with psychological distress at home following elective surgery in a representative group of surgical patients: An explorative panel study. *Vard i Norden, 30*(1), 34–39.

Tait, A. R., Voepel-Lewis, T., Burke, C., & Doherty, T. (2010). Anesthesia induction, emergence, and postoperative behaviors in children with attention-deficit/hyperactivity disorders. *Pediatric Anesthesia, 20*(4), 323–329.

Tartaglia, A., Faulkner, K., & Roberson, A. R. (2009). Ethics in perianesthesia nursing (pp. 98–112). In C. B. Drain & J. Odom-Forren (Eds.), *Perianesthesia nursing: A critical care approach.* St. Louis, MO: Saunders.

Van Staden, C. W., & Krüger, C. (2003). Incapacity to give informed consent owing to mental disorder. *Journal of Medical Ethics, 29*(1), 41–43.

Voepel-Lewis, T., Mitchell, A., & Malviya, S. (2007). Delayed postoperative agitation in a child after preoperative midazolam. *Journal of PeriAnesthesia Nursing, 22*(5), 303–308.

Williams, A. S. (2009). Perianesthesia care of the Alzheimer's patient. *Journal of PeriAnesthesia Nursing, 24*(6), 343–347.

Zisselman, M. H., & Jaffe, R. L. (2010). ECT in the treatment of a patient with catatonia: Consent and complications. *The American Journal of Psychiatry, 167*(2), 127–132.

CHAPTER 18

Families of Perianesthesia Patients

Daphne Stannard, RN, PhD, CCRN, CCNS, FCCM

Perioperative and perianesthesia settings are frightening places for patients and family members. They connote pain, separation from loved ones, and the unknown—be it diagnosis (was it malignant or benign?), clinical trajectory (will I bounce back from this surgery?), and even life course (will my child be able to walk again?). They are also time-sensitive areas, with to-follow cases depending on efficient movement through the entire perioperative continuum. Finally, they are high-intensity nursing care areas that range from caring for a stable phase II patient who is out of bed, sitting up, and eating crackers to a critically ill phase I patient who lacks a stable airway. This chapter will highlight family care in perianesthesia settings.

1. Who should be considered family?

The legal definition of family, based on blood or legitimized relationship (e.g., spouse or durable power of attorney for health care), is purposefully narrow and limiting and is used routinely for informed consents and end-of-life decisions. However, its restrictive quality excludes many types of families and family members, making it an ill-suited definition for routine care issues, such as the person(s) providing emotional support to the patient at the preoperative stage (preop) and postanesthesia care unit (PACU) bedside and those present to hear discharge instructions. When the patient can communicate, the ideal definition of family is whomever the patient defines as her or his family. Currently, federal guidelines are being drafted to ensure that patients may designate

visitors, so that healthcare facilities cannot restrict visitation to immediate family members only (Obama, 2010). When the patient is unable to communicate, a practical definition of family is anyone who shares a history and a future with the patient (Stannard, 2006).

2. Why care for a patient's family?

There is a lifelong and reciprocal relationship between a patient and her or his family. For example, the family is greatly affected by the patient's illness; likewise, a "sick" or dysfunctional family can greatly affect the patient. Nurses who respect this reciprocal relationship understand that caring for a patient's family is simply another way of caring for the patient. By working with patients and their families, perianesthesia nurses can support and strengthen meaningful relationships during times of great stress (Stannard, 2006).

3. What are the top needs of families of critically ill patients?

Many researchers have examined the needs of family members of critically ill patients. Researchers have also studied family needs across the life span and in a variety of specialty critical care and acute care settings. The results of these studies suggest that family members of hospitalized loved ones have predictable sets of needs. The needs experienced by most families can be grouped into three major categories: receiving assurance, remaining near the patient, and receiving information (Leske, 1991). Meeting these needs has been shown to increase family satisfaction. See Table 18-1 for the

TABLE 18-1. Critical Care Family Needs

To have questions answered honestly
To know specific facts regarding what is wrong with the patient
To know prognosis, outcome, or chance for recovery
To be called at home with changes
To receive information once a day
To receive information in understandable terms
To believe that hospital personnel care about the patient
To have hope
To know exactly what or why things are done to the patient
To know that the best care possible is being given to the patient

Source: Hickey, 1990

top 10 family needs of critically ill patients and Table 18-2 for acute care family needs.

4. Should family members of pediatric patients be cared for differently than family members of adult patients?

There is a strong bias in our society that underscores the importance of keeping the pediatric patient and family unit together. Walking through any pediatric hospital, one can readily see how accessible and welcoming the nursing units are to family members. However, this bias also cuts the other way: it is assumed that an adult patient does not need her or his family, except perhaps during times of expected and significant transitions, such as birth and death.

TABLE 18-2. Acute Care Family Needs

To have directions as to what to do at the bedside
To receive more support from their own family unit
To have a place to be alone as a family unit in the hospital
To be informed in advance of any transfer plan
To have flexibility in the time allowed for visitation

Source: Foss & Tenholder, 1993

This societal backdrop is so taken for granted that many adults do not even notice this assumption until they or someone in their immediate family becomes ill. In fact, a recent descriptive study querying PACU nurses from across the United States found that only 8% of adult patients are always allowed to have a visitor in the PACU and 11% are allowed visitors most of the time (DeLeskey, 2009). When possible, it is important to honor the patient's wishes and desires, regardless of the patient's age, and to strive to involve family members in the patient's care, as long as it is feasible and desired by the patient and/or family.

5. How can patient privacy be maintained if family members are around?

Provided that the patient gives consent, under the latest iteration of the Health Insurance Portability and Accountability Act (HIPAA), providers are allowed to disclose protected health information and provide access to individually identifiable health information (such as lab values and vital signs) at their discretion to persons assisting in an individual's care (Levine, 2006; Roberts, 2003). At many facilities, patients sign paperwork upon admission granting family member access to their protected health information. If you are unsure in your facility, contact your privacy officer or admitting department.

HIPAA concerns to one side, it is a reality that patient privacy is harder to maintain in open units—as many preop areas and PACUs are designed. However, it is important to remember that family members care foremost about their loved one, and if a quiet conversation is occurring between a nurse and patient in the next bed spot, the family will generally not focus on the other patient's conversation, but will, instead, focus on their loved one. There are nursing interventions that can be easily employed in a situation such as this if the family needs redirection. Closing the curtain between the two bed spots is a visual cue that patient privacy is important. Giving the family permission to talk and touch their loved one is also important, as some family members need direction as to what to do at a loved one's bedside (Foss & Tenholder, 1993). Finally, involving the family in simple caregiving can also focus their attention on their loved one. Asking a family member to remind the patient to take deep breaths when the pulse oximeter dips, or to provide the patient with ice chips when the patient is advancing in her or his diet, are simple ways of involving the family in care and redirecting attention to their loved one.

TABLE 18-3. Elements of Family-Centered Care

Recognizing the family as a constant in the patient's life
Facilitating family and professional collaboration at all levels of health care
Honoring the racial, ethnic, cultural, and socio-economic diversity of families
Recognizing family strengths and individuality and respecting different methods of coping
Sharing complete and unbiased information with families on a continuous basis
Encouraging and facilitating family-to-family support and networking
Responding to patient and family developmental needs as part of healthcare practices
Adopting policies and practices that provide families with emotional and financial support
Designing health care that is flexible, culturally competent, and responsive to family needs

Source: Adapted from Shields, 2007.

6. The term "family presence" is being used more frequently. What does it mean?

The term family presence has been commonly associated with ensuring family access to their loved one during medical procedures and resuscitation efforts. However, family presence does not have to mean access only during procedures and codes. Family presence can also be used in lieu of the word "visitation," which is falling out of favor since it does not imply active involvement with the patient and her or his care. Active involvement in care is emphasized by the Joint Commission, and it is a central tenet in family-centered care. See Table 18-3 for more information on family-centered care.

7. What is family-centered care?

Family-centered care (FCC) can be defined as a philosophy of care delivery and way of caring for patients and their family members throughout the healthcare system that ensures that care is planned around the whole family, not just the individual, such that all of the family members—including the patient—are recognized as recipients of care (Shields, 2007; Shields, Pratt, & Hunter, 2006). FCC is widely used in pediatrics, but there has been very little literature on this approach to patient and family care in the perianesthesia literature. FCC is an approach to the planning and delivery of health care that is based on partnerships among patients, families, and healthcare providers (Chorney & Kain, 2010).

But a philosophy of care delivery can only go so far, as the nature and intent of family care can vary based on the nurse's and family's stance. Stance toward the family can be defined as the habits, practices, concerns, and skills that the nurse brings to the situation (Stannard, 1998). Situational concerns, such as the patient–family care environment and the patient's clinical status, make some family-oriented interventions and activities possible, while prohibiting others. The environment in a busy PACU on the evening of a late start day, for instance, will not allow the comparable level of attentiveness and quality of family care that can be provided in that same PACU on a quiet morning.

Another situational condition that has been identified as an important factor in nurses' ability to provide family care is the unit culture. The tempo, mood, climate, and culture of any nursing unit make certain kinds of caring practices possible while discouraging others. These factors, as well as the patient population and unit staff, influence how nurses interact with patients and their families. A "family-friendly" unit culture, for example, is a unit culture with a socially embedded ethic of family care. This kind of unit culture has been shown to greatly influence nurses' openness to sharing and learning from one another in developing and extending their family care practices (Benner, Hooper-Kyriakidis, & Stannard, in press). However, the opposite is also true; less than optimal family care or breakdown between nurses and families has been shown to occur frequently in intensive care units (ICUs) with a "family-restraint" culture (Chesla & Stannard, 1997). Although it is more difficult to implement FCC in a family-restraint culture, it is possible to achieve FCC through ongoing educational efforts, support, and healthcare provider sensitization interventions.

8. Why is it important to have family members accompany the patient in the preoperative area?

Most facilities encourage family members to accompany the patient into the preop area and many encourage the family to stay at the patient's bedside and provide emotional support.

Family member presence can be tremendously valuable and can offer the following benefits to staff:

- Family members can assist the patient with basic care needs (such as changing into a gown and/or toileting)

- Family members can provide additional and vital information to the healthcare providers when preparing the patient for the procedure or surgery
- While waiting, the family can provide helpful distraction to ease patient anxiety
- Family members, if present to hear preoperative patient teaching, can help to reinforce this content (such as pain management) postoperatively
- Family presence enables staff to provide education and emotional support to family members, in addition to the education and support that is already provided to patients

From the patient's perspective, family presence in the preoperative area offers the following benefits:

- Given the anxiety surrounding the perioperative events and the uncertainty of the anesthesia and surgery or procedure itself, spending time with loved ones is of paramount importance to many patients
- Patients can wear their eyeglasses, dentures, hearing aids, and significant jewelry (such as a lucky charm) right up until the time that they go into the operating room (OR), at which point the family can take these items and hold them for the patient. This should only be done in facilities where family presence is encouraged early in the PACU phase however, as patients should have ready access to these functional items that are often necessary for orientation
- Encouraging family presence in the preop area enhances patient satisfaction of the entire perioperative experience

Finally, from the family's perspective, family presence in the preop area can:

- Foster a feeling that the family was supported
- Increase the family's understanding of the perioperative process and the various healthcare team members
- Serve to reduce family fear and anxiety, and
- Enhance family satisfaction of the entire perioperative experience

As with any patient and family intervention, however, it is important to respect the role of the family; to encourage collaboration between the patient, family, and the healthcare team; and to honor individual patient and family differences, desires, and expectations. Asking a family member to assist the patient in changing into a hospital gown, for example, may not be appropriate for the patient or a family member depending on relationship, role, religion, and cultural background. Clinician judgment, understanding and acceptance, and clear lines of communication between the patient, family, and nurse are essential.

9. Why is it important to have family members present during induction?

Parental presence during anesthetic induction has been the most heavily studied aspect of FCC in the perioperative setting. More than 40% of hospitals in the United States report having some policy allowing or encouraging parents to be present, and it is likely that there are other clinicians who use parental presence in facilities that lack a formal policy (Kain et al., 2004). While the practice of parental presence during induction may be controversial, it has become widely accepted and expected by many parents. However, there is conflicting evidence in the literature regarding the effectiveness of this intervention, as premedication has been shown to be more effective in reducing child anxiety in some cases and, in others, parental presence has been found to be more effective (Kain et al., 1996; Kain et al., 2006). In general, parental presence during induction has the benefits of:

- Decreasing separation anxiety
- Decreasing the amount of premedication needed, and
- Increasing parent satisfaction (Chorney & Kain, 2010)

However, the option of family presence during induction has only been available essentially to pediatric patients and their families. Mayne and Bagaoisan (2009) studied the presence of a support person during the induction phase of anesthesia in an adult surgical population and found that adult patients and their support persons did not show a significant inclination toward family presence during induction and believed that the presence of a support person in the OR would cause a disruption to the surgical team. This is a pioneering study, and it is possible that, as the FCC movement gains momentum in the perioperative setting, patient, family, and staff attitudes will shift, and this practice will become an option for adult patients as it is for pediatric patients and their families.

10. Why is it important to have family members in the PACU?

There have been many published studies examining family visitation in the ICU and PACU. Because some patients are considered critically ill during the initial stage of phase I recovery (e.g., those with an unstable airway and any unconscious child 8 years of age and under) (American Society of Perianesthesia Nurses, 2008), it is appropriate to examine the ICU visitation literature, as well as research conducted within PACUs.

A crucial aspect of family care is ensuring that a family can be with their ill loved one, as family presence promotes family cohesion and connection; fosters patient well-being and patient and family satisfaction; and provides the family with information. Yet, historically, many acute and critical care areas have severely restricted family access, thereby limiting nurse–family interactions and, in some cases, nurses' development of family care practices (Benner et al., in press). In fact, studies consistently show that PACU nurses support restrictive visitation policies (DeLeskey, 2009; Jackson, Marcell, & Benedict, 1997; Walls, 2009). It is true that some families do better and worse than others in supporting their ill family members at their bedsides. A family member crying uncontrollably at the bedside, for instance, can upset the patient and disrupt care. This kind of interruption in care can cause staff dissatisfaction with family visitation (Garrouste-Orgeas et al., 2008). Another family member, though, may cope quite well given the circumstances and can provide the ill patient with solace and comfort. Likewise, some patients respond well to a family member's presence, while other patients may prefer to be alone. It is for this reason that perianesthesia nurses should think of family presence as an intervention. While titrating a vasoactive drip, for example, the PACU nurse will typically monitor the patient's physiologic responses. Likewise, it behooves the perianesthesia nurse to monitor the patient and family member responses during visitation, especially in the early phase following admission to any nursing unit.

Since the immediate concern for most PACU nurses is the physiologic stability of the patient, the logical starting place for visitation research is the examination of the impact of family visitation on the patient.

Family presence has the following effects on the patient:

- Does not increase septic complications (Fumagalli et al., 2006)
- Reduces cardiovascular complications (Fuller & Foster, 1982; Fumagalli et al., 2006; Kleman et al., 1993; Lazure & Baun, 1995; Schulte et al., 1993; Simpson & Shaver, 1990)
- Decreases procedural pain and anxiolytic medication use (Byers, Bridges, Kijek, & LaBorde, 2001)

- Decreases intracranial pressure (ICP) (Hepworth, Hendrickson, & Lopez, 1994; Prins, 1989)
- Decreases negative behavior in children, but this is not seen for up to 2 weeks postoperatively (Lardner, Dick, & Crawford, 2010)
- Does not compromise patient privacy (Fiorentini, 1993)
- Increases patient satisfaction (Fiorentini, 1993; Noonan, Anderson, Newlon, Patrin, Ladue-Weber, & Winstead-Fry, 1991; Tuller et al., 1997)

Family presence has the following effects on the family:

- Decreases family member anxiety (Bru, Carmody, Donohue-Sword, & Bookbinder, 1993; Burke et al., 2009)
- Increases family satisfaction (Garrouste-Orgeas et al., 2008; Mitchell, Chaboyer, Burmeister, & Foster, 2009; Noonan et al., 1991; Tuller et al., 1997)

Family presence has the following effects on nursing staff:

- Makes job easier (Fiorentini, 1993)
- Increases nurse satisfaction (Tuller et al., 1997)

It is clear from these studies that patients and families want to be together during times of great stress (e.g., recovery from a procedure or surgery) and that nurses are more circumspect about family visitation. The bedside nurse should always be in the position to judge the dynamics of the situation and make the determination as to whether or not a family presence intervention would be appropriate. It is important, however, to ensure that perianesthesia nurses feel they have the proper family education and resources at their disposal, so that the bedside nurse is making an informed judgment.

11. Family members often want to come into the PACU while the patient is still in the immediate recovery period. How should this be handled?

Waiting to see one's loved one following a procedure or surgery is difficult, especially if the wait is long. Some truisms regarding waiting include:

- Unoccupied time feels longer than occupied time
- Anxiety makes waits feel longer
- Uncertain waits seem longer than certain waits
- Unexplained waits seem longer than explained waits
- Solo waiting feels longer than group waiting (Maister, 1985)

While the perianesthesia nurse is actively and skillfully caring for the patient, the family member is waiting, not knowing, and worrying. Studies have shown that family members want information specific to their loved one, particularly if the case is running later than expected (Dexter & Epstein, 2001). Additionally, family members stated in one study that their top need was to see the patient, whereas the PACU nurses rated the families' top need as information (Cormier, Pickett, & Gallagher, 1992). This finding can be explained, in part, by understanding that by seeing the patient, the family has the most important information of all: Their loved one still looks like their loved one and appears to be doing fine. Finally, unexpected visitation restrictions cause distress, anxiety, and increased complaints (Rogers, 2004).

If the perianesthesia unit has restrictions regarding family access during the initial recovery period, it is encouraged to have the family come in for a quick "look-see" following a procedure or surgery. This powerful intervention can diminish patients' and families' initial anxieties by decreasing the amount of time they are apart and providing families with critical, visual information.

12. What are family care considerations once the patient has recovered from anesthesia, but is still in the PACU?

If the PACU is being utilized as an area for extended care patients or boarders, it is important to follow the standards of care established for those patient populations. If a patient has met discharge criteria from the PACU, but is awaiting an ICU bed, the nurse caring for that patient should follow the critical care standards of care, including visitation guidelines, for a critically ill patient and her or his family. The same is true for a medical–surgical patient who is boarded in the PACU; the patient's family should have the same access and visitation privileges afforded to them on a medical–surgical unit, even if the patient is located in the PACU.

13. Is it important to have written family care guidelines for a unit?

Guidelines are preferred to policies and procedures, as guidelines allow more flexibility when dealing with human beings and complex social situations. It is helpful for patients, families, and staff to have posted unit guidelines that specify unit expectations concerning family care.

14. Should families be allowed to be present for procedures and resuscitation efforts?

Because families, by convention, are frequently separated from their loved ones in a critical situation (such as procedures and resuscitation efforts), few clinicians consider this to be an inhumane practice. Yet, research has repeatedly shown that patients and family members want to be with their dying loved ones and be given the option to be present for invasive procedures and resuscitation efforts (Barratt & Wallis, 1998; Duran, Oman, Abel, Koziel, & Szymanksi, 2007; Eichhorn et al., 2001; Mangurten et al., 2006; Mazer, Cox, & Capon, 2006; Meyers, Eichhorn, & Guzzetta, 1998; Meyers et al., 2000; Powers & Rubenstein, 1999).

Family member death (along with birth) is one of the most significant transitions a family will experience, hence, the prevalence of family members expressing the desire to have the option to be present while their loved one is undergoing resuscitation and invasive procedures. These sentiments are slowly beginning to spill into the popular press, which will only increase consumer pressure to allow for family presence (Harder, 2001). This moment in time is akin to the social pressures in the 1950s when obstetricians routinely kept fathers out of the delivery room and were forced to change due to changing public opinion. The nurse will still need to interview the family to ensure that their concerns and wishes are honored. Not all family members will want to bear witness to the patient's crisis care, and their wishes too must be met with appropriate care and information and without judgment or coercion to be present if this is not their family preference (Benner et al., in press).

If a perianesthesia area elects to implement family presence during procedures and resuscitation efforts, staff buyin at all levels is critical. Additionally, part of a family presence initiative during procedures and codes should include a designated staff person to support the family, answer questions, explain details, and intervene if necessary (Howlett, Alexander, & Tsuchiya, 2010). Finally, debriefing sessions and supportive work should be offered to staff who may experience greater emotional burden by having family members present (Stannard, 2006).

15. Should children be allowed to be present in the preop or PACU areas?

Many perianesthesia areas do not allow children to visit, except in pediatric areas. This is largely due to concerns that sibling or child visitation will increase the risk of infection and the need for supervision. Many studies have shown, however, that infection rates are not increased with sibling or child visitation (Meyer, Kennally, Zika-Beres, Cashore, & Oh, 1996; Solheim & Spellacy, 1988; Umphenour, 1980; Wranesh, 1982). Additionally, sibling or child visitation has been shown to decrease regressive behavior in siblings (Faller & Ratcliffe, 1993) and decrease negative behaviors in the child visitors (Nicholson et al., 1993; Oehler & Vileisis, 1990). Should a perianesthesia area want to implement a child visitation program, it would be important to work with Infection Control and Child Life Specialists in the facility.

16. Should pets be allowed to be present in the preop or PACU areas?

Research has substantiated that animals improve human health, both psychologically and physiologically (DiSalvo et al., 2006). With the advent of service dogs, therapy dogs, and pet visitation animals, many facilities now have extensive policies and procedures in place. Should a perianesthesia area want to implement a pet policy, it would be imperative to work closely with Infection Control, as consideration must be given to potential adverse events such as allergies and the possibility of zoonotic disease transmission.

17. What are other common family interventions?

A crucial nursing intervention is ensuring that a family can be with the critically ill loved one. Another critical nursing intervention is the provision of information and support to patients' families. Information has been identified as a crucial component in family coping and satisfaction. Support, in the form of nurses' caring behaviors and interactions, is enormously influential in shaping the care experience for both patients and families. Taken together, these two nursing interventions are highly valued by families and are even more meaningful when family access is ensured.

Encouraging family involvement in caregiving activities is another essential family nursing intervention, and it can range from minor involvement (e.g., asking a family member to pass an alcohol wipe) to major involvement (e.g., inviting a family member to assist with the patient's oral care). Pediatric and neonatal nurses have long involved families in caregiving activities, as participation prepares family members for their caregiving roles once the child returns home. Although the same may be said for adult areas, the societal expectations and ethics of involving parents in their child's care are much stronger than for family members of adult patients. Yet, familiar grooming and caring rituals by family members can evoke a sense of continuity and comfort for adult patients also. Although numerous obstacles for family participation exist (including hesitancy on the part of nurses, unit policies that prohibit family involvement, inadequate staffing, and lack of time),

studies have shown that families both desire and value involvement in their loved ones' care. Simple acts of helping can facilitate patient–family bonding and togetherness, promote patient healing and comfort, decrease a family member's sense of helplessness and anxiety, and assist family members in grasping their loved one's condition (Stannard, 2006).

REFERENCES

American Society of Perianesthesia Nurses. (2010). Perianesthesia nursing standards and practice recommendations: 2010–2012. Cherry Hill, NJ: Author.

Barratt, F., & Wallis, D. N. (1998). Relatives in the resuscitation room: Their point of view. *Journal of Accident & Emergency Medicine, 15*(2), 109–111.

Benner, P., Hooper-Kyriakidis, P., & Stannard, D. (in press). *Clinical wisdom and interventions in acute and critical care: A thinking-in-action approach* (2nd ed.). New York: Springer.

Bru, G., Carmody, S., Donohue-Sword, B., & Bookbinder, M. (1993). Parental visitation in the post-anesthesia care unit: A means to lessen anxiety. *Child Health Care, 22*(3), 217–226.

Burke, C. N., Voepel-Lewis, T., Hadden, S., DeGrandis, M., Skotcher, S., D'Agostino, R., et al. (2009). Parental presence on emergence: Effect on postanesthesia agitation and parent satisfaction. *Journal of Perianesthesia Nursing, 24*(4), 216–221.

Byers, J. F., Bridges, S., Kijek, J., & LaBorde, P. (2001). Burn patients' pain and anxiety experiences. *Journal of Burn Care & Rehabilitation, 22*, 144–149.

Chesla, C. A., & Stannard, D. (1997). Breakdown in the nursing care of families in the ICU. *American Journal of Critical Care, 6*(1), 64–71.

Chorney, J. M., & Kain, Z. N. (2010). Family-centered pediatric perioperative care. *Anesthesiology, 112*, 751–755.

Cormier, S., Pickett, S. J., & Gallagher, J. (1992). Comparison of nurses' and family members' perceived needs during postanesthesia care unit visits. *Journal of Postanesthesia Nursing, 7*(6), 387–391.

DeLeskey, K. (2009). Family visitation in the PACU: The current state of practice in the United States. *Journal of Perianesthesia Nursing, 24*(2), 81–85.

Dexter, F., & Epstein, R. H. (2001). Reducing family members' anxiety while waiting on the day of surgery: Systematic review of studies and implications of HIPAA health information privacy rules. *Journal of Clinical Anesthesia, 13*(7), 478–481.

DiSalvo, H., Haiduven, D., Johnson, N., Reyes, V. V., Hench, C. P., Shaw, R., et al. (2006). Who let the dogs out? Infection control did: Utility of dogs in health care settings and infection control aspects. *American Journal of Infection Control, 34*(5), 301–307.

Duran, C. R., Oman, K. S., Abel, J. J., Koziel, V. M., & Szymanski, D. (2007). Attitudes toward and beliefs about family presence: A survey of healthcare providers, patients' families, and patients. *American Journal of Critical Care, 16*(3), 270–282.

Eichhorn, D. J., Meyers, T. A., Guzzetta, C. E., Clark, A. P., Klein, J. D., Taliferro, E., et al. (2001). Family presence during invasive procedures and resuscitation: Hearing the voice of the patient. *American Journal of Nursing, 101*(5), 48–55.

Faller, H. S., & Ratcliffe, L. (1993). Sibling visitation: How far should the pendulum swing? *Journal of Pediatric Nursing, 8*(2), 92–99.

Fiorentini, S. E. (1993). Evaluation of a new program: Pediatric parental visitation in the postanesthesia care unit. *Journal of Postanesthesia Nursing, 8*(4), 249–256.

Foss, K. R., & Tenholder, M. F. (1993). Expectations and needs of persons with family members in an intensive care unit as opposed to a general ward. *Southern Medical Journal, 86*(4), 380–384.

Fuller, B. F., & Foster, G. M. (1982). The effects of family/ friend visits vs. staff interaction on stress/arousal of surgical intensive care patients. *Heart & Lung, 11*(5), 457–463.

Fumagalli, S., Boniceinelli, L., Lo Nostro A., Valdoti, P., Baldereschi, G., Di Bari, M., et al. (2006). Reduced cardiocirculatory complications with unrestrictive visiting policy in an intensive care unit: Results from a pilot, randomized trial. *Circulation, 113*(7), 946–952.

Garrouste-Orgeas, M., Philippart, F., Timsit, J. F., Diaw, F., Willems, V., Tabah, A., et al. (2008). Perceptions of a 24-hour visiting policy in the intensive care unit. *Critical Care Medicine, 36*(1), 30–35.

Harder, B. (2001). Opening the curtain. *U. S. News & World Reports, 131*(9), 64.

Hepworth, J. T., Hendrickson, S. G., & Lopez, J. (1994). Time series analysis of physiological response during ICU visitation. *Western Journal of Nursing Research, 16*(6), 704–717.

Hickey, M. (1990). What are the needs of families of critically ill patients? A review of the literature since 1976. *Heart & Lung, 17*(6), 670–676.

Howlett, M. S., Alexander, G. A., & Tsuchiya, B. (2010). Health care providers' attitudes regarding family presence during resuscitation of adults: An integrated review of the literature. *Clinical Nurse Specialist, 24*(3), 161–174.

Jackson, L. B., Marcell, J., & Benedict, S. (1997). Nurses' attitudes toward parental visitation on the postanesthesia care unit. *Journal of Perianesthesia Nursing, 12*(1), 2–6.

Kain, Z. N., Caldwell-Andrews, A. A., Krivutza, D. M., Weinberg, M. E., Wang, S. M., & Gaal, D. (2004). Trends in the practice of parental presence during induction of anesthesia and the use of preoperative sedative premedication in the United States, 1995–2002: Results of a follow-up national survey. *Anesthesia & Analgesia, 98*(5), 58–64.

Kain, Z. N., Mayes, L. C., Caldwell-Andrews, A. A., Saadat, H., McClain, B., & Wang, S. M. (2006). Predicting which children benefit most from parental presence during induction of anesthesia. *Pediatric Anaesthesia, 16*(6), 627–634.

Kain, Z. N., Mayes, L. C., Caramico, L. A., Silver, D., Spieker, M., Nygren, M. M., et al. (1996). Parental presence during induction of anesthesia: A randomized controlled trial. *Anesthesiology, 84*(5), 1060–1070.

Kleman, M., Bickert, A., Karpinski, A., Wantz, D., Jacobsen, B., Lowery, B., et al. (1993). Physiologic responses of coronary care patients to visiting. *Journal of Cardiovascular Nursing, 7*(3), 52–62.

Lardner, D. R., Dick, B. D., & Crawford, S. (2010). The effects of parental presence in the postanesthetic care unit on children's postoperative behavior: A prospective, randomized, controlled study. *Anesthesia & Analgesia, 110*(4), 1102–1108.

Lazure, L. L. A., & Baun, M. M. (1995). Increasing patient control of family visiting in the coronary care unit. *American Journal of Critical Care, 4*(2), 157–164.

Leske, J. S. (1991). Overview of family needs after critical illness: From assessment to intervention. *AACN Clinical Issues, 2*(2), 220–226.

Levine, C. (2006). HIPAA and talking with family caregivers: What does the law really say? *American Journal of Nursing, 106*(8), 51–53.

Maister, D. (1985). The psychology of waiting lines (pp. 113–123). In J. Czepiel, M. Solomon, & C. Supernant (Eds.), *The service encounter.* Lexington, MA: Lexington Books.

Mangurten, J., Scott, S. H., Guzzetta, C. E., Clark, A. P., Vinson, L., Sperry, J., et al. (2006). Effects of family presence during resuscitation and invasive procedures in a pediatric emergency department. *Journal of Emergency Nursing, 32*(3), 225–233.

Mayne, I. P., & Bagaoisan, C. (2009). Social support during anesthesia induction in an adult surgical population. *AORN Journal, 89*(2), 307–320.

Mazer, M. A., Cox, L. A., & Capon, J. A. (2006). The public's attitude and perception concerning witnessed cardiopulmonary resuscitation. *Critical Care Medicine, 34*(12), 2925–2928.

Meyer, E. C., Kennally, K. F., Zika-Beres, E., Cashore, W. J., & Oh, W. (1996). Attitudes about sibling visitation in the neonatal intensive care unit. *Archives of Pediatric & Adolescent Medicine, 150*(10), 1021–1026.

Meyers, T. A., Eichhorn, D. J., & Guzzetta, C. E. (1998). Do families want to be present during CPR? A retrospective study. *Journal of Emergency Nursing, 24*(5), 400–405.

Meyers, T. A., Eichhorn, D. J., Guzzetta, C. E., Clark, A. P., Klein, J. D., Taliaferro, E., et al. (2000). Family presence during invasive procedures and resuscitation: The experience of family members, nurses, and physicians. *American Journal of Nursing, 100*(2), 32–43.

Mitchell, M., Chaboyer, W., Burmeister, E., & Foster, M. (2009). Positive effects of a nursing intervention on family-centered care in adult critical care. *American Journal of Critical Care, 18*(6), 543–553.

Nicholson, A. C., Titler, M., Montgomery, L. A., Kleiber, C., Craft, M. J., Halm, M., et al. (1993). Effects of child visitation in adult critical care units: A pilot study. *Heart & Lung, 22*(1), 36–45.

Noonan, A. T., Anderson, P., Newlon, P., Patrin, T., Ladue-Weber, K., & Winstead-Fry, P. (1991). Family-centered nursing in the postanesthesia care unit: The evaluation of practice. *Journal of Postanesthesia Nursing, 6*(1), 13–16.

Obama, B. (2010). *Presidential memorandum - Hospital visitation.* Retrieved from http://www.whitehouse.gov/the-press-office/presidential-memorandum-hospital-visitation

Oehler, J. M., & Vileisis, R. A. (1990). Effect of early sibling visitation in an intensive care nursery. *Journal of Developmental & Behavioral Pediatrics, 11*(1), 7–12.

Powers, K. S., & Rubenstein, J. S. (1999). Family presence during invasive procedures in the pediatric intensive care unit: A prospective study. *Archives of Pediatric Adolescent Medicine, 153*(9), 955–958.

Prins, M. M. (1989). The effect of family visits on intracranial pressure. *Western Journal of Nursing Research, 11*(3), 281–297.

Roberts, D. W. (2003). Privacy and confidentiality: The health insurance portability and accountability act in critical care nursing. *AACN Clinical Issues, 14*(3), 302–309.

Rogers, S. (2004). Why can't I visit? The ethics of visitation restrictions: Lessons learned from SARS. *Critical Care, 8*(5), 300–302.

Schulte, D. A., Burrell, L. O., Gueldner, S. H., Bramlett, M. H., Fuszard, B., Stone, S. K., et al. (1993). Pilot study of the relationship between heart rate and ectopy and unrestricted vs. restricted visiting hours in the coronary care unit. *American Journal of Critical Care, 2*(2), 134–136.

Shields, L. (2007). Family-centered care in the perioperative area: An international perspective. *AORN Journal, 85*(5), 893–902.

Shields, L., Pratt, J., & Hunter, J. (2006). Family-centered care: A review of qualitative studies. *Journal of Clinical Nursing, 15*(10), 1317–1323.

Simpson, T., & Shaver, J. (1990). Cardiovascular responses to family visits in coronary care patients. *Heart & Lung, 19*(4), 344–351.

Solheim, K., & Spellacy, C. (1988). Sibling visitation: Effects on newborn infection rates. *Journal of Obstetric, Gynecologic, & Neonatal Nursing, 17*(1), 43–48.

Stannard, D., (1998). Reclaiming the house: An interpretive study of nurse–family interactions and activities in critical care. *Dissertation Abstracts International, 58*(8), 1–364.

Stannard, D. (2006). Family care (pp. 767–772). In H. M. Schell & K. A. Puntillo (Eds.). *Critical care nursing secrets* (2nd ed.). St. Louis, MO: Mosby Elsevier.

Tuller, S., McCabe, L., Cronenwett, L., Hastings, D., Shaheen, A., Daley-Faulkner, C., et al. (1997). Patient, visitor, and nurse evaluations of visitation for adult postanesthesia care unit patients. *Journal of Perianesthesia Nursing, 12*(6), 402–412.

Umphenour, J. H. (1980). Bacterial colonization in neonates with sibling visitation. *Journal of Obstetric, Gynecologic, & Neonatal Nursing, 9*(2), 73–75.

Walls, M. (2009). Staff attitudes and beliefs regarding family visitation after implementation of a formal visitation policy in the PACU. *Journal of Perianesthesia Nursing, 24*(4), 229–232.

Wranesh, B. L. (1982). The effect of sibling visitation on bacterial colonization rate in neonates. *Journal of Obstetric, Gynecologic, & Neonatal Nursing, 11*(4), 211–213.

CHAPTER 19

Pediatric Patients

Maureen Schnur, MS, RN, CPAN
& Myrna E. Mamaril, MS, RN, CPAN, CAPA, FAAN

It is estimated that over 4 million children in the United States undergo surgery each year (Kain & Caldwell-Andrews, 2005). The experience of surgery is a significant event for both child and family. The nurse providing perianesthesia care to children requires an understanding of age-related physiologic differences, developmental considerations, and an ability to effectively partner with the child's family to achieve best outcomes for the patient. By understanding, recognizing, and eliciting information about the needs of the child and family, the nurse is able to utilize available resources to respond effectively to them. It is important that the child be cared for in the context of her or his unique family with respect to a wide variety of characteristics such as family composition, cultural differences, cognitive abilities, temperament, and parenting and learning styles.

This chapter will discuss essential components of the dynamic pediatric specialty care that spans the preanesthesia through the postanesthesia continuum. It will present basic information about the pediatric patient with the intent to expand the nurse's knowledge base, foster higher levels of comfort during care delivery, provide helpful secrets and tips, and ultimately afford the nurse to have a quick specialized perianesthesia reference available for this unique patient population.

1. What is the definition of a pediatric patient?

Pediatric patients are classified according to age (Hesselgrave, 2009):

- Infancy: neonatal period through 12 months of age
  - Neonate: first 28 days of life
  - Infancy: 1–12 months of age
- Toddler: 1–3 years of age
- Preschooler: 3–6 years of age
- School age: 6–12 years of age
- Adolescence: 13–18 years of age

2. What are important anatomic and physiologic differences to keep in mind when caring for pediatric patients?

- Neonate
  - Head accounts for 25% of the body's length and 33% of weight
  - Ribs are composed mainly of cartilage and project at right angles from vertebral column (more circular)
  - Obligate nose breathers
  - Limited glycogen stores
  - Immature respiratory center in the brain
  - Predisposed to hypothermia due to small muscle mass and inability to shiver

- Fully developed parasympathetic nervous system and underdeveloped sympathetic nervous system
- Large body surface area
- Infant: Growth and development progresses at a rapid rate during the first 12 months of age
  - Body weight doubles at 5 months and triples at 12 months
  - Obligate nose breathers
  - Vocal cords more cartilaginous
  - Limited glycogen stores
  - Immature respiratory center in the brain
  - Predisposed to hypothermia due to small muscle mass and inability to shiver
  - Fully developed parasympathetic nervous system and underdeveloped sympathetic nervous system
  - Chest wall is thin, rib cage is soft and pliable, breathing is predominantly done from diaphragmatic movement
  - Large body surface area
  - Higher circulating blood volume (75 ml/kg)
  - Underdeveloped cervical ligaments with relatively weak neck muscles (very susceptible to hyperextension of neck)
- Toddler
  - Trachea is short in length, contributing to the potential for intubating the right mainstem bronchus
  - Rib cage is very pliable and the chest wall is thin, allowing breath sounds to be transmitted throughout the thorax
  - Underdeveloped bronchial tree and alveolar/capillary gas exchange units
  - Prone to temperature extremes
  - Larger body surface area and increased heat loss through administration of anesthetic gases
- Preschooler
  - Oxygen consumption requirements are about twice that of adolescents or adults (6–8 ml/kg vs 3–4 ml/kg)
  - Cannot sustain rapid respiratory rates for long periods of time due to immature intercostal muscles
  - Smaller functional residual capacity with smaller oxygen reserves, consequently prone to hypoxia

- Liver and spleen in lower abdomen are less protected by rib cage and more prone to injury
- Spinal cord more vulnerable even though vertebral column may withstand traction and tension types of trauma without evidence of deformity
- School age
  - Bones begin to lose flexibility at approximately 6 years of age when bone cortex begins to thicken and become hardened
  - Tracheal shape changes from funnel to cylindrical
  - Lung volume increases to 200 ml by 8 years of age
  - Bronchial tree has attained 16 divisions as in an adult
  - By 10 years of age, size and flexibility of airway matches that of adults
- Adolescents
  - Faster growth rate than any other period except infancy
  - Bone growth ends at age 29, when epiphyses close
  - By age 15, cardiac output is equal to that of an adult
  - By age 15 years, the body's response to shock is similar to that of an adult
  - Sebaceous glands increase production
  - Breast tissue in females develops between 9 and 13 years of age

PREANESTHESIA SCOPE OF CARE

The preanesthesia phase begins when the surgeon informs the parents that their child needs surgery. The goals of the preoperative (preop) assessment are to:

- Evaluate and manage potential or actual health risks
- Provide preop teaching and review the surgical and anesthesia preop instructions, including medications and fasting (NPO) status
- Address parents' concerns and questions
- Determine the need for home care following the surgery or procedure

This phase may be conducted in the preadmission evaluation center or may be in the form of a preop telephone interview. During a phone interview, the nurse asks questions to complete the medical history and to discover any remaining issues needing resolution prior to anesthesia. The nurse determines with the parent whether the patient has individualized needs that warrant special consideration (e.g., needle phobia or sensitivity to noise). In a face-to-face session, the nurse has the opportunity to introduce educational items, such as age appropriate books, anatomic models, and audiovisual and/or written materials that familiarize parents and the child with the perioperative environment. Foremost in preparation for the child's surgery is to communicate significant health information to all healthcare providers so that a perianesthesia plan of care is developed and followed through from the preanesthesia phase of surgery to discharge. This multidisciplinary approach helps guide uniform delivery of care, reduces parent and child anxiety, and optimizes the patient's condition prior to the surgery or procedure.

3. What guidelines are helpful when scheduling patients?

Certain pediatric populations will ideally be prioritized as first or early cases of the day. Scheduling infants and younger children for earlier start times helps to minimize dehydration, the potential for hypoglycemia, and irritability. First case start times for diabetic patients are ideal since insulin schedules are adjusted to account for surgery and to minimize fasting times. For children who have difficulty understanding the concept of waiting, such as those on the autism spectrum, an early and punctual start is recommended. Patients with a potential for malignant hyperthermia (MH) are often scheduled as a first case to optimize a clean technique and thereby avoiding exposure to potential triggers. For scheduling children from families who speak limited English and require an interpreter, choosing time slots when interpreter services are available is recommended. Isolation cases are preferably scheduled as the last case of the day due to room exposure and the terminal cleaning that is required by infection control. Additional considerations include length of stay, inpatient vs outpatient status, and comorbidities.

If surgeries are delayed, it is important to maintain open lines of communication with frequent updates to families. Determine with the anesthesiologist if younger children whose surgery will be significantly delayed might be able to have a drink of clear liquids, and consider providing families with food or parking vouchers to acknowledge the inconvenience caused. Other factors that play an important role in scheduling are how to most efficiently accommodate unplanned urgent cases

and traumas and to determine how scheduling practices can be implemented in a way that promote efficiency, work within facility limitations such as the availability of floor or intensive care unit (ICU) beds, and ensure safe staffing.

4. What are the American Society of Anesthesiologists (ASA) guidelines for fasting?

- 2 hours for clear liquids
- 4 hours for breast milk
- 6 hours for infant formula
- 6 hours for nonhuman milk
- 6 hours for light meal (Aker, 2010)
- Fasting tips:
  - It is important to ask patients who are at an age to verbalize when they last had anything to eat or drink. Many parents are not aware that their child may have had a drink or a snack without asking them. It is also prudent to ask teenagers if they have had any chewing gum and make sure they do not chew gum while they are waiting for surgery.
  - For children who are obese or overweight, fasting times are the same as for children who are not obese. There is no evidence demonstrating a higher risk of aspiration for obese children undergoing general anesthesia (Brusseau, 2010).
  - It is important in children younger than 2 years of age that their blood glucose is monitored, especially if surgery is delayed and they have had nothing by mouth for an extended period of time.

5. What are the key legal considerations to know when caring for pediatric patients?

The healthcare provider caring for the patient preoperatively must ensure that the parent or accompanying caregiver is the legal guardian and that the documentation in the record includes signatures from the legal guardian for consents for surgery or procedure(s) and anesthesia, as well as responsibility for the patient upon discharge to home. Children may become emancipated through marriage, pregnancy, high school graduation, military service, or living independently, and may be recognized as adults and can consent for surgery and invasive procedures according to state legal statutes. If the parent or legal guardian is not with the child, it is permissible in certain situations to obtain consent by telephone when two healthcare providers, such as the surgeon and nurse, are listening simultaneously and informing the parent or legal guardian about the procedure(s), risks and benefits, and the parent or legal guardian gives verbal consent.

6. What are the most common medication errors in pediatrics?

Data collected from 1998 to 2005 from nearly 400 facilities participating in medication error reporting demonstrated that 1.8% of all medication errors reported were in pediatrics. Nearly 20% of these resulted in harm to the patient as compared to 8.7% in the adult patients. In total, half of reported medication errors were during administration. More than half of the pediatric errors noted a contributing factor, including inexperienced staff and distractions. Actions to take may include individual follow-up, staff education, environmental modification, policy or procedure change, and modification of computer software (Hicks, Becker, & Cousins, 2006).

- Medication tips:
  - Make the medication area a "no distraction" zone
  - Strictly follow facility program for an independent double check
  - Keep general weight-based emergency medication lists on the code cart and/or individualized emergency medication charts at each patient's bedside

7. How are intravenous fluid maintenance rates for children calculated?

Maintenance rates are calculated in milliliters per kilogram per hour (ml/kg/hr). For the first 10 kg of body weight, 4 ml/kg/hr is given, and typically is a crystalloid solution (such as lactated ringers). For the next 10 kg of body weight, an additional 2 ml/kg/hr of fluid is given. For children over 20 kg, an additional 1 ml/kg/hr is added to determine the total maintenance rate per hour. In total, this calculation determines the hourly maintenance rate. First published in 1957, this formula is commonly known as the "4-2-1" formula and it is widely used to calculate fluid maintenance rates in pediatrics (Holliday & Segar, 1957). See Table 19-1 for examples of IV fluid maintenance calculations.

8. Why is an accurate weight important in the pediatric patient?

Medications are given to children based on weight. The administration of ordered medication

TABLE 19-1. Examples of IV Fluid Maintenance Calculations

Weight	Calculation	Maintenance IV rate/hour
8 kg	8 kg × 4 ml/hr	32 ml/hr
16 kg	(10 kg × 4 ml/hr) + (6 kg × 2 ml/hr) = 40 + 12 = 52 ml/hr	52 ml/hr
43 kg	(10 kg × 4 ml/hr) + (10 kg × 2 ml/hr) + (23 kg × 1 ml/hr) = 40 + 20 + 23 = 83 ml/hr	83 ml/hr

is a high volume, high risk nursing intervention. Medications are typically calculated in milligrams per kilogram. An inaccurate rate may lead to errors in medication administration discovered after incorrect doses have been given. It is important to remember that parents will likely report weights to the care provider in pounds, therefore, extra care needs to be taken in determining and documenting weights in kilograms using accurate scales. The astute pediatric nurse develops an ability to suspect weight discrepancies upon viewing a child and takes steps necessary to ensure appropriate follow through to correct the weight and determine with the healthcare team if there are any needed interventions.

- Weight tips:
  - To help younger children cooperate with being weighed, include the parent in the weighing process. First, weigh the parent. Then, weigh the parent holding the child. Subtract the weight of the parent to determine the weight of the child
  - If a wheelchair-bound child needs to be weighed, weigh the child while seated in the wheelchair. After the child is transferred to the stretcher, weigh the wheelchair alone and subtract it from the total to obtain the weight. It may be helpful for the parent or caregiver to place a sticker on the wheelchair with the weight of the wheelchair clearly documented in kilogram and/ or pounds.

9. Why is it important to minimize anxiety in children during the preanesthesia period?

A considerable proportion of children experience significant anxiety during the preoperative period, estimated at up to 75%, with induction of anesthesia being the most stressful time. For these children, it is important to understand that they are at risk for exhibiting behavioral signs of stress at home for up to 2 weeks following surgery. These new onset behaviors may occur in up to 55% of children and include changes in appetite, nightmares, separation anxiety, enuresis, and fear of healthcare providers. These children may be at a higher risk for increased anticipatory anxiety in the future, which may result in an increased perception of pain. These behaviors may continue in up to 19% of children for up to 6 months postoperatively (Kain & Caldwell-Andrews, 2005).

10. What are ways to minimize a child's anxiety and fear and engage a child's cooperation with necessary tasks and procedures?

It is essential to include and engage the child's primary adult support system throughout the perianesthesia period as much as possible. Ways that may help decrease anxiety and fear for the child include being patient and letting the child indicate that they are ready for what you are asking them to do. Additionally, maintaining a calm voice and relaxed demeanor, and asking the child or caregiver what they think will work best are other helpful strategies. When speaking to the child, the nurse should be positioned at the child's eye level to foster a nonthreatening atmosphere. Engage the caregiver, child life specialist, patient care assistant, or other assistant available to help the child cope. Encourage the parent to hold the child's hand or hold him or her in a position of comfort—for example, on the parent's lap. Utilize behavioral distraction techniques such as "I Spy" books, counting, and bubble blowing. Encourage the child with supportive phrases such as "great job" and "we're almost done." Allow the child to hold a transitional comfort object—for instance, a blanket or stuffed animal—to help them feel more secure.

- Anxiety reduction tips:
  - Including well-prepared parents who are calm for induction may benefit the child. Parents need to be informed that their child may be upset or go limp as anesthesia takes effect. They need to be prepared in advance that they will be escorted out of the operating room (OR) right after the child is asleep (Astuto et al., 2006; Eaton, Everson, Jirava, & Zwingman-Bagley, 2006).
  - Encourage the child to put an identification (ID) bracelet on an extremity of their doll or stuffed animal. Then let the child put the ID bracelet on their own extremity of choice.
  - Talk in simple words, such as the blood pressure (BP) is a "tight squeeze" on your arm.
  - If the child expresses anxiety with an automated BP and/or there is difficulty securing a reading in a timely manner, consider performing a manual BP.

Use of an anxiolytic, such as oral midazolam preoperatively, may work well to reduce behavioral responses to preop anxiety for the child and prevent stressful memories. Keep in mind that the drug relaxes the patient significantly. Key points to teach the parent(s) include that the child cannot stand or sit on their own and may become limp very quickly. Fall precautions must be taken.

11. What general equipment should be available in the routine perioperative care for pediatric patients?

- Scales for obtaining weights
  - Scales to accommodate the varying age groups: infants, small children, older children, adolescents, and young adults
  - Chair scales
  - Scales to accommodate wheelchairs
  - Patient lift scales
  - Bariatric floor scale if indicated
- Thermometers per facility protocol
  - Axillary, tympanic, oral, and temporal artery
- Various size stethoscopes (infant to adult size)
- Assorted sizes of BP cuffs (from premature to large adult as indicated)
- Pediatric electrocardiogram (ECG) leads that are easy to place on and remove
- Pulse oximeter probes
- Emergency medications that are readily available (see Table 19-2)
- Pediatric code cart that is readily available (see Table 19-3)
- MH cart that is readily available in perioperative area
  - Dantrolene dosing chart per facility guidelines (see Table 19-4)
  - Dosing chart for other medications per facility guidelines (see Table 19-5)

TABLE 19-2. Pediatric Emergency Medications

- Adenosine
- Albuterol
- Amiodarone
- Anticholinergics
  - Atropine
  - Glycopyrrolate
- Atenolol
- Calcium Chloride
- Calcium Gluconate
- Corticosteroids
  - Dexamethasone
  - Hydrocortisone
  - Methylprednisone
- Dexamethasone
- Dextrose (25%, 50%)
- Diphenhydramine
- Dobutamine
- Dopamine
- Ephedrine
- Epinephrine (1:1000, 1:10,000)
- Epinephrine (Racemic)
- Esmolol
- Etomidate
- Furosemide
- Hydralazine
- Insulin, regular
- Ketamine
- Labetolol
- Lidocaine
- Magnesium Sulfate
- Mannitol
- Methylprednisolone
- Methohexital
- Metoprolol
- Midazolam
- Sodium Bicarbonate
- Naloxone
- Neostigmine
- Nitroprusside
- Norepinephrine
- Paralytics
  - Succinylcholine
  - Vecuronium
  - Rocuronium
- Phenylephrine
- Phenytoin
- Procainamide
- Proprofol

TABLE 19-3. Pediatric Code Cart

- Backboard
- Gloves, masks/face shields, precaution gowns
- Equipment for intubation
  - Laryngoscope handles and blades
  - Magill forceps
  - Stylettes
  - Equipment to secure endotracheal tube (ETT)
    - Latex free cloth tape
    - Commercial ETT holder
    - Other method to secure ETT per facility protocol
  - Benzoin
- Multiple sizes of airway support devices:
  - Endotracheal tubes (ETT)
  - Laryngeal mask airways (LMA)
  - Oral airways
  - Nasal airways
  - Face masks
  - Bag valve masks
- Non-rebreather oxygen masks
- Nebulizer (to be hand-held, used with ETT)
- Suction catheters (#6, 8, 10, 12 and 14 French)
- Yankauer suction catheters
- Syringes, needles, blood collection tubes
- Drains - Multiple sizes of nasogastric tubes, feeding tubes and urinary catheters
- Catheter tip syringes
- Equipment for venous access
  - Peripheral: Catheters, butterfly needles, dressing supplies
  - Central
- Intraosseous equipment
- IV solutions as per facility protocol
- Calculators to determine weight based dosages
- Flashlights and batteries
- Consider capability for end tidal carbon dioxide (ETCO2) monitoring

Defibrillator
- Adult and pediatric paddles
- Conductive gel
- EKG paper for recording
- Optional: towel, razor

Malignant Hyperthermia Cart
- Located in perioperative area
- Stocked with 36 vials of Dantrolene (Hommertzheim & Steinke, 2006)

TABLE 19-4. Dantrolene Chart Based on Weight[a]

Weight in Kilograms (kg)	Initial dose (2.5 mg/kg continuous rapid IV push)	No. vials of dantrolene to have on hand for 4 doses	Sterile water necessary for 4 doses	Total ml administered per dose
10	25 mg	5	300 ml	75 ml
20	50 mg	10	600 ml	150 ml
30	75 mg	15	900 ml	225 ml
40	100 mg	20	1,200 ml	300 ml
50	125 mg	25	1,500 ml	375 ml
60	150 mg	30	1,800 ml	450 ml
70	175 mg	35	2,100 ml	525 ml

[a]Dantrolene 20 mg vials mixed are mixed with 60 ml preservative-free sterile water. Each 20 mg vial contains 3 g of mannitol. Frequency of dosing is every 5 minutes, and may take up to 4 doses of a total of 10 mg/kg and occasionally up to as much as 30 mg/kg.
Adapted by Schnur, M. & Simon, R. J., Children's Hospital Boston, 2010

- Appropriate size pediatric gowns
- Assorted diaper sizes and scales for weighing urine output
- Gowns, gloves, and masks for children on isolation precautions
  - Droplet isolation masks along with standard precaution equipment

  - Consider disposable thermometers and/or designated stethoscopes for children on precautions
- Items for distraction such as televisions, toys, books, and games
- Rocking chairs and footstools for caregivers to hold children

TABLE 19-5. Chart for Insulin/Glucose Drips and Sodium Bicarbonate Based on Weight

Weight in kilograms (kg)	Insulin (0.1 unit insulin/kg to mix with 50% glucose as drip)	Glucose 50% (1 mL/kg to mix with insulin as drip)	Sodium bicarbonate (1–2 milliEquivalents (mEq)/kg)
10	1 unit	10 ml	10–20 mEq
20	2 units	20 ml	20–40 mEq
30	3 units	30 ml	30–60 mEq
40	4 units	40 ml	40–80 mEq
50	5 units	50 ml	50–100 mEq
60	6 units	60 ml	60–120 mEq
70	7 units	70 ml	70–140 mEq

[a]Insulin/glucose drips: for hyperkalemia, titrated per physician order to potassium level
[b]Sodium bicarbonate: for metabolic acidosis. In absence of blood gas, administer 1–2 mEq/kg.
Calcium chloride 10 mg/kg or calcium gluconate 10–50 mg/kg for life-threatening hyperkalemia.
Adapted by Schnur, M. & Simon, R. J., Children's Hospital Boston, 2010

- Safe seating for family member(s)
- Access to breast pump and related supplies for nursing mothers
- Availability of changing tables

POSTANESTHESIA SCOPE OF CARE

Postanesthesia nursing care may encompass diverse pediatric clinical settings. The scope of care includes recovering children who have undergone sedation, analgesia, or anesthesia for surgery or invasive procedures. The postanesthesia care unit (PACU) nurse may be practicing in the traditional PACU or may be recovering children in remote areas, such as other specialty settings like radiation oncology, electroconvulsive therapy (ECT), or magnetic resonance imaging (MRI). The PACU nurse must be competent in postanesthesia nursing skills as well as in the pediatric nursing specialty. The ultimate goal during both PACU phase I and phase II is that the child's perioperative experience is not only safe, but also has positive outcomes for the patient and the family.

12. What additional equipment other than general equipment for the perioperative area should be available for routine PACU care for pediatric postoperative patients?

- Approved protective devices to protect surgical sites, tubes, and intravenous (IV) lines
- Multiple sizes of IV catheters, arm boards, and facility-approved protective devices
- Arm restraints for self-protection
- Measuring tapes to determine sizes (e.g., height, reddened areas, abdominal girth)
- Assorted cribs for infants and toddlers
- Side rail pads
- Baby bottles, glucose water, assorted formulas, and pacifiers
- Pillows for comfort and positioning

13. What are important airway implications when caring for pediatric patients?

The past medical history of the child, including reports of snoring, episodes of croup, asthma, and current or recent upper or lower respiratory infection may point to airway implications that should be considered when planning the perioperative trajectory. Children diagnosed with reactive airway disease, asthma, history of respiratory syncytial virus (RSV), bronchiolitis, bronchopulmonary

dysplasia (BPD), tracheomalacia, or congenital malformations of the jaw or mouth are all considered to be at risk for oxygen decompensation and complications during the postoperative period. A birth history of prematurity may place the young child at a higher airway risk for anesthesia. Premature infants may have BPD associated with hyperexpansion, atelectasis, and interstitial thickening. Although computerized tomography (CT) scans reveal abnormalities in more than 90% of children and adolescents with BPD, symptoms tend to resolve over the first few years of life (D'Angio & Maniscalco, 2004). In cases of obstructive sleep apnea (OSA), the best postoperative positions to foster ventilatory compensation may be side-lying or prone, depending on the severity of the OSA.

Assessment and management of the airway is the foremost priority of care in the pediatric patient. With all pediatric patients, the PACU nurse must be vigilant in assessing the rate, depth, and quality of respirations. The average respiratory rate decrease as the child ages. This rate decreases from 45 to 60 breaths per minute in a newborn to 20 breaths per minute by adolescence. The respiratory pattern of the infant may be irregular due to an immature respiratory center. Infants are at increased risk for apnea up to 6 months of age. In infants born prematurely, apnea can be problematic until they reach 60 weeks postmenstrual age. For example, if a patient was born prematurely at 28 weeks, he or she would be at risk for apnea until 32 weeks post-birth. In all cases, the nurse ensures optimal positioning to ensure adequate oxygenation and ventilation.

- Airway tips
  - Children with an active or resolving upper respiratory infection will have increased airway reactivity and are predisposed to atelectasis, mucous plugging, and postoperative arterial hypoxemia.
  - In children who have had a viral lower respiratory tract infection, bronchial reactivity may continue for 6 to 8 weeks. Patients who present with a respiratory tract infection and who are scheduled for elective surgery may need to have their case rescheduled after considering the urgency of the surgery and a careful evaluation of the symptoms (Aker, 2010).

14. What are critical elements of nursing care during the immediate postoperative period?

After airway, the other critical elements of immediate postoperative care include ongoing observation

TABLE 19-6. Pediatric Vital Signs

	Respiratory rate	**Heart rate resting**	**Heart rate awake**	**Blood pressure**
Newborn	45–60	80–160	100–180	65/40
1 year	40	70–120	80–160	95/65
3 years	30	60–90	80–120	100/70
6 years	25	60–90	70–115	90/60
12 years	20	50–90	65–90	110/60

Adapted from Landriscina, 2009.

and frequent vital sign assessment, including temperature, heart rate (HR) and rhythm, respiratory rate (RR) and depth, BP, oxygen saturation (SPO$_2$) and pain assessment (see Table 19-6 for age-appropriate vital signs).

The nurse is vigilant for respiratory depression and/or respiratory distress and intervenes as needed to optimize oxygenation or ventilation, by repositioning the patient, providing reminders and/or stimulation to take deep breaths, and placing the patient on supplemental oxygen. Additionally, the nurse promotes restoration of normothermia and fluid and electrolyte balance.

After measuring PACU admission vital signs and receiving report from the anesthesia care provider, the nurse attends to immediate patient needs such as managing pain, nausea, and/or vomiting, and conducting a head to toe assessment. Depending on the child and the surgery or procedure, the nurse assesses the surgical site noting the condition of any dressing(s) and/or drainage. Urinary catheters, chest tubes, surgical drains, nasogastric tubes, and other drains are checked for patency, amount, appearance, and consistency of drainage. Issues of concern are reported to the surgeon. Physician orders are reviewed to determine patient care priorities, such as initiating medications, administering IV fluids, and collecting blood samples.

The nurse assesses the patient for pain and nausea and implements a plan to optimize comfort. Comfort measures, such as warmed blankets, ice bags for operative areas, popsicles, music, and distraction are provided to the patient as indicated. The family is included in care per facility protocol, as soon as possible, to lessen patient and family anxiety. In many cases, it is possible for the child to be held by the parent upon reunion. The nurse determines when the patient has reached discharge criteria such as airway stability, stable vital signs, normothermia, and adequate oxygenation per

facility protocol and/or in collaboration with the designated anesthesia care provider.

- Vital sign tips:
  - Infants and young children may better tolerate a BP cuff or SPO$_2$ probe on a lower extremity.
  - With infants and small children, obtaining a BP may be less disturbing if a manual cuff is used and the systolic BP is palpated.

15. What vital sign changes are frequently seen in the PACU?

When postoperatively interpreting vital sign changes in pediatric patients, it is important that the nurse gather information based on a global view of the patient's status and consider current, as well as preoperative and intraoperative, vital signs and details related to the surgery or procedure. The nurse physically assesses the patient and monitors HR, RR, and BP (with the appropriate size cuff), SPO$_2$, temperature, urine output, and the overall appearance of the child. Vital signs are interpreted with knowledge of many factors, including the procedure performed, possible complications, estimated blood loss, fluid and electrolyte balance, level of consciousness, past medical history, comorbidities, and lab values if available.

An increased RR in the postoperative pediatric patient may indicate respiratory distress, an increased temperature, fluid excess, pain, or hypothermia. A decreased RR may be due to the effects of opioids and anesthetic agents (Brown, 2009). Children in pain may "splint" or voluntarily reduce their respiratory rates to limit abdominal and thoracic movements that contribute to discomfort (McCaffery & Pasero, 1999).

In the infant, bradycardia may be an ominous sign in cases of hypovolemia, because the infant's heart is not capable of increasing the heart rate to compensate. Thus, in infants and young children, bradycardia may reflect hypoxemia and impending arrest. Bradycardia can also present in pediatric patients who are resting or sleeping, or in cases of hypothermia (Landriscina, 2009). Bradycardia may occur in response to vagal stimulation due to medications such as neostigmine bromide and as a result of increased intracranial pressure (Algren & Arnow, 2007). Sinus bradycardia is often present in young athletes as a result of the increased stroke volume that comes from physical conditioning (Ralson, Hazinski, Zaritsky, Schexnayder, & Kleinman, 2006).

Sinus tachycardia may be present due to discomfort from hunger and/or pain, anxiety, agitation, and/or struggling as the child emerges from anesthesia. Additionally, an increased temperature, the stress response, and side effects of medications, such as atropine or glycopyrrolate, can also cause a sinus tachycardia (Landriscina, 2009). Sinus tachycardia may be a compensatory mechanism for hypovolemia; however, this is not the case in infants as noted previously. Unexplained tachycardia may also be the first sign of MH in the extubated patient. The PACU nurse should have a high index of suspicion for MH, especially if intubation was noted to be challenging due to masseter muscle rigidity (Algren & Arnow, 2007; Hommertzheim & Steinke, 2006; Landriscina, 2009).

Hypotension may result because of the vasodilatory effects of general or regional anesthetic agents and opioids. It is a late sign of shock. Blood pressure may be increased from pain, fluid volume excess, shivering, bladder distention, increased intracranial pressure, and/or carbon dioxide retention. Increased blood pressure may also be caused by medications such as ketamine or epinephrine, including racemic epinephrine (Brown, 2009; Landriscina, 2009). Postoperative hypertension may also be related to comorbidities, such as renal disease and/or previously undiagnosed high blood pressure due to the silent nature of the condition.

- ECG tip:
  - Sinus arrhythmia, in which the heart rate varies with breathing, is common in pediatric patients and is usually benign.

16. What should the nurse providing care to the postoperative pediatric patient know about fluid management?

Total body fluid is the percentage of body weight that is comprised of intracellular and extracellular fluid. Extracellular fluid includes interstitial fluid

and intravascular fluid. In infancy, the total body fluid is 80% of body weight, decreasing to 65% by 3 years of age and reaching adult proportions of 60% by age 15. Due to the higher proportion of body water and a large body surface area, the infant and younger child are more at risk for dehydration and fluid overload (Muscari, 2005).

Postoperative care includes assessing the patient's fluid status, ensuring ongoing IV access if applicable, administering maintenance fluids as indicated, and monitoring urine output. Maintenance fluids are determined based on the child's weight. When present, the central venous pressure catheter and/or arterial line enable the nurse to continuously monitor the hemodynamic status of the more acutely ill patient. When considering the fluid status of the patient, it is vital to consider the patient's medical condition, surgical procedure, IV fluids and blood products administered in the OR, vital signs, and urine output. Additional IV fluid needs or fluid restrictions are determined per physician orders, unit or facility protocol, and/or in collaboration with the anesthesia care provider.

Since oxygen is carried by hemoglobin in the blood, it is important to consider the child's estimated intraoperative blood loss when determining fluid volume replacement strategies. Determination of each child's ability to tolerate blood loss is based on their medical condition, surgical procedure, and respiratory and hemodynamic status. To replace blood loss in children, an isotonic crystalloid solution (such as 0.9% normal saline) or a colloid may be used. Since intravascular volume in children totals approximately one third of their extracellular fluid, replacement with crystalloid is with a ratio of 3 ml crystalloid per 1 ml estimated blood loss. If colloid is used for replacement, the blood loss is replaced milliliter for milliliter. Signs of compromised intravascular volume to monitor during the postoperative stay include tachycardia, hypotension, a narrowed pulse pressure, decreased urine output, pallor, and slow capillary refill (Aker, 2010). See Table 19-7 for average pediatric blood volumes.

TABLE 19-7. Pediatric Blood Volume

Average blood volumes (ml/kg)	
Neonate	80–90
Infant to 3 years	75–80
Child older than 6 years	65–70

17. Why is temperature monitoring and maintenance or restoration of normothermia important?

Normothermia is defined as a core body temperature between 36° and 38°C. The body temperature in infants and children tends to be higher than that of adults and slowly declines to normal body temperature throughout puberty. Infants and young children have an immature thermoregulatory system. They have a larger body surface area compared to body mass. The ability of infants to shiver may not be developed. General and regional anesthesia contribute to decreased heat production. Hypothermia in infants and children may result in hypoventilation and, in extreme cases, apnea and metabolic acidosis. Heat loss may be attributed to the exposure of body cavities during surgery, infusion of cold liquids and inhalation gases, and the decreased ability to maintain thermoregulatory stability. It has been reported in the literature that even mild perioperative hypothermia increases surgical site infections, reduces surgical wound healing, impairs platelet and clotting cascade function, and may prolong the effects of general anesthesia.

Among the various routes available for taking temperatures, the tendency in pediatric settings is to use minimally intrusive thermometers such as tympanic, axillary, and more recently, temporal artery thermometers to determine temperature. The PACU nurse monitors temperature upon arrival and during the PACU stay as necessitated by the patient's temperature, warming methods utilized, and unit or facility protocol. The nurse may promote normothermia by utilizing warming measures. Passive warming measures appropriate for pediatric patients include warmed blankets, socks, and hats. With older children, a warmed blanket may be placed around the head. Skin exposure should be limited. The use of active warming measures, such as a forced air convection device, may be used per facility and unit protocol as indicated.

- Warming tip:
  - Prewarming in the preoperative area may provide comfort while optimizing the patient's temperature prior to entering the OR.

18. What children are at higher risk for developing malignant hyperthermia?

Malignant hyperthermia (MH) occurs in 1 out of 15,000 children and 1 out of 50,000 adults. A partial list of children considered at risk include those with a family history of MH, central core disease, muscular dystrophies, and congenital myopathies (Bertorini, 2004). Keeping a list of medications, doses, and amounts by weight used in the treatment of MH will provide a ready reference tool for staff in the event of an MH emergency. See Tables 19-4 and 19-5 for drugs commonly administered during an MH crisis.

- MH tips:
  - Unexplained tachycardia may be an early sign of MH.
  - Maintain a heightened vigilance for MH with report of masseter muscle (jaw) rigidity with intubation.
  - An elevated temperature is a late sign of MH.

19. What are the recommendations regarding the management of postanesthesia agitation in children?

Postanesthesia agitation (PAA) is also known as emergence delirium, emergence agitation, and postanesthetic excitement. Behaviors associated with PAA include disorientation, nonpurposeful movements, lack of focused eye contact, disorientation, incoherence, inconsolability, restlessness, and agitation. Possible reasons for PAA include physiologic causes, such as hypoxemia or hypercarbia. Evidence to date suggests an association between PAA and the use of the general anesthetic agent sevoflurane and, possibly, desflurane in young children (Aker, 2010).

Upon admission to the PACU and presentation of PAA, the healthcare team assesses for adequate oxygenation and ventilation, protects the patient from injury, and determines the need for intervention. After ruling out possible physiologic causes, the nurse assesses for pain, fear, and anxiety. Since the agitated child is not capable of self-report, pain may be assessed based on the likelihood of pain associated with the patient's procedure in the context of the analgesia and anesthesia received. Although PAA can last up to 45 minutes, it is typically self-limiting. However, undesirable outcomes of PAA include surgical site bleeding or patient injury, loss of IV access or surgical drains, increased pain, and potential injury to members of the healthcare team. Furthermore, additional PACU resources are necessary to manage the patient experiencing PAA, thereby affecting total unit throughput (Aker, 2010).

20. What are the most common emergent events that the PACU nurse should be prepared for in the pediatric postoperative patient?

Laryngospasm may occur in infants and children after extubation. The normal function of the larynx is to protect the airway from aspiration by ensuring a closed glottis, exemplified by the glottic closure that occurs during swallowing. When the superior laryngeal nerve experiences noxious stimulation, such as from excessive secretions after extubation, it can precipitate a vigorous closure of the glottic opening and spasm of the laryngeal musculature, known as laryngospasm. Children exposed to secondhand tobacco smoke, with a current or recent upper respiratory infection, gastroesophageal reflux, a nasogastric tube, or mechanical irritants (such as oropharyngeal secretions) are at higher risk for developing this condition (Aker, 2010).

If an infant or child exhibits signs of high-pitched crowing sounds and chest retractions, and/or becomes less responsive, page the anesthesia care provider immediately to evaluate the patient in the PACU and:

- Gently reposition the patient's head and airway as indicated with such maneuvers as a head extension, chin lift, and jaw thrust.
- Provide high-flow O_2 at the highest concentration available.
- If secretions are present, consider suctioning gently to avoid eliciting a gag reflex.

If the child's laryngospasm continues, the healthcare team should respond with progressively more aggressive measures until the spasm resolves, including the application of gentle positive pressure ventilation or administration of a short-acting agent such as the depolarizing muscle relaxant succinylcholine to enable muscle relaxation and rapid intubation.

In cases of postintubation croup, in addition to cool mist, the patient may be treated with steroids and/or inhalational racemic epinephrine. Due to a potential for a rebound effect following racemic epinephrine administration, the child should stay in the PACU for an extended period or may be admitted according to unit or facility protocol.

21. What are important principles to keep in mind when treating postoperative or postprocedural pain in children?

In the pediatric patient, inadequately treated pain may lead to untoward sequelae, such as altered pain pathways in infants, unnecessary suffering, and increased anticipatory anxiety with subsequent healthcare encounters. Pain that is managed effectively contributes to improved outcomes, including comfort, decreased anxiety, timely discharge, faster healing time, and faster resumption of activities of daily living.

It is essential that pain be assessed according to the child's condition and developmental level on a regular basis, utilizing an age and developmentally appropriate pain scale following the hierarchy of pain assessment:

- Self-report
- Knowledge of the likelihood of the presence of pain
- Behavioral indicators of pain
- Parent proxy
- Physiologic indicators of pain

Self-report is the single most reliable indicator of pain and is the gold standard for pain assessment. There are children as young as 3 years of age who are capable of an accurate self-report. Children should be encouraged to let someone know if they hurt. Even adolescents may assume that the nurse or doctor would know when to treat their pain and may not advocate for themselves. Examples of commonly used self-reporting scales are the Wong-Baker FACES scale and the Numeric Rating Scale (Jacob, 2009).

If a child has had surgery, it is important that the PACU nurse consider the surgery or procedure the child had, the pain relief interventions received, and the expected occurrence of pain based on the available information. Sleep, play, and denial should not be misinterpreted to indicate the absence of pain. The FLACC scale, a behavioral distress scale appropriate for children 2 months to 7 years of age, determines a distress score that is interpreted in light of the patient's situation to determine if the distress is due to anxiety, hunger, pain, or other factors (Jacob, 2009).

For children unable to self-report who are nonverbal and/or cognitively impaired, parent proxy is often a helpful option. This population is challenging to assess for pain. However, several scales are available, including the revised FLACC, Noncommunicating Child's Pain Checklist, and the Individualized Numeric Rating Scale (Jacob, 2009; Malviya, Voepel-Lewis, Burke, Merkel, & Tait, 2006; Solodiuk & Curley, 2003). Some of the items considered in these scales include facial expression, vocalizations, body movements, as well as input from the patient's caregiver.

Pain is documented on a regular basis depending on the condition of the child and facility or unit protocol. For example, pain may be documented by score or observation as frequently as every 5 minutes while intervening actively to achieve comfort or as infrequently as every 4 hours if the patient is on a maintenance schedule of pain management. It is crucial that the pediatric PACU nurse is committed to regular pain assessment that includes the input of the child and family whenever possible, as well as astute nursing observations for subtleties that may otherwise be easily overlooked (such as the quiet child, a slight grimace, guarding, or denial of pain in the context of the child's surgical course). A wide variety of interventions, including the presence of family, comfort measures, complementary therapies such as Reiki, behavioral distraction techniques, guided imagery, and multiple pharmacologic choices, are typically available to the nurse for a multimodal approach to minimizing pain.

- Pain tip:
  - A child may not admit to pain for fear of receiving a shot.

22. What are key points about postoperative nausea and vomiting (PONV) in children?

PONV following anesthesia and surgery can be a common occurrence in children, causing distress, delayed resumption of oral intake, tension on surgical sites, and potential admission or prolonged stay. Wound dehiscence may occur related to the retching and/or vomiting that may occur (Sakellaris et al., 2008). For children undergoing day surgery, it is the fourth leading cause of admission to the hospital, and overall incidence of postoperative vomiting (POV) in children is reported to be 8.9–42% overall (Kovac, 2007).

Certain surgeries are noted to be associated with PONV. For example, patients may be more prone to PONV following adenotonsillectomy due to swallowing blood. PONV may also result from the extraocular stimulation associated with strabismus repair. In plastic surgery of the ears, POV may result due to labyrinthine, otic, and vestibular stimulation. Patients with a history of motion sickness also have a higher risk of PONV (Kovac, 2007).

Risk factors for PONV in children include those 3 years of age or older, receiving strabismus surgery, receiving surgery lasting longer than 3 hours, a history of POV or PONV, motion sickness in family members, and the use of postoperative opioids. Physiologic symptoms related to PONV include sweating, increased salivation and swallowing, pallor, tachypnea, and tachycardia (Kovac, 2007).

For children at moderate-to-high risk for POV, a combination of two to three antiemetics from varying classes of medications is recommended. Common drugs used include odansetron, metoclopramide, dexamethasone, and dolasetron. Anesthesia care providers may consider alternate choices to reduce risk, such as local or regional anesthesia, or the use of propofol, which has antiemetic properties. In some facilities,

TABLE 19-8. Erikson's Stages of Development

Trust versus mistrust: Birth to 1 year
Autonomy versus shame and doubt: 1–3 years
Initiative versus guilt: 3–5 years
Industry versus inferiority: 5–10 years
Identity versus role confusion: Adolescence
Intimacy versus isolation: Young adult
Generativity versus stagnation: Middle age
Integrity versus despair: Old age

acupuncture and/or acupressure are available (Kovac, 2007).

- PONV tips:
  - Ensure adequate hydration, taking special care if the patient will be discharged home.
  - Provide explicit teaching to families of children who are being discharged home that have experienced PONV and ensure they have supplies for the ride home (e.g., an emesis basin, tissues).

23. What are the cognitive and social stages of development that correlate with pediatric physical considerations?

- For Erikson's Stages of Development, see Table 19-8.
- For Piaget's Stages of Learning, see Table 19-9.

TABLE 19-9. Piaget's Stages of Learning

Sensorimotor: Birth to 2 years; learn about their world through their senses
Preoperational: 3–5 years; learn about their world through experience, such as developing a sense of time as it relates to their daily routine of meals, naps, and playtime
Concrete operations: 5 to 10/12 years; learn the rules and use logic in thought such as understanding another person's point of view
Formal operations: Adolescence and adults; learn to use abstract thinking and the use of verbal as well as electronic communication increases

Adapted from Mullen and Pate, 2006.

- The infancy period is characterized by rapid growth and development (see Table 19-10).
- The toddler is becoming more independent, asserting her or his personality, acquiring language, and achieving mobility (see Table 19-11).
- The preschooler is active, shows initiative, and is full of wonder. The preschooler is engaged in life and is constantly asking "why?" (see Table 19-12).
- The school age child is becoming more adept at physical and social activities (see Table 19-13).
- The adolescent years are filled with tumultuous times that are exhibited by great physical, psychological, and emotional changes (see Table 19-14).
- For pediatric caring secrets and tips, see Table 19-15.

24. Why is it important to consider the family when providing care to the pediatric postoperative patient?

When the family or caregiver entrusts a child to a healthcare team, it is the responsibility of the healthcare team to respect that trust and utilize the knowledge of the family, in combination with the skill of the team, to provide safe and individualized care to the child.

Although the healthcare team members are the experts in delivering health care, family members and caregivers are the experts with regard to their child. The family unit is able to provide valuable and individualized information to optimize health care for the child. Upon discharge, the family will be caring for the child. If the child is going home after a day surgery procedure, it is up to the nurse to provide education to the family, assess abilities to provide care, and evaluate understanding of the teaching related to the child's care, while respecting and accounting for privacy and special needs. It is important to educate the family that it is not uncommon for a child to regress after surgery, to be irritable and/or demanding postprocedure, to have changes in appetite, or to experience nightmares for a short period of time.

25. What are effective ways to communicate with families?

The most important communication skill is to be an active listener and to accept each family's uniqueness. It is important to respect traditional

and nontraditional family units. Families come with a wide variety of coping skills and support systems and will have varying needs. Start by introducing yourself to the family and identifying your role. Clarify the role and full name of each member of the family unit present, including the legal guardian(s). Utilize an interpreter approved by your facility if indicated. Unless otherwise determined, utilize titles of respect, such as "Mr." and "Mrs." It is not appropriate to address a mother and father as "Mom" and "Dad." Optimize privacy by speaking in a low voice. If indicated, utilize a more private area or consult room.

26. What additional services for pediatric patients and families can be helpful?

- Tours for pediatric patients and their families
  - On site
  - Virtual
- Child life specialists
- Surgical liaison nurses to update families while the child is in surgery
- Social services
- Interpreters
- Financial counselors
- Physical therapists
- Case managers for specialties, such as orthopedics, transplants
- Spiritual services
- Ethics committees
- Wireless services
- Vending machines in waiting area while the child is in surgery
- Laundry facilities

27. What points of postoperative care should be discussed in the discharge instructions?

Postoperative care is one of the most important components of the child's perioperative course. When the nurse is reviewing discharge instructions with the parent, it is important to determine that the caregiver understands and can give a repeat demonstration to ensure compliance with instructions once the child is cared for in the home. Optimize the timing of postoperative teaching, so that the caregiver is able to pay attention and is not distracted by the child's crying or irritability. It is recommended that an adult sit in the back seat with the patient during the ride

(Text continues on page 188)

TABLE 19-10. Physical, Cognitive, and Social Stages of Development: Infant

Physical development	Cognitive development	Social development	Common fears	Nursing implications
At birth, infants have weak and immature musculature and immature nervous systems. Their neck muscles are unable to support their head in an upright position. As the months pass, the infant's muscles strengthen and the nervous system matures. The infant gains control of the head and will soon be sitting upright. Infants move by crawling, reaching, and eventually standing. The infant does experience physical pain.	The neonate interacts largely by reflex, such as the sucking reflex. Over the course of the first year, the infant shows an increasing response to sounds and sights, showing interest in toys such as rattles and developing the ability to distinguish strangers. The infant begins to demonstrate an understanding of cause and effect and may begin to vocalize.	The infant is very social, often cooing or squealing in delight, smiling at anyone who smiles back at them. Infants are curious. At 6 months of age or older, infants experience separation anxiety from parents that may last until 30 months of age. The infant's personality is developing.	Fear of separation from parent or caregiver. Stranger anxiety.	Observe infant before making contact. Speak softly and smile. Observe for signs and symptoms of hunger, like crying. Keep infant on parent or primary caregiver's lap. Handle infant gently but firmly, always supporting the head and neck. Perform least invasive procedures first. Keep infant warm. Ensure warm hands/equipment before touching (i.e., stethoscope). Provide comfort measures, such as a pacifier. Use distraction techniques with various items such as music, keys, toys or penlight. Persistent crying, irritability, or inability to console or arouse infant may indicate physiologic distress.

TABLE 19-11. Physical, Cognitive, and Social Stages of Development: Toddler

Physical development	Cognitive development	Social development	Emotional responses	Common fears	Nursing implications
The toddler's gross motor skills continue to improve. Walking is mastered, and running, jumping, and climbing are tried. The toddler is very curious and lacks the understanding of dangerous situations. The household needs to be childproofed. The toddler's fine gross motor skills are revealed through activities such as coloring and playing with blocks or dolls.	Toddlers are learning to speak and imitate words, identify body parts, know colors, and understand simple commands.	Toddlers are very energetic and enjoy exploring, simple games, and parallel play. Temper tantrums may be developing. The child at this age believes the world revolves around them. Crying loudly, biting, kicking, and hitting may be normal expressions of frustration.	Children in this age group that undergo urologic procedures often react with anger, and postoperative crying and arching may not be indicative of pain, but may indicate anger as they react to invasion of their genitals. This is especially evident in boys. Distraction and discussion about going home often helps and getting them dressed in their own clothing postoperatively as soon as possible may assist them as a positive diversionary measure. Breath holding can occur in this age group leading to sudden oxygen desaturation. Children that breath hold in the PACU often have a history of it when they are angry or crying. It is an important question to ask preoperatively in order to be prepared postoperatively.	Being left alone. Fear of separation from parents. Interacting with strangers. Interruptions in usual routine. Loss of control. Getting hurt/fear of injury. Fear of intrusive procedures. Fear of the toilet. Fear of going down the drain. Fear of the dark.	Gain trust of child and parent/caregiver. Physically, position nurse at the child's eye level to be less intimidating. Avoid separating the child from the parent/caregiver if possible. Address child by name. Smile and speak in calm quiet tone. Encourage child to participate in care. Respect modesty. Promote holding a familiar/transitional object in times of stress. Be truthful; avoid words and phrases that may be frightening such as: "put to sleep, stick, needle." Provide safe limits for expression of negative feelings. Expect and accept regressive behavior. Offer choices to enhance their feeling of control. Prepare immediately before surgery or procedure.

TABLE 19-12. Physical, Cognitive, and Social Stages of Development: Preschool

Physical development	Psychological development	Social development	Emotional responses	Common fears	Nursing implications
The preschooler's gross motor skills and hand-to-eye coordination continue to improve. They have much energy and love to move, run, jump, hop, skip, and dance to music.	Preschoolers are developing initiative and like to pretend and imitate others. They like to color "inside the lines," play "make believe," and talk a lot. They love to tell stories and may have a difficult time distinguishing between reality and fiction. Piaget calls this preconcrete thinking. They are just beginning to understand time. Preschoolers may regress to the toddler stage under stress.	Preschoolers may be loud as they are still learning what is the appropriate volume of speech. They may believe they have superhuman powers. Preschoolers love to learn and enjoy playing games and working on large puzzles. Preschoolers are beginning to think by the rules.	Children in this age group have some understanding of what is going to occur. Preoperative tours are often helpful and also prepare families for what to expect on the day of surgery. Encouraging children to make choices at this age is also important. The light of the pulse oximeter can become a fascinating toy, as opposed to a scary clip. Storytelling by nurses and anesthesia care providers are great distractions.	Fear of the unknown and the dark. Fear of being left alone. Fear of being lost or abandoned. Fear of separation from parents or caregiver. Fear of injury, pain, mutilation, loss of function. Fear of pain as a punishment. Fear of loss of control. Fear of adults that look or act "mean."	Speak quietly in clear simple language, avoid baby talk; avoid scary terms such as "cut," "shot," "germs," "put to sleep." Physically, position nurse at the child's eye level as it is less intimidating. Encourage the child to hold transitional objects, such as favorite toys. Encourage hands-on practice with equipment. Provide distraction techniques such as guided imagery. Offer child treatment choices. Respect the child's modesty. Keep the child warm. Prepare the child for uncomfortable procedures and make a plan for distraction, a position of comfort, availability of a favorite toy, or other intervention that will lessen anxiety. Optimize parental visitation.

TABLE 19-13. Physical, Cognitive, and Social Stages of Development: School Age

Physical development	Psychological development	Cognitive development	Social development	Emotional responses	Common fears	Nursing implication
School-aged children continue to improve their large muscle and fine muscle skills. They demonstrate industry and participate in gymnastics, dancing, and team sports that reflect the increasing growth and development of their muscles and nervous systems. They draw, paint, and play musical instruments.	Children of this age group are generally happy and excited about life. School-aged children have a need to develop a sense of achievement and competence, such as engaging in team activities such as sports, scouting, or church events. They are usually eager, enthusiastic, and willing to cooperate. It is important for children to master skills and develop self-confidence and self-esteem.	Children during this period learn through concrete operational thought. Children are constantly learning new concepts such as letters, colors, words, and numbers. They are gaining knowledge and are able to make abstract associations.	Children enjoy same sex peer groups. They like activities such as games, parties, and team sports. During this period, children develop close friendships and best friends. Children understand what is acceptable behavior in public. School-aged children know the difference between right and wrong.	School-aged children may have shared stories of surgical experiences with siblings or friends. Preconceived ideas may affect their emotions and fears. Preoperative tours are a benefit to this age group. Asking questions may promote a better understanding of worries and concerns.	Fear of the unknown. Fear of separation from parent or caregiver. Fear of loss of control. Fear of pain, loss of body function. Fear of body injury, mutilation. Fear of rejection of peers. Failure to live up to others' expectations. Anger over dependence. Fear of physical disability, disfigurement or not being able to participate in sports. Fear of procedures involving genitals. Guilt about illness.	Listen attentively. Acknowledge fears. Respect dignity and need for increasing privacy. Provide honest, factual information. Offer optimized parental visitation. Help establish coping skills and distraction techniques.

TABLE 19-14. Physical, Cognitive, and Social Stages of Development: Adolescent

Physical development	Psychological development	Cognitive development	Social development	Emotional responses	Common fears	Nursing implications
Adolescents continue to develop, increasing strength and coordination in their large muscles and fine motor movement is still developing. The sexual development process takes approximately 4 years. Adolescents adjust to their ever changing bodies. Height and weight increases with muscle mass.	The adolescent years are a time of emotional struggle for, independence as the teenager searches for his or her personal identity. Adolescents feel a sense of invincibility. Emotions are labile and may be volatile.	The adolescent is able to synthesize information and draw a conclusion. They continue to master academic subjects and engage and think abstractly.	The adolescent is rapidly maturing into adulthood. Friendships continue and they may begin to date. The peer group is very important and experimentation may occur. At this age, many enter the workforce.	The teenager often stays up late into the night, and postoperatively may appear to be slow to arouse from anesthesia because he or she slept very little the night before surgery. Since teens also like to feel in control, respect the teen's growing independence and include them in determining the best time for the parents to rejoin them at the bedside. The various levels of maturity in the teen population results in a wide spectrum of needs and responses.	Fear of being left out or socially isolated. Fear of inheriting parent's problems (i.e., alcoholism, mental illness). Fear of infection. Fear of loss of control. Fear of loss of privacy. Fear of altered body image, disfigurement. Fear of separation from peer group. Fear of pain.	Speak in a respectful, friendly manner as one would to an adult. Obtain history from patient if possible. Be sensitive and interview privately when questioning about tobacco, drug, or alcohol use. Consider pregnancy testing for menstruating females or per facility policy. Assess for body piercings. Respect independence. Allow parent or caregiver to be involved if patient wishes. Explain things clearly and honestly; allow time for questions. Respect patient's modesty. Address patient's concerns of body integrity or disfigurement. Provide discharge instructions to the patient and parent or caregiver. Implement interventions aimed at gaining control, increased coping measures, and learning distraction techniques.

TABLE 19-15. Pediatric Caring Secrets and Tips

Caring tips	Nursing actions

Play therapy	• Encourage children to participate in their care as much as possible.
	• Encourage child to put bracelet on stuffed animal and then let him or her choose which extremity to place the ID bracelet on self.
	• Use children's bandages with action figures or customize a regular bandage by drawing a happy face with an ink pen/marker or using small character stickers.
	• Introduce children to medical equipment and make it an adventure or a fun game such as:
	  a. Show them an oxygen mask with high flow O_2 and ask them to listen to the O_2 mask to hear the wind saying it might be like hearing the sound of a seashell. Bend the O_2 tubing when O_2 is free flowing and hear the whistling sound it makes referring to it as an astronaut's mask.
	  b. Place a pulse oximeter on the finger of a child and ask them to take deep breaths to reach 100%. Refer to it as a special flashlight.
	  c. Show a stethoscope and let them touch and feel it. Let them hear your heartbeat, their parent's heartbeat or their own heartbeat.
	  d. Show them the thermometer and encourage them touch and feel it. Let them take your temperature, their parent's temperature or their own.
	  e. Show them an anesthesia mask. Let them choose the flavor and apply it to their mask.
	  f. When provider is auscultating for bowel sounds, refer to listening to the rumble in the tummy.
	• Create a simple coloring book that tells a story about what they can expect during their hospital experience and let them color in the book.
	• Give out large colorful action character stickers.
	• Create a badge of courage, hospital certificate, or a personalized photo of the child to give to them at discharge with the hospital or ambulatory care center's logo or with a caring message.

Communication secrets	• Be honest with the child to maintain trust in the healthcare system. • Always inform the child what you are going to do before you do it, letting them know in simple terms what to expect. • Address the child by the preferred name using a calm demeanor. • Consult parents about their perceptions about how the child is responding to nursing care provided, especially when medicating for pain. • Ensure the caregiver understands discharge instructions and when and where to call if questions arise or an emergency occurs.
Equipment	• For snap-on ECG leads, be careful to snap the ECG lead to the electrode pad first and then place it on the child's chest. • Be aware that for many children, removal of ECG pads is upsetting. Gently lifting a small portion of the pad while working the pad off slowly wiping an alcohol pad back and forth between the skin and adhesive will lessen the pulling on the child's skin. • It is helpful to loop and anchor the wire leading from the O_2 saturation probe to lessen the chance that it will be pulled off.

Caring tips	Nursing actions
Modesty and privacy	• Provide patient explanation before all procedures. • Replace clothing promptly. • Provide privacy during weighing patient. • Always pull privacy curtains if patient will be exposed (e.g., turning). • Ensure hospital gowns are the correct size and provide pajama bottoms or second hospital gown to use as a bathrobe when appropriate. • Avoid covering the child's face.
Bundling care	• Combine care interventions to minimize disturbance to the child • Prioritize minimization and prevention of stress around procedures including needles to avoid development of needle phobia
Transportation	• Encourage parent of older infants or young children to bring strollers. • Provide a wagon outfitted with safety straps to transport young child to operating room and/or upon discharge when appropriate. • Ensure that safety belts are in place on facility wheelchairs. • For patients going home on the day of surgery, ensure that the caregiver has arranged for transportation home during the preoperative assessment to optimize a timely discharge once the patient has recovered.
Postop nutrition	• Provide multiple flavors of popsicles, Italian ice, or Jell-O. • Customize cups with stickers. • Tip for at home: make snow cones or crushed ice drinks with different flavors (i.e., ginger ale, lemon lime).
Surgery-specific tips	
Myringotomy and tubes	• Warmed wet facecloths applied to the ear(s) may help relieve ear discomfort. • Teach parent to time administration of eardrops 30 minutes after providing the child pain medication. If possible, warm ear drops up in a pants pocket or a pan of water (not the microwave) and instill the drops in the less affected ear first, then the more affected ear.
Abdominal	• Place a pillow under the child's knees to lessen stress on the child's incision and to promote comfort. Place a pillow between the knees if child wants to be in a side-lying position. • Teach the child to roll to the side and push up with their hand to get into a sitting position to get out of bed rather than trying to sit up straight from the supine position to alleviate pressure on the surgical site.
Circumcision/ hernia	• Teach the caregiver to avoid picking the child up in a manner that let their legs drop such as by picking the child up by placing hands under the axillae, but rather, encourage them to support the legs when picking the child up. • Teach the parent to avoid allowing the child to use riding toys.
Tonsillectomy	• Child may be comforted by applying a bag of ice to the neck area. o Ensure that there is no possibility of strangulation by ties on ice bag.
Knee surgery	• For families going home, elevation of extremity may be more effective if less compressible items, such as bulk packages of paper towel rolls or couch cushions, often readily available in the home, are used as a base to provide elevation to the lower extremity. Pillows could be used on top for comfort.

(Continued)

TABLE 19-15. Pediatric Caring Secrets and Tips *(Continued)*

Caring tips	Nursing actions
Pain management	• Administer oral medications whenever possible for same day surgery patients. • Optimize nonopioids and nonpharmacologic techniques. • For children who are hesitant to take oral medications but are able to cooperate, allowing them to gather themselves and to choose a plan for what works best for them such as to take it all at once with a "chaser" of their choosing such as apple juice or a lick of a popsicle, or to take it in small amounts at a time with a chaser after each sip followed by the chaser of their choice. • For children going home that have had surgeries expected to be on the more painful end of the spectrum (i.e., tonsillectomy, orthopedic surgery), educate the parent as to the importance of maintaining pain management during the night, especially the first night at home to avoid an escalation in the child's pain.
Fall prevention	• Ensure that facility provided slippers or socks have adequate treads on soles (some have double treads for sole and top of foot to protect against falls if the sock is not on properly). • Caution parent(s) to stay close to their child and take precautions such as ensuring side rails are up, alerting nurse if leaving the bedside, and not allowing the child to freely walk or run in work areas such as hallways and patient care areas.

The authors would like to thank the pediatric PACU nurses at Children's Hospital Boston and at the Johns Hopkins Children's Center for sharing their expertise in developing this table.

home. If the child vomits or starts to cry, the second person can immediately attend to the patient while the other adult is driving. Reinforce that the patient should not lie down in the car. Educate the caregivers about the importance of utilizing car or booster seats and/or seat belts for the ride home.

Provide instructions regarding the effects of anesthesia and medications, as well as pain assessment and management strategies, fall risk, care of the operative site (i.e., dressing, cast, brace), and resumption of diet and the possibility of nausea and/or vomiting. For teenagers, it is important to stress any limitations on physical activity and restrictions on driving, especially when taking pain medications.

When discussing postoperative care after the patient is discharged to the home, it is important to emphasize the following if applicable:

• Monitor the child with close observation, which may include staying in the same room with the child during the night.
• Keep the child quiet on a sofa or bed.
• Do not let the child participate in contact sports or ride bicycles.
• Provide a safe environment at home to prevent injury to the surgical site.

• Discuss advancing the diet as tolerated and ordered, beginning with liquids and then trying soft food that is easily digested.
• Instruct parents about the signs and symptoms of infection and how to maintain the surgical site dressing.
• For extremity surgery, ask the parents to demonstrate back the assessment of distal circulation and what to look for when there are signs of deteriorating perfusion to the fingers or toes.
• Foremost, ensure that the parents know who, when, and where to call in an emergency or if they are concerned about their child's recovery.
• Discharge instruction tips:
  ◦ For younger children, it is best to go over discharge teaching with the family, if possible, while the child is still sleeping. The family will need to focus on the patient once he or she awakens, and it is more challenging for them once the patient is awake to listen as attentively to instructions.
  ◦ For adolescents, wait to give instructions until the patient is able to listen. Review any restrictions, such as on driving, if applicable.

REFERENCES

Aker, J. G. (2010). Pediatric anesthesia (pp. 1174–1206). In J. J. Nagelhout & K. L. Plaus (Eds.), *Nurse Anesthesia* (4th ed.). St. Louis, MO: Saunders Elsevier.

Algren, C. L., & Arnow, D. (2007). The child who is hospitalized: Pediatric variations of nursing interventions (pp. 1083–1139). In M. J. Hockenberry & D. Wilson (Eds.), *Wong's Nursing Care of Infants and Children* (8th ed.). St. Louis, MO: Mosby Elsevier.

Astuto, M., Rosano, G., Rizzo, G., Disma, N., Raciti, L., & Sciuto, O. (2006). Preoperative parental information and parents' presence at induction of anaesthesia. *Minerva Anesthesiology, 72,* 461–465.

Bertorini, T. E. (2004). Perisurgical management of patients with neuromuscular disorders. *Neurology Clinics of North America, 22,* 293–313.

Brown, T. L. (2009). Pediatric variations of nursing interventions (pp. 694–698). In M. J. Hockenberry & D. Wilson (Eds.), *Wong's Essentials of Pediatric Nursing* (8th ed.). St. Louis, MO: Mosby Elsevier.

Brusseau, R. (2010). The obese pediatric patient (pp. 151–162). In J. Weiner-Kronish & V. Ortiz (Eds.), *Perioperative Anesthesia for the Obese Patient: Complications and Challenges of the Obese Patient.* London: Informa Healthcare.

D'Angio, C. T., & Maniscalco, W. M. (2004). Bronchopulmonary dysplasia in preterm infants: Pathophysiology and management strategies. *Paediatric Drugs, 6*(50), 303–330.

Eaton, S., Everson, C., Jirava, J., & Zwingman-Bagley, C. (2006). Parents influence and advance pediatric policy. *Nursing Administration Quarterly, 30*(2), 147–152.

Hesselgrave, J. (2009). Developmental influences on child health promotions (p. 73). In M. J. Hockenberry & D. Wilson (Eds.), *Wong's Essentials of Pediatric Nursing* (8th ed.), St. Louis, MO: Mosby Elsevier.

Hicks, R. W., Becker, S. C., & Cousins, D. D. (2006). *MEDMARX Data Report: A Chartbook of Medication Error Findings from the Perioperative Settings from 1998–2005.* Rockville, MD: USP Center for the Advancement of Patient Safety.

Holliday, M. A., & Segar, W. E. (1957). The maintenance need for water in parenteral fluid therapy. *Pediatrics 19*(5), 823–832.

Hommertzheim, R., & Steinke, E. E. (2006). Malignant hyperthermia – The perioperative nurse's role. *American Operating Room Nurses Journal, 83*(1), 151–166.

Jacob, E. (2009). Pain assessment and management in children (pp. 158–192). In M. J. Hockenberry & D. Wilson (Eds.), *Wong's Essentials of Pediatric Nursing* (8th ed.), St. Louis, MO: Mosby Elsevier.

Kain, Z. N., & Caldwell-Andrews, A. A. (2005). Preoperative psychological preparation of the child for surgery: An update. *Anesthesiology Clinics of North America, 23,* 597–614.

Kovac, A. L. (2007). Management of postoperative nausea and vomiting in children. *Paediatric Drugs, 9*(1), 47–69.

Landriscina, D. (2009). Care of the pediatric patient (pp. 697–716). In C. B. Drain & J. Odom-Forren (Eds.), *Perianesthesia Nursing: A Critical Care Approach.* St. Louis, MO: Saunders.

Malignant Hyperthermia Association of the United States (2008). *Emergency therapy for malignant hypothermia.* Retrieved from http://medical.mhaus.org

Malviya, S., Voepel-Lewis, R., Burke, C., Merkel, S., & Tait, A. R. (2006). The revised FLACC observational pain tool: Improved reliability and validity for pain assessment in children with cognitive impairment. *Paediatric Anaesthesia, 16,* 258–265.

McCaffery, M., & Pasero, C. (1999). *Pain: Clinical Manual* (2nd ed.). St. Louis, MO: Mosby.

Mullen, J. E., & Pate, M. F. D. (2006). *Core curriculum for pediatric critical care nursing* (2nd ed.). Philadelphia: Saunders Elsevier.

Muscari, M. E. (2005). *Pediatric Nursing* (4th ed.). Philadelphia: Lippincott Williams and Wilkins.

Ralson, M., Hazinski, M. F., Zaritsky, A. L., Schexnayder, S. M., & Kleinman, M. E. (Eds.). (2006). *PALS provider manual.* Dallas, TX: American Heart Association.

Sakellaris, G., Georgogianaki, P., Astyrakaki, E., Mikalakis, M., Dede, O., Alegakis, A., et al. (2008). Prevention of postoperative nausea and vomiting in children – A prospective randomized double-blind study. *Acta Paediatrica, 97,* 801–804.

Solodiuk, J., & Curley, M. A. Q. (2003). Pain assessment in nonverbal children with severe cognitive impairments: The Individualized Numeric Rating Scale (INRS). *Journal of Pediatric Nursing, 18*(4), 295–299.

CHAPTER 20

Pregnant Patients

Molly M. Killion, RNC-OB, MS, CNS

Although pregnancy is usually a naturally occurring state in women of childbearing age, it is not without risk. There are risks that may occur due to pregnancy and childbirth, but also the possibility of exacerbation of an underlying disease process. Undergoing surgery during pregnancy is no exception. There are factors that must be considered when caring for the pregnant or immediately postpartum surgical patient. Pregnancy is a time when the nurse is responsible for two patients (or more in the case of twins or higher order multiples) but is only able to see one of them before the birthing event. This makes care of the mother a delicate balance while also caring for her unborn child(ren). Coordination of care among surgery, anesthesia, pediatrics/neonatology, and/or obstetrics/perinatology is critical to providing safe and informed care for mother and baby (American College of Obstetricians and Gynecologists, 2003). Please note that the information about pregnancy contained in this section is meant to serve as an adjunct to regular preoperative and postoperative care, not to replace it.

1. What are the normal physiologic changes associated with pregnancy?

Over the course of a pregnancy, a woman's circulating blood volume increases by 30–45%. This increase peaks between 28 and 34 weeks gestation and is 1,200–1,600 ml greater than before pregnancy. Cardiac output increases by 30–40% with a 20% increase by 8 weeks gestation and peaks around 20–24 weeks gestation. Stroke volume increases 30% and heart rate increases by 10–15 beats per minute. Systemic vascular resistance decreases 30% by 8 weeks gestation, and there is a mild decrease in mean blood pressure. Oxygen consumption is higher with total consumption increasing approximately 20% during pregnancy with an increased sensitivity to carbon dioxide. Pregnancy is often referred to as a hypercoagulable state with factors VII, VIII, X, and fibrinogen all increased. Taking precautions to decrease the risk of deep vein thrombosis (DVT) is critical. There is an increase in the glomerular filtration rate (Abbas, Lester, & Connolly, 2005; Creasy & Resnik, 2009). There are also changes to many other systems and organs and, thus, lab values in pregnancy are often slightly different than in the nonpregnant population (Mandeville & Troiano, 1999).

2. What effects does the gravid (pregnant) uterus have?

As a woman's uterus grows, so too does her work of breathing. Dyspnea may accompany many normal pregnancies. Maternal tidal volume increases by about 40%, causing maternal hyperventilation and hypocapnia (Hacker, Moore, & Gambone, 2004). Encouraging a postsurgical pregnant woman to cough and breathe deeply is important. Mild respiratory alkalosis is a normal blood gas finding in pregnancy. Dependent edema occurs from the full uterus exerting pressure on the vessels of the lower extremities, as well as the aorta, iliac veins, and inferior vena cava. Keeping a pregnant woman from a supine position can help to maximize blood flow by decreasing aorto-caval compression. A side-lying or side-tilt position to keep the uterus off midline will help to alleviate pressure on the maternal great vessels, and it does not matter if the side tilt is toward the left or the right (Blackburn, 2007; Creasy & Resnik, 2009).

3. What is the ideal time to perform surgery on a pregnant patient?

The best time to perform surgery on a pregnant patient is in the second trimester. During the first trimester, the fetus is much more susceptible to teratogens or spontaneous abortion. In the third trimester, the uterus has grown in size and is more likely to contract. A pregnant woman is susceptible to needing any surgery that a nonpregnant person would require (Creasy & Resnik, 2009). Whenever possible, elective surgeries should be delayed until the postpartum period. If that is not feasible, there are some considerations unique to pregnancy. The exception to this is fetal surgeries.

4. When would fetal surgery be indicated?

Surgery may be indicated when there is a problem affecting the fetus that could benefit from being surgically repaired while still in utero. This is a highly specialized field, and there are only a limited number of centers that offer these procedures. Indications for fetal surgery include resection of teratomas, laser ablation of uterine vessels causing Twin-to-Twin Transfusion Syndrome, release of an amniotic band, and others.

5. Is preoperative care different for pregnant patients?

When bringing a pregnant patient in for surgery, the same work-up and preoperative visit should be given to her as to anyone else receiving the same type of surgery. In addition to the standard preparations, there are other special considerations (American College of Obstetricians and Gynecologists, 2003).

- For all pregnant patients, consideration should be given to obtaining obstetrics/maternal fetal medicine, pediatrics/neonatology, and anesthesia consults to ensure the patient understands the risks and benefits to both her and her unborn child of having surgery, and the risks to her newborn if an early delivery were required.
- If the fetus is viable (around the 24th week of gestation), consideration should be given to finding out if the woman would want intervention to save the baby in the case of fetal distress.
  - If she does, the surgery should ideally occur at a center where a safe delivery can be

accomplished and there is a nursery to care for the newborn appropriate to the gestational age.
- A staff member trained in fetal monitoring may need to be in attendance to monitor the baby preoperatively, intraoperatively, and postoperatively.
- Instruments and supplies to perform an emergency cesarean section should be available to go with the patient into the operating room (OR) and should also be available at the bedside in the postanesthesia care unit (PACU) or recovery area.

6. When is fetal monitoring indicated preoperatively?

- For previable pregnancy, consider confirming fetal viability (positive heart beat) prior to surgery either through Doppler or ultrasound.
- For viable pregnancy, consider obtaining a nonstress test (approximately 20 minutes of fetal heart rate tracing which must be interpreted by a practitioner trained in fetal heart rate interpretation) prior to surgery.

7. What medications are considered safe for use in pregnancy?

- Sodium citrate or other antacid is recommended prior to surgery. Pregnant women become more susceptible to aspiration and regurgitation as pregnancy progresses. It is not clear at what point in the pregnancy this occurs. This is likely the result of increased intra-gastric pressure from the gravid uterus and decrease in esophageal sphincter tone causing regurgitation (Huges, Levinson, & Rosen, 2002).
- Narcotics are safe in pregnancy and should not be withheld if needed.
  - The FDA categories for use in pregnancy (A through D and X) can be useful when a medication clearly has no risk (category A and sometimes B). However, some medications with increased risk may need to be used to care for the mother or if alternatively lower risk options are not available (Briggs, Freeman, & Yaffe, 2008). Using a pharmacology resource that deals specifically with medication usage in pregnancy and lactation may give more comprehensive information and assist in prescribing and administering medications to this population.

8. What are important postoperative nursing interventions when caring for a pregnant patient?

- Coughing and deep breathing or other respiratory exercises are critical due to increased risk of atelectasis.
- Uterine tilt to the right or left is important to maximize uterine blood flow and blood flow to the fetus, which optimizes fetal oxygenation.
- Consider enlisting help from obstetric colleagues (such as having an OB nurse present at the bedside) whenever a patient pregnant with a viable pregnancy is present in the PACU.
- Fetal monitoring should be done when indicated.
  ◦ For previable pregnancy, consider confirming fetal viability (positive heart beat) after surgery either through Doppler or ultrasound.
  ◦ For viable pregnancy, at a minimum, consider obtaining a nonstress test (approximately 20 minutes of fetal heart rate tracing, which must be interpreted by a practitioner trained in fetal heart rate interpretation) after surgery but continuous fetal monitoring and a trained practitioner available for interpretation (every 15–30 minutes) may be warranted.
  ◦ For the uterus, if contractions are occurring and a decision is made that the team would intervene to achieve delivery in the case of fetal distress, the fetal heart rate should be continuously monitored by someone trained in interpretation and the tocodynamometer should also be placed to monitor uterine contractions (Blackburn, 2007; Huges, Levinson, & Rosen, 2002).

9. What is preterm labor and what is the significance of it?

Preterm labor is defined as uterine contractions before 37 weeks that cause cervical change. Preterm contractions are uterine contractions before 37 weeks that do not cause cervical change. Stress, dehydration, certain medications, and uterine manipulation can all cause the uterus to contract. If a woman is experiencing preterm contractions, she may progress to unstoppable preterm labor and give birth to a premature infant. It is difficult to differentiate between preterm contractions and preterm labor and, therefore, many clinicians treat it conservatively with uterine relaxants before any cervical change has occurred (Blackburn, 2007; Creasy & Resnik, 2009).

- Medications: If a woman is having preterm contractions between 24 and 34 weeks with concern for preterm birth, consideration should be given to administering steroids to boost fetal lung surfactant production, such as betamethasone (Celestone), and transport to an obstetrics unit should be evaluated. There is some controversy as to the gestational age cutoff of receiving steroids for this purpose. The administration of this steroid can help to boost the fetus' production of lung surfactant in hopes of decreasing respiratory problems after birth (Brownfoot, Crowther, & Middleton, 2008). If the mother needs to be transported to another facility, betamethasone should be administered prior to transport whenever indicated, safe, and possible.

10. What are commonly used uterine relaxants, and what does the perianesthesia nurse need to know about safe administration?

- Brethine (Terbutaline) can cause tachycardia in both the woman and her unborn child. Use with caution in the presence of fetal or maternal tachycardia.
- Indomethacin can be used rectally or orally. Usually only used for short courses as it can cause a constriction of the fetus' ductus arteriosis (as can all nonsteroidal anti-inflammatory drugs).
- Magnesium sulfate is controversial as to the efficacy, but it is still used in practice. Therapy is usually initiated with a bolus-loading dose and then a continuous infusion as the maintenance dose. This medication must only be administered on an infusion pump and frequent vital signs (including oxygen saturation and respiratory rate) are critical. Signs and symptoms of magnesium toxicity include respiratory compromise. Magnesium is excreted by the kidneys, so strict urine output measurement is required. Calcium gluconate is the antidote and should be readily available if a patient is receiving magnesium therapy.
- Nifedipine is usually given as a loading dose, then as a maintenance dose every 4–6 hours. Consider having blood pressure hold parameters to prevent hypotension.
- Nitroglycerin may be given sublingually or intravenously to cause temporary uterine relaxation. Usually used as a "rescue dose" when urgent uterine relaxation is needed (Briggs, Freeman, & Yaffe, 2008). Use with caution in maternal hypotension.

11. How can evidence of bleeding be different in a pregnant patient, and what are the management considerations?

Pregnancy is generally thought of as a high-flow, low-resistance cardiovascular state. By the end of pregnancy, blood volume and cardiac output will increase about 50%, whereas systemic vascular resistance decreases. If a pregnant woman is bleeding late in pregnancy or early in the postpartum period, she can lose up to 35% of her circulating blood volume before signs of shock present. Tachycardia is an early sign of blood loss and hypotension may be delayed (Mandeville & Troiano, 1999).

Placental blood flow is around 50 ml/min toward the end of the first trimester and 500–600 ml/min by the end of the third. The arteries that supply the placenta are almost maximally dilated to be able to supply this large blood flow. Changes in maternal blood pressure can impede placental blood flow, and these vessels are minimally responsive to pharmacologic pressor agents (Huges, Levinson, & Rosen, 2002).

Replacing circulating volume can be accomplished by infusing fluids, volume expanders, and blood products. Vasopressors, which decrease uterine blood flow (i.e., epinephrine), should be avoided. Ephedrine and phenylephrine have not been shown to diminish uterine blood flow and are considered safe (Huges, Levinson, & Rosen, 2002).

12. What is gestational hypertension, and how does it differ from preeclampsia?

Gestational hypertension is generally described as new onset hypertension in pregnancy without proteinuria or edema. Preeclampsia is new onset hypertension in the presence of proteinuria. It is broken into two groups based on severity of symptoms, mild or severe. There is a third category, eclampsia, which is characterized by the presence of the symptoms of preeclampsia with seizure activity. This is referred to as an eclamptic seizure (American College of Obstetricians and Gynecologists, 2002; Mandeville & Troiano, 1999).

There are many possible complications associated with preeclampsia and eclampsia, such as thrombocytopenia, extreme hypertension leading to organ damage, a decrease in the glomerular filtration rate due to decreased renal blood flow, hepatic hemorrhage, and seizure with the related complications that it brings (Blackburn, 2007).

Hypertension should be treated when diastolic values get above 110 mmHg with a nonselective alpha- and beta-adrenergic antagonist such as labetalol or a vasodilator such as hydralazine. However, the goal of treatment is to keep the diastolic around 90–95 mmHg. Decreasing maternal blood pressure to a "normal" level will appear as hypotension to placental perfusion and circulation, which can impede fetal blood flow and oxygenation. Magnesium sulfate may be given as seizure prophylaxis as a continuous infusion of 1–2 g/hr after a loading bolus of 4–6 g. If preeclampsia or eclampsia is suspected or diagnosed, involvement of the obstetric team is imperative as the best treatment of severe preeclampsia or eclampsia is birth of the fetus and placenta. Continuous fetal heart rate monitoring and transfer to an obstetric service are recommended. Note: Preeclampsia most commonly begins in the antepartum period, but may also present intrapartum or postpartum (Mandeville & Troiano, 1999).

13. What are the special considerations with a pregnant patient who experiences a cardiac arrest?

A pregnant woman who experiences cardiac arrest in pregnancy requires some special considerations to standard basic life support (BLS) and advanced cardiac life support (ACLS) practice. Less than 20 weeks of gestation, the uterus is too small to cause additional problems and standard BLS/ACLS is reasonable. After 20 weeks, the gravid uterus will press on the aorta and inferior vena cava, which affects blood flow and cardiac output. If within 4–5 minutes of the arrest there is no maternal response, steps should be taken to evacuate the uterus to maximize cardiopulmonary resuscitation of the mother. Less than 24–25 weeks of gestation, this is only done to rescue the mother and will most likely cause neonatal death. More than 24–25 weeks, birth of the baby will also help to preserve the neonate's life and neurologic well-being (American Heart Association, 2005). Any pregnant woman more than 20 weeks in the PACU or ICU should have instruments and supplies available to perform an emergency cesarean section in a timely manner. For those women whose pregnancies have reached viability, a pediatric team should also be aware of her presence in the hospital and have their emergency resuscitation gear readily available.

14. What is the most common obstetric complication in the immediate postpartum period?

The most common obstetric complication in the immediate postpartum period is bleeding from uterine atony, which requires treatment with fundal massage (firm pressure or massage to the top of the uterus, which can be palpated through the abdomen to increase uterine tone and expel blood or clots within the uterus) and uterotonic medications (medications that increase uterine tone by causing contractions of the uterus).

15. What are commonly used uterotonics (medications used to increase uterine tone and decrease bleeding), and what does the perianesthesia nurse need to know about safe administration?

Uterotonics should only be used in the postpartum period. Causing prolonged uterine contractions when a woman is still pregnant can cause serious complications, including fetal and maternal death (Briggs, Freeman, & Yaffe, 2008; US National Library of Medicine, 2009; Mandeville & Troiano, 1999).

- Carboprost tromethamine (Hemabate) is contraindicated in patients with active cardiac, pulmonary, renal, or hepatic dysfunction; use with extreme caution in patients with asthma or cardiac disease. Can be given intramuscularly.

- Methylergometrine (Methergine) can cause rebound hypertension; use with caution in patients with hypertension (including preeclampsia) or pre-existing cardiac ischemic disease. Intramuscular is the standard route of administration.

- Misoprostol (Cytotec) is usually given rectally for fastest effect but can be given buccally or orally; used in very small doses for cervical ripening for induction of labor.

- Oxytocin (Pitocin) can be given intramuscularly but most commonly given intravenously. It should not be given undiluted intravenously but in 500–1,000 ml maintenance fluid such as lactated ringers; used in small doses (milliunits/min) for induction and augmentation of labor.

REFERENCES

Abbas, A. E., Lester, S. J., & Connolly, H. (2005). Pregnancy and the cardiovascular system. *International Journal of Cardiology, 98*, 179–189.

American College of Obstetricians and Gynecologists. (2002). Diagnosis and management of preeclampsia and eclampsia: ACOG practice bulletin number 33. *American College of Obstetricians and Gynecologists, 99*(1),159–67."

American College of Obstetricians and Gynecologists. (2003). Nonobstetric surgery in pregnancy: ACOG committee opinion number 284. *American College of Obstetricians and Gynecologists, 102*(2), 431.

American Heart Association. (2005). Part 10.8: Cardiac arrest associated with pregnancy. *Circulation, 112,* IV-150–IV-153.

Blackburn, S. T. (2007). *Maternal, fetal, & neonatal physiology: A clinical perspective* (3rd ed.). St. Louis MO: Saunders Elsevier.

Briggs, G. G., Freeman, R. K., & Yaffe, S. J. (2008). *Drugs in pregnancy and lactation* (8th ed.). Philadelphia: Lippincott Williams and Wilkins.

Brownfoot, F. C., Crowther, C. A., & Middleton, P. (2008). Different corticosteroids and regimens for accelerating fetal lung maturation for women at risk of preterm birth. *Cochrane Database of Systematic Reviews, 4.* doi: 10.1002/14651858.CD006764.pub2

Creasy, R. K., & Resnik, R. (2009). *Maternal-fetal medicine: Principles and practice* (6th ed.). Philadelphia: Saunders Elsevier.

Hacker, N. F., Moore, J. G., & Gambone, J. C. (2004). *Essentials of obstetrics and gynecology* (4th ed.). Philadelphia: Elsevier Saunders.

Huges, S. C., Levinson, G., & Rosen, M. A. (2002). *Shnider and levinson's anesthesia for obstetrics* (4th ed.). Philadelphia: Lippincott Williams and Wilkins.

Mandeville, L. K., & Troiano, N. H. (1999). *AWHONN high-risk and critical care intrapartum nursing* (2nd ed.). Philadelphia: Lippincott.

US National Library of Medicine. (2009). Drugs and lactation database. Retrieved from http://toxnet.nlm.nih.gov/cgi-bin/sis/htmlgen?LACT

Surgery-Specific Principles

CHAPTER 21

Abdominal Surgery

Linda Wilson, RN, PhD, CPAN, CAPA, BC, CNE, H. Lynn Kane, RN, MSN, MBA, CCRN, & Fabien R. Pampaloni, RN, BSN

The purpose of this chapter is to review questions related to abdominal surgery. This chapter will review surgeries of the gastrointestinal track, stomach, small bowel, postoperative nursing considerations, and drainage devices. Specific diseases such as peptic ulcers, gastroesophageal reflux disease, Crohn's disease, and diverticular disease will also be presented. Anesthetic techniques, patient outcomes, discharge instructions, and other important aspects of abdominal surgery will be explored.

1. What are the five major parts of the gastrointestinal tract?

The gastrointestinal tract is composed of the esophagus, stomach, small intestine, large intestine, and lower rectum and anus. Because of the many organs (pancreas, liver, gallbladder) and surgical procedures involved in the gastrointestinal tract, it is important to understand its functions (Drain, 1994).

2. What surgeries involve the very first part of the gastrointestinal tract, in this case, the esophagus?

Surgery on the esophagus includes repair of hiatal hernia and various forms of tracheoesophageal fistulas, excision of esophageal diverticula, treatment of stenosis of the lower end of the esophagus, esophagomyotomy, esophagectomy, and cardiomyotomy (Drain, 1994).

3. What are some of the postoperative nursing considerations following surgeries involving the esophagus?

Postoperative care depends on the kind of incision used to expose the operative site: abdominal or thoracic. Surgery on the esophagus frequently involves a thoracic incision. Procedures on the esophagus are performed under general anesthesia. Frequently, a tracheostomy is performed. Immediately upon arrival to the Phase I Post Anesthesia Care Unit (PACU), one major priority is airway management and safety. If the patient arrives to the PACU with the head of the bed flat, unless raising the head is contraindicated, the PACU registered nurse (RN) will usually, gradually, and incrementally raise the head of the bed to assist the patient as he or she emerges from the anesthetic. Once the patient's continued airway patency is ensured, the patient may be placed in a semi-Fowler's position postoperatively to relieve tension on the suture line and to promote drainage. The semi-Fowler's position may aid in the drainage of blood from the pleural space and prevent tension from blood from impinging on the suture lines. The incision is generally long and painful. Analgesics must be given in adequate doses to promote rest and adequate respiratory effort. An epidural catheter often is in place for postoperative analgesia. Patient-controlled analgesia may be used. Transcutaneous electrical nerve stimulation (TENS) may also provide incisional pain relief. A nasogastric tube will be in place and should be properly monitored. It should not be manipulated by the nurse. Chest tubes should be adequately managed. A large sterile dressing should be in place, and it should be checked frequently for drainage and reinforced as necessary. The PACU RN may mark the outline area of drainage to indicate the level as patient is received (e.g., date, time, or PACU start), thus providing a visible determination of, and the extent of, any additional drainage. Excessive bloody drainage should be reported to the surgeon (Drain, 1994).

4. What surgeries imply the second part of the gastrointestinal tract, in this case, the stomach?

"Surgery on the stomach involves procedures to treat ulcers (antrectomy and vagotomy, gastric resection, gastrectomy); removal of portions of the stomach, for malignancy; and rerouting of the gastrointestinal system at this point to treat pyloric obstruction" (Drain, 1994, p. 454).

5. What are some of the postoperative nursing considerations following surgeries involving the stomach?

All postoperative care of the patient is generally the same. The anesthesia technique may be general anesthesia. For specific patient cases, regional anesthesia may be indicated. The use of regional anesthesia provides analgesia to the patient by numbing the area, while avoiding the potential side effects resulting from the use of general anesthesia. Immediately upon arrival to the Phase I PACU, one major priority is airway management and safety. If the patient arrives to the PACU with the head of the bed flat, unless raising the head is contraindicated, the PACU RN will usually, gradually, and incrementally raise the head of the bed to assist the patient as he or she emerges from the anesthetic. Once the patient's continued airway patency is ensured, the patient may be placed in a semi-Fowler's position postoperatively to relieve tension on the suture line and to promote drainage. The abdominal incisions are fairly high, long, and painful, and particular attention must be paid to pulmonary toilet. This type of patient must be encouraged more frequently than any other to expand the lungs and to cough and must generally have assistance to change position. Assistance in splinting the wound with the hands or with a firm pillow is most appreciated by the patient. These procedures generally produce considerable postoperative pain, and analgesics should be used generously but judiciously. Patient controlled or epidural analgesia may be effective for upper abdominal incisional and visceral pain (Drain, 1994).

6. What are some of the postoperative concerns following surgeries involving the stomach?

Blood loss and urinary retention are major concerns in patients who undergo stomach surgery. A nasogastric tube will be placed and should be closely monitored. Small volumes of bright, bloody drainage from the nasogastric tube can be expected for the first 2–3 hours, because it is not uncommon to have bleeding at the anastomotic site in these

procedures. However, bright bleeding that does not decrease after this period or bleeding that becomes excessive (more than 75 ml/hr) should be reported immediately to the surgeon. Observe the nasogastric tube and its drainage closely because blood easily clots and clogs the tube; notify the surgeon immediately if the tube stops draining or appears obstructed with blood. Because blood loss may be highly significant in this patient, cardiovascular status must receive careful scrutiny. Vital signs are checked frequently, and a certain amount of hypotension and tachycardia is to be expected. If hypotension and tachycardia persist or maintain a downward trend, the surgeon should be notified. Blood replacement may have to be instituted. Hemoglobin and hematocrit levels should be reassessed at regular intervals (e.g., every 4–6 hours postoperatively) and the surgeon should be notified of specific decreases. Little or no drainage should be expected from the incision unless drains are in place. If drainage appears, the dressing should be reinforced, and the surgeon notified. The first and initial dressing is considered a surgical dressing and is, therefore, replaced only by the surgeon. Surgical dressings that are saturated are reenforced by the PACU RN with documentation of the number and type of sterile dressings applied to reinforce the area. The patient may need an evaluation of the surgical dressing in combination with other clinical parameters and potential complications. Drains with copious output may need a drainage device applied over them to protect the patient's skin and allow for accurate measurement of drainage (Drain, 1994; Meeker & Rothrock, 1999).

7. What does a bulb drainage device or a Hemovac do?

A bulb drainage device or Hemovac may be used to ensure drainage during the immediate postoperative phase and for postoperative day (POD) #1 (or as needed into the postoperative period until the drainage is minimal). The bulb and Hemovac devices provide continuous, less aggressive suction to the surgical site. Surgical incisions drain to the absorptive sterile dressings. Residual bleeding resulting from adjacent, underlying tissue may accumulate under, or nearby, the surgical incision; therefore, a bulb drainage or Hemovac provides a mechanical outlet via the drain inserted so that fluid is evacuated.

Urinary retention is commonly a problem, and many surgeons prefer to insert a Foley catheter while the patient is in the operating room. Accurate measurements of output should be ascertained. If a urinary catheter is not in place, the patient should be checked frequently for bladder distention, which may indicate an overfull bladder and urinary retention. In Phase I PACU, the patient may or may not void, especially as he or she emerges from the effects of an anesthetic and the stressful experience of the surgery itself.

The PACU RN records the patient leaving the PACU. Additional documentation may indicate that the patient is due to void approximately 1800–2000 ml. If the patient is unable to void, usually a bladder scanner is used to evaluate the specific amount of urinary retention. An indwelling urinary catheterization order may be needed along with a corresponding physician's order (Drain, 1994). The patient may require the use of an indwelling urinary catheter, and its use may be justified. Surgeons have usually been proponents of discontinuing all tubes as soon as possible to restore the patient to the preoperative level. In recent years, CAUTI (catheter-associated urinary tract infection) is a major focus for all acute care centers. The National Database of Nursing Quality Indicators (NDNQI) includes CAUTI as a nurse sensitive indicator (Montalvo, 2010). The recent change for some clinicians is the change in clinical culture to discontinue the Foley catheter as soon as possible postoperatively. The existence of an indwelling urinary catheter may be justified clinically; that clinical need is now usually documented daily in many acute care hospitals.

8. What surgeries involve the third part of the gastrointestinal tract, in this case, the small bowel?

"Operations on the small bowel include exploratory laparotomy with lysis of adhesions and resection for obstruction or perforation" (Drain, 1994, p. 455).

9. What are some of the postoperative nursing considerations following surgeries involving the small bowel?

Care following small bowel procedures is essentially the same as the other parts of the gastrointestinal tract. The patient may have a long gastrointestinal tube in place that should be cared for and monitored closely. No excessive drainage from incisions should be noted, unless drains have been placed. Fluid and electrolyte balance must be monitored carefully. Remember that the loss of sodium and bicarbonate ions will be great, resulting in imbalance, and that fluid losses during surgery may be significant, but fluid overload must be avoided (Drain, 1994).

10. What is the postoperative care for a patient with an ileostomy?

The patient with an ileostomy will enter the PACU with a bag in place over the stoma, and returns may be expected almost at once; these should be recorded. Particular attention must be paid to this stoma, the drainage, and the collection device; no leakage onto the skin should be allowed, because this causes significant skin damage. Under the collection device, the peristomal skin is protected with a skin barrier that includes pectin- and karaya-based wafers or paste (Drain, 1994).

11. What surgeries imply the fourth part of the gastrointestinal tract, in this case, the large bowel?

Surgery on the large bowel includes appendectomy, colostomy (for obstruction), sigmoid colon resection, herniorrhaphy, removal of tumors or correction of deformities, total proctocolectomy with ileoanal anastomosis, and abdominoperineal resection (Drain, 1994).

12. What are some of the postoperative nursing considerations following surgeries involving the large bowel?

Herniorrhaphy is frequently done under spinal anesthesia with appropriate sedation. All other surgical procedures are usually performed under general anesthesia. On return to the PACU, patients are kept flat and on one side until the reflexes have returned. They may then assume a position of comfort unless otherwise specified by the surgeon. Postoperative care is essentially the same as for small bowel surgery (Drain, 1994).

13. What is the postoperative care for a patient with a colostomy?

If the patient returns from surgery with a colostomy, some special care is required. "It is unusual for the colostomy to start functioning immediately postoperatively; however, spillage must be prevented from contaminating the incision or excoriating the skin. A pouch or collection device may be in place over the colostomy" (Drain, 1994, p. 456). The skin around the stoma should be protected with an appropriate skin barrier if drainage is present. Check the color of the stoma. It should be bright red and moist; its appearance should be documented in the nursing record (Drain, 1994).

14. What surgeries imply the fifth part of the gastrointestinal tract, in this case, the lower rectum and anus?

Surgery on the lower rectum and anus includes excision of pilonidal cysts, rectal fissures, fistulas, rectal abscesses, tumors, and hemorrhoids (Drain, 1994).

15. What are some of the postoperative nursing considerations following surgeries involving the lower rectum and anus?

Postanesthesia nursing care is the same as for any patient undergoing anesthesia, which may be local, regional, or general. Dressings should be checked frequently for excessive drainage of infected material and to aid in healing. Urinary retention may be a problem because of the proximity of the bladder and operative site may make urination difficult. Pain can be exquisite, but patients are often embarrassed by the location of the operative site and may not ask for analgesia. The nurse should be alert to signs and symptoms of pain and discomfort and administer analgesia using multimodal pain therapies and intervention as necessary for relief (Drain, 1994).

16. A patient is undergoing primary colon resection. What would be the major intraoperative expected outcomes?

Maintaining the patient's hemodynamic and thermodynamic stability is a priority. In addition, skin integrity must be maintained at all time. It is also important to make sure that the patient does not experience neurovascular compromise related to positioning and is free of infection (Meeker & Rothrock, 1999).

17. What patient population is subject to gastroenterology procedures?

The patient population undergoing these procedures consists of patients with known or suspected cancer (pancreatic, hepatic, gallbladder, gastric), patients at risk of developing Barrett's esophagus or colonic polyps, and patients with gastroesophageal reflux. In addition, these patients may have other comorbidities (diabetes, coronary artery disease, stroke, renal disease, hepatitis, pregnancy) that need to be considered in the anesthetic preoperative evaluation. Another segment of the adult gastrointestinal patient population consists of liver transplant patients. (Cole & Schlunt, 2004, p. 392)

18. What medications of choice are used for gastrointestinal surgery anesthesia?

Fentanyl and midazolam are a common combination used in gastrointestinal procedure areas; droperidol, meperidine, and others are used as well. Guidelines for the administration of droperidol in gastrointestinal procedures are included in the Guidelines for the Use of Deep Sedation and Analgesia for GI Endoscopy Procedures published by the American Society for Gastrointestinal Endoscopy. Droperidol has been reported to cause torsade de pointes in patients and its use by

anesthesia care providers has diminished. (Cole & Schlunt, 2004, p. 392)

19. Are inhalation agents advised during gastrointestinal surgery?

Propofol and inhalation agents, including nitrous oxide, have been used for endoscopic procedures. Propofol has been used in combination with other drugs for upper endoscopies and colonoscopies but without any distinct advantages over other drug regimens. However, its use during endoscopic retrograde cholangiopancreatography (ERCP) and endoscopic gastric duodenum examination with ultrasound-guided biopsy (EUS) has resulted in shorter recovery times, allowed patients to transfer independently, and allowed a faster return to baseline oral intake and activity level. Propofol has been administered for these procedures by other physicians and nurses with advanced airway skills and even by patient-controlled sedation. (Cole & Schlunt, 2004, p. 393)

20. How does one assess proper sedation according to the patient's past medical history?

Anesthesiologists are usually consulted when any of the following pertinent items in the history are obtained: an obvious/known difficult airway, a previous failed sedation by the gastroenterology team, problems associated with prior anesthetic exposure, morbid obesity, stridor, snoring, sleep apnea, gastroesophageal reflux/aspiration risk, and procedures performed in the prone position. Patients may be tolerant to sedative medications if they are chronic users of benzodiazepines, narcotics, alcohol, or other drugs. Patients with neurologic diseases may be more susceptible to sedative medications and may hypoventilate. Patients with psychiatric disorders or extremely anxious patients may not cooperate during the procedure. Patients who have had a previous unsatisfactory experience with sedation for this procedure may request general anesthesia. Patients who have a known difficult airway or who have features suggestive of a difficult airway/difficult mask (small mouth opening; head and neck cancer patients, particularly after radiation therapy; patients with cervical fusions and limited airway/extension of the neck) are frequently scheduled with an anesthesiologist from the beginning. (Cole & Schlunt, 2004, p. 393)

21. What are the considerations when choosing general, regional, or local anesthesia?

The choice of general anesthesia does have some limitations as well as some advantages. Increased time scheduled for the procedure allows for a thorough preoperative evaluation, as well as induction and positioning of the intubated patient in the prone position. The procedure room must incorporate enough space for the addition of anesthesia personnel and equipment. The cost per procedure is increased. However, in a small study of 65 patients, the use of general anesthesia resulted in fewer complications. In addition, patients who have had an unsuccessful sedation in the past may successfully complete the procedure with propofol sedation or with a general anesthetic. (Cole & Schlunt, 2004, p. 393)

22. What are the considerations when choosing spontaneous respirations versus orotracheal sedation in gastrointestinal endoscopy?

The size of the patient and his or her airway condition are crucial factors in choosing the appropriate sedation techniques. If, according to the anesthesiologist's opinion, the patient is a good candidate for sedation with spontaneous respirations (i.e., small stature, good airway), then the procedure is executed in the prone position. If, on the other end, the patient is not a good candidate for sedation with spontaneous respirations (i.e., obese, difficult airway, gastroesophageal reflux), orotracheal intubation is preferred (Cole & Schlunt, 2004).

23. What postanesthesia complications can occur after gastrointestinal surgery?

In general, most postanesthesia complications with gastrointestinal surgery happen several days following the operation. They are life threatening and immediate intervention is needed. A good example is the esophageal perforation following instrumentation of the esophagus; the patient is instructed to report to the surgeon any pain and fever after the surgery as they are signs and symptoms of a perforated esophagus. If the situation presents, an esophagram is immediately ordered to rule out any life-threatening complications. Surgery is the preferred treatment. Another postanesthesia complication is blood loss at the surgical site or internal blood loss. Patients are closely monitored for signs and symptoms of this serious complication (e.g., hypotension, tachycardia) (Brown & Brown, 1997).

24. What is the surgical treatment of choice for patients suffering from peptic ulcers?

Pyloroplasty is the surgical treatment of choice. It consists on the formation of a larger passageway between the prepyloric region of the stomach and the first or second portion of the duodenum with excision of the peptic ulcer. This technique is also used to remove cicatricial bands in the pyloric ring to relieve spasm and to permit rapid emptying of the stomach (Meeker & Rothrock, 1999).

25. What surgical repair is available to patients suffering from gastroesophageal reflux disease (GERD)?

Laparoscopic Nissen fundoplication is usually done when a patient has failed to respond to previous medical treatment. It is a fairly uncommon procedure as only a small percentage of GERD patients need surgical attention. GERD is usually controlled or treated by basic antireflux regimen of antacids and a specific diet (Ignatavicius & Workman, 2010).

26. What specific postanesthesia care should be provided to an infant following surgery for pyloric stenosis?

The first priority is the position. The infant should be placed and kept on the right side or on the abdomen until the risk of emesis and aspiration has subsided. An upright position is advised next. Contamination of the wound by urine or feces is a concern and proper diaper placement is crucial. The placement of a pediatric urine collector is useful to avoid contamination of the wound and to calculate an accurate urine output postsurgery. Feedings can usually resume 4–6 hours postoperatively unless specific surgeon orders have been given (Drain, 1994).

27. What surgery is also known as the Whipple procedure?

The Whipple procedure is also known as radical pancreaticoduodenectomy.

The process is the removal of the head of the pancreas, the entire duodenum, a portion of the jejunum, the distal third of the stomach, the lower half of the common bile duct, and a portion of the pancreatic duct, with reestablishment of continuity of the biliary, pancreatic, and gastrointestinal systems. (Ignatavicius & Workman, 2010, p. 1382)

28. What surgical management is available for patients suffering from Crohn's disease?

Once all nonsurgical options have failed, the surgical treatment of choice for patients with Crohn's disease is the resection (partial or total) of the diseased area. The procedure can be performed as minimally invasive surgery (MIS) via laparoscopy, which leaves the patient with less scaring and more manageable postoperative pain. Both small bowel resection and ileocecal resection can be achieved using this procedure (Ignatavicius & Workman, 2010).

29. What surgical treatment of choice is available for patients suffering of diverticular disease?

Inflammation of the diverticulum can put the patient at risk for peritonitis, pelvic abscess, bowel obstruction, fistula, persistent fever and pain, or uncontrollable bleeding. If rupture happens, an emergency surgery is in order. The most common surgery to treat a ruptured diverticulum is the colon resection, with or without a colostomy. Postoperative care is the same for any patients undergoing abdominal surgery (Ignatavicius & Workman, 2010).

30. What postsurgical concern is to be considered after a hemorrhoidectomy?

Due to the rectal spasms and anorectal tenderness, urinary retention is a major concern for patients with hemorrhoidectomy. To prevent bladder distention, detailed urinary output should be recorded by the nurse, and a Foley catheter should be ready to be inserted if urinary retention is suspected. Another rare but potential complication is hemorrhage as it could be internal and not visible. Careful vital signs monitoring is requested (Ignatavicius & Workman, 2010).

31. What are the general discharge instructions for the patient undergoing gastrointestinal surgery?

Due to the swelling inside the gastrointestinal tract, the patient may feel a pressure or tightness that should dissipate in 6–8 weeks. The discharge nurse should advise the patient to avoid carbonated drinks for 3–4 weeks in order to alleviate internal bloating. Solid foods should be gradually added to the patient's daily diet, and the importance of chewing should be underlined. To prevent and avoid infection, proper teaching is needed to keep the incisional area clean and dry. Signs and symptoms of complication (e.g., persistent fever, bleeding, increasing pain, persistent nausea and vomiting, chills, persistent cough or shortness of breath) must be immediately reported to the doctor (Meeker & Rothrock, 1999).

32. What surgical treatment of choice is available for patient suffering of cholelithiasis?

Cholelithiasis is a common occurrence in patients with chronic gallbladder disease. In the past, cholecystectomy was the surgery of choice, but more recently, biliary lithotripsy is selected by surgeons. Biliary lithotripsy has many advantages, including no surgical incision, less pain, a shorter postoperative period, and a reduction in cost to the patient. In addition, the patient has a 50% reduction in postoperative pulmonary complications. Biliary lithotripsy consists in breaking the gallstones down into small fragments, with the patient receiving either local anesthesia and sedation or general anesthesia (Drain, 1994).

33. What are the possible complications during biliary lithotripsy procedure?

Complications of this procedure are associated with the type of anesthetic technique and its inherent complications and from the shock wave therapy used during the procedure. The most common problems from this procedure include nausea, vomiting, abdominal pain, hemoptysis, and diarrhea. The postanesthesia care for a patient recovering from biliary lithotripsy is the same as for the upper abdominal surgical patient (Drain, 1994).

34. What procedures are available to the patient diagnosed with pancreatic cancer?

The proper procedure is based on the staging of the disease. The Whipple procedure is often preferred to treat cancer of the head of the pancreas. "This procedure entails a gastrectomy, a pancreaticojejunostomy, a choledochojejunostomy, and a gastrojejunostomy. It is also common for the surgeon to perform a splenectomy during this procedure" (Ignatavicius & Workman, 2010, p. 1382).

35. What postsurgical concerns are to be considered after a Whipple procedure?

Because of the intensive surgical intervention needed during a pancreaticoduodenectomy, the patient is usually admitted to the surgical critical care unit for recovery. Preventive measures are required to avoid complications such as pancreatitis, hepatic failure, infection, fistulas (pancreatic, gastric, and biliary), renal failure, acute respiratory distress syndrome, pulmonary embolism, thrombophlebitis, or heart failure. Upon arrival to the PACU or ICU (intensive care unit), the patient is placed in the semi-Fowler's position to reduce tension on the suture line and anastomosis site. This position also allows the lungs to expand in order to avoid pulmonary complications. Because of the extensive duration of the procedure, maintaining adequate fluid and electrolyte balance is fundamental. In addition, glucose levels should be monitored frequently to prevent hypoglycemia or hyperglycemia due to the stress and manipulation of the pancreas (Ignatavicius & Workman, 2010).

36. In treating appendicitis, what is the difference between laparoscopy versus laparotomy approach?

Today, most appendectomy procedures are done via laparoscopy, a MIS procedure with several small incisions near the umbilicus through which a small endoscope is placed. Patients undergoing MIS procedures are usually discharged the day of the surgery and recover quickly. In the case of an atypical appendicitis or peritonitis (medical emergency), a laparotomy is then advised. Patients undergoing a procedure with a laparotomy have a longer hospitalization and recovery time due to larger abdominal incisions (Ignatavicius & Workman, 2010).

REFERENCES

Brown, M., & Brown, E. M. (1997). *Comprehensive postanesthesia care*. Baltimore, MD: Williams & Wilkins.

Cole, D. J., & Schlunt, M. (2004). *Adult perioperative anesthesia—the requisites in anesthesiology*. Philadelphia: Elsevier Mosby.

Drain, C. B. (1994). *The postanesthesia care unit*. Philadelphia: W. B. Saunders Company.

Ignatavicius, D. D., & Workman, M. L. (2010). *Medical-surgical nursing—patient-centered collaborative care*. St. Louis, MO: Saunders Elsevier.

Meeker, M. H., & Rothrock, J. C. (1999). *Care of the patient in surgery*. St. Louis, MO: Mosby, Inc.

Montalvo, I. (2010). The national database of nursing quality indicators (NDNQI): Future plans and goals for NDNQI. Retrieved from http://www.medscape.com/viewarticle/569395_5.

CHAPTER 22

Cardiac Surgery

Gail Gustafson, RN, MSN, CRNP

Cardiac surgery is the field of surgery that treats cardiovascular disease through surgical intervention and postoperative management. This includes any surgery where the chest is opened and surgery is performed on the heart muscle, valves, arteries, or other heart structures. Although cardiac surgery is a very large field that includes many types of surgeries, postoperative management is still very similar.

1. What are the indications for cardiac surgery?

Patients with coronary artery disease, valvular dysfunction, congenital heart defect, aneurysm, and cardiomyopathy may receive cardiac surgery. As the ability to do noninvasive procedures such as coronary stenting increases, the population that actually receives cardiac surgery are sicker and older.

2. What is the importance of preoperative assessment for cardiac surgery?

It is extremely important that a patient has a good preoperative evaluation. The perioperative and postoperative course can be adjusted to reduce morbidity and mortality by establishing a good historic reference and identifying the risk factors before surgery. The source of most postoperative complications are existing preoperative problems or a consequence of the operation and cardiopulmonary bypass.

3. What is included in the preoperative workup?

The preoperative evaluation includes the chief complaint, history of present illness, past medical history, previous cardiac interventions, past surgical history, family history, social history, review of systems, allergies, medications, physical exam by system, current medications, and preoperative laboratory results and studies.

It is important to have a standardized systematic preoperative assessment to ensure all topics will be thoroughly covered. Once the preoperative workup is completed, any abnormalities are discussed with the surgeon. Depending on abnormalities that are found, this can increase the risks associated with surgery and postoperative recovery.

4. What are some of the major risk factors for complications in cardiac surgery?

The more risk factors a patient has, the higher the risk for cardiac surgery. Some of the risk factors include multiple procedures (cardiac and noncardiac), age, gender, race, body surface area, diabetes, hemoglobin A1c, renal insufficiency, hemodialysis, endocarditis, hypertension, chronic lung disease, immunosuppressive therapy, peripheral vascular disease, cerebrovascular disease or accident, previous cardiac interventions, myocardial infarction, cardiac presentation on admission (angina symptoms), congestive heart failure, cardiogenic shock, resuscitation, arrhythmia, atrial fibrillation or flutter, inotropic agent, number of diseased vessels, left main disease greater than 50%, ejection fraction, aortic stenosis, mitral stenosis, aortic insufficiency, mitral insufficiency, tricuspid insufficiency, number of reoperations, status of procedure (urgent, emergent, salvage), and the presence of intraaortic balloon pump (Ferguson et al., 2000).

5. Is there a standard risk that can be applied as a calculator?

Preoperative prediction tools have been developed and trialed to calculate a patient's risk for a longer and more complicated postoperative course. There is no standard risk calculator used. Frequently, the estimate that more risk factors equals more operative risk for patients receiving cardiac surgery is used.

6. What is coronary artery bypass grafting (CABG) surgery?

CABG (pronounced like cabbage) is used when there is a blockage that prevents blood flow in the coronary artery. The surgeon may use the saphenous vein from the leg, which runs down the inner aspect of each leg from groin to ankle. New techniques such as endoscopic vein harvesting has significantly decreased the infection rates and postoperative pain associated with the removal of this vein. The surgeon may also choose to use an artery that sits along the chest wall called the internal mammary artery. The surgeon will attach one end to the blocked artery below the blockage and the other end to the aorta. This allows a bypass or new highway for blood to circulate to the heart muscle.

7. What is valve surgery?

Valve surgery may include replacement or repair. This occurs when a valve is dysfunctional either from stenosis or regurgitation and does not allow the blood to continue in a forward direction. In stenosis, the valve becomes too small and the blood cannot move forward. In regurgitation, the valve will not completely close and the blood then leaks forward and backward, thus prohibiting adequate forward flow.

8. What is congenital surgery?

Congenital surgery can involve any part of the heart structure. This surgery may close a hole, such as with an atrial septal defect or ventricular septal defect. Congenital surgery can also become extremely complicated and involve removing and replacing many vessels of the heart. The goal of surgery for congenital defects is to allow a path from which unoxygenated blood can be carried to the lungs, and oxygenated blood can be carried from the lungs to the heart muscle and the rest of the body.

9. What is aneurysm repair surgery?

Aneurysm repair surgery can be minimal and involve placement of a patch to add strength to a weakened vessel, or it may be extensive and involve replacement of many vessels. This is generally done with a Dacron device that is shaped like a tube and comes in varied sizes.

10. What other surgeries are performed in cardiac surgery?

Cardiac surgery may also include placement of a left ventricular pacemaker lead, ventricular remodeling, aortic conduit, ventricular assist device, or heart transplantation. New surgeries as well as new techniques to perform the old surgeries are being developed every day.

11. What happens during cardiac surgery?

Cardiac surgery involves opening the chest. This can be done via sternotomy, thoracotomy, or a minimally invasive approach that goes through the rib cage. Cardioplegia may be utilized either warm (37°C) or cold (4°C) to slow or stop the heart. With cold cardioplegia, the heart is not beating and needs much less oxygen. With warm cardioplegia, the heart is still beating, which makes surgery more technically difficult for the surgeon. During cardiac surgery, the patient may require the use of a cardiopulmonary bypass.

12. What is cardiopulmonary bypass?

Cardiopulmonary bypass is a machine that does the work of the heart and lungs by moving the blood like the heart and oxygenating the blood like the lungs. This machine works by having a large plastic tube placed through the right atrial appendage into the inferior vena cava. The blood then goes through this machine and can either heat or cool the blood as well as provide oxygen. The blood is then returned to the patient via another tube into the patient's aorta. In this method, the blood bypasses the heart and recirculates back into the patient's body, thus allowing the heart to be opened and operated on. During a bypass, the patient's blood is heparinized to achieve an activated clotting time (ACT) greater than 450 to prevent the blood from clotting while it runs through the bypass machine.

13. What care is specific to the operating room during heart surgery?

Intraoperative care affects postoperative care and this begins management of the patient as they go through the physical changes related to cardiac surgery. Before coming off bypass, heparin is reversed with protamine at a dose of 10 mg per 1000 units of heparin to achieve a normal ACT. While it is essential to have the patient's blood thinned during surgery, it can cause extremely serious effects once surgery is completed. While coming off bypass, the hemodynamics and oxygenation of the patient are closely monitored. The bypass machine has been delivering, as well as oxygenating the blood. It is essential to monitor that the heart and lungs are able to adequately resume these jobs while the patient comes off bypass.

14. How is the heart assessed in the perioperative period?

The surgeon will assess the patient's heart contractility before, during, and after a cardiac operation by measurements of ejection fraction, ventricular wall motion, and cardiac output. This may be done by direct visual observation, transesophageal echocardiogram (TEE), or invasive monitoring. For monitoring, hemodynamics pulmonary artery (PA) catheters are frequently, but not always, used in the operative and intensive care unit (ICU) setting. All patients must have an arterial line and a central venous catheter.

15. What is the importance of a transesophageal echocardiogram (TEE) during surgery?

An intraoperative echocardiogram may be performed via TEE to look for new wall motion abnormalities, which may be indicative of ischemia, as well as adequate cardiac output while coming off bypass. A TEE is also performed after valve surgery to evaluate for success of the repair.

16. What is the use of cardiac assistance devices in cardiac surgery?

Patients who have difficulty coming off bypass may have an intra-aortic balloon pump (IABP) placed and maintained during the postoperative course to improve coronary perfusion and cardiac output. If the use of an inotropic support and IABP does not allow a patient to come off bypass and maintain good cardiac output, a ventricular assist device may also be placed. This device may be placed in the right, left, or both ventricles depending on which ventricle is failing.

17. What intraoperative hand-off information is important for postoperative care?

Upon admission to the postoperative area, the surgical anaesthesia staff will give a report of the patient's preoperative workup, surgical procedure, and intraoperative course. All of this information is important because it affects management during the patient's postoperative course. The intraoperative report includes what happened prebypass, on bypass, and coming off bypass. This may include the echocardiogram results and the hemodynamics

that allowed the patient to have the best cardiac output. The most recent blood values will be obtained in order to adjust medications like insulin, to manage the ventilator, and to monitor postoperative bleeding. Admission labs for a nonbleeding patient will include arterial blood gas, hemoglobin, potassium, glucose, and I-calcium. For a bleeding patient, admission labs will also include aPTT, PT, CBC, fibrinogen, and possibly a thromboelastogram so that a coagulopathy may be appropriately treated.

18. What is the estimated postoperative recovery time for cardiac surgery patients?

With new techniques and quicker, less invasive surgeries without the need for cardiopulmonary bypass, recovery can be as quick as 3–4 days for CABG and 4–6 days for valve surgery.

19. What would a stable postoperative cardiac surgery patient look like?

The patient would either be extubated in the operating room (OR) or would be extubated within 6 hours of arrival to the postoperative area. The patient would have come off bypass without inotropic support and would therefore not have a need for a PA catheter. The chest tubes placed in the OR would have minimal drainage and will be removed postoperative day 1. Pacer wires would not be needed and therefore not placed. The patient would be able to ambulate, have all invasive lines removed, and restart preoperative medications on the first postoperative day.

20. What are some of the causes of postoperative hemodynamic instability in the cardiac surgery patient?

Causes include hypovolemia (the most frequent and easily treated), as well as bleeding, cardiogenic shock, and cardiac tamponade. Causes of hemodynamic instability are not exclusive of each other.

21. Why is it important to treat hypovolemia?

Volume replacement is the treatment for hypovolemia. As patients rewarm, the venous system dilates and the need for ongoing volume replacement is important to prevent hypovolemia. Volume therapy recommendations are individualized and can be guided by the intraoperative report and current hemodynamics. Hypovolemia can be even more pronounced in a patient who has left ventricular hypertrophy (LVH). About 15–20% of patients with hypertension have LVH, which increases twofold in obese patients (Cabezas et al., 1997).

22. What is important information about a bleeding patient?

Bleeding can lead to hypovolemia, cardiogenic shock, and cardiac tamponade. Generally, bleeding more than 100 cc/hr for 2 hours is considered too much. It is important to determine if bleeding is medical or surgical, and to use coagulation labs including CBC, PT, aPTT, fibrinogen, and thromboelastogram to evaluate clotting function.

23. How should a bleeding patient be treated?

If a patient received a preoperative medication affecting platelet function or if platelets are less than 100,000 and bleeding is a problem, the patient should receive platelets. PTT elevation usually means a deficit in factor VIII and DDAVP would be given. An elevated PT/INR would be treated with FFP. A low fibrinogen level in a bleeding patient would be treated with cryoprecipitate. Until the patient stops bleeding, any loss will have PRBC replacement. If a patient has not received the maximum protamine needed to inactivate the operative heparin, then this may also be given. The surgeon must always be notified for postoperative bleeding. If a patient's blood work does not demonstrate the presence of a coagulopathy, this may be an indication of surgical bleeding and may require a return to the OR for evaluation and possible surgical repair.

24. When is cardiogenic shock anticipated?

Cardiac complications are not a surprise after cardiac surgery. There are many complications that can occur to the heart after cardiac surgery. Cardiogenic shock is the result of inadequate cardiac output. Left ventricular (LV) or right ventricular (RV) failure may also be causes of cardiogenic shock and may be the result of myocardial stunning and reperfusion injury. LV failure is usually reflected as low cardiac output, pulmonary congestion, and hypotension. RV failure may be reflected by an increased central venous pressure and pulmonary artery diastolic pressures. Patients with pulmonary hypertension are at high risk of developing RV failure.

25. What is the importance of the cardiac output?

Cardiac output can be measured by invasive monitoring such as a PA catheter or clinical exam. To determine cardiac output, multiply stroke volume by heart rate. The optimum heart rate after cardiac surgery is 80–100 bpm. If the rate is slower, it may compromise the cardiac output. In the absence of invasive monitoring to measure cardiac output, we must rely on clinical exam. Skin temperature, capillary refill, pulse rate, blood pressure, urine output, and level of consciousness are reliable markers of cardiac output and are easily assessed.

26. How can the heart rate be adjusted after cardiac surgery?

A patient may have epicardial pacing wires placed in the OR before chest closure. These wires may be atrial and ventricular and can be attached to a pacemaker to increase the patient's heart rate. Slowing a heart that is too fast is equally important because a fast beating heart may cause unnecessary work on a heart that is trying to recover from surgery and may lead to myocardial ischemia.

27. What are considerations when assessing stroke volume?

Stroke volume is dependent on three important factors: preload, afterload, and contractility. All of these factors are linked when looking at a struggling heart, and it is important to understand how the factors affect each other and the underlying cardiac output. Addressing medical reasons for low cardiac output includes too high or too low of a heart rate, too high or too low blood pressure, and too much or not enough volume. The intravenous medications used in the immediate postoperative area serve to improve these three factors influencing stroke volume and cardiac output. If these attempts do not improve cardiac output, then surgical complications should be considered, including coronary graft occlusion, valve malfunction, tamponade, bleeding, and coronary spasm.

28. What is preload?

Preload is the force distending the ventricle. The greater the stretch (within certain limits), the greater the force of contraction (known as the Frank-Starling curve). The heart, like an elastic band, has the ability to stretch. An increase in preload will result in an increase in cardiac output. Factors affecting preload include blood volume, heart rate, body position, respiratory affects on intrathoracic pressure, venous return of blood, atrial contraction, and valve regurgitation.

29. What is afterload?

Afterload is the force that the ventricles push against to eject the blood. This is largely dependent on blood pressure and vascular resistance, but may also be affected by myocardial stiffening. Increasing afterload increases myocardial oxygen consumption and may decrease stroke volume and cardiac output.

30. What is contractility?

Contractility is the ability of the heart muscle to contract independent of preload and afterload, but dependent on the catecholamine and inotropic state. A positive inotropic response will increase contractility. Drugs such as norepinephrine and epinephrine have a positive inotropic effect. Sympathetic stimulation can also increase circulating catecholamines and the heart rate. Cardiopulmonary bypass may cause a surge of catecholamines in the patient, but this may only be temporary. The indication for inotropic support postcoronary pulmonary bypass surgery is depressed cardiac output in the face of an adequate preload and acceptably low afterload (mean BP). In one large study of 1500 elective cardiac surgery patients, over more than 30% required inotropic support postbypass (Müller et al., 2002).

31. What arrhythmias occur after cardiac surgery?

Arrhythmias such as ventricular fibrillation and ventricular tachycardia, atrial arrhythmias such as atrial fibrillation, and heart blocks can all occur after cardiac surgery. Atrial fibrillation is the most common postoperative arrhythmia. The loss of atrial kick with atrial fibrillation may result in up to a 30% decrease in cardiac output. Amiodarone is commonly given as a postoperative prophylaxis for atrial fibrillation. Arrhythmias may best be treated by following an important rule: If the patient is hemodynamically unstable, use electricity (cardioversion or defibrillation), and if the patient is hemodynamically stable, use drugs like amiodarone. Heart blocks, which are more common after valve surgery, may be treated with a pacemaker or medication. This may depend upon the availability of epicardial wires, which can be placed by the surgeon at the end of the operation.

32. Why is an EKG important after cardiac surgery?

Ischemia is a concern after cardiac surgery and postoperatively, an EKG is routinely obtained to monitor for early signs. A patient that just had surgery may have coronary spasm, plaque rupture causing a new coronary occlusion, or blockage of a new bypass graft. Troponin levels may be obtained to evaluate for ischemia, but, unless significantly elevated, it is difficult to differentiate between new ischemia and tissue damage related to recent surgery. EKG changes associated with hemodynamic instability is a cardiac emergency and the patient should go immediately for coronary angiography. The same rules apply here as to a new myocardial infarction (MI): Time saves lives, and it

is important to get blood flow to the coronary as soon as possible.

33. What is cardiac tamponade?

Cardiac tamponade starts as hemodynamic instability, but can quickly progress to cardiac arrest and asystole. In tamponade, the heart cannot adequately contract due to external forces, usually blood around the heart. The initial symptoms may be a sudden decrease in chest tube drainage, pulsus paradoxus, an increase in central venous and pulmonary diastolic pressures, and a decrease in cardiac output. A chest x-ray must be obtained immediately to look for a widened mediastinum. An echocardiogram can also be obtained to rule out tamponade. A blocked chest tube preventing drainage can be a simpler fix, but generally, enough volume to cause a tamponade will need surgical intervention.

34. What are the neurologic complications that can occur with cardiac surgery?

The most severe neurologic complications include stroke, seizure, and brain damage. Neurologic complication is second only to heart failure as a cause of morbidity and mortality following cardiac surgery (Gardner et al., 1985). A patient older than the age of 60 years and/or a prior history of TIA, CVA, or vascular surgery will receive a preoperative carotid ultrasound. If there is severe disease, the patient will receive a preoperative consult by a vascular surgeon and carotid surgery, if appropriate prior to cardiac surgery. A patient who undergoes cardiopulmonary bypass is at higher risk for neurologic complication. Many factors, including preoperative neurologic abnormalities, hypoxia, hypothermia, anesthetics, and thrombosis from cardiac manipulation and cross clamp can cause intraoperative neurologic complications. Cerebral ischemia can occur when cerebral oxygen is insufficient to meet the cerebral oxygen consumption. It is especially important to get an early neurologic exam after cardiac surgery and, once obtained, the patient is closely monitored for any change in exam. Neurologic complications can occur at anytime during the postoperative course.

35. What are the pulmonary complications after cardiac surgery?

The postoperative pulmonary goal for the cardiac surgery patient is to be extubated as soon as possible. Preoperative pulmonary function tests can assist in the estimation of the likelihood of success or failure at early postoperative extubation. The risks of intubation include ventilator-acquired pneumonia and failure to wean from the ventilator, which may lead to tracheostomy and long-term ventilator management. Ventilator management is a frequent contributor to extended ICU stay and hospitalization (Hortal et al., 2009).

As the patient rewarms, CO_2 production increases. Managing the patient when they are cold with a slight respiratory alkalosis may prevent hypercapnia and acidosis when the patient reaches normal body temperature.

36. What is the formula to estimate the effects of changes in ventilator settings on arterial blood gas?

The following formula can be used to estimate changes in ventilator settings on pCO_2:

$$\text{Present } pCO_2 \times \text{minute ventilation} = \text{desired } pCO_2 \times \text{new minute ventilation}$$

Every blood gas obtained should be analyzed for evidence of respiratory and/or metabolic acidosis or alkalosis. Arterial blood gas base excess or deficit can be evaluated if every 10 mmHg change in pCO_2 is accompanied by a reciprocal change in arterial pH of .08, the decimal is disregarded, and then take two thirds of the difference between the expected pH and the actual pH. This is the base excess or deficit.

37. What are considerations that need to be included in the extubation protocol?

Most institutions have an extubation protocol that is initiated early in all patients to minimize the time on the ventilator. The extubation protocol may use a rate wean, in which the rate of breaths of the ventilator is slowly decreased to the point that a patient is able to take breaths unassisted. A pressure support wean may also be used, which allows the amount of assistance that the ventilator gives to each patients breath to be slowly decreased to the point that the patient is initiating breaths unassisted. When a patient gets to the minimal setting and they are initiating their own breaths with normal ABGs, mechanics are obtained.

38. What are pulmonary mechanics?

Pulmonary mechanics include a forced vital capacity (FVC), an outward measurement of air movement and a negative inspiratory force (NIF), an inward measurement of air movement. These two measurements equal the actions necessary for breathing. In addition, the rapid shallow breathing index (RSBI) is obtained. This is a measurement that calculates the frequency (RR) × tidal volume, and RSBI less than 105 is considered to be a predictor of extubation success. The predictability

of success increases as the RSBI decreases. The potential for pulmonary complications does not end once a patient is extubated.

39. What are the considerations related to pneumonia?

Cardiac surgery patients can develop pneumonia related to many factors. Aspiration pneumonia may occur if the patient does not have adequate ability to swallow prior to oral intake being initiated. After endotracheal tube removal, a bedside swallow test may be obtained by the nurse. If the patient is high risk or does not pass the nurses criteria for swallowing, a speech therapist should evaluate the patient. A cine-esophagram may need to be performed, which is an x-ray obtained while the patient swallows a radiopaque contrast material to evaluate if he or she has silent aspiration. Another pneumonia risk may be related to a patient's poor cough effort associated with incisional pain. Use of an incentive spirometer or flutter valve can help a patient achieve adequate pulmonary toilet and ward off any possible pneumonia. Ventilator-associated pneumonia (VAP) is also a major cause of mortality post-cardiac surgery. Risk factors for VAP include mixed ICU, days on mechanical ventilation, number of blood products transfused, IABP, use of vasopressors, peripheral vascular disease, renal disease, reoperation, ascending aorta surgery, and length of surgery.

40. What should be done for postoperative incisional pain?

Pain control is extremely important and can help quicken recovery, as well as reduce the risk of developing certain complications after surgery, such as pneumonia and blood clots. If pain is well controlled, the patient will be better able to complete important tasks such as walking and deep breathing exercises.

Pain may be treated with oral narcotics such as acetaminophen and oxycodone (such as Tylox or Percocet). If the patient cannot yet take oral medication, intravenous narcotics using a patient-controlled analgesia device or infusion pump may be used. Other forms of pain relief include acetaminophen, NSAIDS, anesthetic (Marcaine), or epidural.

41. What are the renal complications after cardiac surgery?

Preoperative evaluation of kidney function can be used to assess and adjust intraoperative and postoperative care to further reduce detrimental effects of surgery. A patient with preoperative renal insufficiency, diabetes, advanced age, renal artery stenosis, and long bypass runs will be more likely to have postoperative renal complications that may lead to a need for temporary or even permanent dialysis. BUN and creatinine levels in the initial postoperative period are not indicative of renal failure and may be more related to volume shifts and the effects of cardiopulmonary bypass. Renal failure can be separated into three stages: prerenal, intrinsic renal, and postrenal.

42. What care is necessary in prerenal failure?

In prerenal failure there is presence of normal tubular and glomerular function with depressed GFR (glomerular filtration rate) from decreased renal perfusion. Early support and improvement in renal blood flow by maintaining adequate cardiac output and blood pressure is essential to prevent long-term kidney damage and progression to intrinsic renal failure most commonly acute tubular necrosis (ATN).

43. What are the causes and care of intrinsic renal failure?

Intrinsic renal failure includes damage to the kidney itself that can affect the glomerulus or tubule. ATN (acute tubular necrosis) must be suspected in patients who have experienced a period of hypotension or decreased perfusion after cardiac surgery. Ischemic renal injury is the most common cause of intrinsic renal failure, but toxins may also be a cause and close management of nephrotoxic agents needs to be made postoperatively.

44. What is postrenal failure?

Postrenal failure is usually an obstruction beyond the kidney. A common cause after cardiac surgery is an improperly placed or kinked Foley catheter. This should be suspected when there is sudden oliguria, which can be diagnosed and usually treated by repositioning and flushing the catheter. Clots may also cause an obstruction, but ongoing hematuria may require continuous bladder irrigation and urology consultation.

45. What causes gastrointestinal complications?

Gastrointestinal complications are not common, but when they occur, they can carry a high morbidity and mortality rate. The major cause of gastrointestinal complications is ischemia caused by hypotension, low cardiac output, and cardiopulmonary bypass. This complication may be precipitated by a metabolic acidosis, and although this can have many causes, a lactate level, abdominal x-ray, and CT should be performed. Other gastrointestinal

complications include pancreatitis, gastroduodenal ulceration and inflammation, emboli/thrombosis, gastrointestinal bleeding, cholecystitis, and liver failure. Calcium chloride is frequently used in cardiac surgery, but the use of more than 800 mg per square meter of body surface area is an independent risk factor for pancreatitis.

46. What causes infectious complications after cardiac surgery?

The standard postoperative empiric antibiotic includes a 24-hour course of vancomycin (if the patient is allergic to penicillin), but these should not be given to a patient who has an infectious diagnosis like endocarditis. The infections that are most prevalent in postoperative cardiac surgery include mediastinitis, catheter-related bloodstream infections, urinary tract infection (UTI), bacteremia, saphenous vein site infection, and ventilator-associated pneumonia.

Risk factors for increased risk of mediastinitis include advanced age, obesity, preoperative hospital stay, current smoker, diabetes, low albumin, and preoperative and nasal presence of MRSA. The risks for the cardiac surgery patient are not only related to their incision.

REFERENCES

Cabezas, M., Comellas, A., Ramon Gomez, J., Lopez Grillo, L., Casal, H., Carrillo, N., et al. (1997). Comparison of the sensitivity and specificity of the electrocardiography criteria for left ventricular hypertrophy according to the methods of Romhilt-Estes, Sokolow-Lyon, Cornell, and Rodriguez Padial. *Revista Espanola de Cardiologia, 50*(1), 31–35.

Ferguson, T. B., Dziuban, Jr., S. W., Edwards, F. H., Eiken, M. C., Shroyer, A. L. W., Pairolero, P. C., et al. (2000). The STS National Database: current changes and challenges for the new millennium. *The Annals of Thoracic Surgery, 69*, 680–691.

Gardner, T. J., Horneffer, P. J., Manolio, T. A., Pearson, T. A., Gott, V. L., Baumgartner, W. A., Borkon, A. M., Watkins, Jr., L., & Reitz, B. A. (1985). Stroke following coronary artery bypass grafting: A ten-year study. *The Annals of Thoracic Surgery, 40*(6), 574–581.

Hortal, J., Muñoz, P., Cuerpo, G., Litvan, H., Rosseel, P. M., & Bouza, E. (2009). Ventilator-associated pneumonia in patients undergoing major heart surgery: An incidence study in Europe. *Critical Care, 13*(3), R80.

Müller, M., Junger, A., Bräu, M., Kwapisz, M. M., Schindler, E., Akintürk, H., et al. (2002). Incidence and risk calculation of inotropic support in patients undergoing cardiac surgery with cardiopulmonary bypass using an automated anaesthesia record-keeping system. *British Journal of Anaesthesia, 89*(3), 398–404.

CHAPTER 23

Plastic and Reconstructive Surgeries

Ruth J. Lee, RN, MS, MBA, Renee Blanding, MD, MPH, & Michelle A. Shermak, MD, FACS

INTRODUCTION

The word plastic derives from the Greek work *plastikos* and means to mold or shape (American Society of Plastic Surgeons [ASPS], 2010b). Many modern plastic surgery techniques evolved from devastating wartime reconstructive needs: Sir Harold Gillies in England, one of the pioneers of modern plastic surgery, took care of victims of trench warfare who suffered from disfiguring facial, trunk, and extremity injuries requiring both functional and aesthetic coverage (Gillies, 1983).

Plastic and reconstructive surgery is becoming more prevalent and more of a topic of interest. While plastic surgical procedures are generally separated into cosmetic and reconstructive surgeries, there is often a blurred boundary between the two. While breast augmentation may seem to be cosmetic, in a teenage girl with developmental deformity and significant asymmetry, breast augmentation serves a reconstructive purpose. Similarly, in a massive weight loss patient with severe skin excess, an abdominoplasty serves a much greater purpose beyond a straightforward aesthetic definition.

While much of plastic surgery is performed in the hospital setting, more procedures are moving into an ambulatory surgery setting, converting the recovery room into an area with much higher turnover. This chapter will review several of the common plastic surgery procedures performed and the perianesthesia nursing needs of the plastic surgery patient.

RECONSTRUCTIVE PLASTIC SURGERY PROCEDURES

1. What are some of the common reconstructive plastic surgery procedures performed in a hospital setting?

According to the ASPS, in 2008, 4.9 million reconstructive surgery procedures were performed. The top five procedures were: tumor removal, laceration repair, scar revision, hand surgery, and breast reduction. Other reconstructive procedures performed included breast reconstruction, burn care, maxillofacial surgery for oncologic or traumatic reconstruction, dog bite repair, birth defect reconstruction, and tumor removal (ASPS, 2010a).

2. What plastic surgery methods are used on these common procedures?

For reconstructive cases, plastic surgeons follow the reconstructive ladder when considering how to address cases. The lowest rung of the ladder is primary closure. The next step is skin grafting, split thickness, or full thickness. Grafting also may involve allografting, which is human skin temporarily applied for wound coverage to stabilize the wound bed. This is done when the donor sites for skin grafting are limited or when the wound bed is not completely clean so that the graft may die. Grafting is following in complexity by flap procedures. Local flaps involve movement of adjacent tissue to reconstruct a defect such as moving local skin into a facial defect for cancer reconstruction or moving adjacent gastrocnemius or soleus muscle into a traumatic lower extremity tibia defect. The highest rung of the reconstructive ladder is free flap reconstruction, moving fat, fascia, muscle and/or skin, and attaching its blood supply to a recipient site which is distant, like the TRAM (transverse rectus abdominus myocutaneous) or DIEP (deep inferior epigastric perforator) abdominal tissue flaps for breast reconstruction. A reconstructive procedure not covered by the traditional reconstructive ladder is vacuum assisted closure (VAC), which optimizes an open wound healing in from the edges and depths of the wound from negative pressure applied through a sponge dressing and provided by an attached unit (Drain & Odom-Forren, 2008; Townsend, Mattox, Evers, & Beauchamp, 2007).

3. What occurs during a skin graft procedure?

The skin graft provides coverage for wounds that cannot be primarily closed, but have a bed that can provide adequate nutrition to a skin graft. For split thickness skin grafting (STSG), a layer of epidermis and underlying partial thickness dermis are harvested for transfer, often from the thigh. Full-thickness skin graft (FTSG) includes all of the epidermis and underlying dermis and is used for more durable coverage with minimal postoperative contraction such as treatment needed for a contracted neck after a burn injury (Drain & Odom-Forren, 2008). STSG donor sites are dressed in various ways, including semipermeable dressings, petroleum gauze, or silver products, and management of the wound depends on the coverage. FTSG donor sites, often including the groin area, are primarily closed. Allograft, or cadaver skin, is often dressed like STSG wounds. Allograft provides temporary coverage as the patient will ultimately reject the skin due to immune differences (Drain & Odom-Forren, 2008).

4. What are the primary differences between an STSG and FTSG? Why are they clinically important?

An STSG can be meshed to expand its size; the recipient site revascularizes the graft easily but is also vulnerable to surface trauma because of the graft's variable thickness. Postoperative STSG wounds tend to contract because of the minimal dermal element. The donor site from an STSG does not require primary closure and heals by regeneration of the epithelium (Drain & Odom-Forren, 2008).

An FTSG contains the epidermis and all of the dermis and provides more structural integrity when compared to an STSG. Because of the absence of the dermis, a primary closure of the wound edges of the donor site must occur. FTSG is preferred

when contraction of the skin in the healing process, such as that seen with STSG, would be detrimental. Body regions that mandate FTSG include the neck and joint surfaces like the axilla (Drain & Odom-Forren, 2008; Rothrock & McEwen, 2006).

5. What are some of the postoperative nursing considerations for patients with skin grafts?

Nursing considerations may be simplified into the three Ps: pressure, position, and pain. Avoid excessive pressure, which may interrupt the blood supply and cause subsequent ischemia. The position of the graft site is important; elevation reduces swelling and minimizes separation of the graft. Additionally, the graft site should be immobilized to avoid trauma and promote adherence of the graft. Pain management may be more pronounced in FTSGs, and is important postoperatively for comfort and to decrease agitation; excessive and prolonged pain after the administration of pain medicine may signal tissue ischemia and should be reported to the surgical team. The site should also be inspected for progressive edema, temperature, or cyanosis or blanching of the skin, which may indicate an interruption in the vascular supply. Skin grafted wounds cannot tolerate shear forces or hematoma or seroma, so dressings tend to be thick and compressive, and wounds near joint surfaces require immobilization (Drain & Odom-Forren, 2008).

6. What are some causes for graft failure?

Skin graft healing depends upon ingrowth of blood vessels from the wound bed into the graft, so anything that would interfere with consistent contact of the graft against the wound will compromise healing. Common causes for graft failure include infection, hematoma or seroma formation, and movement of the graft (Townsend et al., 2007).

7. What are flaps, and what are the clinical indications for flap surgery?

Flaps are tissue transfer procedures. For pedicled flaps, a portion of the tissue, whether it be muscle, fascia, and/or skin, is detached from its donor site while the remaining portion, the base or pedicle, remains attached to its defined blood supply, which is most often proximally based in considering the extremities. Flaps, in contrast to skin grafts, provide their own blood supply, which must remain unharmed. Much of the tissue in the human body has a well-defined blood supply. Flaps are indicated when large tissue defects require coverage. Examples of such scenarios include paralyzed, immobilized, or malnourished individuals with pressure sores with exposed infected bone, or in cases where there is exposed hardware or bone that requires coverage that is ample and can carry its own blood supply, which will also provide antibiotic coverage and more healing potential to the wound. There are several types of pedicled flaps. The type used depends on the blood supply and the type of tissue and the method of transfer used for the flap (Drain & Odom-Forren, 2008; Townsend et al., 2007).

If a wound has no viable options for adjacent tissue coverage, then more distant tissue must be imported into the wound with microvascular anastomosis from the imported tissue to vessels in the wound bed (Drain & Odom-Forren, 2008; Townsend et al., 2007).

8. What are the postoperative nursing considerations for flap procedures?

Flaps may be monitored for color, warmth, and appearance, and sometimes a Doppler is necessary to monitor vascularity. Necrosis of the tissue is a serious complication of flap procedures and may occur within hours of the procedure. Postoperatively, meticulous management of the patient's blood pressure should occur as hypotension may decrease perfusion to the flap and hypertension may cause bleeding due to damage to the delicate vessels repaired under the microscope. It is also important to closely observe the appearance of the flap. A pale, cool flap may indicate arterial occlusion, whereas venous blockage within the flap presents with darker, purple color and edema. The surgeon should be alerted immediately if changes in the flap occur during the postoperative period, which could occur as early as minutes after surgery (Drain & Odom-Forren, 2008; Rothrock & McEwen, 2006; Townsend et al., 2007).

COSMETIC PLASTICS SURGICAL PROCEDURES

9. What are the five most common surgical cosmetic procedures?

According to the ASPS, the five most common cosmetic procedures in 2008 were breast augmentation, rhinoplasty (nasal surgery), liposuction, blepharoplasty, and abdominoplasty. Other cosmetic surgery performed included rhytidoplasty (face-lift), browlift, mastopexy (breast-lift), breast implant removal, otoplasty (ear pinning), gynecomastia surgery (breast reduction in men), and mentoplasty (chin advancement) (ASPS, 2010a). With a growing population interested in weight loss, more body lifting procedures are being performed, including brachioplasty (arm-lift), upper and lower back-lift, buttock-lift, gluteal augmentation, and thigh-lift.

10. Which cosmetic procedure was the most common?

Over 300,000 breast augmentations were performed during 2008 (ASPS, 2010).

11. What is the purpose of breast augmentation?

The purpose of breast augmentation is to increase the size and/or modify the shape of the native breast, or to correct defects from congenital, developmental abnormalities, or from tumor removal. The breast implant, either saline or silicone, can be placed directly under the breast tissue or under the pectoralis major (chest) muscle; an endoscope may be used to insert the implant. Inframammary, axillary, periareolar incisions, or incisions from prior scars, like those from mastectomy, may be used (Rothrock & McEwen, 2006; Townsend et al., 2007).

12. Are silicone implants safe to use?

Silicon implants are absolutely safe to use. In the early 1990s, the U.S. Food and Drug Administration (FDA) removed silicone implants from use for cosmetic purposes due to concerns about development of autoimmune disease or connective tissue disease from leaking silicone. Many retrospective studies subsequently dispelled this concern, while also disproving causal links to cancer. Additionally, the silicone implants that are currently used have a thicker shell and more dense gel, which are believed to decrease the rate of implant rupture. All patients who consent to it are enrolled in a clinical trial for surveillance by the breast implant manufacturers (Rothrock & McEwen, 2006).

13. How does breast reconstruction differ from breast augmentation procedures?

Breast reconstruction most commonly occurs after a mastectomy and can be performed using native tissue in the form of various flaps or with the use of implants. A combination of the two can also be used. Multiple surgical revisions including the use of tissue expanders may occur to achieve the desired result. In breast reconstruction, the skin and breast must be replaced, whereas in breast augmentation there is native breast tissue present. According to the 2008 statistics reported by the ASPS, breast reconstructions are performed nearly as much as breast reductions (ASPS, 2010; Nathan & Singh, 2001).

14. What complications might occur following breast augmentation?

Hematoma formation, infection, implant exposure, capsular contracture (tight scar tissue from implant failure), deep venous thrombosis, and pulmonary emboli may occur following breast augmentation, but rates of complication are low (Alderman et al., 2009, Gabriel et al., 1997).

15. What is the role of the perianesthesia nurse for augmentation mammoplasty procedures?

The perianesthesia nurse should palpate the superior aspect of the pectoralis muscle and inspect the surgical site for symmetry to rule out hematoma formation. The dressing should be inspected for bleeding and hematoma formation as well. Because the risk of pneumothorax is greater in the axillary approach or with the use of numbing intercostal blocks, monitoring oxygenation with a pulse oximeter and auscultation of the lungs should occur to determine unequal or decreased breath sounds. Chest tube setup and drainage equipment should be readily available in case of this rare issue (Alderman et al., 2009; Doherty, 2010).

16. What is a rhinoplasty?

Rhinoplasty is a procedure performed to reshape the nose and open the airway; this procedure can be performed under general or local anesthesia with sedation (Drain & Odom-Forren, 2008; Doherty, 2010).

17. Are there postoperative concerns for rhinoplasty patients?

The patient's head should be elevated 30° to 45° to reduce to swelling and facilitate drainage. Postoperative nasopharyngeal bleeding and secretions can occur; therefore, suction and airway equipment should be readily available (Drain & Odom-Forren, 2008; Doherty, 2010). The passage of blood in the stomach during the procedure may predispose the patient to nausea and vomiting; antiemetic therapy may have to be implemented.

18. What is liposuction?

Liposuction is a surgical contouring technique involving the removal of subcutaneous body fat. It may be used on multiple areas of the body including the abdomen, hips, arms, and back. Traditional techniques such as suction-assisted lipectomy (SAL), involve placement of tumescent solution with lidocaine and epinephrine into the fatty tissue prior to placing a cannula or tube attached to a vacuum source. Ultrasound-assisted liposuction (UAL) or VASER liposuction involves the application of ultrasound energy to break up the fat prior to aspiration. With power-assisted liposuction (PAL), the cannula reciprocates and mechanically breaks up the fat as it is being aspirated (Drain & Odom-Forren, 2008; Logan & Broughton, 2008).

19. What does tumescent mean and how does it relate to liposuction?

Tumescent literally means "swollen." First, small incisions are made at the surgical site and the area undergoing liposuction is made swollen by the infiltration of a solution consisting of lactated ringers, lidocaine, and epinephrine. The liposuction occurs by connecting cannulas to suction for aspiration (Kucera et al., 2006; Rohrich, Leedy, Swamy, Brown, & Coleman, 2006).

20. What is the advantage to the tumescent technique?

This technique has the advantage of decreased blood loss as a result of epinephrine in the solution and improved pain control with less anesthetic requirement because of large volumes containing dilute concentrations of lidocaine (Kucera et al., 2006).

21. What role does lidocaine play in liposuction?

Because lidocaine is infiltrated in large volumes, concern has been raised about the impact of the local anesthetic, particularly after reported deaths following liposuction. The typical tumescent solution is diluted by a factor of 10 to 20 times, and the vasoconstriction due to the epinephrine limits the introduction of the lidocaine in the circulation. There are certain drugs that have the potential to affect the metabolism of lidocaine (Iverson & Pao, 2008; Rohrich et al., 2006; Townsend et al., 2007).

22. What complications can occur following liposuction?

Pulmonary emboli, fat emboli, hemorrhage, blind perforation of the viscera, and infection may occur. Pulmonary emboli and fat emboli are very serious and may present within a short time after surgery in the recovery room, manifesting as hypoxia and tachycardia. This requires supplemental oxygen, hydration, and an emergency call to the surgeon. Visceral perforation is also very serious and more typically occurs in areas of latent hernias and present as tachycardia, fever, and abdominal pain and infection. Several factors influence the complication rate, aspiration of large volumes (greater than 5 liters total aspirate) with prolonged operation time and accompanying hypothermia increases the risk of complication. Additionally, performing more than one procedure at a time may result in a higher complication rate (Iverson & Pao, 2008; Lehnhardt et al., 2008; Logan & Broughton, 2008).

23. What is the role of the perianesthesia nurse following liposuction procedures?

Knowledge of the type of tumescent technique and the intravenous volume as well as the aspirated volumes is helpful. Monitor the patient for cardiac arrhythmias due to the use of lidocaine and epinephrine. Plasma levels of lidocaine can peak 10 to 12 hours after infiltration when epinephrine is used in the solution (Iverson & Pao, 2008). The patient should be observed for signs of hypovolemia and fluids should be replaced as indicated. Pain and drainage should be monitored. Any evidence of hypoxia could indicate a serious problem, like a fat embolus. Some patients have a urinary catheter in place, which helps better assess fluid status.

24. Are there contraindications to liposuction?

Liposuction is contraindicated in patients with severe cardiovascular disease, coagulation disorders, and during pregnancy. It should not be performed in scarred areas of the torso, which might be hiding hernias, or in areas of radiation, which increases the risk of visceral perforation. Liposuction should not be performed to treat obesity, but rather, localized fatty deposits in the subcutaneous space. Men typically carry their fat around their abdominal organs in the peritoneal cavity, and they may therefore be poor candidates for liposuction (Logan & Broughton, 2008; Mysore, 2008).

25. What can patients expect following liposuction?

Patients should expect to wear compression garments and binders to reduce bruising, hematomas, and pain (Mysore, 2008). Early on, there may be bloodstained drainage from the access incisions. Patients often become dehydrated or may have some blood loss, requiring fluid supplementation. Patients must ambulate early to protect against deep venous thrombosis and pulmonary embolism.

26. What is blepharoplasty?

Blepharoplasty is eyelid surgery. This procedure is commonly performed for facial rejuvenation or for obstructed visual fields from overhanging skin (Lelli & Lisman, 2010). Excess skin and fat are removed, and adjustments to muscle and tendons (ptosis surgery) may also occur.

27. What complications can occur after blepharoplasty?

Complications occurring acutely, possibly manifesting themselves in the recovery room, include corneal abrasions and vision, threatening retrobulbar hemorrhage. Such complications require immediate attention, and may require the assistance of an ophthalmologist. The intermediate and late complications occurring between weeks 1 through 6 and beyond include lid malposition, strabismus, dry eye, and corneal exposure; changes in eyelid height, scarring, and edema represent later findings (Lelli & Lisman, 2010).

28. What should the perianesthesia nurse look for following blepharoplasty?

Vision changes, excessive pain, bleeding, or swelling are important clinical clues to early postoperative complications that may result in permanent blindness. The plastic surgeon should be alerted in these circumstances. The normal postoperative course will include the elevation of the head and application of ice to reduce swelling and assist the management of pain. An ophthalmic ointment may be ordered by the surgeon to aid in dryness of the eye (Lelli & Lisman, 2010).

29. What is abdominoplasty?

Abdominoplasty literally means plastic surgery of the abdomen, which includes a broad spectrum of procedures and involves surgical correction of abdominal deformities involving lax muscle or skin. The panniculectomy procedure involves the direct removal of the pannus or apron deformity such as that seen in hypermorbid obesity or in massive weight loss, which includes redundant skin and adipose tissue. Damaged muscles due to laxity or previous abdominal surgeries may also repair with abdominal muscle plication (Logan & Broughton, 2008; Rothrock & McEwen, 2006; Townsend et al., 2007).

30. What are some complications following abdominoplasty?

Minor complications include seroma or hematoma formation not requiring intervention, cellulitis, pain, and small wound dehiscence. Major complications include hematoma and seroma formation requiring surgical intervention, abscess requiring hospitalization and intravenous antibiotics, large hematoma or seroma, significant skin necrosis, deep venous thrombosis, and pulmonary embolism (Logan & Broughton, 2008; Nemen & Hansen, 2007; Stewart et al., 2006).

31. What is the role of the perianesthesia nurse following abdominoplasty?

Dressings and contour should be inspected for signs of increased bleeding, and an abdominal drain output should be recorded. Urine output should be monitored to rule out bleeding or dehydration. Patients should be kept warm as hypothermia puts patients at risk for postoperative infection and wound healing problems. Patients should be flexed at the waist to avoid undue tension on the abdomen, unless another procedure was performed during the abdominoplasty that would be hurt with this positioning. The patient should be treated with antiemetics, if necessary, to avoid retching, which may increase intraabdominal pressure and predispose to wound dehiscence. Additionally, the patient should be given instructions on ambulation, coughing, and deep breathing. The patient should be given directions regarding the compression garment and should be educated about the signs of postoperative bleeding and infection. Compression should be firm but not tight (Logan & Broughton, 2008; Rothrock & McEwen, 2006; Townsend et al., 2007).

BURNS

Patients with major burns with ventilator dependence are often transported directly from the burn unit to the operating room and directly back to the unit for postoperative care. Patients with less severe injuries and patients who are undergoing reconstruction secondary to past burn injury will be recovered in the postanesthesia care unit. Knowledge of burn injury and care for these patients is critical.

32. What kind of procedures do burn care patients have?

Acute burn patients undergo excision of burns and skin graft procedures depending on the extent of the injury. Emergent burn surgery is required in compartment syndromes; emergent chest escharotomies (deep incisions through the burned skin) are performed to relieve chest wall restriction and to allow breathing, whereas upper and lower extremities escharotomies help optimize circulation. Sometimes these procedures are performed in the burn intensive care unit (ICU), often early on arrival.

33. How are burns classified?

Burns are classified according to the depth of injury. A first-degree burn presents with pain and redness; only the epidermis is involved. Sunburns and blisters are examples of first-degree burns. A second-degree burn presents with pain, redness, and blistering; the epidermis and the superficial layer of the dermis are involved. Depending on the extent of the burn, excision of the burned skin layers and grafting may have to occur to promote proper healing of the injury. With a third-degree burn, the epidermis, and dermis are damaged. Third-degree burns may require excision down to fascia and routinely involve skin grafting, which may be sagged with allograft placement performed initially. A fourth-degree burn extends to bone, muscle, and tendon (National Burn Association, 2010).

34. What influences the mortality of a patient with a burn?

According to the American Burn Association, advanced age, burn size, and inhalation injury increase the mortality (National Burn Association, 2010).

35. What are the most common types of burn injury?

- Fire/flame (42%)
- Scald (31%)
- Contact with hot object (9%)
- Electrical (4%)
- Chemical (3%) (National Burn Association, 2010)

36. What should the perianesthesia nurse know when caring for the burn patient?

The skin represents the largest thermoregulatory organ in the body. Burn injury represents a disruption in the body's ability to maintain a normal body temperature; therefore, avoidance of hypothermia is important. This can be accomplished by the use of convective heat warmers and fluid warmers. Significant blood loss can occur during the excision of burns; fluid resuscitation may have to be continued in the recovery phase. Inspection of the burn dressing should occur; the graft site should be protected from pressure and excessive movement, and bleeding through the dressings may indicate the need for better hemostasis, to be performed at bedside or with a return to the operating room (OR). Burn patients also need to be monitored for oxygenation in light of significant resuscitation that may lead to pulmonary edema or exacerbation of pulmonary damage from the initial fire.

PLASTIC SURGERY TRAUMA

Trauma cases requiring plastic surgery involve the face, upper and lower extremities, and trunk. Soft tissue trauma such as lacerations and animal bites tend to be treated in the emergency room unless the degree of tissue injury is extensive or the individual is a child (Townsend et al., 2007). Patients with facial fractures have sustained their injuries from high-energy forces such as motor vehicle accidents, blunt trauma, penetrating trauma, and falls, and depending on the injury, may present with cranial nerve involvement or cervical spine injury. A detailed evaluation is critical preoperatively and following surgery. Plastic surgeons also assist general surgeons, vascular surgeons, neurosurgeons, and other surgical subspecialists in stability and closure of complex wounds (Doherty, 2010).

37. What are the most common facial fractures requiring plastic surgery?

Nasal fractures are the most common facial fractures. Mandibular fracture ranks second. Midface fractures of the maxilla, zygomatic complex, and frontal sinus may also occur (Doherty, 2010).

38. How are nasal fractures treated?

Most nasal fractures are treated with closed reduction, splinting, and intranasal packing. Recovery of the patient with nasal fracture is similar to the care of the rhinoplasty patient (Doherty, 2010).

39. What are the clinical considerations for patients with mandibular fractures?

The mandible is the largest and strongest of the facial bones; the force required to fracture the mandible can also damage the cervical spine. Airway compromise may occur in certain mandibular fractures because of the loss of support to the posterior oropharynx. Airway management is critical. Pain is also very important to manage. With open wounds and after surgery, perioral hygiene with mouth rinses is important (Defazio Quinn & Schick, 2004; Doherty, 2010; Townsend et al., 2007).

40. What is intermaxillary fixation (IMF), and why is it important in facial fractures?

IMF is necessary to reestablish the proper dentoskeletal relationships. A critical part of managing the fracture involves restoring occlusion of the maxillary and mandibular dentition. Arch bars are placed before fracture exposure and plating. The proper occlusal alignment will guide proper reduction of the bone fracture. IMF may provide closed reduction as a stand-alone procedure in management of mandible fracture or used as an adjunct for open reduction internal fixation with plates. IMF can result in significant weight loss after surgery (Doherty, 2010; Townsend et al., 2007).

41. What should the perianesthesia nurse anticipate postoperatively in patients with mandibular and maxillary fractures?

Postoperatively, the arch bars prevent mouth opening and the patients will have to be educated on the puree diet, mouth rinses, and antibiotics (Townsend et al., 2007). In addition to suction and airway equipment, it is imperative that a pair of wire cutters be placed at the bedside to release the arch bars in the case of an airway emergency. Oversedation should be avoided because of the potential risk for respiratory depression. A thorough neurologic exam should occur to rule out nerve injury. Due to the close relationship of the maxilla and orbit, visual light perception should be monitored (Defazio Quinn & Schick, 2004).

PLASTIC SURGERY EMERGENCIES

As in all surgical procedures, uncontrolled bleeding may occur with plastic surgery. Postoperatively, this may be detected in the recovery room and often requires a reexploration in the operating room. Complications from flap procedures should be anticipated. A baseline exam upon entry to the recovery room serves as a critical frame of reference if the patient's status deteriorates. Compartment syndrome, ischemia, and amputations of digits are some of the most common plastic surgery emergencies (Townsend et al., 2007).

42. Which types of amputations are suitable for replantation?

The thumb, multiple digits, transmetacarpal, wrist, forearm, and single digits in children are suitable for replantation. Replanting digits often results in postoperative stiffness and could put the patient at risk for significant infection, so noncritical fingers may be amputated, particularly if the injury is significant and the patient has multiple comorbidities, including tobacco use (Beasley, Aston, Bartlett, Gurtner, & Spear, 2007).

43. What are the absolute contraindications to replantation?

Significant associated injuries, multiple injuries or crush within the amputated part, systemic illness, tobacco use, and advanced age have been reported to be contraindications to replantation (Beasley et al., 2007).

44. What are the relative contraindications to replantation?

Advanced age, avulsion injuries, prolonged warm ischemia time, massive contamination, and single digit amputation in an adult are relative contraindications (Beris et al., 2009).

45. Which type of injury has a better outcome?

Sharp, guillotine-like amputations are more favorable to success because the tissue, away from the site, sustains very little damage. Crush injuries and avulsion injuries have a less favorable outcome due to the extensive damage of the vessels and nerves (Beasley et al., 2007; Beris et al., 2009).

46. What role does ischemia time play in the amputation?

Muscles are the least tolerant of ischemia and undergo irreversible changes after 6 hours. Because the digits lack muscle, the permitted duration of warm ischemia is up to 12 hours. If the amputated digit is cooled, the period of ischemia extends past 30 hours (Beasley et al., 2007; Beris et al., 2009).

47. What should the perianesthesia nurse keep in mind when caring for patients who have undergone replantation?

The role of the perianesthesia is critically important to a successful outcome following replantation because the replanted digit will require careful observation for an extended period of time. The perfusion of the digit should be monitored for 48 hours by inspection of the color of the fingertip and capillary refill. The replanted part should be elevated and kept in a warm room. A heater and glow lamp may have to be used to aid in maintaining normothermia (Beasley et al., 2007; Beris et al., 2009).

48. What should the perianesthesia nurse suspect when the digit is pale or blue?

Paleness represents slow capillary refill and arterial thrombosis and vasospasm of arterial inflow. A swollen and blue fingertip with increased capillary return indicates venous congestion caused by constricted dressings or thrombosis of the venous anastomoses. Monitoring of the digit is critically important because thrombosis at the vascular anastomoses is the leading cause of microsurgery failure (Beasley et al., 2007; Beris et al., 2009).

49. What additional parameters should be monitored by the nurse?

Temperature and pulse oximetry should be employed to aid in determining the viability of the digit. A temperature drop of 3.6°F or an absolute temperature of 86°F mandates reexploration of the anastomoses. Meticulous control of the blood pressure is warranted. Hypotension will influence perfusion and hypertension may compromise the vascular anastomosis. The use of vasoconstrictors should not be used to maintain the blood pressure unless it is absolutely necessary. The surgical team should be alerted on issues pertaining to extreme changes in these parameters (Beasley et al., 2007).

50. What are the complications of replantation?

Malunion, nonunion, joint stiffness muscle contractures, poor sensation, and cold intolerance are noted complications from replantation (Beris et al., 2009).

REFERENCES

Alderman, A., Collins, D. E., Streu, R., Grotting, J. C., Sulkin, A. L., Neligan, P., et al. (2009). Benchmarking outcomes in plastic surgery: National complication rates for abdominoplasty and breast augmentation. *Plastic and Reconstructive Surgery, 124*(6), 2127–2133.

American Society of Plastic Surgeons. (2010a). *2009 report of the 2008 statistics: National clearinghouse of plastic surgery statistics.* Retrieved from http://www.plasticsurgery.org/Media/stats/2008-US-cosmetic-reconstructive-plastic-surgery-minimally-invasive-statistics.pdf

American Society of Plastic Surgeons. (2010b). *Why the "plastic" in plastic surgery?* Retrieved from http://www.plasticsurgery.org/Patients_and_Consumers/Plastic_Surgery_FAQs/Why_the plastic_in_plastic_surgery.html

Beasley, R. W. Aston, S. J., Bartlett, S. P., Gurtner, G. C., & Spear, S. L. (2007). 6th Ed. Replantation in the upper extremity. *In Grabb and Smith's Plastic Surgery.* (pp.872–883) Heidelberg, Germany: Spring Berlin.

Defazio Quinn, D. M., & Shick, L. (2004). Plastic and reconstructive surgery. In D. M. Defazio Quinn & L. Schick (Eds.), *PeriAnesthesia nursing core curriculum: Preoperative, phase I and phase II PACU nursing.* Philadelphia: Saunders.

Doherty, G. M. (2010). Plastic and reconstructive surgery. In H. C. Vasconez & A. Habash (Eds.), *Current diagnosis and treatment: Surgery* (13th ed., pp. 1092–1131). New York: McGraw Hill.

Drain, C. B., & Odom-Forren, J. (2008). Care of the plastic surgical patient. In C. B. Drain & J. Odom-Forren (Eds.), *Perianesthesia nursing: A critical care approach* (pp. 600–606). Philadelphia: Saunders.

Gabriel, S. E., Woods, J. E., O'Fallon, M. W., Beard, M. D., Kurland, L. T., & Melton, J. L. (1997). Complications leading to surgery after breast implantation. *The New England Journal of Medicine, 336*(10), 677–682.

Gillies, H. D. (1983). *Plastic surgery of the face: based on selected cases of war injuries of the face, including burns.* London: Gower Medical Publishing Limited.

Iverson, R. E., & Pao, V. S. (2008). Liposuction. *Plastic and Reconstructive Surgery, 121*(4), 1–11.

Kucera, I. J., Lambert, T. J., Klein, J. A., Watkins, R. G., Hoover, J. M., & Kaye, A. D. (2006). Liposuction: Contemporary issues for the anesthesiologist. *Journal of Clinical Anesthesia, 18*(5), 379–387.

Lehnhardt, M., Homann, H. H., Daigeler, A., Hauser, J., Palka, P., & Steinau, H. U. (2008). Major and lethal complications of liposuction: A review of 72 cases in Germany between 1998 and 2002. *Plastic and Reconstructive Surgery, 121*(6), 396e–403e.

Lelli, G. J., & Lisman, R. D. (2010). Blepharoplasty complications. *Plastic and Reconstructive Surgery, 125*(3), 1007–1017.

Logan, J. M., & Broughton, G. (2008). Plastic surgery: Understanding abdominoplasty and liposuction. *American Operating Room Nurses, 88*(4), 587–600.

Mysore, V. (2008). Tumescent liposuction: Standard guidelines of care. *Indian Journal of Dermatology, 74,* S54–S60.

Nathan, B., & Singh, S. (2001). Postoperative compression after breast augmentation. *Aesthetic Plastic Surgery, 25*(4), 290–291.

National Burn Association. (2010). National burn repository: Report of data from 2000–2009. (Retrieved from http://www.ameriburn.org/ 2010NBRAnnualReport.pdf

Neman, K. C., & Hansen, J. E. (2007). Analysis of complications from abdominoplasty: A review of 206 cases at a university hospital. *Annals of Plastic Surgery, 58*(3), 292–298.

Rohrich, R. J., Leedy, J. E., Swamy, R., Brown, S. A., & Coleman, J. (2006). Fluid resuscitation in liposuction: A retrospective review of 89 consecutive patients. *Plastic and Reconstructive Surgery, 117*(2), 431–435.

Rothrock, J. C., & McEwen, D. R. (2006). Plastic and reconstructive surgery. In S. K. Chandler (Ed.), *Alexander's care of the patient in surgery* (pp. 863–905). Philadelphia: Saunders.

Stewart, K. J., Stewart, D. A., Coghlan, B., Harrison, D. H. Jones, B. M., & Waterhouse, N. (2006). Complications of 278 consecutive abdominoplasties. *Journal of Plastic Reconstructive Anesthetic Surgery, 59*(11), 1152–1155.

Townsend, C. M., Mattox, K. L., Evers, M. B., & Beauchamp, D. (2007). Plastic surgery. In J. L. Burns, S. J. Blackwell (Eds.), *Sabiston textbook of surgery*. Philadelphia: Saunders.

SECTION

I

SECTION

II

SECTION

III

CHAPTER 24

Dental and Maxillofacial Surgeries

Carol Sallese Maragos, MSN, CRNP, CORLN

Dental and maxillofacial surgeries are usually performed in an urgent or emergent situation because of the underlying problem. As the patient wakes up from their surgery, protecting their airway is of key importance due to swelling of the mouth and/or airway. In addition, patients who have their teeth wired shut are at high risk for aspiration should they vomit after surgery. A pair of wire cutters needs to be kept at the bedside should the patient vomit or need their mouth opened urgently. It is imperative that the postoperative nurse keep a diligent eye on these patients recovering from surgery.

Patients who have surgery due to an accident leading to their injury may need additional emotional support. The mental replay of the traumatic event and the potential for facial disfigurement may cause heightened anxiety in the patient. The nurse should be aware of the many hospital and community resources available to the patient.

ORAL INFECTIONS

1. What causes infections?

A majority of infections is caused by anaerobic organisms, and about one third is caused by aerobic and anaerobic organisms (Carlson & Hudson, 2005).

2. What should be assessed when a toothache is suspected?

Ask the patient the following questions: When did the pain start and where does it hurt? Do you have a fever? Are you taking any antibiotics? How far are you able to open your mouth? Do you have difficulty breathing and/or swallowing?

Patients can present with symptoms ranging from mild to life threatening. The skin may appear reddened, a lump or swelling may be present in the gum around the infected tooth, the area may be warm, and there may be pain (Carlson & Hudson, 2005).

3. What criteria need to be present for the patient to be hospitalized?

If the patient exhibits signs of toxicity, which include paleness, tachycardia, tachypnea, fever, malaise, shivering, sweating, lethargy (Carlson & Hudson, 2005), the patient will need to be hospitalized. The patient may also show signs of central nervous system toxicity, including change in level of consciousness, headache, neck stiffness, vomiting, eyelid swelling, and ophthalmoplegia (Carlson & Hudson, 2005).

4. What is the treatment for oral infections?

IV antibiotics are usually required. It is best to culture the infection first to obtain the correct speciation of organisms and sensitivities for determining the appropriate antibiotics. Surgical decompression of the infection needs to accompany antibiotic administration in order to eradicate the infection (Carlson & Hudson, 2005).

5. Are oral infections ever fatal?

Yes, oral infections have been known to be fatal if the patient exhibits any of the following: airway compromise, dysphagia (difficulty swallowing), a change in vision or a change in eye movement or both, voice quality changes, lethargy, and decreased level of consciousness (Carlson & Hudson, 2005). The patient's airway must be monitored closely. If the patient requires the establishment of an emergency airway, the surgeon has several choices: fiberoptic awake oral intubation, nasoendotracheal intubation, tracheostomy, or cricothyroidotomy (Carlson & Hudson, 2005).

6. What is Ludwig's angina?

Ludwig's angina is bilateral cellulitis of the submandibular and sublingual spaces. It can be a life-threatening condition because it can lead to airway compromise.

7. What are the signs and symptoms of Ludwig's angina?

The patient's floor of mouth may feel "wooden," the neck may be swollen with induration, there may be respiratory distress, tongue swelling, drooling, dysphagia, and trismus, or the patient may present with airway compromise (Pasha, 2006).

8. What is the treatment for Ludwig's angina?

The ABCs of resuscitation should always be at the top of your mind. If the patient is having respiratory difficulty, they will need to have a tracheostomy tube inserted. This will usually be done as an emergent case in the operating room. While in the operating room (OR), the patient may have the area in question probed and possibly drained. The patient will also need antibiotics. The tracheostomy tube is usually temporary and the patient will be decannulated when there is no longer a risk of airway obstruction.

9. When teeth need to be extracted, what are the postoperative considerations?

Most teeth may be removed in the dentist's office under local anesthesia; however, a trip to the OR may be warranted based on the patient's age, an inability to withstand local anesthesia, an inability to lie still, the number of teeth to be removed, and how impacted the teeth may be. Postoperatively, the patient's head should be kept elevated at least 30°, hydration should be maintained, pain effectively managed with acetaminophen and narcotics, "dry socket" syndrome should be prevented by applying pressure to the socket with the patient biting on a gauze pad, and the patient should avoid infection by taking the antibiotics as directed.

ORIF MANDIBLE

10. Where on the mandible do fractures commonly occur?

The condylar neck is the most common site, while the angle is the second (especially with an unerupted third molar), and the parasymphysis region near the mental foramen is the least common (Pasha, 2006).

11. What are the main causes for mandibular fractures?

Mandibular fractures are very common in males age 18 to 30 years, with the main cause being assault, with motor vehicle accidents, sports, falls, and gunshot wounds being other causes.

12. What are the different types of mandibular fractures?

There are three classifications of fracture types: compound (open wound, exposed bone) versus simple (closed wound, skin and mucosa intact); fracture pattern including comminuted, oblique, transverse, spiral, and greenstick (incomplete fracture through only one cortical surface); and fractures secondary to bone disease such as osteoporosis and osteogenic tumors (Pasha, 2006).

13. What is the treatment for mandibular fractures?

The goal for treating mandibular fractures is to restore occlusion, establish bony union and return of function, and to prevent temporomandibular joint (TMJ) ankylosis. These fractures do not need immediate repair; however, they should be repaired within the first week of occurring. A delay in treatment increases complications (Pasha, 2006).

Maxillo-mandibular fixation (MMF) is indicated for initial stabilization of the occlusion prior to exposure of the fracture, minimally displaced fractures, and selected condylar fractures. Arch bars are the strongest MMF and are usually the treatment of choice. You may also see interdental eyelet wires (Ivy loops), or circumferential wiring of dentures or teeth (Pasha, 2006). Rubber bands may then be applied to allow for exercise. The bars stay on for about 2–8 weeks, depending on the age and the degree of injury. Children with arch bars have them removed in 3–4 weeks, adults in 4–6 weeks, and the elderly in 8 weeks or more (Pasha, 2006).

14. What should the nurse teach the patient about MMF?

Since the patient's mouth will be wired closed, they will only be able to take in a liquid diet. The patient should be told to maintain adequate nutrition to promote the healing process. The patient will be given a pair of disposable wire cutters to keep with them at all times should they experience vomiting. The patient will need to cut the wires so that if they vomit, there is less likelihood for aspiration. The patient will usually go home with an antibiotic and antiseptic mouthwash. The patient needs to adhere to the prescription so as to avoid infection.

15. Are there any other treatment modalities?

If the patient has an unfavorable and comminuted fracture, multiple fractures, if they have poor pulmonary reserve and/or seizures, if they are elderly, noncompliant, or pregnant, they would do better with an open reduction internal fixation (ORIF) of the fracture (Pasha, 2006). This can be performed either transorally or externally. These patients will be allowed to eat a soft diet as tolerated. They will need antibiotics, analgesics, and close follow-up care.

16. How does a peritonsillar abscess develop?

Peritonsillar abscesses form due to recurrent tonsillitis or chronic tonsillitis that is not properly treated (Wiatrak & Woolley, 2005). The proper therapy is to perform drainage of the abscess by needle aspiration or by incision and drainage. In addition, the tonsils may need to be removed.

17. How does a parapharyngeal space abscess develop?

A parapharyngeal space abscess develops when infection or pus drains from the tonsils or from a peritonsillar abscess through the superior constrictor muscle. The abscess can be found between the superior constrictor muscle and the deep cervical fascia, which usually causes displacement of the tonsil on the lateral pharyngeal wall toward the midline.

It is sometimes difficult to detect fluctuance because of the thickness of the overlying sternocleidomastoid muscle. The patient exhibits a fever, low white blood cell count, and pain. Trismus and a stiff neck occur when there is inflammation of the adjacent pterygoid and paraspinal muscle (Wiatrak & Woolley, 2005).

18. How are parapharyngeal space abscesses treated?

The first course of treatment includes aggressive use of IV antibiotics, fluid management, and close observation. Surgical intervention may be employed when the infection does not show signs of resolving (Wiatrak & Woolley, 2005).

REFERENCES

Carlson, E. R., & Hudson, J. W. (2005). Odontogenic infections. In C. W. Cummings, B. H. Haughey, J. R. Thomas, L. A. Harker, and P. W. Flint (Eds.), *Otolaryngology: Head and neck surgery* (4th ed.). Philadelphia: Elsevier.

Pasha, R. (2006). *Otolaryngology head and neck surgery clinical reference guide* (2nd ed.). San Diego: Plural.

Wiatrak, B. J., & Woolley, A. L. (2005). Pharyngitis and adenotonsillar disease. In C. W. Cummings, B. H. Haughey, J. R. Thomas, L. A. Harker, and P. W. Flint (Eds.), *Otolaryngology: Head and neck surgery* (4th ed.). Philadelphia: Elsevier.

CHAPTER 25

The Endocrine System

Kathleen DeLeskey, DNP, RN

INTRODUCTION

The endocrine system is made up of glands that produce body hormones. They include the hypothalamus, pituitary, pineal, thyroid, parathyroid, thymus and adrenal glands, as well as the pancreas, ovaries, and testes. The endocrine glands differentiate systems in the developing fetus, stimulate human growth and development, coordinate the human reproductive system, maintain the internal body environment, and initiate responses to emergency demands by excreting the appropriate hormones. Alterations in hormonal regulation may result in both intracellular and extracellular disorders that may threaten the well-being of patients, particularly during stressful events such as surgery. Caring for postoperative patients who have been or may be at risk for diseases related to the endocrine system when the body is exposed to surgical trauma requires extra vigilant attention by the caregiver (Lewis, Heitkemper, & Dirksen, 2007).

1. What is diabetes insipidus and how will it affect my postoperative patient?

Diabetes insipidus (DI) results from the inadequate production of antidiuretic hormone (ADH) or a decreased renal response to ADH. ADH is produced in the posterior pituitary gland, so diseases affecting the pituitary may result in DI. Fluid and electrolyte imbalances occur as a consequence of increased urine output. Central (neurogenic) DI is caused by an organic lesion that interferes with ADH synthesis, transport, or release. Nephrogenic DI is a result of a decreased response by the kidneys to ADH.

Psychogenic DI is associated with increased water consumption and may result from psychiatric problems. Clinical manifestations of DI include polydipsia and polyuria. Intercranial surgery may precipitate DI, which tends to take place in three phases. The initial acute phase manifests with a sudden onset of polyuria. DI is often permanent in these cases. If fluid intake does not keep up with urinary loss, severe fluid volume deficit with hypernatremia and hypovolemic shock may result.

2. What is the postoperative risk to my patient who has hyperthyroidism?

Patients who have hyperthyroid disease can be at risk from stress. The stress of surgical trauma may induce a thyrotoxic crisis, sometimes called thyroid storm, in which all the manifestations of hyperthyroidism become acute. Signs and symptoms of thyrotoxic crisis include tachycardia, heart failure, agitation, nausea and vomiting, restlessness, delirium, seizures, and coma. Management of respiratory distress, fever reduction, and fluid replacement are critical. Provision of a quiet, cool environment may help the agitation. Frequent and thorough assessment of patients with hyperthyroid disease is essential to recognizing thyrotoxic crisis early and treating it quickly.

3. How do I care for my patient who has undergone thyroidectomy?

Thyroidectomy is the removal of all or part of the thyroid gland. The parathyroid glands are usually spared to prevent hypocalcemia. Because the thyroid gland is located in proximity to the airway, postoperative management focuses on maintaining good air exchange. Irritability and twitching can be caused by hypocalcemia. One complication that can arise following thyroidectomy includes laryngeal nerve damage. Postoperative management includes the following:

- Monitor carefully for respiratory distress owing to bleeding and aspiration or swelling
- Observe for signs that indicate low calcium levels
- Use humidified oxygen to cool the airway and minimize edema
- Maintain semi-Fowler's position and good head support
- Monitor vital signs to identify bleeding
- Observe for frequent swallowing, which may indicate bleeding
- Observe for swelling of the neck and voice changes
- Keep a tracheostomy set nearby for emergency use

4. Will patients having thyroidectomy be affected by thyrotoxic crisis?

Thyroidectomy is the definitive treatment for hyperthyroid disease that is unresponsive to other modes of treatment. Postoperative complications in patients undergoing thyroidectomy include airway impairment from swelling or risk of aspiration. If inadvertent damage to the parathyroid glands occurred during surgery, hypocalcemia, hemorrhage, infection, or thyrotoxic crisis may result. Signs and symptoms of parathyroid damage include stridor, which may be indicative of tetany and will need treatment. Caring for postoperative thyroidectomy patients includes:

- Frequently assessing airway for signs of swelling, hemorrhage, choking, or bloody drainage.
- Placing the patient in semi-Fowler's position and supporting the head with pillows
- Avoiding neck flexion
- Checking for signs of tetany (tingling or twitching of toes, fingers, or around the mouth)
- Observing for Chvostek's sign and Trousseau's sign
- Controlling postoperative pain

5. What should I do if my surgical patient has hypothyroid disease?

Hypothyroidism is caused by inadequate amounts of circulating thyroid hormone. The disease causes fatigue and lethargy. It is associated with a decrease in cardiac contractility, resulting in decreased cardiac output. Hemodynamic stability may be impacted in patients with other cardiovascular diseases or in patients who experience acute blood loss during surgery. Monitor vital signs frequently as the stress response from surgery may impact cardiac output. Hypothermia can cause an increase in metabolic rate and this should be avoided by warming postoperative patients. Assess fluid status carefully to avoid overhydrating and stressing the cardiac system. Hypothyroidism may also cause hypersensitivity to opioids and anesthetic medications, so caution should be used when these are administered.

In patients with severe hypothyroidism, a sudden progression to a coma state can be precipitated by opioids, barbiturates, or surgical trauma. Hypothermia, hypotension, and hypoventilation are characteristic signs of impending coma. Observe for all signs and symptoms that indicate possible instability and be prepared to provide appropriate treatment.

6. What should I know about my patient with hyperparathyroidism who has undergone surgery to remove parathyroid tissue?

Patients who undergo parathyroid surgery are at increased risk for hypocalcemia. Low calcium results in renal disturbances including calculi, ulcers in the gastrointestinal tract, and demineralization of bones. Careful monitoring of airway and breathing owing to the proximity of the surgical site to the airway is critical. Additionally, fluid and electrolytes must be monitored to maintain adequate hydration and renal output. Any complications like nausea and vomiting that can exacerbate dehydration should be reported immediately. Signs and symptoms of hypocalcemia include irritability, twitching, and spasms of hand and feet (den Brinker et al., 2008).

7. What is diabetic ketoacidosis (DKA)? Is my postoperative patient at risk for DKA?

Diabetic ketoacidosis (DKA) is an acute complication of diabetes mellitus marked by ketonuria, hyperglycemia, dehydration, and acidosis. Besides insulin deficiency, two of the factors commonly associated with DKA are fasting and dehydration. Patients experiencing severe hyperglycemia can progress quickly to DKA, coma, and death. Most postoperative patients have fasted before surgery and may continue to be dehydrated postoperatively if intraoperative fluid replacement was insufficient. Clinical manifestations of DKA include polydipsia, polyuria, drowsiness, and acetone breath. Abdominal pain, tremors, and vomiting may also occur. Blood glucose is always elevated and may reach 1000 mg/dL. Surgical trauma is a direct stressor to the body and may cause an increase in blood glucose, so diabetic patients should be carefully monitored for blood glucose levels. Nondiabetic postoperative patients displaying these symptoms should be evaluated for diabetes since undiagnosed diabetics are at higher risk. Nurses should evaluate for dehydration, metabolic acidosis, and the resulting changes in vital signs. Treatment includes IV fluids to replace losses, insulin to displace glucose into the cells, and evaluation and treatment of electrolyte imbalances.

8. What should I do if my postoperative patient has diabetes type I?

Type I diabetes mellitus, or insulin dependent diabetes mellitus (IDDM), is common among hospitalized patients owing to the organ damage that occurs from long-term, poorly controlled blood glucose. Besides normal postoperative care, consideration for IDDM patients focuses on maintaining stable blood glucose levels. Postoperative diabetic patients should have bedside glucose monitoring done within the first few minutes upon admission to the postanesthesia care unit (PACU). Abnormal levels should be treated immediately. Hyperglycemia or hypoglycemia impacts metabolic processes and healing. Nurses need to observe for signs of abnormal blood glucose.

- Hyperglycemia symptoms include high blood glucose, polydipsia, and polyuria.
- Hypoglycemia symptoms include shakiness, dizziness, sweating, hunger, headache, pale skin color, seizure, confusion, and tingling around the mouth.

Normal blood glucose should be maintained throughout the recovery period and treatment should be initiated as needed.

9. Is it important to check the blood sugar of my postoperative diabetic patient if they do not use insulin?

Yes. Patients with noninsulin dependent diabetes mellitus (NIDDM) or type II diabetes possess the same risks as type I diabetics for injury caused by hypoglycemia and hyperglycemia. Stress can induce changes in metabolic processes. The anxiety triggered by the anticipation of surgery and the trauma to tissue caused by surgery are both significant stressors, so normally stable diabetics can have unusual changes in blood glucose levels.

Maintaining a normal blood glucose level facilitates healing and prevents the risks associated with unstable blood glucose.

10. What are the implications of long-term diabetes on my postoperative patient?

Long-term diabetic patients demonstrate numerous abnormalities that can impact postoperative recovery. Blood vessels usually sustain damage, which presents earliest in the retina and kidneys. Coronary collaterals do not form as readily in diabetics, rendering them more susceptible to cardiac events. In addition, poor circulation causes impaired wound healing. Nurses must be vigilant in assessing postoperative diabetic patients. Maintaining glucose control is extremely important. Adequate urinary output and tissue edema must be noted. Supplemental oxygenation may assist in delivering adequate oxygen to surgically traumatized tissue. Diabetic patients are predisposed to pressure ulcers caused by positioning, so repositioning may be required if the patient is unable to reposition independently.

11. What do I do if my postoperative patient has Addison's disease?

Addison's disease may be referred to as adrenal insufficiency because the adrenal glands do not produce enough of the hormone cortisol. There may also be a shortage of aldosterone. Among other things, cortisol helps maintain blood pressure and cardiovascular function and regulates metabolism. Tuberculosis (TB) negatively impacts the adrenal glands, so patients with TB may be suspect.

Patients with Addison's disease who are undergoing surgery need to be treated with hydrocortisone and saline to maintain hemodynamic stability. Addison's disease progresses slowly, and a traumatic event like surgery can cause symptoms to become more noticeable. Postoperatively, assess vital signs carefully to identify changes, particularly hypotension. Other symptoms may include muscle weakness, fatigue, nausea, vomiting, or diarrhea. Addisonian crisis may be marked by severe hypotension, low blood glucose, and hyperkalemia and must be treated quickly.

12. How should I care for my patient who has undergone transsphenoidal hypophysectomy?

Transsphenoidal hypophysectomy is the removal of the pituitary gland using a surgical approach through the nasal cavity instead of an intracranial approach. The benefits of the transsphenoidal approach are decreased blood loss and a lower infection rate. Major complications include the development of meningitis, leaking cerebrospinal fluid (CSF), transient diabetes insipidus (DI), and syndrome of inappropriate antidiuretic hormone (SIADH). Postoperative nursing care includes:

- Frequently monitoring vital signs and visual acuity
- Regularly completing neurologic assessment to identify increasing intercranial pressure
- Using humidified oxygen to maintain oral and nasal mucosa
- Identifying signs and symptoms of DI, which include polyuria and hypotension
- Observing for clear fluid coming from the nose, which may indicate a CSF leak
- Controlling postoperative pain
- Observing for signs of infection

13. How does SIADH affect a postoperative patient?

SIADH is the excessive release of antidiuretic hormone (ADH), causing the renal system to retain body fluids rather than excrete them. The result is less urine output, increasing intravascular fluid, hyponatremia from excess water, hypertension, hemodilution, and fluid overload. SIDAH is usually associated with diseases of the hypothalamus or pituitary gland. It is also important to note that ADH is produced in response to stressors including surgical trauma, general anesthetics, narcotics, or malignancy. Signs and symptoms of SIADH include weakness, muscle cramps, and nausea, which are nonspecific, particularly in a fresh postoperative patient. More specific signs include higher intake than output, rising blood pressure, low serum osmolality, high urine specific gravity, and hyponatremia. Eventually, peripheral edema, confusion, and seizures will ensue. Nursing care includes lung assessment, hydration status, level of consciousness assessment, meticulous recording of intake and output, and monitoring of electrolytes.

14. What is the best IV solution to use for my diabetic surgical patient?

Diabetic patients must be assessed for blood glucose levels before, during, and following surgery. Although most have been NPO due to safe anesthesia restrictions, stress and trauma cause changes in metabolism and glucose levels. Intravenous fluid that does not contain glucose should be considered when patient blood glucose remains stable.

Normal saline (NS) and lactated ringers (LR) meet the criteria for nonglucose containing crystalloid solution for IV use, and both are isotonic. Waters and colleagues (2001) studied the differences between patients who received LR and NS in nondiabetic patients undergoing major surgical procedures and found patients who received NS during surgery tended to be more acidotic and needed more blood products than those who received LR.

It is important to remember that NS also contains a high sodium level and a decreased potassium level. The most important criteria is to assess blood glucose level frequently and to maintain a stable level for good wound healing (Hoffman, Charbel, Edelman, Misra, & Ausman, 1998).

15. How will diabetic neuropathy impact my surgical patient?

Nerve damage caused by diabetes is called diabetic neuropathy. Diabetic neuropathy is a sign of poor peripheral circulation, thus the healing of surgical wounds located at peripheral sites may be at risk. Patients with neuropathy should maintain adequate saturated oxygen and good circulation to all extremities to promote healing. Warming blankets cause vasodilation, which increases blood flow and oxygen delivery to healing tissues.

Sensorimotor neuropathy (peripheral neuropathy) causes pain, numbness, and tingling in the extremities, particularly feet. Autonomic neuropathy leads to problems in the digestive system, the genitourinary system, lightheadedness, and loss of other gut sensations.

Caring for patients with diabetic neuropathy requires careful assessment and positioning of extremities to avoid pressure ulcers or other skin damage. A study by Kitamura, Hoshino, Kon, and Ogawa (2000) found that patients with diabetic neuropathy are also at greater risk for hypothermia during and following surgery. Careful assessment of body temperature in the perioperative period should be done to avoid hypothermia (American Diabetes Association [ADA] 2010; Bloomfield & Noble, 2006).

16. What is hyperosmolar hyperglycemic nonketotic syndrome (HHNS)?

HHNS is a complication seen in diabetic patients, most commonly those with diabetes type II. Symptoms include hyperglycemia, dehydration, and hyperosmolarity without ketosis. The stress related to surgery can be a precipitating factor for HHNS. Prolonged periods of hyperglycemia lead to osmotic diuresis with loss of water, sodium, and potassium resulting in severe dehydration and blood viscosity. Ultimately, circulation to organs is impaired and tissue hypoxia develops. The ensuing shift of body fluids also produces neurologic symptoms. Clinical manifestations include fatigue, nausea, vomiting, polyuria, and dehydration that may proceed to hypothermia, muscle weakness, seizures, and coma. Careful assessment of the patient's level of consciousness, skin turgor, and cardiovascular status is crucial to caring for patients at risk for HHNS. Maintenance of fluid and electrolyte balance and blood glucose control may help to avoid the severe symptoms that can occur (Medras, Tworowska, Jozkow, Dumanski, & Dubinski, 2005).

17. How should I care for a patient undergoing surgery for pheochromocytoma?

Pheochromocytoma is a neoplasm that is most often found in the adrenal medulla that secretes excessive catecholamines. The excessive production of catecholamines causes severe hypertension, which is resistant to medication. Blood pressure must be controlled prior to surgical removal of the tumor. Reduction of patient anxiety is essential, so a calm, quiet environment is helpful. The maintenance of adequate tissue perfusion is vital to proper healing, so vital signs and intake and output should be carefully monitored. Following surgery, the sudden drop in catecholamines can cause vasodilation and hypotension. The effects of pheochromocytoma may cause psychotic behavior in some patients, so postoperative neurologic status should be assessed (Nettina, 2006).

18. What should I know about Graves' disease in my postoperative patient?

Graves disease is most commonly caused by hyperthyroidism. Currently, the treatments for hyperthyroidism are radioactive iodine, antithyroid drugs, surgery, or some combination of these. All the treatment options have their own risks and benefits. Bilateral, subtotal thyroidectomy is sometimes chosen as the surgical treatment. In addition to common risks associated with surgery, thyroidectomy presents other serious risks. Due to its proximity to the airway, thyroid patients must be carefully monitored for airway edema. Post-thyroidectomy patients may also have laryngeal nerve damage or hypothyroidism. Tetany may also occur and should be assessed carefully. Signs and symptoms of tetany are Trousseau's sign, Chvostek's sign, laryngeal stridor, and numbness or tingling around the mouth or in the extremities. Any signs of tetany should be reported immediately (Lewis et al., 2007).

19. What are Trousseau's sign and Chvostek's sign?

Both Trousseau's sign and Chvostek's sign are usually found with hypocalcemia or hypomagnesemia.

Trousseau's sign is manifested by nerve excitability causing spasm of the carpopedal muscle, which is exacerbated by ischemia. When a blood pressure cuff is inflated above the level of the systolic pressure, within 3 minutes the wrist and metacarpophalangeal joints flex and fingers will hyperextend and the thumb will flex into the palm of the hand. Patients with positive Trousseau's sign may also experience finger twitches and stiffness.

Chvostek's sign manifests as twitching or contracture of facial muscles when the facial nerve is gently tapped. Upon tapping, the entire side of the face that was tapped can demonstrate involuntary movement. This sign is also due to extra-excitability of nerves. Both of these signs may be indicative of abnormal electrolytes and should be observed in patients undergoing procedures that induce abnormal electrolytes, especially calcium.

20. How should glucose be controlled during surgery for patients with implanted insulin pumps?

There is no research data at this time that supports or negates controlling glucose level during surgery using an implanted insulin pump. According to White, Montalvo, and Monday (2004), there is no perfect way to care for these patients nor are any two patients with diabetes exactly alike. Preoperative diabetic patients must have glucose levels measured and reported to the anesthesia provider. Immediately postoperatively, glucose should be checked and treated as needed. Maintaining stable blood glucose creates an environment more conducive to healing and expedites the recovery of blood flow and tissue.

21. What is the dawn phenomenon in diabetic patients?

The dawn phenomenon is an increase in blood glucose, or hyperglycemia, that occurs specifically in the early morning. Although there is controversy about the frequency of this phenomenon, 54% of type I diabetics and 55% of type II diabetics experience it. There are theories about its cause, however, the exact physiologic pathway is unknown. The very existence of such a frequent phenomenon underscores the importance of assessing the blood glucose in diabetic patients preoperatively and postoperatively, especially when the surgery takes place in the early morning.

22. What is the Somogyi effect in diabetic patients?

The Somogyi effect is the body's response to hypoglycemia that occurs at night during sleep. When hypoglycemia occurs at night, the body responds rigorously by producing extra glucose, resulting in the dawn phenomenon. Hypoglycemia that occurs at night may not wake the patient up and, therefore, can be dangerous. It is induced by too much insulin, or lack of glucose. Postoperative patients should be monitored at night, particularly if they have had insulin and are NPO, or are under the effects of anesthesia. Nighttime sweating or headaches may be symptoms of hypoglycemia.

23. What should I know about the use of etomidate as an anesthetic agent during surgery?

Etomidate has been used as an induction agent in critically ill patients, owing to its ability to minimize hemodynamic changes. Unfortunately, it also causes adrenocortical dysfunction when used in this capacity. In response to acute illness, patients become hypermetabolic due to the activity of the adrenal glands. When the adrenal glands are rendered useless, patients are at higher risk for hypoxia and mortality. Etomidate has also been found to inhibit platelet activity, leading to a longer surgical period and increased blood loss. Furthermore, one dose of etomidate impairs adrenal function for up to 24 hours. When patients arrive in the PACU following etomidate use, patients must be carefully monitored for changes in blood pressure or heart rate, respiratory function and outcome, bleeding, and increased blood glucose. Without adrenal activity, the body's ability to respond quickly to any traumatic insult is impeded (Bloomfield & Noble, 2006; den Brinker et al., 2008; Edelman, Hoffman, & Charbel, 1997; Guldner, Schultz, Sexton, Fortner, & Richmond, 2003; Hoffman et al., 1998; Malerba et al, 2005; Roberts & Redman, 2002).

24. How do I care for a patient who uses anabolic steroids?

It is important that the perianesthesia nurse be aware of the major side effects of anabolic steroid abuse in the postoperative period. Abuse is most common among those involved in competitive sports. Reported consequences that may impact postoperative recovery include changes in mood, hypertension, left ventricular hypertrophy, impaired diastolic filling, and polycythemia. Fluid and electrolyte imbalances are also common. Changes in the myocardium may lead to unexpected arrhythmias. Increased risk for thromboembolism also exists, so deep vein thrombosis should be prevented. The mortality among abusers is four times higher than nonabusers. Careful assessment is critical to avoid untoward outcomes following anesthesia and surgery in patients who potentially abuse anabolic steroids. Additionally, steroid users frequently use the parenteral route

and share needles. Healthcare workers need to use careful precautions in this population to avoid exposure to bloodborne infections (Gonzalez, McLachlan, & Keaney, 2001; Kam & Yarrow, 2005; Medras et al., 2005).

25. How will postoperative shivering impact my hyperthyroid patients?

Hyperthyroidism is a result of an overfunctioning thyroid gland with production of excess thyroid hormone. The high hormone level leads to an increase in heart rate and often, blood pressure. Postoperative shivering is a critical event due to increased oxygen consumption at the cellular level when surgical patients are just arousing from anesthesia and require adequate oxygenation. Shivering also causes the release of catecholamines, which induce increased cardiac output, heart rate, and blood pressure. When both shivering and hyperthyroid disease are present, patients are at risk for excessively high cardiac output, blood pressure, and heart rate. Perianesthesia nurses should be alert to assess for tachycardia and hypertension in this population.

REFERENCES

American Diabetes Association. (2010). Living with diabetes: Neuropathy (nerve damage). Retrieved from http://www.diabetes.org/living-with-diabetes/complications/neuropathy/

Bloomfield, R., & Noble, D. W. (2006). Etomidate, pharmacological adrenalectomy and the critically ill: A matter of vital importance. *Critical Care, 10*(4), 161.

den Brinker, M., Hokken-Koelega, A. C., Hazelzet, J. A., de Jong, F. H., Hop, W. C., & Joosten, K. F. (2008). One single dose of etomidate negatively influences adrenocortical performance for at least 24 h in children with meningococcal sepsis. *Intensive Care Medicine, 34*(1), 163–168.

Edelman, G. J., Hoffman, W. E., & Charbel, F. T. (1997) Cerebral hypoxia after etomidate administration and temporary cerebral artery occlusion. *Anesthesia and Analgesia, 85*(4), 821–825.

Gonzalez, A., McLachlan, S., & Keaney, F. (2001) Anabolic steroid misuse: How much should we know? *International Journal of Psychiatry in Clinical Practice, 5*(3), 159–167.

Guldner, G., Schultz, J., Sexton, P., Fortner, C., & Richmond, M. (2003). Etomidate for rapid-sequence intubation in young children: Hemodynamic effects and adverse events. *Academic Emergency Medicine, 10*(2), 134–139.

Hoffman, W. E., Charbel, F. T., Edelman, G., Misra, M., & Ausman, J. I. (1998). Comparison of the effect of etomidate and desflurane on brain tissue gases and pH during prolonged middle cerebral artery occlusion. *Anesthesiology, 88*(5), 1188–1194.

Kam, P. C., & Yarrow, M. (2005). Anabolic steroid abuse: Physiological and anaesthetic considerations. *Anaesthesia, 60*(7), 685–692.

Kitamura, A., Hoshino, T., Kon, T., & Ogawa, R. (2000). Patients with diabetic neuropathy are at risk of a greater intraoperative reduction in core temperature. *Anesthesiology, 92*(5), 1311–1318.

Lewis, S., Heitkemper, M. M., Dirksen, S. R., O'Brien, P. G., & Bucher, L. (2007). *Medical–surgical nursing* (7th ed). Mosby: Elsevier, MI.

Malerba, G., Romano-Girard, F., Cravoisy, A., Dousset, B., Nace, L., Levy, B., et al. (2005). Risk factors of relative adrenocortical deficiency in intensive care patients needing mechanical ventilation. *Intensive Care Medicine, 31*(3), 388–392.

Medras, M., Tworowska, P., Jozkow, A., Dumanski, A., & Dubinski, A. (2005). Postoperative course and anabolic-androgenic steroid abuse—a case report. *Anaesthesia, 60*(1), 81–84.

National Endocrine and Metabolic Diseases. (2009). Adrenal insufficiency and Addison's disease. NIH publication #04-3054. Retrieved from http://endocrine.niddk.nih.gov/pubs/Addison/Addison.htm

Nettina, S. M. (2006) Lippincott manual of nursing practice (8th ed). Lippincott, Willams & Wilkins: Baltimore.

Oyelana, O. O. (2008). Theoretical approach in the management of Type I diabetes mellitus: A care study of Mr. O. B. *West African Journal of Nursing, 19*(1), 62–67.

Roberts, R. G., & Redman, J. W. (2002) Etomidate, adrenal dysfunction and critical care. *Anaesthesia, 57*(4), 413.

Stedman's (Ed.), (2008). Medical dictionary for the health professions and nursing (6th ed). Lippincott Williams & Wilkins: Baltimore. The Free Dictionary. (2009, July 27). *Pituitary gland*. Retrieved from http://www.thefreedictionary.com/pituitary+gland

Urbano, F. L. (2000) Signs of hypocalcemia: Chvostek's and Trousseau's signs. *Hospital Physician, 36*(3), 43–45.

Waters, J. H., Gottlieb, A., Schoenwald, P., Popovich, M. J., Spring, J., & Nelson, D. R. (2001). Normal saline versus Lactated Ringer's solution for intraoperative fluid management inpatient undergoing abdominal aortic aneurysm repair: An outcome study. *Anesthesia and Analgesia, 93*(4), 817–822.

White, W. A., Montalvo, H., & Monday, J. M. (2004). Continuous subcutaneous insulin infusion during general anesthesia: A case report. *AANA Journal, 72*(5), 353–357.

Wikipedia. (2009, October 28). *General anesthesia*. Retrieved from http://en.wikipedia.org/wiki/General_anaesthesia#Shivering

CHAPTER 26

Ear, Nose, and Throat (ENT) Surgeries

Carol Sallese Maragos, MSN, CRNP, CORLN

INTRODUCTION

ENT stands for ear, nose, and throat. The more sophisticated term is otolaryngology/head and neck. Though there are many procedures performed by otolaryngologists, ranging from basic to complicated, we will focus on the more common procedures performed.

TONSILLECTOMY AND ADENOIDECTOMY

1. What is a tonsillectomy and adenoidectomy (T&A)?

A tonsillectomy is the removal of the palatine tonsils, which are located on either side of the oropharynx. The procedure is performed either on an outpatient basis, or the patient is admitted for a one night stay to monitor the respiratory status. An adenoidectomy may be performed at the same time, which involves removal of the adenoids that are located in the nasopharynx.

2. What are the indications for performing a T&A?

T&A may be performed for recurrent tonsillitis; hypertrophy of the tonsils causing airway obstruction, dysphasia, and speech distortion; and peritonsillar abscess (Sigler & Schuring, 1993).

3. What should I look for when caring for the patient postoperatively?

Bleeding is not a very frequent occurrence; however, if it does occur, it usually happens in the first 24 hours after surgery, and from 10 to 14 days postoperatively. Signs that the patient may be bleeding from the tonsillectomy site include frequent swallowing, taste of blood in the mouth, and a warm feeling in the back of the throat. On examination, blood is visualized in the oral cavity and oropharynx. Bleeding from the nasopharynx may occur from the adenoidectomy site. Usually the bleeding may be controlled by a nasal decongestant; however, if the bleeding persists, the patient may require nasal packing. The surgical team needs to be notified when bleeding occurs to determine if surgical control of the bleeding is indicated (Sigler & Schuring, 1993). It is important to have oral suction available postoperatively if bleeding occurs.

4. Is it true that a tonsillectomy is usually a very painful procedure?

Tonsillectomy can be a very painful procedure, especially in the adult. The pain comes from the movement of saliva over the incisional area. It is very important to provide adequate pain relief in order for the patient to want to swallow. Pain management may entail administering pain medication around the clock for the first several days as opposed to providing pain medication when the patient asks for it.

5. When can patients eat after T&A?

Patients are usually started off on a clear liquid diet and advanced to soft as tolerated. The patient is to avoid eating hard, crunchy, and scratchy foods. Patients can easily become dehydrated posttonsillectomy when it hurts too much to swallow. Pain control is vital in order to make the patient comfortable enough to want to swallow. IV fluids are maintained until the patient is able to swallow a sufficient amount of fluids. Cool fluids are usually better tolerated than warm fluids. In addition, increased swallowing decreases muscle spasms, thus decreasing pain (Sigler & Schuring, 1993).

FUNCTIONAL ENDOSCOPIC SINUS SURGERY (FESS)

6. What does FESS stand for?

FESS is the acronym for functional endoscopic sinus surgery, a procedure performed to restore natural sinus drainage and function (Cohen & Kennedy, 2006; Salamone & Tami, 2004). With the advent of more sophisticated endoscopic surgical experience and instrumentation, functional endoscopic sinus surgery has become the gold standard for the treatment of chronic rhinosinusitis (CRS) (Maragos, 2009).

7. What are the indications for FESS?

Indications for FESS include the treatment of CRS, treatment modality for allergic fungal sinusitis, nasal polyposis with or without aspirin sensitivity, chronic sinus headaches, impaired sense of smell, inverted papillomas, sinonasal paraganglioma, chronic hyperplastic sinusitis, cerebrospinal fluid leaks, nasolacrimal duct obstruction, choanal atresia, dysthyroid orbitopathy, traumatic optic neuropathy, and posterior medial orbital lesions (Dutton, 2010; Miller, Agrawal, Sciubba, & Lane, 2008; Reh & Lane, 2009).

8. What should I look for when assessing the patient postoperatively?

Major complications from functional endoscopic sinus surgery include hyposmia and anosmia (complete lack of smell), exposure of orbital fat, vascular damage, blindness, exposure of dura, cerebrospinal fluid leak, intracranial injury, intraoperative damage to the optic nerve, and hemorrhage resulting in irreversible compressive optic neuropathy and/or central retinal artery occlusion, injury to the extraocular muscles or their nerves resulting in persistent diplopia, or death occur in up to 1.5% of cases (Miller et al., 2008; Jackman, Palmer, Chiu, & Kennedy, 2008). Minor complications consist of bleeding, infection, crusting, synechia formation (abnormal union of body parts) (Sillers & Lay, 2006), ostial stenosis, tooth or lip numbness, or recurrence of disease occur in 1.1 to 20.8% of cases.

SEPTOPLASTY

9. What is the definition of septoplasty?

Septoplasty involves straightening the nasal septum to restore nasal breathing, and it is performed with or without rhinoplasty (Sigler & Schuring, 1993).

10. What are the indications for septoplasty?

Indications for septoplasty include obstruction of the nasal airway, mouth breathing, headaches, recurrent rhinosinusitis, nasal bleeding, and crooked nose (Sigler & Schuring, 1993).

11. What are the postoperative considerations for septoplasty?

Expect to see packing in one nostril or both, depending on the closure and the surgeon's preference. Splints may be inserted into the nose to prevent the formation of nasal synechiae (bands of scar tissue that may form between the surgical site and the lateral nasal wall) (Sigler & Schuring, 1993). Complications that may develop include septal hematoma, nasal bleeding, persistent obstruction caused by incomplete removal of the septum or by intranasal scarring, collapse of the nasal structure, and intranasal synechiae.

12. When testing a patient's hearing, how do you perform a Weber test?

A Weber test needs to be performed with a tuning fork tuned to 512 Hz. Strike the tuning fork on a hard surface and place in the center of the patient's forehead. Ask if the sound is heard midline or is louder on one side. A negative Weber test is when the patient hears the sound in the midline, which means that bone conduction is equal in both ears. If the sound is heard louder in the right ear, it is referred to as a Weber right, indicating unilateral right conductive hearing loss and unilateral sensorineural hearing loss. If the sound is louder in the left ear, it is just the opposite (Backous & Niparko, 2005).

13. What is the purpose of a Rinne test?

The Rinne test checks for bone conduction. To conduct the test, strike the tuning fork on a hard surface and hold in front of the ear, then place behind the ear on the mastoid process. A positive Rinne is when the sound is heard longer in front of the ear (air conduction) and a negative Rinne is when the sound is heard longer on the mastoid process (bone conduction) (Backous & Niparko, 2005). Unilateral sensorineural hearing loss lateralizes to the better ear, and unilateral conductive hearing loss lateralizes to the diseased ear.

TYMPANOPLASTY

14. What is the definition of tympanoplasty?

This is a general term used for describing five types of procedures for repairing the tympanic

membrane (Sigler & Schuring, 1993). Type I is
used to repair a tear or hole in the tympanic
membrane. Type II repairs the tympanic membrane and a graft is placed on the long process
of the incus in cases with malleus dislocation or
necrosis. Type III is performed to repair the tympanic membrane and a graft is applied directly
on the stapes head in cases with necrosis of the
malleus and incus. Type IV repairs the tympanic
membrane and a graft is applied on the nonsta-
tionary stapes footplate in cases with necrosis of
the malleus, incus, and stapes superstructure.
Type V has been replaced by stapes surgery.

15. What are the indications for performing a
tympanoplasty?

A tympanoplasty is performed to repair perforations, retraction pockets, and plaques in the tympanic membrane; to prevent recurrent infections;
to provide adequate aeration of the middle ear;
and to improve hearing.

16. What are common postoperative considerations?

The nurse should be aware of potential complications, which include sensorineural hearing loss,
tinnitus, mouth dryness, graft failure, vertigo,
facial nerve injuries, infections, and taste disturbance. Report these to the surgical team if they
develop in the patient.

COCHLEAR IMPLANT

A cochlear implant is inserted to provide auditory
sensation to patients with severe to profound
binaural congenital or acquired sensorineural
hearing loss. These patients cannot benefit from
conventional hearing aids.

17. How does a cochlear implant work?

A microphone in the implant picks up speech
and environmental sounds, which are then sent
to a processing unit that filters the broad range
of acoustic stimuli. The auditory stimuli are converted into an electrical code, which is transmitted to an external transmitter unit. The unit is
worn over an internal receiver, which is held in
place by a set of magnets found in each unit.
The magnets work through the skin. The internal
receiver translates the electrical code into electrical stimuli, which are transmitted to the cochlea
by an electrode. Each of the many electrodes
that are implanted at varying points along the
cochlear partition is individually stimulated to
discharge a particular portion of the cochlear
nerve fibers.

TRACHEOSTOMY

18. What are the indications for performing a
tracheostomy?

A tracheostomy is performed for patients requiring
prolonged intubation, for airway compromise and
airway protection related to aspiration, edema, coma,
paralysis, and tumor. If a patient remains intubated
with an endotracheal tube, the tube may cause
temporary or permanent damage to the vocal cords
and/or trachea. Any patient who is intubated longer
than 14 days should be considered for a tracheostomy.

19. What is the difference between an open tracheostomy and a percutaneous tracheostomy?

Both an open and percutaneous tracheostomy are
performed for the same reasons; however, percutaneous tracheostomies are performed on patients
who may be too sick to move from their hospital bed
to the operating room. These patients are usually in
the intensive care unit. A percutaneous tracheostomy is performed using the same technique as for
central line insertion. A bronchoscope is inserted
into the trachea by the anesthesia team, then the
surgeon inserts the guide wire through the front of
the neck between the second and third tracheal ring.
Dilating catheters are inserted over the guidewire
until a large enough opening has been created. The
tracheostomy tube is then inserted into the trachea.

20. How often do patients need to be suctioned?

Patients may need to be suctioned very frequently,
about every 1 to 2 hours in the immediate postoperative phase. Before the surgery, the patient's airway is
protected from dust by the cilia in the nose. Now,
being a neck breather, the patient does not have that
mechanism and, therefore, the dust goes directly into
the bronchus. The body's response to this is to
produce mucous. The patient's response is to cough
out the mucus and foreign particles. At first, the
patient may have a weak cough and may be unable
to clear secretions on her or his own. Eventually over
time, the patient might be able to go without suctioning, but this is long after they have left the hospital.
Therefore, it is imperative for the nurse to follow the
provider's orders and suction according to the
patient's needs. It is not acceptable to just listen for
rattling in the airway. Patients can easily develop a
silent mucus plug if not suctioned properly.

21. What is the purpose of instilling saline into the
trachea before suctioning?

The patient needs a lot of humidification to keep
the mucus moist. Dried secretions are very hard to

remove from the airway; therefore, some providers recommend instilling saline before suctioning as this helps to moisten the mucus for easier removal, and it encourages the patient to cough out the mucus. However, this practice is controversial. Up to 5 ml of normal sterile saline may be instilled before each episode of suctioning. Maintaining humidification via a tracheostomy collar is critical in making sure that secretions can easily be removed.

22. When I suction a fresh tracheostomy, there is bloody mucus. Is this expected?

Bloody tinged sputum is expected in a fresh tracheostomy patient due to surgery. The blood may be bright red or dark. The nurse should become concerned about bleeding when dark blood turns to bright red (a sentinel bleed), when the bleeding increases, and when the blood is pumping. The provider needs to be contacted immediately. Tracheal bleeding may also result from deep suctioning when the catheter hits against the tracheal wall and/or the carina. Care should be taken to suction the length of the tracheostomy tube to 1 cm below the end of the tracheostomy tube.

23. What should I do if I cannot pass the catheter into the inner cannula?

There are several reasons why a catheter may not pass easily: mucus is plugging the tube, the catheter is too big for the tube size, the tube is not properly placed in the trachea, and a fenestrated inner cannula is in the tube.

24. What else should I assess when caring for the tracheostomy patient?

Assess secretions for quantity, color, odor, and consistency. Check the stoma and neck plate for skin integrity, color, pain, drainage, bleeding, swelling, and crepitus. The skin around the stoma can easily become red and irritated due to the mucus buildup and constant wiping. Meticulous skin care must be performed on these patients to avoid skin breakdown.

25. Is there anything special that should be kept at the bedside for tracheostomy patients?

Yes, there are several critical items that need to be available in case of accidental decannulation or plugging. These items include a tracheostomy tube of the same size and one smaller, small scissors for cutting sutures that may be holding the tracheostomy tube in place, tracheal dilator or Kelly clamp, tracheal hook, 10-ml syringe, obturator, suction equipment, and Ambu bag. These can easily be stored in one large bag and placed within easy reach.

26. When is the first tracheostomy change performed?

The first tracheostomy change can occur several days after placement of the tracheostomy. The surgical team will usually perform this at the bedside. If it is a percutaneous tracheostomy, the tube is usually changed no sooner than 7 days to allow the tract to mature.

27. If a patient with a tracheostomy arrests, what should I do?

Make sure that the patient has a cuffed tracheostomy tube in place and that the cuff is inflated. If the patient has a cuffless trach tube in place, obtain a cuffed tracheostomy tube of the same size or one size smaller. The surgical or anesthesia team will replace the current tracheostomy tube for a cuffed tracheostomy tube before attaching to the ventilator. An Ambu bag should also be available should the patient need to be ventilated.

28. What should I do if the tracheostomy tube accidentally comes out?

The first thing to do is maintain the airway. Provide oxygen, position the patient so that the stoma is open and not compromised, call the primary team who placed the tube, try to replace the tube if at all possible, and keep the patient safe.

29. What is a T-tube?

A T-tube is a tracheal tube shaped like the letter T. It is used for patients with tracheal stenosis and tracheal malacia. The top part of the T-tube is placed in the trachea to maintain patency of the trachea. The tube does not have an inner cannula and, therefore, the patient needs to maintain meticulous care of the tube to maintain a patent airway. The upper and lower limbs of the T-tube need to be suctioned with a flexible suction catheter. A red rubber catheter is ideal, as long as the patient is not latex allergic. Humidification is very important for these patients as well.

30. What are considered reportable issues?

The nurse should contact the provider should any of the following occur: increase in the respiratory effort or change from baseline, inadequate air exchange through the tracheostomy tube, change in stoma site or secretions, bleeding from or around the tracheostomy, and accidental decannulation.

DIFFICULT AIRWAY

31. What constitutes a difficult airway?

There is no one mechanism for determining if a patient has a difficult airway. The anesthesia team sees the patient preoperatively, evaluating the patient for a previous history of difficult intubation, such as the presence of a large overbite, large tongue, narrow mouth opening, or short chin; and the patient's Mallampati score (Mark, Akst, & Michaelson, 2005), class 1–4, with class 4 being the most difficult type of airway. The Mallampati examination requires the patient to open his or her mouth fully to view the internal structures.

- Class 1 indicates that the patient's uvula, soft palate, and tonsils are in full view.
- Class 2 shows the hard and soft palate, upper portion of the tonsils, and uvula.
- Class 3 reveals the soft and hard palate and base of the uvula.
- Class 4 shows only the hard palate.

32. What is the management of difficult airway patients?

Preoperative planning is the best strategy, as long as it is known that the patient is a difficult airway. The patient may require the use of a LMA (laryngeal mask airway) instead of an endotracheal tube. However, if prolonged anesthesia is necessary, an awake fiberoptic intubation will be performed. If the patient requires a tracheostomy tube, an awake tracheostomy with local anesthesia will be performed.

33. What symptoms are associated with head and neck cancer?

Symptoms that are commonly experienced by head and neck cancer patients include persistent cough, persistent sore throat, change in voice, sensation of a lump in the throat (globus), difficulty swallowing (dysphagia), frequent choking on food, swelling of the jaw or inability to fit dentures, painful swallowing (odynophagia), difficulty breathing, noisy breathing, persistent ear pain, lump in the neck, unplanned weight loss, and bad breath.

34. What type of pathology is associated with head and neck cancer?

The main type of cancer is squamous cell cancer, because squamous cells are found in the tissue that forms the surface of the skin, the lining of the hollow organs of the body, and the passages of the digestive and respiratory tracts, though the other types found are undifferentiated carcinoma, lymphoma, lymphoepithelioma, spindle cell carcinoma, and verrucous cancer.

TOTAL LARYNGECTOMY

35. What is the definition of total laryngectomy?

A total laryngectomy is the removal of the larynx (voice box). The larynx is important for communication, and is a safety organ that prevents food or liquids from entering the trachea. The entire section from the hyoid bone down to the first or second tracheal rings is removed, and the remaining trachea is sewn to the skin forming an ostomy. This opening is the new airway and makes the patient a neck breather. The opening is a permanent hole and, therefore, does not and should not close.

36. What does it mean if the patient is a "neck breather"?

Since the trachea is now sewn to the neck creating a permanent stoma, the patient is no longer able to breathe out of their nose and/or mouth. It is a very important point to keep in mind that the patient is a neck breather should they require oxygen or airway resuscitation.

37. What is a TEP?

A TEP, or tracheoesophageal puncture, is a puncture made at the time of surgery that may be made in the party wall, which is the posterior tracheal wall, as well as anterior esophageal wall. This puncture then allows for the insertion of a voice prosthesis. The voice prosthesis is used by the patient for speaking. The one-way valve in the voice prosthesis allows air to enter the valve from the trachea as the patient occludes the stoma. The air enters the esophagus and is pushed up through the hypo- and oropharynx where it vibrates, thus producing the voice. Before the surgery, the patient is evaluated by the surgeon and speech language pathologist to determine if the patient will be able to care for a voice prosthesis. Some surgeons prefer to place the voice prosthesis at the time of surgery. The prosthesis may not be used for 1 to 2 weeks until the tract has matured.

38. What are other speaking options?

The voice prosthesis is the most common speaking option following a total laryngectomy. Another speaking option is the electrolarynx, which is a device used on the skin or mucous membranes to cause vibration. The patient forms words with their mouth and the electrolarynx produces sound. Patients may also utilize esophageal speech, which is a hands-free method of communication. Other electronic devices are available that talk for the patient.

39. Why is there a catheter sticking out of the patient's neck after total laryngectomy?

A red rubber catheter may be inserted into the TEP site instead of placing the voice prosthesis directly after surgery. This catheter serves two purposes: the first is to mature the tract, and the second is a method for providing enteral nutrition. This catheter prevents the need for inserting a gastrostomy tube.

40. Can laryngectomy patients swallow safely after surgery?

Yes, laryngectomy patients are able to swallow after surgery once the healing of the incisions has healed. Remember that there is now no communication between the esophagus and trachea. When the patient swallows, the food goes directly into the esophagus. Even if the patient has a TEP, the one-way valve prevents foods and liquids from entering into the trachea and lungs.

41. What are the indications for total laryngectomy?

The purpose of performing a total laryngectomy is to completely remove cancer of the larynx, that is either primary or metastatic.

42. What are the risk factors for developing larynx cancer?

Tobacco use (smoking and chewing), alcohol abuse, poor nutrition (a diet lacking in vitamin A and B), gastroesophageal reflux disease (GERD), human papilloma virus (HPV), weakened immune system, Epstein-Barr virus, exposure to wood dust, cement dust, chemicals, pesticides, and asbestos are risk factors for developing cancer in the larynx.

43. How are head and neck cancers staged?

First, the cancer needs to be classified according to the tumor size (T), number and size of nodes present (N), and if there is metastasis (M). Then the cancer is placed into one of four categories:

- Stage 1 cancers are small, localized, and usually curable.
- Stage II and III cancers typically are locally advanced and/or have spread to the lymph nodes.
- Stage IV cancers usually are metastatic and are generally considered to be inoperable.

44. What are the important postoperative considerations for laryngectomy patients?

Maintaining a patent airway is vital since the patient has only one avenue for breathing through the neck. Prior to the surgery, the patient was able to breathe through his nose and mouth, but after the surgery, the trachea is sown to the skin. Nothing should be placed over the stoma that would prevent the patient from breathing, such as bed linens. If the patient requires oxygen or resuscitation, the airway device needs to be placed over the stoma, not over the mouth or nose.

45. What is the importance of stoma care?

Stoma care is very important as it prevents a mucous plug from blocking the airway. As the patient coughs, mucus may collect on the tracheal wall or on the stoma. If the mucus is not removed, new mucus will deposit on top of the old mucus, producing a plug or web, thus decreasing the patient's ability to breathe.

46. How do I perform stoma care?

You will need a pair of tweezers or pickups, hydrogen peroxide, saline, 3 × 3 inch gauze pads or larger, and cotton tip applicators. Try to remove the mucus with the tweezers or pickups. If the mucus does not come away easily, wet the mucus with hydrogen peroxide to soften it. After cleaning, gently wipe the hydrogen peroxide away with saline.

47. A patient had a total laryngopharyngectomy and flap reconstruction. What happens if the patient vomits?

It is very important to prevent the patient from vomiting, as the pressure of the stomach contents coming over the incision line could rupture the sutures. Therefore, as soon as the patient identifies that they are having nausea, antiemetics should be administered. Be sure to alert the surgical team if the patient vomits.

48. What equipment should be available for tracheostomy and laryngectomy patients needing transport to another department within the hospital?

A patient with a tracheostomy tube or stoma who is being transported within the hospital should be suctioned first at the bedside. Then, they need to be placed into one of four transportation classifications (see Table 26-1).

TABLE 26-1. Transportation Classification Level

Level	Definition	Ventilator requirements[a]	Staff required to transport[b]	Monitor[c]	Equipment needed
IV	Patient requires specialized monitoring and interventions, as they have a high potential for instability.	Vented: FiO_2 >40%, PEEP >5 Set RR >20 Nonvented: FiO_2 >50%, RR >25	Minimum of two clinicians: one physician/ NP/PA, and one unit nurse; two critical care team members; RT if vented patient	EKG SaO_2 BP RR	Cardiac monitor, trach equipment, suction supplies, Ambu bag and mask, oxygen, IV, medications
III	Patient requires specialized monitoring and interventions.	Vented: FiO_2 ≤40%, PEEP ≤5 Set RR ≤20 Nonvented who need some assistance to maintain airway patency: FiO_2 ≤50%, RR ≤25	Minimum of two clinicians: one physician/ NP/PA or one unit nurse (plus unlicensed personnel); two critical care team members	EKG, SaO_2, BP, RR	Cardiac monitor, trach equipment, suction supplies, Ambu bag and mask, oxygen, IV, medications
II	Requires minimal intervention by nursing unit level staff. Able to maintain airway patency and ventilation spontaneously.	Does not require airway secretions management.	One of the following: RN, LPN, clinical nursing intern, technician, critical care transport technician	Only based on medical and nursing care needs	Airway management equipment: Trach equipment Suction supplies Ambu bag and mask Oxygen
I	Requires no intervention by nursing unit level staff.	None	None	None	None

[a]PEEP, positive end-expiratory pressure; RR, respiratory rate
[b]NP, nurse practitioner; PA, physician assistants; RT, registered technician; RN, registered nurse; LPN, licensed practice nurse
[c]EKG, electrocardiogram; BP, blood pressure

SUPRAGLOTTIC LARYNGECTOMY

49. What does a supraglottic laryngectomy entail?

This procedure is performed on patients whose cancer is confined to the supraglottis (above the vocal cords) with no evidence of lymph node, vocal cord, cartilage, or involvement outside the glottis. Basically, the larynx above the vocal cords, including the epiglottis and hyoid bone, are removed. The glottic area may be pulled up to the base of the tongue with sutures to offer better protection from aspiration.

50. Following a supraglottic laryngectomy, will the patient have a stoma?

The patient who has undergone a supraglottic laryngectomy will not have a stoma as the vocal cords have been preserved. They will, however, have a tracheostomy until their edema has subsided and airway difficulty is no longer a threat.

SUPRACRICOID LARYNGECTOMY

51. What does a supracricoid laryngectomy entail?

A supracricoid laryngectomy is performed by removing the thyroid cartilage, bilateral true and false vocal cords, and one arytenoid and paraglottic space. It may be reconstructed with a cricohyoidopexy (CHP) or cricohyoidoepiglottopexy (CHEP) if the epiglottis is spared (Pasha, 2006). The patient will have a temporary tracheostomy tube instead of a stoma. The goal for this surgery is for the patient to be able to produce voice and to swallow.

52. What are the indications for this type of surgery?

Certain T3, T4 glottic and supraglottic cancers may involve the preepiglottic space, paraglottic space, ventricle, limited thyroid cartilage, or epiglottis.

53. What are the postoperative considerations?

The patient may be an aspiration risk, especially if the epiglottis is removed. Postoperatively, the surgeon may have the patient spit all secretions into a cup to avoid aspiration on saliva. The tracheostomy tube will likely stay in place after the patient goes home, so the patient will need to be taught tracheostomy care and suctioning.

THYROIDECTOMY

54. What does a total thyroidectomy and a lobectomy entail?

The thyroid gland is divided into left and right lobes. A total thyroidectomy is the removal of both lobes of the thyroid gland. A lobectomy is removal of just one thyroid lobe.

55. What are the indications for a thyroidectomy?

A thyroidectomy is performed for the following indications: presumed malignancy, compressive symptoms, an extension into the mediastinum, failed medical management for Graves' disease or hyperthyroidism, pregnancy in Graves' disease or Hashimoto's thyroiditis, metastasis from thyroid carcinoma, and cosmesis.

56. What are most common postoperative issues?

There are several complications that may develop postthyroidectomy. A hematoma may develop within the surgical bed after surgery at the time of extubation when venous pressure increases (Gourin & Johnson, 2003) and when the patient coughs or strains. Usually, before the incision is closed and after hemostasis has been performed, the surgeon will ask the anesthesiologist to induce a Valsalva's maneuver to increase the venous pressure, thus allowing the surgical team to identify areas of bleeding (Gourin & Johnson, 2003). The nurse should examine the neck for an enlarged area around the incision. Palpate it to see if it is hard or soft. If it is soft and ballotable, it may be a seroma that may or may not have to be drained. It will likely be drained when it causes compressive symptoms. If the area feels hard, it is probably a hematoma. A suture or staple removal kit should always be at the bedside if the incision has to be opened immediately at the bedside to evacuate the hematoma.

Another complication is recurrent laryngeal nerve (RLN) injury or paralysis resulting in voice hoarseness, though this may not be detected immediately postoperatively. The incidence of permanent RLN paralysis is approximately 1 to 1.5% for total thyroidectomy (Pelliterri & Ing, 2005). After surgery, the vocal cords may lie in the paramedian position and as they lateralize, hoarseness and aspiration become apparent (Gourin & Johnson, 2003). When the superior laryngeal nerve and RLN are injured at the same time, the vocal cord will be positioned more laterally, resulting in worsened voice quality and glottic competence. Patients may have difficulty with aspiration and pneumonia on occasion. If there is immediate postoperative stridor and dyspnea, this may indicate bilateral RLN injury, which may require immediate reintubation and a possible tracheostomy. Speech therapy is initiated for evaluation of voice quality and swallowing difficulty (Pelliterri & Ing, 2005).

PARATHYROIDECTOMY

57. What is the definition of parathyroidectomy?

Humans typically have four parathyroid glands that surround the thyroid gland. There is a superior and inferior parathyroid gland found on each side. One or more of these glands may be removed surgically for varying reasons.

58. Why would the parathyroid glands need to be removed?

Hyperparathyroidism is the typical indication for removal of a parathyroid gland. A person needs only one parathyroid gland to maintain normal calcium balance. Symptoms of primary hyperparathyroidism include renal stones, painful bones (osteitis fibrosa cystic), abdominal moans (gastric ulcer, pancreatitis), psychiatric overtones (depression), and fatigue overtones (Randolph, 2003); although some patients are asymptomatic. An elevated serum calcium level may be found on routine screening. Calcium levels greater than 11.4 mg/dl may indicate hyperparathyroidism, or it may indicate multiple melanoma.

59. What are postoperative considerations?

The patient may have persistent hypercalcemia if the suspicious gland is missed; if there are more than four glands; if there is a second adenoma; a failed recognition of parathyroid hyperplasia; or incorrect diagnosis and residual disease (Pasha, 2006). A serum parathyroid hormone (PTH) check will be completed during surgery and often in the postanesthesia care unit (PACU) to make sure the level decreases and drops back down to baseline. On the other hand, hypocalcemia and hypomagnesemia may develop, especially if the patient has low calcium–bone stores. The treatment for this may be lifelong repletion of calcium and vitamin D.

NECK DISSECTION

60. What does a neck dissection involve?

A neck dissection involves systematic removal of lymph nodes with surrounding fibrofatty tissue from the various compartments of the neck. It is for eradicating metastasis from the lymph nodes.

61. What is the difference between a neck dissection and radical neck dissection?

During a radical neck dissection, the lymph nodes from Sections 1 through 5 are removed, including the sternocleidomastoid muscle (SCM), cranial nerve XI (spinal accessory nerve), and internal jugular vein (IJ). Removal of the SCM results in no functional deficit to the patient; however, a cosmetic deformity results when the operative side of the neck becomes flattened. When cranial nerve XI is sacrificed, the patient is at risk for developing shoulder immobility (the cranial nerve XI innervates the trapezius muscle).

A modified neck dissections also takes lymph nodes from Sections 1 through 5, but spares one or more of the three vital structures: the SCM, cranial nerve XI, and IJ. A selective neck dissection removes one or more section of lymph nodes only.

62. What are the different levels of neck dissection?

There are six compartments of the neck where lymph nodes are found.

- Level 1 contains the body of the mandible, anterior belly of the contralateral digastric muscle, anterior and posterior bellies of the ipsilateral digastrics muscle, and stylohyoid muscle.
- Level 2 consists of the area containing the upper jugular lymph nodes.
- Level 3 contains the middle jugular lymph nodes.

- Level 4 contains the lower jugular lymph nodes.
- Level 5 consists of lymph nodes in the posterior triangle and contains the lymph nodes of the anterior compartment of the neck.

63. What are the postoperative considerations for patients undergoing neck dissections?

Patients will usually have at least one neck drain, so stripping, emptying, and recording the output will be important. The patient may require drain care teaching when they have to go home with the drain. The surgeon will usually want the drain pulled when there is less than 25 ml of output in a 24-hour period.

64. How are surgical drains cared for?

Surgical drains can become clotted off if they are not stripped on a regular basis. Stripping involves pulling the drain tubing contents from the drainage site to the bulb. Follow the orders as to how often you need to strip the drains, but it is usually every 4 hours.

65. What can happen if a nurse does not strip the drain?

If the drain does not get stripped, the tubing may get clogged with blood clots or particulate matter. Therefore, fluid does not move away from the operative site. It may appear that the drainage has decreased, when in actuality, fluid is still accumulating around the site. The drain may be pulled prematurely, and the patient may develop a fluid collection at the drainage site. This excess fluid may also be a source for infection.

PAROTIDECTOMY

66. What is the definition of parotidectomy?

A parotidectomy is the removal of the superficial and/or deep lobe of the parotid gland.

67. What is the reason for the removal of the parotid gland?

The parotid may need to be removed for benign neoplasm (which are most common) or malignant tumors (which make up 6% of all head and neck malignancies) (Simental & Carrau, 2005).

68. What are important postoperative considerations?

Keep the head elevated above the level of the heart to drain lymphatic fluids and to reduce swelling. The eye on the affected side may be weakened and, therefore, may not completely close. In this case, the eye can then easily dry out, which may lead to corneal abrasions. Untreated corneal abrasions can lead to permanent blindness. Administer frequent eye drops as ordered throughout the day, and apply an ophthalmic lubricant at night. A moisture chamber, either made by hand with plastic wrap and tape, or a commercially available chamber, is applied at night to seal in moisture around and over the eye. The chamber can be removed during the day.

69. What are important considerations for facial nerve damage after parotid surgery for malignancy?

Cranial nerve VII, otherwise known as the facial nerve, runs directly through the parotid gland. Of the five branches of the facial nerve, the zygomatic branch innervates the eye. The facial nerve is responsible for closing the eye. If the eye has scleral show, the eye is at risk for developing corneal abrasions, which could lead to blindness. If the sclera shows when the patient tries to close his eyes, the provider will order saline eye drops to be instilled every 1 to 2 hours during the day and lubricant to be applied at night. A moisture chamber may also be applied at night to prevent eye dryness. A moisture chamber, either made by hand with plastic wrap and tape or a commercially available chamber, is applied at night to seal in moisture around and over the eye. Patients with facial droop may need surgical enhancement with muscle transfers and gold weight placement in the upper lid to allow for complete closure. Since the sensory nerve may also be damaged, men should shave with electric razors only, and the face should be protected from extreme temperatures (Wirkus, 2007).

70. What is Frey's syndrome and why does it develop?

Frey's syndrome, or gustatory sweating, occurs as transected postganglionic secretomotor parasympathetic fibers regenerate and follow the sympathetic nerve sheaths of denervated facial sweat glands (Simental & Carrau, 2005). The mastication causes facial sweating as a result in cholinergic neurotransmission. The patient will experience perspiration, flushing, and a feeling of warmth over the preauricular and temporal areas while eating and/or smelling aromas (Wirkus, 2007). If the patient prefers not to have to dab the sweat during meals, the patient may apply glycopyrrolate or 20% aluminum chloride (deodorant) to facial skin. Also, injecting botulism toxin may benefit the patient (Wirkus, 2007). The patient may opt for surgery that involves placing barrier tissue in the parotid space to prevent nerve regeneration. Another technique to relieve gustatory sweating is a transcanal neurectomy of the tympanic plexus.

71. Are there any other complications from parotidectomy?

Another common complication of parotidectomy includes formation of a salivary fistula (sialocele) (Wirkus, 2007). Saliva may drain through the wound or collect beneath the flap, thereby compromising the wound.

FLAPS

72. Are there different types of flaps?

There are basically two major types of flaps: free flaps and rotational flaps.

73. What influences the choice of location from where to acquire the flap?

The surgeon will look at the following when deciding where to take the flap: amount of skin color and soft tissue, pedicle length and vessel quality, innervation capacity, availability of bone quantity and quality, donor site location and donor site, and the health of the vessel (Byrne & Goding, 2005).

74. What are the postoperative considerations with flaps?

It is very important for the outgoing nurse to show the incoming nurse where to place the Doppler wand to check for vascular flow. Therefore, the nurses need to go to the patient's bedside so that the proper location of flap checks can be identified.

During a flap check, the nurse needs to assess the flap site for skin temperature, color, capillary refill, and the presence of edema. The nurse should not hesitate to contact the surgical team with any concerns about the flap. The highest risk for flap failure is during the first 72 hours after surgery, and therefore, the flap needs to be checked every 1 hour for the first 24 hours. As the days progress, monitoring can be decreased and, often, discontinued on postoperative day 6.

When a patient has a flap in the head and neck area, nothing compressing should be placed around the neck. This includes ties for a tracheostomy tube and straps to hold oxygen or humidification in place.

Vasopressors should be avoided at all costs. The increase in vascular pressure may cause dehiscence of the vessel anastomosis. If the patient is hypotensive, IV fluids are given. An acceptable urine output is nothing less than 15 cc/hr. A hematocrit of 25 to 30 is ideal.

The provider may order for the patient's head to be positioned a certain way. A sign stating this should be posted in the room for the patient and staff to be reminded of this important order. If the head is turned in the opposite direction, the vessel anastomosis may come apart, resulting in bleeding and flap failure.

75. What are the postoperative complications with flaps?

The most common complication with flaps is thromboses at the venous anastomosis site, resulting in venous congestion. Signs to look for are increased flap turgor, rapid capillary refill with brisk bleeding, appearance of darker blood, and mottling and darkening of the flap skin. Color changes occur later during this ischemic time. An arterial pulse may still be palpable (Byrne & Goding, 2005).

Arterial insufficiency, on the other hand, appears as paleness and coolness, loss of skin turgor, absence of capillary refill and loss of bleeding to pinprick. A Doppler signal is usually absent. The longer the ischemic time, the more difficult it becomes to salvage the flap (Byrne & Goding, 2005).

The donor site should also be assessed for drainage color and amount, pain, skin color, pulses, and presence of tingling or numbness.

76. Are leeches really used for venous congestion?

Yes, medicinal leeches have been shown to relieve venous congestion and to aid in salvaging the flap. Leeches may be applied one or more at a time, depending on the amount of congestion and size of the flap. Leeches secrete hematin, a local anesthetic, and hirudin, an anticoagulant, when it latches on. Therefore, patients do not feel the leeches. Leeches will usually fall off when they become engorged, and a new one is put in its place. The engorged leech is then euthanized in alcohol. Leeches do not latch on to dead skin. Expect oozing from the attachment site. Leeches may harbor gram-negative beta-lactamase producing organisms. Therefore, the start of antibiotic prophylaxis with the initiation of leech therapy is important. The antibiotic of choice is Bactrim.

REFERENCES

Backous, D. D., & Niparko, J. (2005). Evaluation and surgical management of conductive hearing loss. In C. W. Cummings, B. H. Haughey, J. R. Thomas, L. A. Harker, & P. W. Flint (Eds.), *Otolaryngology: Head and neck surgery* (4th ed.). Philadelphia: Elsevier.

Byrne, P. J., & Goding, G. S. (2005). Skin flap physiology and wound healing. In C. W. Cummings, B. H. Haughey, J. R. Thomas, L. A. Harker, & P. W. Flint (Eds.), *Otolaryngology: Head and neck surgery* (4th ed.). Philadelphia: Elsevier.

Cohen, N., & Kennedy, D. (2006). Revision endoscopic sinus surgery. *Otolaryngologic Clinics of North America, 39*(3), 417–435.

Dutton, J. (2010). *Endoscopic sinus surgery.* Retrieved from http://www.american-rhinologic.org/patientinfo.sinussurgery.phtml.

Gourin, C. G., & Johnson, J. T. (2003). Postoperative complications. In G. W. Randolph (Ed.), *Surgery of the thyroid and parathyroid glands*. Philadelphia: Saunders.

Jackman, A. H., Palmer, J. N., Chiu, A. G., & Kennedy, D. W. (2008). Use of intraoperative CT scanning in endoscopic sinus surgery: A preliminary report. *American Journal of Rhinology, 22*(2), 170–174.

Maragos, C. S. (2009). Improving quality of life with FESS. *OR Nurse, 3*(6), 24–29.

Mark, L., Akst, S., & Michaelson, J. (2005). Difficult airway/intubation: Implications for anesthesia. In C. W. Cummings, B. H. Haughey, J. R. Thomas, L. A. Harker, & P. W. Flint (Eds.), *Otolaryngology: Head and neck surgery* (4th ed.). Philadelphia: Elsevier.

Miller, N. R., Agrawal, N., Sciubba, J. J., & Lane, A. P. (2008). Image-guided transnasal endoscopic resection of an orbital solitary fibrous tumor. *Ophthalmic Plastic and Reconstructive Surgery, 24*(1), 65–67.

Pasha, R. (2006). *Otolaryngology head and neck surgery clinical reference guide* (2nd ed.). San Diego: Plural.

Pellitteri, P. K., & Ing, S. (2005). Disorders of the thyroid gland. In C. W. Cummings, B. H. Haughey, J. R. Thomas, L. A. Harker, & P. W. Flint (Eds.), *Otolaryngology: Head and neck surgery* (4th ed.). Philadelphia: Elsevier.

Randolph, G. W. (2003). Surgical anatomy of the recurrent laryngeal nerve. In G. W. Randolph (Ed.), *Surgery of the thyroid and parathyroid glands*. Philadelphia: Saunders.

Reh, D. D., & Lane, A. P. (2009). The role of endoscopic sinus surgery in the management of sinonasal inverted papilloma. *Current Opinion in Otolaryngology & Head and Neck Surgery, 17*(1), 6–10.

Salamone, F., & Tami, T. (2004). Acute and chronic sinusitis. In A. Lalwani (Ed.), *Current diagnosis and treatment in otolaryngology head and neck* (pp. 285–292). New York: McGraw-Hill.

Sigler, B. A., & Schuring, L. T. (1993). *Ear, nose and throat disorders*. St. Louis, MO: Mosby.

Sillers, M., & Lay, K. (2006). Symptom outcomes following endoscopic sinus surgery. Operative techniques. *Otolaryngology: Head and Neck Surgery, 17*(1), 6–12.

Simental, A., & Carrau, R. L. (2005). Malignant neoplasms of the salivary glands. In C. W. Cummings, B. H. Haughey, J. R. Thomas, L. A. Harker, & P. W. Flint (Eds.), *Otolaryngology: Head and neck surgery* (4th ed.). Philadelphia: Elsevier.

Wirkus, J. (2007). Parotid masses: Face the facts. *ORL-Head and Neck Nursing, 25*(1),10–16.

CHAPTER 27

Genitourinary Surgery

Pamela E. Windle, MS, RN, NE-BC, CPAN, CAPA, FAAN

The genitourinary system is very important in the care of postoperative patients in perianesthesia settings. This chapter is a short review of the basic anatomy and physiology of certain structures of the renal system, and the kidney function is imperative to ensure positive outcomes as well as the return to its normal values. Tests are indicators of the progression of patient's safe emergence from anesthesia and surgery. In the renal system, the assessment of the kidney function is important for maintaining homeostasis, which also plays an important part in the regulation of the cardiovascular system. Included also are simple problems encountered by nurses and residents; however, the clinical correlation between the physiology of the renal system and a simple guide for nursing care is explained throughout this chapter.

1. What is the structure of the kidney?

The kidneys are a pair of bean-shaped organs located in the retroperitoneal space of the abdomen. It receives its blood supply from a single renal artery. This renal artery branches to the afferent arteriole of the nephron, which carries blood to the glomerulus. The right kidney is slightly lower than the left due to the placement of the liver.

2. What are the three macrostructures of the kidney?

- The cortex includes the proximal tubules, cortical portion of Henle's loop, glomeruli, distal tubules, and cortical collection ducts.

- The medulla includes the renal pyramids and the medullary part of the collecting ducts.

- The renal sinus and pelvis includes the calyx, the functional unit of the kidney; the papillae, the renal tissue projections located at the ends of renal pyramids; the renal lobe, composed of the pyramid and the surrounding cortical tissue; and the corticomedullary junction, a division between the cortex and medulla formed by the base of the pyramids.

3. What is the functional unit and two main functions of the kidney?

The nephron is the functional unit of the kidney. Nephrons remove metabolic substances and waste products and retain essential electrolytes and water through the formation of urine. The two main functions are elimination of waste products and regulation of fluid and electrolyte balance. Renal function can be measured by assessing the serum levels of blood urea nitrogen (BUN) and creatinine. Urea is a byproduct of dietary protein metabolism and creatinine is a breakdown product of muscle metabolism. Both of these substances are excreted by the kidney and will be elevated in patients with renal dysfunction.

4. What are the important electrolytes involved in the kidney and the normal values of each?

- Sodium: 135–145 mEq/L
- Potassium: 3.5–5.5 mEq/L
- Calcium: 8.5–10.5 mg/DI
- Magnesium: 1.3–2.1 mEq/L
- Phosphorus: 2.7–4.5 mg/dL
- Chloride: 98–106 mEq/L

5. What are the important laboratory tests used to assess renal function?

- BUN: normal range: 10–20 mg/dL

- Serum creatinine (Cr): normal range: 0.5–1.2 mg/dL (slightly higher in males than females)

- Urinalysis: Check for appearance, color, and clarity; specific gravity (1.010–1.025) and urine concentration; identify the presence of red blood cells (0–2), glucose (0), and proteins (albumin, 0–8 mg/dL). Proteins should never be excreted by a normal or healthy kidney. Presence of protein indicates glomerulonephritis or trauma to urinary drainage system.

- Cr clearance: Measures the creatinine amount produced against creatinine excreted. Collect urine for 24 hours and keep the bottle in an ice bucket. The normal range is 110–120 ml/min. Below 50 ml/min indicate significant renal dysfunction.

- BUN/Cr ratios: Useful to assess type of acute kidney disease (prerenal or intrarenal).

6. What are the renal imaging or radiologic tests involved?

Renal angiography is a small catheter with radiopaque dye that is threaded through the femoral artery into the aorta and renal artery for visualization. Watch out for swelling and bleeding. Encourage increased fluids to facilitate excretion of the dye. Tests include renal biopsy, where bed rest is maintained for at least 4 hours postprocedure, and activities are avoided that increase abdominal venous pressure such as coughing. The patient is observed for bloody urine.

Flat plate KUB (Kidney Ureter Bladder) is an antero-posterior (AP) abdominal x-ray that uses radiation to take a picture of structures inside the abdomen to check for gastrointestinal conditions, such as: a bowel obstruction, and can detect the presence of kidney stones or foreign bodies. Other diagnostic tests include: kidney ureter bladder CT scan; IV pyelogram, which visualizes the entire urinary system and isolates abnormalities; renal ultrasound, which focuses on a particular organ with high frequency sound waves and measures shape and sizes; renal angiogram, which evaluates renal artery stenosis and checks renal circulation and the great vessels; renal computed tomography, which evaluates retroperitoneal lymph nodes; renal MRI allows direct imaging (transverse, coronal, and sagittal) plane and evaluates renal and prostate abnormalities; and renal biopsy.

7. What is renal failure?

Renal failure (RF) is a sequelae or syndrome of varying critical etiologies or illness, caused by low cardiac output and hypoperfusion of the kidney that can damage and initiate RF. Acute renal failure (ARF) shows an acute deterioration in kidney function due to the inability to eliminate waste products and regulate fluid balance, which could occur rapidly within days or weeks, but can be irreversible.

8. What are the types of acute renal failure (ARF) or acute kidney failure (AKF)?

Prerenal failure is the most common type of renal failure and occurs before the blood enters the kidney, which causes diminished renal perfusion and potential ischemia result. Prerenal causes include dehydration, shock, vasodilatation, impaired cardiac function, renal vascular obstruction, and hepatorenal syndrome.

Intrarenal (parenchymal) or intrinsic failure acute tubular necrosis (ATN) is common with possible causes of nephrotoxic damage, ischemic insult, and inflammatory damages such as glomerulonephritis (Glomerular, interstitial, vascular, acute tubular necrosis, and allergic interstitial nephritis). Postrenal or postobstructive failure is due to a partial or complete obstruction of the lower urinary tract, such as structural defects of ureters, tumors, renal stones, urethral strictures benign prostatic hyperplasia (BPH), blood clots, or an atonic bladder. The Glomerular filtration rate (GFR) is the best test to measure the level of kidney function as well as the stage of kidney disease. The obstruction causes an increased hydrostatic pressure in the tract and decreased GFR. The patient with obstruction usually presents as oliguric or anuric, exhibits signs and symptoms of fluid excess, bounding pulse, crackles in lung bases, increased right atrial pressure, peripheral edema, and sudden weight gain (ureter, bladder, and urethra).

9. What are the potential causes of prerenal failure?

Prerenal failure is caused by any condition that decreases blood flow to the kidneys due to hypovolemia and low cardiac output. The signs and symptoms related to hypovolemia are oliguria, hypotension, tachycardia, orthostatic blood pressure changes, central venous pressure (CVP) less than 5 mm-Hg, a dry mucous membrane, flat jugular veins, and lethargy progressing to coma.

The signs and symptoms related to low cardiac output are hypotension, tachycardia, peripheral and systemic edema, clammy skin, elevated pulmonary artery diastolic pressure (PADP) , pulmoartery wedge pressure (PWP) greater than 18 mm-Hg due to the heart's inability to pump the blood out into the systemic circulation.

10. What is the major cause of death in ARF patients?

The major cause of death in ARF patients is hyperkalemia, which can be caused by high potassium intake or low renal potassium excretion.

11. What causes metabolic acidosis?

Metabolic acidosis is a state commonly associated with acute and chronic renal failure due to potential for acid-base imbalance caused by the inability of the kidneys to excrete hydrogen.

12. What are the defining characteristics for metabolic acidosis state?

In a metabolic state, assess the patient for Kussmaul's respirations, watch for potential headache, fatigue, cardiac dysrhythmias, ABGs with pH below 7.35 with bicarbonate level below 22 mEq/L, possible seizures, and CNS depression that progress to possible coma.

13. Describe chronic renal failure (CRF), the causes and treatment of CRF, and the three stages of CRF.

Chronic renal failure (CRF) is a slow, progressive, and irreversible process that progress to end stage renal disease (ESRD). Most cases are caused by diabetes and hypertension. Treatment includes dialysis or transplantation. The 3 stages of chronic renal failure are (CRF): Stage 1, Diminish renal reserve; Stage 2, Renal insufficiency; and Stage 3, ESRD, a complete loss of kidney function.

14. What are nonconservative therapy options for ARF?

There are three main treatment options for ARF: hemodialysis, peritoneal dialysis, and continuous renal replacement therapy (CRRT). Hemodialysis pumps blood through an artificial kidney that removes solutes by dialysis along a concentrated gradient, and water is removed by ultrafiltration through a pressure gradient. Peritoneal dialysis (PD) is a repetitive instillation and removal of fluids into and from the peritoneal cavity. A patient can perform their own PD. CRRT uses gradual and continuous removal of fluids and electrolytes through dialysis. CRRT is indicated for patients who cannot tolerate intermittent hemodialysis. CRRT can effectively remove myoglobin which is too large to be cleared by traditional hemodialysis filters. It provides better hemodynamic stability than intermittent hemodialysis and provides 24/7 volume status maintenance, where nutrition and medication can be given.

15. What are the common reasons for renal replacement therapy?

The reasons include fluid overload, hyperkalemia, metabolic acidosis, severe hypotension, and uremia.

16. What are the indications for renal replacement therapy?

- Oliguria: urine output less than 200 mL/12 hr
- Anuria or extreme oligoria: urine output less than 50 mL/12 hr
- Hyperkalemia: potassium greater than 6.5 mEq/L
- Acidemia: pH less than 7.1
- Azotemia: urea greater than 30 mg/dL
- Pulmonary edema
- Uremic pericarditis
- Uremic encephalopathy
- Uremic neuropathy/myopathy
- Hyperthermia
- Dysadrenia: sodium less than 115 or greater than 160 mEq/L
- Drug overdose with dialyzable toxin

17. What are the options to treat renal replacement therapies?

Treatment options include peritoneal dialysis, hemodialysis, and hemofiltration.

18. How is hemodialysis processed?

Hemodialysis is a process, whereby the dialysis machine replaces the kidneys in performing the functions of removing excess blood electrolytes, waste products, and fluid. Blood is removed from the body and transported to a dialyzer, which removes excess electrolytes and toxins through diffusion. Solute drag is created from the ultrafiltration process, then blood exits the dialyzer and an electric pump returns it to the patient's circulation. This process usually last for 3 to 4 hours and is usually done daily or three times per week per individualized patient.

19. When is hemodialysis indicated?

Patients with ARF usually require hemodialysis. Some indications include overdose, abnormal laboratory values, some medical conditions, and chronic renal failure. Permanent access includes AV fistula, AV graft, and AV shunt. The goal is to keep these clean at all times to provide patency of the device and prevent infection and not to perform blood pressure readings, as well as venipunctures on the affected limb.

20. What are the contraindications for hemodialysis?

Contraindications are patients with unstable hemodynamic profile, or who cannot tolerate anticoagulant medication and when vascular access cannot be obtained.

21. What role do family members play with patients going through hemodialysis?

The family needs to provide constant support and guidance, making sure the patient goes for his or her dialysis as required by the physician.

22. What are potential complications of CRRT?

Some potential complications are air embolism, ischemia, hemorrhage, and temperature alterations.

23. What important preoperative nursing assessments should be performed in preparation for patients undergoing renal surgery?

- Check the patient's history of hypertension, pulmonary function, and urinary problems.
- Perform medication reconciliation for the patient's medications.
- Record accurate weight, height, and vital signs for the patient.
- Perform head-to-toe assessment and check for any swelling on the patient.
- Check if the patient is taking antibiotics being excreted through the kidneys, and if so, adjust the dosage.
- Explain to the patient the "need to void" after surgery and instruct the patient not to attempt to void around the catheter because exertion of pressure can cause the bladder muscle to contract, causing painful bladder spasms.

24. What are pertinent surgical procedures?

- Extracorporeal shock wave lithotripsy: Noninvasive approach for obstructive renal stone disease, where external shock waves are directed at the renal and ureteral calculi. Remnants usually pass in urine through forced diuresis; sometimes ureteral stents are placed to maintain patency.
- Cystoscopy: A direct visualization of the urethra and bladder by means of a tubular lighted telescopic lens with flexible or rigid

instrumentation. A biopsy or instillation of bladder medications is commonly performed.
- Cystotomy: An incision into the bladder
- Circumcision: Surgical incision to remove constricting foreskin
- Bladder and urinary stents: Stents inserted to provide and maintain patency of the organs
- Prostatectomy (laparoscopic or open): Transurethral resection of prostate (TURP); retropubic prostatectomy, which is a radical procedure for carcinoma of prostate using a lower abdominal approach; laparoscopic, which is a lengthy procedure requiring magnification of laparoscopic image; and laser TURP, which is used for patients with blood thinner and ablation of bleeders.
- Transurethral resection of bladder tumor or bladder neck (TURBT): A resection of lesions and contractures. Watch for extravasations of irrigating fluids caused by bladder perforation.
- Partial or radical cystectomy: A lengthy procedure requiring removal of entire bladder if malignant.
- Nephrectomy (laparoscopic or open): The removal of the kidney may include excision of ureter or adrenal gland. Intraoperative concerns for open procedure include positioning of patient, which causes compression of the dependent side and might compromise arterial and venous circulation and potential injury to peritoneum. Laparoscopic procedure concerns include hemorrhage and potential injury to the spleen, liver, and pleura.
- Nephrostomy: An opening into the kidney for temporary or permanent drainage
- Adrenalectomy (laparoscopic or open): A removal of neoplasms; corrects hypersecretion of adrenal hormones. Intraoperative concerns include damages to the liver, spleen, and pancreas; fluid volume imbalance; and hypotension.
- Ureterolithotomy or nephrolithotomy (laparoscopic or open): A surgical removal of large and adherent renal and ureteral calculi
- Urinary diversion (laparoscopic or open) such as abdominal stoma, ileal conduit: Bladder replacement with colon, ileum, or sigmoid sections, and continent diversion (Kock pouch and Indiana pouch)
- Bladder neck suspensions (laparoscopic or open): Corrects urinary stress incontinence. Examples are Marshall-Marchetti-Krantz and endoscopic

techniques using pubovaginal (PB) sling, Burch procedure, Raz sling, and the Stamey procedure.

- Penile implant: Corrects erectile dysfunction through implant or venous diversion

- Penectomy resection (partial or total): Depends on the extent of the tumor and location of the carcinoma of the penis

- Urinary sphincter: Artificial implantation that corrects persistent incontinence and urinary leakage, which is most commonly performed on the postprostatectomy patient, where a mechanical inflation pump device is placed around the bladder neck or urethra.

- Orchiectomy: The removal of diseased testis either through the inguinal or scrotal approach

- Vasectomy: A scrotal approach used for elective sterilization for men.

- Vasovasostomy or epididymovasostomy: A surgical procedure to reverse previous vasectomy and to correct vas deferens or epididymis stenosis.

25. What are the important PACU nursing assessments that should be performed after renal surgery?

- Assess for dyspnea and auscultate for crackles for volume overload.

- Assess for peripheral dependent edema, weight gain, CHF, pericardial friction rub, and extra heart sounds (S3 or S4).

- Assess fluid volume and administer fluids replacement to maintain blood volume and monitor hourly urine output.

- Identify the presence of a Foley catheter, and assess color and amount of urine.

- If other catheters are present (ureterostomy or suprapubic), identify the position, as well as color and amount of urine.

- Observe swelling or ulcerations around the genitalia.

- Assess for possible acute renal failure.

- Observe for signs of hemorrhage and shock. Furosemide (Lasix) might be indicated, and minimize narcotic use due to decreased renal function.

26. What are some possible renal complications?

- Acute renal necrosis
- Acute kidney injury
- Prerenal azotemia
- Postrenal azotemia

- Atelectasis
- Hypertension
- Urinary obstruction
- Bleeding/hemorrhage
- Foley obstruction
- Bacterial infection
- Ureteral stricture
- Renal colic
- Bladder neck obstruction
- Calculi
- Urinary retention
- Improper trocar placement causing vascular injury or organ perforation
- Cardiac dysrhythmias
- Acute/chronic renal failure

27. What are the common perianesthesia nursing concerns or issues that occur after renal surgery?

- Leaking of urine around catheter
- Hematuria
- Difficult Foley placement: Nursing hints include using lots of lubricating jelly, using French size 14 and 16 (when using Caudae, inflate the balloon after inserting Foley completely even up to the Y-port visually)
- Spasms
- Hypovolemic or hyponatremic shock
- Bleeding/hemorrhage
- Persistent pain (acute and/or chronic)
- Foley not draining
- Dehydration
- Scrotal swelling
- Infection
- Sterility

28. What is the specific nursing care for renal and ureteral surgeries?

Excision of tumors, obstructions to urine flow such as stones, reconstruction of urine outflow tracts, repair of lacerations or deformities, excision of a kidney, or kidney transplant are specific renal and ureteral surgeries. Watch for the risk of fluid volume deficit from the intake restrictions before and after surgery. Accurate intake and output is very important; notify the surgeon for low urine output. Patients with drains or stomas need a small plastic bag over the area for collection of drainage, which should be emptied frequently. Skin care is also important; urine should not be allowed to remain on the skin to avoid any infection. Observe for blood loss from damage to an intrarenal surgery and extravasation of the irrigation solution used during surgery. Always encourage adequate fluid intake unless restricted. Strict intake and output for renal patients.

29. What are some postoperative nursing interventions to watch for?

- Monitor arterial blood gases to assess abnormal results, degree of acidosis, identify causes of metabolic acidosis, and provide necessary electrolytes to keep electrolyte balance.

- Dressing applied after urinary tract surgery is often soaked with blood and urine. It is important to reinforce dressing as necessary and to keep the skin clean and dry to prevent any excoriation, breakdown, and infection.

- Assess for abdominal distention caused by overfilling of the bladder due to an inability to void or a malfunction of the catheters. Use a bladder ultrasound scan to assess for bladder volume.

30. What to watch for when patients have oliguria?

Oliguria indicates significant fluid deficit or dehydration, so insertion of indwelling catheter and measuring hourly output is important. Check the indwelling catheter for patency, make sure the catheter is not obstructed, and that there is no postoperative urinary retention or occlusion by physically checking the patient's abdomen and/or bladder or checking with a bladder scan.

31. How much urine output should be expected postoperatively?

Urine output should be 30 mL/hr or 1 mL/kg/hr. Optimal fluid intake is very important postoperatively. Fluid intake should be increased to a total of 3000 ml in a 24-hour period.

32. What is the common fluid therapy for postoperative oliguria?

The initial fluid is 1 L of 0.9% normal saline, then 500 mL/hr for 2 hr, 250 mL/hr for 4 hr, 166 mL/hr for 6 hr, then the maintenance fluid order of usually 125 mL/hr.

33. What are the common postoperative diuretics used to prevent oliguria?

Diuretics are categorized based on the sites of action on the renal tubules and the secretion of urine.

- Potassium sparing diuretics act on the distal convoluted tubule, which increases urine output without the loss of potassium. Examples include triamterene (Dyrenium), amiloride (Midamor), and triamterene and hydrochlorothiazide (Dyazide).

- Osmotic diuretics act on the tubules, which increases plasma osmolality and draws fluid from intracellular space into the extracellular space. Examples include mannitol and urea.

- Thiazide diuretics are secreted in the proximal convoluted tubule with the effect at the loop of Henle. These diuretics are commonly used for diabetic insipidus, edema, and hypertension. Examples include benzthiazide (Exna), chlorothiazide (Diuril), and hydrochlorothiazide (Esidrix, HydroDIURIL, Oretic).

- Loop diuretics are secreted into the tubule and acts on the medullary segment where chloride transport is prohibited, interferes with the concentration and dilution mechanism of the kidneys, the result of which is isotonic urine production. These diuretics are highly potent and act rapidly. Examples include bumetanide (Bumex), ethacrynic acid (Edecrin), and furosemide (Lasix).

- Aldosterone antagonists act on the aldosterone receptors in the conducting ducts, which enhance the reabsorption of sodium and chloride and increase potassium excretion in the renal tubules. An example includes spironolactone (Aldactone). This is usually used for liver cirrhosis, congestive heart failure, and nephritic syndrome.

- Carbonic anhydrase inhibitors act in the proximal renal tubules and result in diminished excretion of hydrogen ions and increased excretion of bicarbonate and produces alkaline urine. An example includes acetazolamide (Diamox). This is usually used for reduction of intraocular pressure and for seizures.

34. What are the common side effects of diuretics?

Some concerns or side effects include pulmonary edema, when there is an increase extracellular fluid volume. Therefore, the PACU nurse should watch for early signs of wheezing, crackles, or rales upon chest auscultation. Other concerns are hyperkalemia due to frequent potassium supplement; hypokalemia; and hypovolemia. The PACU nurse should watch for muscle weakness, ventricular dysrhythmias, hypotension, tachycardia, and monitor ventilation and $PaCO_2$ level.

35. Why is ECG monitoring important for postoperative renal patients?

Continuous ECG monitoring is important for ARF because of hyperkalemia, which may lead to cardiac arrest. Watch out for high peak T waves, depressed ST segments, and any heart block.

36. What are some important management techniques for patient's with indwelling urinary catheter?

Inappropriate, prolonged catheter usage can cause infection or catheter-associated urinary tract infection (CAUTI). A study of patients with a 7-day catheter showed that 50% developed bacteriuria, catheter blockage, serious infections, sepsis, and death (Wound Ostomy and Continence Nurses Society, 2008). The best prevention is to remove the catheter as soon as possible and to allow the patient to void freely.

37. Describe other alternatives for bladder management.

Fewer complications is the key reason to discontinue indwelling catheters. Several options for bladder management of patients with urinary retention or incontinence include using urinals, external catheters for men, and absorbent products for urinary incontinence or intermittent catheterization for urinary retention.

38. What are the causes of urinary tract infections (UTIs)?

UTIs are caused by pathogenic microorganisms in the urinary tract. The types of UTIs are cystitis, prostatitis, urethritis, pyelonephritis, and interstitial nephritis.

39. What coping or support mechanisms are needed for families?

A holistic approach is needed to care for a patient with renal problems. Family support is required, but most importantly, a patient assessment on the ability to cope with the disease is needed. The patient could either go into chronic renal failure, which requires long-term dialysis or waiting for renal transplantation. Independence and compliance with the treatment regimen is important for its success. The verbalization of stress and/or an inability to cope is needed so family members can provide trust and confidence when with the patient.

40. What specific outpatient teachings should be given to the patient and caregiver or family prior to going home with a Foley or leg bag?

The patient and family or caregiver should check for patency, that it is not obstructed, and should make sure urine is flowing. Hygiene is important, and the caregiver or family should be taught to clean aseptically with soap and water.

41. What specific discharge instructions should a renal patient be aware of?

Patients should call their physician immediately if they are experiencing any type of pain, bladder spasms, or difficulty with urination.

Thank you to Dr. Lambros Stamatakis, Senior Urology resident, Baylor College of Medicine, Houston, Texas, for reviewing this chapter.

REFERENCES

Alspach, J. (Ed.) (1998). *Core curriculum for critical care nursing*. Philadelphia: Saunders.

American Association of Critical-care Nurses. (2008). *Care of the patient with renal disorders* (E-learning module). Retrieved from www.aacn.org/wd/elearning/content/ecco/module7-renal.pcms?menu=elearning

Drain, C. B., & Odom-Forren, J. (2008). *Perianesthesia nursing: A critical care approach* (5th ed.). St. Louis, MO: Saunders.

Moore, R. G., Bishoff, J. T., Loening, S., & Docimo, S. G. (Eds.). (2005). *Minimally invasive urologic surgery*. New York: Taylor & Francis.

Newman, D. (2009). CAUTIon: Carefully manage indwelling urinary catheters. *Nursing Management, 40*(7), 50–52.

Pagana, K. D., & Pagana, T. J. (2008). *Mosby's diagnostic and laboratory test reference* (9th ed.). St. Louis, MO: Mosby.

Parsons, P. E., & Wiener-Kronish, J. P. (2007). *Critical care secrets* (4th ed.). Philadelphia: Mosby Elsevier.

Schell, H., & Puntillo, K. (2006). *Critical Care Nursing Secrets* (2nd ed.). Philadelphia: Mosby Elsevier.

Schick, L., & Windle, P. (2010). *Perianesthesia nursing core curriculum: Preprocedure, phase I and phase II PACU nursing* (2nd ed.). St. Louis, MO: Saunders.

Sirivella, S., Gielchinsky, I., & Parsonnet, V. (2000). Mannitol, furosemide and dopamine infusion in postoperative renal failure complicating cardiac surgery. *Annals of Thoracic Surgery, 69*(2), 501–506.

Wound Ostomy and Continence Nurses Society. (2008). *Catheter associated urinary tract infections (CAUTI): Fact sheet*. Retrieved from http://www.wocn.org/pdfs/WOCN_Library/Fact_Sheets/cauti_fact_sheet.pdf

CHAPTER 28

Gynecology and Obstetrics Surgeries

Denise O'Brien, MSN, RN, ACNS-BC, CPAN, CAPA, FAAN

While most perianesthesia nurses care for patients undergoing gynecologic procedures, care of patients for nonobstetric and obstetric procedures is less common. This chapter focuses on specific gynecologic and obstetric issues, beginning with a brief discussion on the menstrual cycle and other gynecologic issues. The primary focus of the chapter centers on operative procedures for gynecologic concerns and information useful to the perianesthesia nurse caring for the gynecologic patient. The final section of the chapter discusses the obstetric issues, including information on normal pregnancy, operative procedures for the pregnant patient, and issues associated with delivery of the parturient. Perianesthesia nurses whose primary role does not include caring for the pregnant patient will find the discussion helpful in increasing their knowledge and understanding of the patient who happens to be pregnant.

1. What is a normal menstrual cycle?

The usual onset of menarche is between the ages of 9 to 17.7 years with the median age 12.8 years (Griswold, 2004). Cycles vary in frequency from 21 to 40 days, and regularity is normal. Bleeding lasts 3 to 8 days and the usual blood loss averages 30 to 80 mL. The classic cycle of 28 days occurs in only 15% of menstrual cycles.

2. What is an abnormal menstrual cycle?

Menstrual cycles have wide variability (Griswold, 2004). The complete absence of menses is called amenorrhea. Menses that occur infrequently, at intervals greater than 35 days, are labeled as oligomenorrhea. The opposite extreme, menses at intervals of 21 to 24 days or fewer, is known as polymenorrhea. When regular bleeding is excessive in duration and flow (greater than 80 mL/cycle or lasting longer than 7 days), it is defined as hypermenorrhea or menorrhagia. Metrorrhagia describes irregularly occurring bleeding that is excessive in flow and length. Irregular, heavy bleeding is called menometrorrhagia. Hypomenorrhea is regular bleeding in less than the normal amount. Bleeding at any time between otherwise normal menses is defined as intermenstrual bleeding.

3. Does the menstrual cycle and hormones influence anesthesia outcomes?

During menses, pain thresholds have been found to be lower (Hurley & Adams, 2008). When women are in low progesterone and high estradiol states, their pain thresholds were not different from men. Additionally, during the low estradiol phase of the menstrual cycle, females were found to have higher pain scores to persistent noxious stimulation. This has been attributed to a reduction in endogenous opioid receptor activation in brain regions associated with analgesia when compared with the high estradiol state. Age also modifies the pain threshold; advancing age is positively associated with pain threshold.

Studies investigating the relationship of PONV to the stage of the menstrual cycle have shown inconsistent results (Habib & Gan 2004). Some studies report an increased susceptibility to PONV during the first seven days of the menstrual cycle; however, this has not been confirmed in other studies. A systematic review of the results of all available studies published in the early 2000s, suggested that the phase of the menstrual cycle had no impact on the occurrence of PONV.

4. When should women start having pelvic examinations and Pap smears?

Current recommendations state that screening should start within 3 years after first having vaginal intercourse or by age 21 (Zieve & Storck, 2010). After age 21, women should have a pelvic exam and Pap smear every 2 years to check for cervical cancer. Over the age of 30 or after 3 negative Pap smears, the Pap smear may be needed every 3 years. After a total hysterectomy, Pap smears are not necessary. Sexually active women should be also screened for chlamydia infection. This can be done during a pelvic exam. Additional detailed information may be found at: http://www.cancer .org/docroot/CRI/content/CRI_2_6X_Cervical_ Cancer_Prevention_and_Early_Detection_8 .asp?sitearea=&level

5. Who should be tested preoperatively?

Routine pregnancy testing for all women of child-bearing age is not supported by the American Society of Anesthesiologists (ASA) (ASA, 2002/2003). The ASA amended the advisory in 2003 to recommend that testing may be offered to those women "for whom the result would alter the patient's management."

6. Is informed consent for pregnancy testing necessary?

Prior to obtaining a specimen (urine or blood) for pregnancy testing, the patient should be asked regarding the possibility of pregnancy, informed of the potential risks of anesthesia relating to pregnancy, and the request for the pregnancy test (Bierstein, 2006; Palmer, Van Norman, & Jackson, 2009; Van Norman, 2008). Once informed, the patient needs to consent to the pregnancy test or may refuse to be tested. The discussion and patient decision is then documented. Institutional policy may vary as to whether the operative procedure will proceed if the patient refuses, and the patient's surgeon must be notified of the patient's refusal to be tested. It is unethical to test the woman who refuses testing.

7. Who receives the results?

Results are given to the patient alone (Palmer et al., 2009). Reporting of positive results may be challenging especially with the adolescent patient. The individual's rights to privacy and confidentiality must be respected. State laws may vary regarding the adolescent's legal status; if the results are positive, the insti-

tution should have plans in place to address who will inform the patient and what services are immediately available to support the patient, regardless of the age of the patient. The decision to proceed with the operative procedure may vary depending on the urgency of the procedure and the surgeon's and anesthesia care provider's preference.

8. What are defined as external procedures?

Procedures include hymenectomy, hymenotomy, excision and drainage of Bartholin cysts, bartholinectomy, excision of external lesions, and vulvectomy.

These procedures enlarge or open the hymen at the vaginal orifice; drain infected cysts; remove various growths (warts, papilloma, or malignant lesions); and treat premalignant or malignant lesions of the vulva with the excision of the labia majora, labia minora, and surrounding structures, and skin grafting, respectively (Krieger, 2010).

9. What are the potential complications and postoperative implications of these procedures?

Bleeding and infection are potential complications. Pain management and perineal care will be required. Sitz baths may be ordered for cleanliness and comfort.

10. What instructions will the patient and family need?

Patient education includes identifying signs of infection or excessive bleeding, when to contact the physician (unrelieved pain, infection, bleeding, drainage), and expected pain, instructions on sitz baths, and perineal care.

11. What procedures are included in the transvaginal approach?

Dilatation and curettage (D & C) and cervical procedures (conization, colposcopy, loop electrosurgical excision procedure [LEEP], laser) are completed through the vaginal approach (Krieger, 2010). Tension-free vaginal taping (TVT) to correct stress incontinence uses a transvaginal approach and two small abdominal incisions.

12. Why is a D & C done, and what is included in the procedure?

D & C may be performed to diagnose and treat abnormal uterine bleeding, manage abortion (incomplete, missed, or induced), stenosis, or cancer of the uterus (Weislander, Dandade, & Wheeler, 2007). The procedure, under anesthesia, includes dilatation of the cervix, examination of the cervix, sounding of uterus, and scraping (curetting) of the uterine cavity. Perforation and bleeding are potential complications of the procedure. Patients undergoing these procedures will usually be outpatients. Postoperative teaching includes when to contact the surgeon for excessive bleeding (generally saturating more than 1 perineal pad per hour) and pain management (mild analgesics are usually adequate for cramping discomfort) (Krieger, 2010).

13. What are the most common cervical procedures?

Colposcopy, often done in the office setting, allows the gynecologist to visually evaluate the cervix with a microscope and obtain biopsies and specimens for evaluation and surveillance (Schorge et al., 2008d, 2008e). Other cervical procedures may require sedation and anesthesia in the outpatient surgical setting. These include cryotherapy, LEEP, and carbon dioxide laser vaporization of cervical tissue. Postoperatively, cramping is common. Watery vaginal discharge or light bleeding is expected and requires perineal pad. Tampons should not be used. Infection is a risk and intercourse should be avoided for 4 weeks following surgery. Patients may return to work and other regular activities dependent on their symptoms.

14. Why is a conization of the cervix done?

Cervical conization uses a cone-shaped tissue biopsy to remove ectocervical lesions and a portion of the endocervical canal (Schorge et al., 2008f). This safe and effective method treats cervical intraepithelial neoplasia (CIN), carcinoma in situ (CIS), and adenocarcinoma in situ (AIS). Laser or LEEP conization may also be done for these lesions. Bleeding is the greatest risk after conization. Patients need to be instructed to follow up with their surgeons if bleeding exceeds 1 pad per hour. Other postoperative instructions are similar to the other cervical procedures.

15. What is a hysteroscopy, and why is it done?

Hysteroscopy, which uses a lighted endoscope inserted through the vagina and cervix, and into the uterus, for evaluation and treatment of abnormal uterine bleeding (AUB) and evaluation and treatment of infertility (Schorge et al., 2008f). It may be combined with dilatation and curettage for treating AUB. Endometrial ablation is accomplished by a variety of hysteroscopic techniques, including ND: YAG laser, rollerball, thermal balloon ablation, hysteroscopic thermal ablation, impedance-controlled electrocoagulation, microwave, and cryoablation. A distention medium is used to separate the uterine walls for viewing of the endometrium; carbon dioxide, saline, and low-viscous solutions (sorbitol, mannitol, glycine) may be used. Significant complications include uterine perforation

and hemorrhage. Fluid overload from the distention medium can result in water intoxication, or hypernatremia. Recovery after an endometrial ablation is typically rapid; spotting or light bleeding is common and stops within a few days after the procedure.

16. How are uterine leiomyomas removed?

Leiomyomas (fibroid masses) may be removed by hysteroscopy. This is the operative method of choice for smaller masses when fertility preservation is desired or for treatment of AUB. An open operative approach or possibly hysterectomy may used to treat larger masses (Schorge et al., 2008f). Bleeding is common during the myomectomy. Postoperative bleeding, spotting or light bleeding, may occur for 1 to 2 weeks after the procedure.

17. What is water intoxication (dilutional hyponatremia), which may be associated with hysteroscopy?

If an excessive amount of distending media results in vascular intravasation, the patient can experience hyponatremia and pulmonary edema (Weislander et al., 2007). The procedure should be completed quickly; if the fluid deficit exceeds 1 L, electrolytes should be checked. When the fluid deficit reaches 1500 mL or the serum sodium is less than 125 mmol/L, the procedure must be terminated. These risks can be prevented with close monitoring of fluid use intraoperatively.

18. What is a tension-free vaginal taping (TVT) procedure?

TVT procedures are the most commonly performed procedure for the treatment of stress urinary incontinence (Schorge et al., 2008c, 2008g).

The procedure provides midurethral support and offers a 5-year cure rate of approximately 85%. Appropriate patient selection improves success; urodynamic evaluation is necessary before scheduling the procedure. The procedure, performed with the patient in a high lithotomy position, requires 2.5 cm skin incisions in the abdomen above the symphysis and a midline vaginal incision. Mesh tape, attached to needles and an introducer, is threaded around the urethra and the tension set. Hemorrhage, bladder perforation, or bowel injury can complicate the procedure. Short-term complications, often seen initially in the postanesthesia care unit, include incomplete bladder emptying, requiring drainage with an indwelling catheter or intermittent self-catheterization (ISC) for several days. Post void residuals need to be less than 100 mL before the ISC is discontinued. The vaginal incision should be healed before intercourse is resumed. Adequate healing is necessary before the resumption of exercise and strenuous physical activity, with the standard recommendation of waiting for 2 months.

19. What are common operative treatments for infertility (Schorge et al., 2008b)?

If tubal patency is questionable, reconstruction of the tube is an option. The approaches include hysteroscopic cannulation, surgical reanastomosis, and neosalpingostomy. For correction of uterine factors that include leiomyomas, endometrial polyps, and intrauterine adhesions, either hysteroscopic or open procedures may be required to remove the tissue interfering with fertility.

20. What is laparoscopy?

Using a transperitoneal endoscopic technique, the skilled surgeon visualizes the pelvic structures to diagnose and manage gynecologic disorders without laparotomy (Weislander et al., 2007). Carbon dioxide (CO_2) is instilled with a pneumatic insufflator into the peritoneal cavity to distend the abdominal wall to provide visualization of the structures. The rate, pressure, and volume of the CO_2 is continuously monitored. Resection, biopsy, coagulation, aspiration, and manipulation are accomplished by passing a variety of instruments through cannulas; laser (CO_2 or ND: YAG) may also be used. Procedures may be minor or major, and performed through small abdominal incisions. The technique requires skill and experience to be performed safely. Morbidity is low and recovery tends to be relatively short.

21. Any specific issues with postoperative care?

Recovery is generally short, although more extensive laparoscopic procedures may require hospitalization of 1 to 2 days (Weislander et al., 2007). Pain is usually minimal; oral analgesics should manage the pain. The most common complaint after laparoscopy is referred shoulder pain due to subdiaphragmatic accumulation of the CO_2 used for insufflation during the procedure. Mild analgesics and supine positioning may help minimize this pain.

22. What are common complications after these procedures?

Complications include intestinal perforation, urologic injury, air embolus, surgical site infection (superficial and deep), abdominal wall vascular injury, incisional hernia, and major vascular injury (MVI) (Weislander et al., 2007). In a review of the literature, 84% of patients with retroperitoneal hemorrhage experienced abdominal or groin pain, whereas a minority displayed the classic periumbilical or flank ecchymosis (Cullen's and Grey-Turner's sign, respectively) (Moore, Vasquez, Lin, & Kaplan, 2005).

Complications during the operative procedure may lead to open laparotomy in approximately 2.1% of laparoscopic cases (Weislander et al., 2007). Most common reasons for complications are injuries to major vessels or the intestine. Vascular injuries are most likely to occur during blind placement of a Veress needle and trocars than during the procedure itself. Mortality associated with injuries to the aorta, inferior vena cava, and iliac arteries and veins is between 9% and 17%. Immediate conversion to an open procedure is usually required with transfusion. Bleeding may be concealed in large retroperitoneal hematomas.

Intestinal injuries are uncommon but associated with mortality rates of 2.5% to 5% (Weislander et al., 2007). Injuries to the colon and small bowel may be from sharp instruments or thermal burns. Recognition is often delayed until postoperation when patients present with low-grade fever, leucopenia, or normal leukocyte count. In reviews of bowel injuries after laparoscopy, patients commonly presented with pain at the trocar site near the injury, abdominal distention, and diarrhea, whereas signs associated with peritonitis (severe pain, nausea, vomiting, ileus) were uncommon. Other complications include bladder injuries, ventral hernias, subcutaneous emphysema, gas embolisms, and postoperative shoulder pain (see previous).

23. What are the procedures for tubal sterilization?

Methods used for tubal sterilization include postpartum partial salpingectomy, unipolar coagulation, bipolar coagulation, spring clip, silicone rubber band, or interval partial salpingectomy (Cunningham et al., 2010d). Commonly, the approach is laparoscopic, although minilaparotomy may also be used. Lowest failure rates are found with postpartum partial salpingectomy and unipolar coagulation.

Newer tubal sterilization techniques, using a transcervical hysteroscopic approach, are available and offer advantages of effectiveness and placement without general anesthesia or laparoscopy. The Essure device is an expanding spring device made of titanium, stainless steel, and nickel that contain Dacron fibers that induce an inflammatory response and final fibrosis of the intramural tubal lumen (Weislander et al., 2007). The Adiana device causes tubal occlusion through a combination of radio-frequency tubal endocoagulation and the implantation of a silicone matrix (Smith, 2009). Evaluation of the effectiveness of these newer techniques continues.

24. Vaginal, abdominal, or laparoscopic hysterectomy: What's the difference between these procedures and the indications?

Hysterectomy is performed for benign (e.g., symptomatic leiomyomas, pelvic organ prolapse, AUB,
endometriosis, chronic pain, premalignant neoplasia) and malignant conditions (Schorge et al.,
2008f). The approach may be abdominal, vaginal,
or laparoscopic, determined by physical properties
of uterus and pelvic, surgical indications, presence
or absence of adnexal pathology, surgical risks,
costs, recovery, and quality of life issues. Abdominal hysterectomy may be preferred for large pelvic
organs, extensive adhesions, if oophorectomy is
needed, if urogynecologic procedures are planned.
While the abdominal approach usually requires less
operating time and specialized instrumentation and
expertise than laparoscopic approaches, the recovery time is longer, pain is increases, and there is a
greater risk of infection and fever. Postoperative
bleeding and bladder injury are lower with abdominal incisions compared with the vaginal approach,
but transfusion and ureteral injury may be greater.
Smaller pelvic organs, minimal adhesions, no
significant adnexal pathology, and minimal pelvic
organ prolapse support the vaginal approach to
hysterectomy. Recovery is faster, there is lower
cost, and pain is less than with abdominal incisions.
Laparoscopic approaches require longer operating
times, more expensive equipment, and extensive
surgical skill. The indications are similar to vaginal
hysterectomy as is the postoperative outcomes;
however, the laparoscopic approach offers greater
visualization and access to the abdomen and pelvis.
Risk of ureteral injury is higher than either the
abdominal or vaginal approach. Postoperative care
for abdominal hysterectomy is similar to that of any
major abdominal procedure. Length of stay may be
up to 4 days. Complications include fever, which
may be due to pelvic, abdominal wall, or urinary
tract infection, abscess, hematoma, or pneumonia.
Patients who have vaginal hysterectomies recover
normal bowel function, ambulate easier, and have
less pain than patients who have abdominal
hysterectomies.

25. Why are pelvic and periaortic lymph node
dissections performed?

Patients with uterine, ovarian, and cervical cancer
commonly have pelvic lymphadenectomy (lymph
node removal) procedures (Schorge et al., 2008h).
This procedure is one of the hallmarks of surgical
staging for these conditions and includes complete removal of all nodal tissue in a defined area. Typically, a

minimum of 4 pelvic nodes, up to 11 nodes from
multiple sites, will be removed. Enlarged nodes may
be removed for debulking and to improve survival
benefit in some cancers. These procedures may be
accomplished with open or laparoscopic approaches.

26. In a pelvic exenteration, what organs are
resected? What are the potential complications?
What is included in postoperative care? What are
the outcomes?

Total pelvic exenteration is indicated for persistent
or recurrent cervical cancer after radiation therapy;
also, although less commonly, the procedure may
be indicated in some instances of recurrent endometrial adenocarcinoma, uterine sarcoma, or
vulvar cancer; locally advanced carcinoma of the
cervix, vagina, or endometrium when radiation is
contraindicated, and melanoma of the vagina or
urethra (Schorge et al., 2008h). The bladder, rectum, uterus, cervix, and surrounding tissues are
removed. When less radical surgery, chemotherapy,
or radiation options are exhausted, pelvic exenteration may be indicated as a curative procedure. Preoperative evaluation is extensive, searching for any
signs of metastatic disease. Counseling is required
to prepare the patient for the results of the extensive procedure. Quality of life issues may be significant; sexual function and body image are altered.

Preoperative preparation includes bowel cleansing, locating urinary and intestinal stoma sites, and
administering antibiotics and deep vein thrombosis
prophylaxis. Patients are blood typed and cross-
matched for replacement red cells. Intraoperative
positioning will be in a low lithotomy position. The
surgical approach is both abdominal and perineal.
Postoperatively, the patient may require intensive
care unit admission. Complications include fever,
wound breakdown, ileus, bowel obstruction, intestinal fistulas, anastomotic leaks or stricture, and venous thromboembolism. Postoperative care needs
include drain and stoma care, hemodynamic monitoring (potential for extensive fluid loss and third
spacing), and pain management (Krieger, 2010).

27. Why is the omentum removed?

In advanced ovarian cancer, metastases to the
omentum are expected (Schorge et al., 2008h).
Tumor debulking and cancer staging are the
primary reasons for removal of the omentum.
It may also be used in patients without obvious
metastatic disease. Of note, if a total omentectomy
has been performed, gastric decompression is
continued for 48 hours to avoid gastric dilation.
This protects ligated gastric vessels from postoperative dislodgement.

28. What are the special considerations associated with vulvectomy?

Vulvectomy, which includes the en bloc removal of the vulva and surrounding tissues, poses particular postoperative challenges (Schorge et al., 2008h). The vulvar wound is initially kept dry and clean. Brief sitz baths or irrigation of the perineum, followed by air-drying will help with healing after a few days. Underwear should not be worn, and garments should be loose-fitting to avoid tension and pressure on the incision. The most common complication is separation of a portion of the incision. Debridement may be needed with healing by secondary intention allowed.

Scarring and altered sensation may affect sexual satisfaction. Counseling may help address the significant sexual dysfunction that results from the procedure.

29. What are the risks for deep vein thrombosis? What is recommended for prophylaxis?

The American College of Obstetricians and Gynecologists (ACOG) published evidence-based recommendations for the prevention of deep vein thrombosis and pulmonary embolism in 2007 (ACOG, 2007). ACOG does not recommend discontinuing hormone therapy or oral contraceptives preoperatively. However, patients undergoing major operative procedures who are on oral contraceptives should receive heparin prophylaxis to reduce their risk of perioperative venous thromboembolism. Risk classification is used to determine appropriate prophylaxis for surgical patients (Geerts et al., 2004). The recommendations for moderate-to-high risk patients range from the use of graduated compression stockings to pneumatic compression devices, to pharmacologic prophylaxis with unfractionated heparin and low-molecular weight heparin based on the patients' risk factors including length of operating time, condition, and age. Low-risk patients require no specific prophylaxis but early ambulation is recommended.

30. What are the normal physiologic changes of pregnancy that are of concern to anesthesia care providers?

Maternal uptake and elimination of inhaled anesthetics are altered by the increase in alveolar ventilation and decrease in functional residual capacity (Barash, Cullen, Stoelting, Calahan, & Stock, 2009). The decreased FRC and increased basal metabolic rate may increase the risk of arterial hypoxemia during periods of apnea (e.g., during intubation of the trachea). Vascular engorgement of the airway increases the risk of bleeding during instrumentation. Delayed gastric emptying has long been associated with the pregnant patient, but controversy exists as to when risk increases for aspiration. Other factors, such as pain, anxiety, and opioid administration, may have led to the belief that delaying emptying began early in pregnancy.

31. How is an ectopic pregnancy identified and managed?

When the blastocyst implants anywhere other than the uterus, it is defined as an ectopic or extrauterine pregnancy. Improved diagnosis with radioimmunoassay of beta hCG and high resolution transvaginal sonography have reduced the risk of mortality and morbidity significantly (Schorge et al., 2008a). Signs and symptoms may include normal pregnancy signs (breast tenderness, nausea, urinary frequency) and shoulder pain from subdiaphragmatic blood irritating the phrenic nerve during inspiration or syncope and dizziness from hypovolemia due to bleeding. Prior to rupture, physical findings may be minimal to absent. Treatment consists of laparoscopic salpingostomy or salpingectomy depending on the state of the contralateral fallopian tube and desire to preserve fertility. Recurrent ectopic pregnancies are possible.

32. What medications typically used during the perioperative period are safe for the pregnant patient?

Most drugs readily cross the placenta (Barash et al., 2009). Opioids can produce neonatal respiratory depression. Fentanyl does not produce severe depression. Ketamine also produces analgesia without depression of the neonate. To minimize risk to the fetus, delay any nonurgent surgery until after first trimester or after delivery. Fetal heart tones should be monitored after the 16th week.

33. What is recommended for anesthesia and positioning for nonobstetric procedures on pregnant patients?

Nonobstetric surgery during pregnancy is uncommon, performed in 1.5% to 2.0% of all pregnancies (Holschneider, 2007). Both the mother and the fetus must be considered when planning surgical care. Procedures should be limited to emergencies; if nonemergent surgery must occur during pregnancy, the second trimester is recommended. Avoid imaging that exposes the fetus to radiation when possible; risk varies with exposure and gestational age. Anesthesia is considered generally safe; regional anesthesia is recommended when appropriate for the procedure. Perioperative monitoring and maintenance of oxygen-carrying capacity, affinity, arterial PO_2, and placental blood flow can reduce the risk of intrauterine asphyxia for the fetus. Displacing the uterus (left lateral positioning) helps prevent venocaval compression and hypotension. Oxygen supplementation and volume and blood pressure maintenance maximize fetal oxygenation. If a vasopressor is needed for the mother, ephedrine is the best option since it produces less vasospasm. Continuous fetal monitoring is recommended for the latter half of gestation to detect preterm labor and appropriate intervention during and after the surgical procedure.

34. What is cerclage for incompetent cervix?

To prevent preterm birth, cerclage placement may be used, generally between 12 and 16 weeks of pregnancy (Cunningham et al., 2010a, 2010f).

Cerclage consists of a ring or loop that encircles the incompetent cervix uteri, or a stitch into the cervix (Krieger, 2010). Women with a history of recurrent midtrimester losses, or a short cervix, or at risk for preterm labor with cervical incompetence may benefit from cerclage.

35. Should fetal monitoring be intermittent or continuous for labor?

For women with low-risk pregnancies, electronic fetal monitoring is recommended on admission for labor if the membranes have ruptured; continuous monitoring is used if fetal heart rate abnormalities are identified (Cunningham et al., 2010c). External monitoring is available for women whose membranes are intact. Complications of internal electronic fetal monitoring reported include fetal injury by the electrode, entanglement with cord leading to severe cord compression, placental penetration by catheter causing hemorrhage, or uterine perforation during catheter insertion. Internal monitoring may increase infection risk in both the fetus and the mother.

36. What are the signs of labor?

True or active labor is distinguished by contractions that are regular in rhythm, with shortening intervals between contractions and increasing intensity (Cunningham et al., 2010c). Discomfort is located in the back and abdomen with no relief with sedation. Cervical dilatation is observed.

37. What is preeclampsia and eclampsia? Who is at risk of developing this disease of pregnancy?

During pregnancy, the presence of hypertension and proteinuria signal that the patient has preeclampsia (Rogers, Cox, & Crombleholme, 2010). When seizures develop in this patient, eclampsia is diagnosed. Edema is no longer a required element. Onset can occur anytime after 20 weeks of gestation and up to 6 weeks postpartum. Delivery of the fetus and placenta cures this unique disease. Approximately 7% of pregnant women in the United States will develop preeclampsia–eclampsia. Women at risk are

primiparas, which increases with multiple pregnancies; those with chronic hypertension; diabetes; renal disease; collagen-vascular and autoimmune disorders; and gestational trophoblastic disease. Of the women who develop preeclampsia, 5% will progress to eclampsia. Maternal death can result from uncontrolled eclampsia. Patients with mild preeclampsia may have minimal complaints; in severe cases, the patient may have dizziness and headache with hypertension. A form of severe preeclampsia is identified as HELLP syndrome. The syndrome includes hemolysis, elevated liver enzymes, and low platelets. If the patient progresses to eclampsia, seizures occur. Treatment includes early recognition of subtle changes in blood pressure and weight during prenatal visits. Bed rest is recommended for mild preeclampsia. When the patient convulses, the treatment of choice is 4 to 6 g of magnesium sulfate, followed by 2 to 3 g/hr maintenance. Upon stabilization of the mother, delivery needs to proceed to save the fetus and the mother. After delivery, magnesium sulfate infusions are continued for at least 24 hours. Resolution of the preeclampsia–eclampsia is indicated by urinary output of over 100 to 200 mL/hr and the magnesium sulfate is discontinued.

38. What are the most common complications associated with operative delivery by cesarean section?

Postpartum hemorrhage, endometritis, and wound infection can occur after cesarean section (Incerpi, 2007). For women with previous cesarean section deliveries, the risk of rupture is increased if a classic uterine incision was used. While rare, rupture is a major emergency requiring surgical intervention.

39. What types of anesthesia is used for analgesia during labor and anesthesia for delivery?

Labor anesthesia includes epidural analgesia (for pain relief during labor and vaginal delivery, and converted to epidural anesthesia if cesarean delivery is required), spinal analgesia, combined spinal–epidural analgesia, paracervical block, and pudendal nerve block (Barash et al., 2009; McDonald & Yarnell, 2007). Operative deliveries may be accomplished with spinal or lumbar epidural anesthesia and, rarely, general anesthesia. General anesthesia is chosen if contraindications to regional anesthesia exist or occur during emergency situations.

40. What is the Apgar score?

Virginia Apgar introduced this scoring system in 1952 to identify neonates who require resuscitation and to assess the effectiveness of such efforts (Raab, 2007). Each of the five elements (heart rate, respiratory rate, muscle tone, reflex irritability, and color) are assigned a value of 0–2 at 1 minute, and again 5 minutes after delivery. The total score of each element is used to evaluate the condition of the newborn. Changes in the score between 1 minute and 5 minutes measures effectiveness of resuscitative efforts; low scores at 5 minutes are associated with high infant mortality.

41. What is assessed in the initial newborn examination?

Assessment of the newborn includes airway patency, chest wall movement (respiratory effort), respiratory rate, breathing pattern, breath sounds, heart rate and rhythm, abdomen (soft, nondistended), umbilical stump (number of vessels), skin color, genitalia, alertness, activity, tone and movement of extremities, and anomalies or birth trauma (nerve injuries) (Raab, 2007).

42. What are the most common causes of abnormal bleeding during pregnancy and delivery?

Causes of bleeding include placenta abruption (placental separation from implantation site before delivery), placenta previa (placenta implanted over or very near internal cervical os), prolonged third stage, uterine atony after delivery, and uterine inversion (Cunningham et al., 2010e). Risk factors for placenta abruption include increased age and parity, preeclampsia, chronic hypertension, preterm ruptured membranes, multifetal gestation, low birth weight, hydramnios, cigarette smoking, thrombophilias, cocaine use, prior abruption, and uterine leiomyoma. Maternal age, multiparity, prior cesarean delivery, smoking, and unexplained elevated screening levels of maternal serum alpha-fetoprotein (MSAFP) increase the risk for placenta previa. Management of the bleeding varies with the source of bleeding. Emergent cesarean delivery may be necessary in some cases of preterm bleeding; bleeding after delivery may require uterine massage, oxytocics, removal of retained placenta, or surgical intervention depending on the cause and status of the mother.

43. What are the risks of trauma for the pregnant patient?

Trauma (motor vehicle accidents, falls, direct assaults to the maternal abdomen, other causes) complicate approximately 7% of all pregnancies (Holschneider, 2007). The most common causes of fetal death are maternal death and abruptio placentae. While motor vehicle accidents account for most injuries, physical abuse is another cause. Stabilizing the mother's condition is key; protecting the fetus from unnecessary drug and radiation exposure is also important. Fetal heart rate and uterine contractions should be monitored after the trauma, for a minimum of 4 hours, up to 48 hours. Frequent uterine

contractions, vaginal bleeding, abdominouterine tenderness, postural hypotension, and fetal heart rate abnormalities require further evaluation.

Since intravascular volume increases up to 8 L in pregnancy, losses of up to 35% of the blood volume can occur without typical signs of hypovolemia and shock (Cothren, Biffl, & Moore, 2010). Pregnant patients may desaturate more rapidly and require oxygen supplementation to prevent maternal and fetal hypoxia during evaluation and treatment. The patient is positioned in the left lateral decubitus position or tilted on a backboard to the left to avoid venocaval compression. Evaluation of the mother by a member of the obstetric team while resuscitation continues may optimize fetal outcomes. Ultrasound of the abdomen can be used to identify abdominopelvic trauma and status of the fetus. Radiography must be considered from a risk–benefit standpoint; x-rays should be limited to the clinically necessary and the pelvis shielded with a lead apron when possible.

44. How does resuscitation during pregnancy differ from resuscitation of the nonpregnant patient?

The critically ill pregnant patient, who arrests, requires positioning in the left lateral position, 100% oxygen supplementation, intravenous access and fluid bolus, and consideration of reversible causes of cardiac arrest and identification of preexisting medical conditions that may complicate resuscitation (American Heart Association [AHA], 2005).

Since the hormonal changes associated with pregnancy alter the gastroesophageal sphincter, the patient is at increased risk of regurgitation and aspiration. Continuous cricoid pressure during positive pressure ventilation is recommended for any unconscious pregnant woman. Chest compressions are performed higher on the sternum to adjust for the gravid uterus elevation of the diaphragm and abdominal contents. Standard defibrillation doses are used; no evidence exists that defibrillator shocks affect the fetal heart adversely. Fetal or uterine monitors should be removed before defibrillation.

MODIFICATIONS OF ACLS FOR THE PREGNANT PATIENT

45. What is included in postdelivery monitoring?

The first few hours immediately following delivery are critical; complications, either obstetric or postanesthetic, may be serious. Monitoring in an appropriately staffed and equipped postanesthesia care unit is essential (American Society of PeriAnesthesia Nurses [ASPAN], 2008). Observe for vaginal bleeding and monitor vital signs, including blood pressure, heart rate, respiratory rate, oxygenation, and temperature,

TABLE 28-1. Modifications of ACLS for the Pregnant Patient

Airway	Secure airway with continuous cricoid pressure before and during endotracheal intubation. Plan to use smaller (0.5–1 mm) endotracheal tube.	Gastroesophageal sphincter insufficiency Airway edema
Breathing	Support oxygenation and ventilation (100% oxygen supplementation). Verify tube placement with exhaled CO_2 detector and clinical assessment. Reduced ventilatory volumes should be used.	Decreased functional residual capacity, increased oxygen demand Esophageal detector devices can fail to detect proper placement in late pregnancy. Elevated diaphragm reduces lung capacity.
Circulation	Follow ACLS medication guidelines. Vasopressors, if used, may cause fetal demise.	These drugs cause decreased uterine blood flow; no alternatives exist.
Differential diagnosis	Same reversible causes as in nonpregnant patients, also look for pregnancy-specific diseases and procedural complications.	Magnesium sulfate overdose: Treat with calcium gluconate (1 ampule/1 g). Acute coronary syndromes: Fibrinolytics are relatively contraindicated; choice is percutaneous coronary intervention for ST-elevation myocardial infarction. Preeclampsia/eclampsia: Untreated, increased risk of maternal and fetal morbidity and mortality Aortic dissection: Increased risk for spontaneous aortic dissection Life-threatening massive pulmonary embolism and ischemic stroke: Use fibrinolytics Amniotic fluid embolism: Use cardiopulmonary bypass Trauma and drug overdose

Modified from Part 10.8: Cardiac Arrest Associated With Pregnancy.
Source: AHA, 2005.

every 15 minutes for at least 1 to 2 hours or until the patient meets discharge criteria for general or regional anesthesia (American Academy of Pediatrics & American College of Obstetricians and Gynecologists, 2007). Additional monitoring may be required for patients with histories of preeclampsia or eclampsia, medical or surgical complications, or comorbidities (cardiac, respiratory, endocrine, renal, trauma).

46. How frequently should the uterus be massaged after delivery?

Uterine massage, accomplished by placing a hand on the lower abdomen and repetitively massaging or squeezing the uterus to stimulate uterine contraction, is recommended every 10 minutes for 60 minutes after delivery (Hofmeyr, Abdel-Aleem, & Abdel-Aleem, 2008). This reduces blood loss and the need for oxytocics.

47. What are the most commonly used drugs to reduce postpartum bleeding?

Oxytocin, ergonovine, and methylergonovine are used in the normal third stage of labor (Cunningham et al., 2010b). Oxytocin, 20 units added to 1 L of intravenous solution, is typically administered after delivery of the placenta and continued in postanesthesia phase. The infusion should be carefully monitored to avoid tetanic uterine contractions and increased pain. Ergot alkaloids are powerful myometrial stimulants resulting in contraction that may persist for hours. These agents can precipitate severe hypertension. Prostaglandins are another option for bleeding during third stage labor. Hemabate (carboprost 250 mcg and tromethamine 83 mcg/1 mL) is one such drug that may be used for the treatment of refractory postpartum uterine bleeding. It is given as a deep intermuscular injection and may be repeated.

REFERENCES

American Academy of Pediatrics & American College of Obstetricians and Gynecologists. (2007). *Guidelines for perinatal care* (6th ed.). Washington, DC: Authors.

American College of Obstetricians and Gynecologists. (2007). ACOG practice bulletin: Prevention of deep vein thrombosis and pulmonary embolism, no. 84. *Obstetrics & Gynecology, 110*(2), 429–440.

American Heart Association. (2005). Part 10.8: Cardiac arrest associated with pregnancy. *Circulation, 112.* Retrieved from http://circ.ahajournals.org/cgi/content/full/112/24_suppl/IV-150

American Society of Anesthesiologists. (2002). Practice advisory for preanesthesia evaluation: A report by the American Society of Anesthesiologists Task Force on Preanesthesia Evaluation. *Anesthesiology, 96*(2), 485–496. Retrieved from www.asahq.org/publicationsAndServices/preeval.pdf

American Society of PeriAnesthesia Nurses. (2008). 2008–2010 Standards of perianesthesia nursing practice. Cherry Hill, NJ: Author.

Barash, P. G., Cullen, B. F., Stoelting, R. K., Calahan, M. K., & Stock, M. C. (2009). *Handbook of clinical anesthesia* (6th ed.). Philadelphia: Lippincott Williams & Wilkins.

Bierstein, K. (2006). Preoperative pregnancy testing: Mandatory or elective? *American Society of Anesthesiologists Newsletter, 70,* 37.

Cothren, C. C., Biffl, W. L., & Moore, E. E. (2010). Trauma (Chapter 7). In F. C. Brunicardi, D. K. Andersen, T. R. Billiar, D. L. Dunn, J. G. Hunter, J. B. Matthews, & R. E. Pollock (Eds.), *Schwartz's principles of surgery* (9th ed.). New York: McGraw Hill Health. Retrieved from http://www.accessmedicine.com.proxy.lib.umich.edu/content.aspx?aID=5019216

Cunningham, F. G., Leveno, K. J., Bloom, S. L., Hauth, J. C., Rouse, D. J., & Spong, C. Y. (2010a). Abortion (Chapter 9). In F. G. Cunningham, K. J. Leveno, S. L. Bloom, J. C. Hauth, D. J. Rouse, & C. Y. Spong, *Williams obstetrics* (23rd ed.). Atlanta: American College of Obstetricians and Gynecologists. Retrieved from http://www.accessmedicine.com.proxy.lib.umich.edu/content.aspx?aID=6053136

Cunningham, F. G., Leveno, K. J., Bloom, S. L., Hauth, J. C., Rouse, D. J., & Spong, C. Y. (2010b). Normal labor and delivery (Chapter 17). In F. G. Cunningham, K. J. Leveno, S. L. Bloom, J. C. Hauth, D. J. Rouse, & C. Y. Spong (Eds.), *Williams obstetrics* (23rd ed.). Atlanta: American College of Obstetricians and Gynecologists. Retrieved from http://www.accessmedicine.com.proxy.lib.umich.edu/content.aspx?aID=6023669

Cunningham, F. G., Leveno, K. J., Bloom, S. L., Hauth, J. C., Rouse, D. J., & Spong, C. Y. (2010c). Intrapartum assessment (Chapter 18). In F. G. Cunningham, K. J. Leveno, S. L. Bloom, J. C. Hauth, D. J. Rouse, & C. Y. Spong (Eds.). *Williams obstetrics* (23rd ed.). Atlanta: American College of Obstetricians and Gynecologists.

Retrieved from http://www.accessmedicine.com.proxy.lib.umich.edu/content.aspx?aID=6024239

Cunningham, F. G., Leveno, K. J., Bloom, S. L., Hauth, J. C., Rouse, D. J., & Spong, C. Y. (2010d). Sterilization (Chapter 33). In F. G. Cunningham, K. J. Leveno, S. L. Bloom, J. C. Hauth, D. J. Rouse, & C. Y. Spong (Eds.). *Williams obstetrics* (23rd ed.). Atlanta: American College of Obstetricians and Gynecologists. Retrieved from http://www.accessmedicine.com.proxy.lib.umich.edu/content.aspx?aID=6032717

Cunningham, F. G., Leveno, K. J., Bloom, S. L., Hauth, J. C., Rouse, D. J., & Spong, C. Y. (2010e). Obstetrical hemorrhage (Chapter 35). In F. G. Cunningham, K. J. Leveno, S. L. Bloom, J. C. Hauth, D. J. Rouse, & C. Y. Spong (Eds.). *Williams obstetrics* (23rd ed.). Atlanta: American College of Obstetricians and Gynecologists. Retrieved from http://www.accessmedicine.com.proxy.lib.umich.edu/content.aspx?aID=6034497

Cunningham, F. G., Leveno, K. J., Bloom, S. L., Hauth, J. C., Rouse, D. J., & Spong, C. Y. (2010f). Preterm birth (Chapter 36). In F. G. Cunningham, K. J. Leveno, S. L. Bloom, J. C. Hauth, D. J. Rouse, & C. Y. Spong (Eds.). *Williams obstetrics* (23rd ed.). Atlanta: American College of Obstetricians and Gynecologists. Retrieved from http://www.accessmedicine.com.proxy.lib.umich.edu/content.aspx?aID=6035539

Geerts, W. H., Pineo, G. F., Heit, J. A., Bergqvist, D., Lassen, M. R., Colwell, C. W. et al. (2004). Prevention of venous thromboembolism: The Seventh ACCP Conference on Antithrombotic and Thrombolytic Therapy. *Chest, 126*(Suppl. 3), 338S–400S.

Griswold, D. (2004). Menstruation and related problems and concerns. In E. Q. Youngkin & M. S. Davis (Eds.), *Women's health: A primary care clinical guide* (3rd ed.). Upper Saddle River, NJ: Pearson Prentice Hall.

Habib, A. S., & Gan, T. J. (2004). Evidence-based management of postoperative nausea and vomiting: A review. *Canadian Journal of Anaesthesia, 51*(4), 326–341.

Hofmeyr, G. J., Abdel-Aleem, H., Abdel-Aleem, M. A. (2008). Uterine massage for preventing postpartum haemorrhage. *Cochrane Database of Systematic Reviews, 16*(3), CD006431.

Holschneider, C. H. (2007). Surgical diseases and disorders in pregnancy (Chapter 27). In A. H. DeCherney & L. Nathan (Eds.), *CURRENT diagnosis & treatment obstetrics & gynecology* (10th ed.). New York: McGraw-Hill. Retrieved from http://www.accessmedicine.com.proxy.lib.umich.edu/content.aspx?aID=2385789

Hurley, R. W., & Adams, M. C. B. (2008). Sex, gender, and pain: An overview of a complex field. *Anesthesia & Analgesia, 107*(1), 309–317.

Incerpi, M. H. (2007). Operative delivery (Chapter 30). In A. H. DeCherney & L. Nathan (Eds.), *CURRENT diagnosis & treatment obstetrics & gynecology* (10th ed.). New York: McGraw-Hill. Retrieved from http://www.accessmedicine.com.proxy.lib.umich.edu/content.aspx?aID=2387143

Krieger, L. (2010). Gynecological and reproductive care. In L. Schick & P. E. Windle (Eds.), *Perianesthesia Nursing Core Curriculum* (2nd ed., pp. 1007–1028). St. Louis: Saunders Elsevier.

McDonald, J. S., & Yarnell, R. W. (2007). Obstetric analgesia and anesthesia (Chapter 29). In A. H. DeCherney & L. Nathan (Eds.), *CURRENT diagnosis & treatment obstetrics & gynecology* (10th ed.). New York: McGraw-Hill. Retrieved from http://www.accessmedicine.com.proxy.lib.umich.edu/content.aspx?aID=2386037

Moore, C. L., Vasquez, N. F., Lin, H., & Kaplan, L. J. (2005). Major vascular injury after laparoscopic tubal ligation. *Journal of Emergency Medicine, 29*(1), 67–71.

Palmer, S. K., Van Norman, G. A., & Jackson, S. L. (2009). Routine pregnancy testing before elective anesthesia is not an American Society of Anesthesiologists standard. *Anesthesia & Analgesia, 108*(5), 1715–1716.

Raab, E. L. (2007). Essentials of normal newborn assessment and care (Chapter 11). In A. H. DeCherney & L. Nathan (Eds.), *CURRENT diagnosis & treatment obstetrics & gynecology* (10th ed.). New York: McGraw-Hill. Retrieved from http://www.accessmedicine.com.proxy.lib.umich.edu/content.aspx?aID=2382132

Rogers, V. L., Cox, S., & Crombleholme, W. R. (2010). *Obstetrics & obstetric disorders* (Chapter 19). In S. J. McPhee, M. A. Papadakis, & L. M. Tierney, Jr. (Eds.), *CURRENT medical diagnosis & treatment 2010*. New York: McGraw-Hill. Retrieved from http://www.accessmedicine.com.proxy.lib.umich.edu/content.aspx?aID=9353

Schorge, J. O., Schaffer, J. I., Halvorson, L. M., Hoffman, B. L., Bradshaw, K. D., & Cunningham, F. G. (2008a). Ectopic pregnancy (Chapter 7). In J. O. Schorge, J. I. Schaffer, L. M. Halvorson, B. L. Hoffman, K. D. Bradshaw, & F. G. Cunningham (Eds.), *Williams gynecology*. Atlanta: American College of Obstetricians and Gynecologists. Retrieved from http://www.accessmedicine.com.proxy.lib.umich.edu/content.aspx?aID=3152827

Schorge, J. O., Schaffer, J. I., Halvorson, L. M., Hoffman, B. L., Bradshaw, K. D., & Cunningham, F. G. (2008b). Treatment of the infertile couple (Chapter 20). In J. O. Schorge, J. I. Schaffer, L. M. Halvorson, B. L. Hoffman, K. D. Bradshaw, & F. G. Cunningham (Eds.), *Williams gynecology*. Atlanta: American College of Obstetricians and Gynecologists. Retrieved from http://www.accessmedicine.com.proxy.lib.umich.edu/content.aspx?aID=3158038

Schorge, J. O., Schaffer, J. I., Halvorson, L. M., Hoffman, B. L., Bradshaw, K. D., & Cunningham, F. G. (2008c). Urinary incontinence (Chapter 23). In J. O. Schorge, J. I. Schaffer, L. M. Halvorson, B. L. Hoffman, K. D. Bradshaw, & F. G. Cunningham (Eds.), *Williams gynecology*. Atlanta: American College of Obstetricians and Gynecologists. Retrieved from http://www.accessmedicine.com.proxy.lib.umich.edu/content.aspx?aID=3159435

Schorge, J. O., Schaffer, J. I., Halvorson, L. M., Hoffman, B. L., Bradshaw, K. D., & Cunningham, F. G. (2008d). Preinvasive lesions of the lower genital tract (Chapter 29). In J. O. Schorge, J. I. Schaffer, L. M. Halvorson, B. L. Hoffman, K. D. Bradshaw, & F. G. Cunningham (Eds.), *Williams gynecology*. Atlanta: American College of Obstetricians and Gynecologists. Retrieved from http://www.accessmedicine.com.proxy.lib.umich.edu/content.aspx?aID=3161509

Schorge, J. O., Schaffer, J. I., Halvorson, L. M., Hoffman, B. L., Bradshaw, K. D., & Cunningham, F. G. (2008e). Cervical cancer (Chapter 30). In J. O. Schorge, J. I. Schaffer, L. M. Halvorson, B. L. Hoffman, K. D. Bradshaw, & F. G. Cunningham (Eds.), *Williams gynecology*. Atlanta: American College of Obstetricians and Gynecologists. Retrieved from http://www.accessmedicine.com.proxy.lib.umich.edu/content.aspx?aID=3162156

Schorge, J. O., Schaffer, J. I., Halvorson, L. M., Hoffman, B. L., Bradshaw, K. D., & Cunningham, F. G. (2008f). Surgeries for benign gynecologic conditions (Chapter 41). In J. O. Schorge, J. I. Schaffer, L. M. Halvorson, B. L. Hoffman, K. D. Bradshaw, & F. G. Cunningham (Eds.), *Williams gynecology*. Atlanta: American College of Obstetricians and Gynecologists. Retrieved from http://www.accessmedicine.com.proxy.lib.umich.edu/content.aspx?aID=3166442

Schorge, J. O., Schaffer, J. I., Halvorson, L. M., Hoffman, B. L., Bradshaw, K. D., & Cunningham, F. G. (2008g). Surgeries for female pelvic reconstruction (Chapter 42). In J. O. Schorge, J. I. Schaffer, L. M. Halvorson, B. L. Hoffman, K. D. Bradshaw, & F. G. Cunningham (Eds.), *Williams gynecology*. Atlanta: American College of Obstetricians and Gynecologists. Retrieved from http://www.accessmedicine.com.proxy.lib.umich.edu/content.aspx?aID=3168017

Schorge, J. O., Schaffer, J. I., Halvorson, L. M., Hoffman, B. L., Bradshaw, K. D., & Cunningham, F. G. (2008h). Surgeries for gynecologic malignancies (Chapter 43). In J. O. Schorge, J. I. Schaffer, L. M. Halvorson, B. L. Hoffman, K. D. Bradshaw, & F. G. Cunningham (Eds.), *Williams gynecology*. Atlanta: American College of Obstetricians and Gynecologists. Retrieved from http://www.accessmedicine.com.proxy.lib.umich.edu/content.aspx?aID=3169013

Smith, R. D. (2009). Contemporary hysteroscopic methods for female sterilization. *International Journal of Gynecology & Obstetrics, 108*(1), 79–84.

Van Norman, G. A. (2008). Ethical issues in informed consent. *Perioperative Nursing Clinics, 3*(3), 213–221.

Wieslander, C. K., Dandade D., & Wheeler J. M. (2007). Therapeutic gynecologic procedures (Chapter 48). In A. H. DeCherney & L. Nathan (Eds.), *CURRENT diagnosis & treatment obstetrics & gynecology* (10th ed.). New York: McGraw-Hill. Retrieved from http://www.accessmedicine.com.proxy.lib.umich.edu/content.aspx?aID=2391387

Zieve, D., & Storck, S. (2010). *Pap smear*. Retrieved from http://www.nlm.nih.gov/medlineplus/ency/article/003911.htm

CHAPTER 29

Neurologic Surgery

Lisa Day, PhD, RN, CNRN

Neurologic surgery patients require specialized care in the immediate postoperative period. The nurse caring for the postoperative craniotomy patient requires knowledge and skill in completing a thorough neurologic examination and in monitoring for and managing seizures and increased intracranial pressure. In addition, some patients require cerebrospinal fluid drainage or administration of specialized medications. This chapter will answer some common questions about providing the best postanesthesia care after brain surgeries including craniotomy for vascular lesions and tumors, and transsphenoidal surgeries.

1. What types of neurologic lesions in the brain are typically treated surgically?

The most common neurologic lesions in the brain that are treated surgically are neoplasms and vascular abnormalities such as arteriovenous malformations or fistulas, and aneurysms (Clatterbuck & Tamargo, 2004). Seizures that are refractory to medical treatment can be treated surgically by removing brain tissue that contains the seizure locus (Erickson & Cole, 2007). Blood from a subdural hematoma can also be evacuated surgically. Cerebral edema that is unresponsive to medical treatments can be treated surgically by removing a bone flap to relieve pressure on the brain (Diedler et al., 2009).

2. What are the general surgical approaches to the brain?

The surgical approach will depend on the location and type of lesion. General approaches to craniotomy include transtentorial (above the tentorium) for access to lesions in the cerebrum, and infratentorial (below the tentorium) for access to the skull base, cerebellum, brainstem, and cerebellar pontine angle (CPA). More specific transtentorial approaches include front sphenotemporal for access to the frontal and temporal areas; subtemporal, for access to the temporal and middle fossa areas; anterior parasagittal, for access to the midline frontal area; and posterior parasagittal, for access to the midline parietal area (Clatterbuck & Tamargo, 2004). More specific infratentorial approaches include midline and lateral suboccipital craniotomy for access to the posterior fossa (Clatterbuck & Tamargo, 2004). Other lesions of the pituitary gland may be accessed by a transsphenoidal approach.

3. What is a craniotomy?

Craniotomy is a surgical approach to treatment of a brain lesion that involves removing a flap of skull bone and surgically opening the dura mater to gain access to the brain tissue. The dura is the tough, fibrous meningeal covering closest to the skull bone.

4. What is transsphenoidal surgery?

The transsphenoidal approach is used to remove tumors of the pituitary gland. Because of the pituitary's position, it can be accessed microscopically and/or endoscopically through the sphenoid sinus rather than by a more invasive transtentorial craniotomy (Nakaji, Maughan, White, King, & Teo, 2005). With the transsphenoidal approach, an incision is made above the upper lip in front of the hard palate (sublabial approach) or inside the nares (endonasal approach) (Elias & Laws, 2000). Through this opening, the surgeon dissects through the sphenoid sinus floor, exposes the sella turcica and opens the dura mater; with the aid of a microscope, the tumor is removed. To prevent CSF leakage, the dura may be closed using a fat tissue graft harvested from the abdomen. Postoperatively, the patient will have nasal packing, may have an abdominal incision and drain to bulb suction, and may have a lumbar catheter. The purpose of the lumbar catheter is to drain cerebrospinal fluid (CSF) in order to relieve pressure and prevent CSF leakage at the surgical site.

5. What are the risks of transsphenoidal surgery?

Because of the location of the incision into the dura, transsphenoidal surgery can result in CSF leak through the sphenoid sinus. Because of the pituitary gland's close proximity to the optic chiasm, pituitary surgery may result in visual impairment. Because of the role of the pituitary gland in regulating the function of many different hormones, pituitary surgery can result in hormonal imbalance; the most immediately concerning of these is the loss of an antidiuretic hormone, resulting in diabetes insipidus (Elias & Laws, 2000).

6. What should be included in baseline and serial neurologic exams after craniotomy?

Most complications that require a return to surgery occur within the first 6 hours following a craniotomy (American Association of Neuroscience Nurses [AANN], 2006). It is important to maintain close observation of neurologic status during the first 12 to 24 hours after a craniotomy. The neurologic exam should always include the patient's level of consciousness or arousability, mental status or cognition, and motor and sensory components. In addition, depending on the location of the surgery, the exam may also include evaluation of cranial nerve function. For example, if the surgery involved the skull base or cerebellar-pontine angle, it will be important to monitor the function of the patient's cranial nerves IX–XII and assess the patient's ability to swallow before giving anything by mouth.

7. What neurologic findings during recovery from anesthesia are concerning?

It is of the utmost importance that the nurse knows the findings of the patient's baseline preoperative neurologic exam and what the neurosurgeon and anesthesiologist expects during the immediate postoperative phase. Unless the neurosurgeon says otherwise, the nurse should expect a gradual recovery of

consciousness, cognition, and motor and sensory function to full preoperative status. In general, any new and/or unexpected focal finding is of concern. A focal finding is a deficit that points to involvement in a specific area of the brain; for example, a weakness in the left arm points to a lesion in the right hemisphere. Other focal findings include aphasia, facial weakness, or cranial nerve deficit. Also concerning is any unexpected delay in recovery of consciousness or arousability.

8. How is the Glasgow coma score used to assess the postcraniotomy patient's neurologic status?

The Glasgow coma score (GCS) assigns a numeric value to arousability and so is useful in tracking arousability over time. The GCS is based on a point total in the following three categories: eye opening, motor response, and verbal response. The examiner records the number corresponding to the best response in each category. Thus, the GCS provides a means of quantifying one component of a complete neurologic exam but fails to capture many other important aspects. For example, if the patient has a right hemiplegia but obeys commands with full motor strength on the left side, he or she will receive full points on the GCS motor response score.

9. What are the main risks during the immediate postoperative period after craniotomy?

The main risks following craniotomy are cerebral edema or hydrocephalus resulting in increased intracranial pressure (ICP), seizures, and bleeding at the surgical site. The risks depend on the surgical approach and the underlying lesion. For example, the patient who is postcraniotomy for tumor resection is at higher risk for cerebral edema and seizures than the patient who is postcraniotomy for clipping a cerebral aneurysm. This has to do with the tumor's effect on the blood–brain barrier and that the invasive nature of most tumors requires more manipulation of brain tissue during removal.

10. What can be done to prevent increased intracranial pressure (ICP) caused by cerebral edema?

Pharmacologic means, fluid restriction, and nursing interventions should all be employed to reduce the risk of cerebral edema postcraniotomy in those patients at risk. The greatest risk of cerebral edema occurs during the first 3 days postcraniotomy; during this time, patients at risk are given steroids (dexamethasone) and may be placed on a fluid restriction. Depending on the severity of risk, the surgeon may order lidocaine administered via the endotracheal tube before suctioning in order to suppress the cough. Adequate sedation and analgesia are also important, as is maintenance of normothermia by use of antipyretics if necessary (Latorre & Greer, 2009). Patients are routinely given stool softeners to prevent straining. The head of bed should be kept at 30° or higher elevation and the neck kept straight to promote jugular venous drainage (Hickey, 2009).

11. What are signs and symptoms of increasing intracranial pressure?

The most common clinical sign of increasing intracranial pressure is a progressive decline in mental status, which will eventually result in coma (Latorre & Greer, 2009). The patient may complain of a headache and/or nausea and may vomit. In some patients, depending on the cause of increasing ICP, dilation of one pupil may be an early sign. Later signs include Cushing's triad, a widening pulse pressure (elevation of systolic blood pressure), bradycardia, and irregular breathing pattern (Hickey, 2009). Also, a late sign is bilateral dilated, nonreactive pupils.

12. What can be done to treat increased intracranial pressure caused by cerebral edema?

If the means used to prevent increased intracranial pressure fail, treatment focuses on reducing the volume in one of the three fluid compartments of the brain: tissue, blood, or cerebrospinal fluid; or by removing part of the skull to allow more room for brain contents (Diedler et al., 2009). Thus, increased intracranial pressure can be treated with a ventricular drain, hypertonic saline, mannitol, hypothermia, and/or hemicraniectomy in which a piece of the skull is removed to relieve pressure on the brain tissue.

13. How do mannitol and hypertonic saline work to reduce intracranial pressure?

Mannitol and hypertonic saline (3 or 23% NaCl) both act as osmotic diuretics that work by increasing the osmolarity of the blood. The increased blood osmolarity pulls fluid out of the brain cells, thus reducing cerebral fluid and increasing blood volume. The increased blood volume then works on the kidney to increase glomerular filtration, and urine output is increased, ultimately reducing blood volume.

14. What can be done to prevent seizures after craniotomy?

Patients at the highest risk for seizures after craniotomy are given prophylactic anticonvulsant medications. The most common drug used is phenytoin, although other drugs with fewer side effects may be just as effective at suppressing seizures (Lim et al., 2009).

15. How is an intravenous loading dose of phenytoin given?

Phenytoin is a drug commonly given postcraniotomy to patients at risk for seizures. It is important to remember that phenytoin is only compatible with normal saline and should not be mixed in any other solution or run in a line with any other drug. Because it has a long half-life, phenytoin is typically given first as a loading dose of 15 to 20 mg/kg, then in three daily doses of 100 mg or one daily dose of 300 mg in an extended release formula. Intravenous (IV) doses of phenytoin should be administered no faster than 50 mg/minute; faster rates can result in cardiac dysrhythmias and hypotension. An inline 0.22–5 micron filter should be used due to the high potential for precipitation. If phenytoin is given through a peripheral IV, it will cause pain at the infusion site; slowing the infusion or further dilution can reduce pain. Extravasations of phenytoin can result in serious tissue damage and necrosis. All of these concerns have prompted some pharmacists to recommend giving an IV loading dose of phosphenytoin, a similar drug that has fewer adverse effects, before starting a daily dose of phenytoin (Turkowski, 2009). Others have moved away from phenytoin all together and prefer other antiseizure medications such as levetiracetam (Lim et al, 2009).

16. What should the PACU nurse do if a patient has a seizure?

The PACU nurse should observe the behavior and protect the patient from injury. Notify the surgeon and expect an order for an IV benzodiazepine (lorazepam or diazepam), and to check serum levels if the patient is on an antiepilepsy drug. If the patient is not on an antiepilepsy drug, expect an order to start a loading dose.

17. What types of devices are used to drain cerebrospinal fluid (CSF) after neurologic surgery?

Intraventricular catheters and lumbar catheters are used to drain cerebrospinal fluid after neurologic surgery. The surgeon also may place a drain into the surgical bed or cavity to drain protein-rich exudate after tumor removal. These cavity drains sometimes also drain CSF depending on their proximity to the ventricles.

18. What types of patients require cerebrospinal fluid drainage after neurologic surgery?

Any patient at risk for hydrocephalus or at risk for cerebrospinal fluid leak may require CSF drainage as well as intracranial pressure monitoring. Patients at risk for hydrocephalus include those postsubarachnoid hemorrhage and postremoval of a tumor in or near the ventricles. Patients' posttranssphenoidal pituitary surgery are at risk for CSF leak and will often have a lumbar catheter to drain controlled amounts of CSF in order to reduce the pressure at the surgical site (Elias & Laws, 2000).

19. How is cerebrospinal fluid drainage managed with an external ventricular drain (EVD)?

An EVD is a catheter placed into the lateral ventricle of the brain through a burr hole in the skull. The catheter is attached to a gravity drainage collection system. Drainage amount is controlled by raising or lowering the collection bag or buretrol and by opening and closing the stop-cock.

20. How is cerebrospinal fluid drainage managed with a lumbar catheter?

A lumbar catheter is placed through the lumbar spine into the subarachnoid space. It is attached to a gravity drainage collection system. Drainage amount is controlled by raising or lowering the collection bag or buretrol and by opening and closing the stop-cock (AANN, 2007).

21. How is intracranial pressure monitored?

Intracranial pressure can be monitored with an external ventricular drain connected to a fluid-filled transducer or with a fiber optic subarachnoid bolt. An indirect measure of ICP can be obtained with a lumbar catheter or cavity drain.

22. What types of patients require intracranial pressure monitoring after craniotomy?

Craniotomy patients at high risk for increased intracranial pressure may need ICP monitoring after surgery. This is especially true if the patient's preoperative neurologic exam was poor and following his or her clinical signs will be difficult or not very informative.

REFERENCES

American Association of Neuroscience Nurses (2006). *Guide to the care of the patient with craniotomy post-brain tumor resection.* Glenview, IL: Author.

American Association of Neuroscience Nurses (2007). Care of the patient with a lumbar drain (2nd ed.). Glenview, IL: Author.

Clatterbuck, R. E. & Tamargo, R. J. (2004). Surgical positioning and exposures for cranial procedures. In H. R. Winn (Ed.), *Youmans' neurological surgery* (pp. 623–630, 5th ed.). Philadelphia: Saunders.

Diedler, J., Sykora, M., Blatow, M., Juttler, E., Unterberg, A., & Hacke, W. (2009). Decompressive surgery for severe brain edema. *Journal of Intensive Care Medicine, 24*(3), 168–178.

Elias, W. J. & Laws, R. E. (2000). Transsphenoidal approaches to lesions of the sella. In H. H. Schmidek (Ed.), *Operative neurosurgical techniques: Indications, methods and results* (pp. 373–384). Philadelphia: Saunders.

Erickson, K. M., & Cole, D. J. (2007). Anesthetic considerations for awake craniotomy for epilepsy. *Anesthesiology Clinics, 25*(3), 535–555.

Hickey, J. V. (2009). *The clinical practice of neurological and neurosurgical nursing* (6th ed.). Philadelphia: Lippincott.

Latorre, J. G. S., & Greer, D. M. (2009). Management of acute intracranial hypertension: A review. *The Neurologist, 15*(4), 193–207.

Lim, D. A., Tarapore, P., Chang, E., Burt, M., Chakalian, L., Barbaro, N., et al. (2009). Safety and feasibility of switching from phenytoin to levetiracetam monotherapy for glioma-related seizure control following craniotomy: A randomized phase II pilot study. *Journal of Neurooncology, 93*(3),349–354.

Nakaji, P., Maughan, H., White, W. L., King, W. L., & Teo, C. (2005) Endoscopic-assisted transsphenoidal surgery: Operative techniques, *8*(4),193–197.

Turkowski, B. B. (2009). *Drug information handbook for nursing* (11th ed.). Hudson, OH: Lexi-Comp.

CHAPTER 30

Surgical Oncology

JoAnn Coleman, DNP, RN, MS, ACNP, AOCN

Surgery is the oldest treatment for cancer and, generally, the only cure for patients with cancer of solid organs. Advances in surgical techniques and a better understanding of the patterns of spread of individual cancers have dramatically changed the surgical treatment of cancer. Modern anesthetic techniques, increased knowledge of antibiotic therapy, blood component administration, improved technology, and surgical skill have greatly increased the safety of major oncologic surgery and allowed surgeons to perform successful resections for an increased number of patients. Surgery is now used in combination with other forms of treatment. Multimodality therapy has led to more conservative and less radical procedures for some cancers as seen in the options for the treatment of breast cancer. There is also a trend toward an increased use of more aggressive major operations for other cancers. New technologies allow for less extensive surgery, with the potential for minimal pain, less use of blood component replacement, decreased hospital stay, and a more rapid recovery. Minimally invasive surgical procedures using laparoscopy, robot-assisted laparoscopy, and video-assisted thoracoscopy are examples of new technologies. Nursing plays a major role in the care of patients having surgery for cancer, providing patient education, care, and support throughout the perioperative period. Nurses are challenged to keep abreast of the changes in surgical cancer care along with new technology and multimodality therapy.

1. What is the purpose of surgery in the patient with cancer?

Surgical therapy remains the primary method of treatment for most solid malignancies. In some cases, it is the only chance for cure. It is estimated that more than 90% of patients with cancer have some type of surgical procedure for diagnosis, treatment, or management of the disease. Curative resections involve the removal of tumor along with a margin of normal tissue and regional lymph nodes. This type of resection offers the best chance of cure and provides histologic information for prognosis. Surgery may be performed for control of cancer. This is done to reduce the size of a tumor as the extensive local spread of cancer may preclude the removal of all gross disease. Surgery may also be performed for recurrence of disease or metastatic cancer from a primary cancer such as liver resection for metastatic colon cancer or neck dissection for a nodal metastasis from head and neck cancer.

Palliative surgery is performed to promote patient comfort and quality of life without curing the disease. The goal of palliative surgery is to relieve symptoms of obstruction, bleeding, pressure, and pain. Surgery is also performed to prevent cancer in high-risk individuals. Removal of precancerous lesions prevents the subsequent development of cancer. Examples of preventive surgery for cancer include:

- Total proctocolectomy (removal of the entire colon and rectum) in a patient with familial adenomatous polyposis or with ulcerative colitis to prevent colorectal cancer

- Prophylactic mastectomy for a patient at high risk for breast cancer
- Orchidectomy in a male patient with cryptorchidism, which places the person at risk for development of testicular cancer

Reconstruction operations aim to improve structure, function, and appearance, and to repair or reduce anatomic defects from cancer surgery or therapy. Examples include breast reconstruction after mastectomy and facial reconstruction for head and neck cancers. Devices for other treatment modalities may be inserted in surgery such as placement of vascular access devices, Ommaya reservoirs, gastrostomy or jejunostomy tubes, and brachytherapy catheters (Coleman, 2004).

2. What is the role of surgery for the patient with cancer?

Surgery is considered part of a multidisciplinary approach to cancer therapy. The combination and careful timing of surgery along with chemotherapy, radiation therapy, immunotherapy, and other novel therapeutic approaches are essential to optimal treatment planning. Nurses must be aware of the various surgeries for cancer as well as the latest evidence related to other cancer therapies. Any initial surgery may prove to be critical in terms of either allowing future treatment options or rendering certain therapies unfeasible.

- Diagnosis: The role of surgery in the diagnosis of cancer is the acquisition of tissue for histologic diagnosis. A tissue diagnosis is important in the planning of treatment for specific cancers.
- Staging: The pathologic examination of tissue is performed to determine the size of the primary tumor, presence of positive lymph nodes, and extent of metastases. Surgical staging is most often performed for tumors that are otherwise inaccessible, or for those difficult to evaluate by any other means. Surgical staging provides a systematic approach to the diagnosis and treatment of malignancies.
- Extent or severity of a patient's cancer: Knowing the stage of the cancer helps the physician plan a patient's treatment and estimated prognosis.
- Treatment:
  ○ Surgery may be the first, and usually the most important, treatment.
  ○ Primary: The removal of the malignant tumor and a margin of adjacent normal tissue

  ○ Adjuvant: The removal of tissues to decrease the risk of cancer incidence, progression, or recurrence
- Therapeutic or supportive device: Placement of therapeutic and supportive hardware, such as gastrostomy tube, ventricular reservoir, external or implantable vascular access devices, and radioactive implants
- Assess tumor response to previous treatment by second-look procedures: procedure performed within a predetermined time frame after initial therapy
  ○ Identify and resect sites and volume of residual tumor
  ○ Reconstruct affected body parts
  ○ Repair or reduce anatomic defects from cancer surgery to improve function and/or cosmetic appearance (e.g., fecal or urinary diversion, breast reconstruction, fistula excision, skin flap development, and prosthesis placement)
- Treat complications of other cancer therapies: Examples include perforation and bleeding from radiation therapy
- Prevention/prophylaxis: Surgery is performed to prevent cancer in high-risk individuals (e.g., total proctocolectomy for patients with familial polyposis, prophylactic mastectomy for patients with predisposing family cancer genetics such as BRCA2 gene, prophylactic total pancreatectomy for patients with family history of pancreas cancer and high grade dysplasia throughout the pancreas)
- Oncologic emergencies (e.g., pericardectomy, pericardial window for neoplastic cardiac tamponade, long-term indwelling implanted catheters or pleuroperitoneal shunts and pleurectomy [decortication] for malignant pleural effusion, surgical decompression for spinal cord compression) (Coleman, 2004; Gillespie, 2005).

3. Why is staging important in the patient with cancer?

Staging describes the extent or severity of a patient's cancer. Knowing the stage of the disease helps the physician (or surgeon) plan a person's treatment and estimate prognosis. Staging systems for cancer have evolved over time and continue to change as scientists learn more about cancer. Some staging systems cover many types of cancer, while others focus on a particular type. The common elements considered in most staging systems are the location of the primary tumor, tumor size, and number of tumors; lymph node involvement; cell type and tumor grade; and presence or absence of metastasis.

There are three different types of staging.

- Clinical staging determines how much cancer there is based on the physical examination, imaging tests, and biopsies of affected areas.
- Pathologic staging can only be done on patients who have had surgery to remove or explore the extent of the cancer. This type of staging combines the results of both the clinical staging (physical exam, imaging test) with the results from the surgery.
- Restaging is used to determine the extent of the disease if a cancer comes back after treatment. This is done to determine what the best treatment option would be at the time.

The TNM Staging System is one of the most commonly used staging systems. This system was developed and is maintained by the American Joint Committee on Cancer (AJCC) and the International Union Against Cancer (UICC). The TNM classification system was developed as a tool for physicians to stage different types of cancer based on certain standard criteria American Joint Committee on Cancer, (2010).

The TNM staging system is based on the extent of a tumor (T), spread to lymph nodes (N), and metastasis (spread to other parts of the body) (M). A number is added to each letter to indicate the size or extent of the tumor and the extent of spread.

- Most cancers can be described as stage 0, stage I, stage II, stage III, or stage IV. Stage 0 is a very early stage of cancer and Stage IV is evidence of metastatic cancer from the primary site.
- Physical exams, imaging procedures, laboratory tests, pathology reports, and surgical reports help provide information to determine the stage of the cancer.

4. What are some key considerations for the different stages in cancer?

- Determining the stage of a cancer helps physicians to make treatment recommendations, form a likely outcome scenario for what will happen to the patient (prognosis), and communicate effectively with other physicians treating the patient.
- Stages I, II, III, and IV represent progressively more advanced cancers characterized by larger tumor sizes, more tumors, aggressiveness with which the cancer grows, and extent to which

the cancer has spread to adjacent tissues and body organs (NCI, 2004).

5. What are the different types of surgical interventions?

- Aspiration biopsy: A procedure in which the cells and tissue fragments are removed by aspiration through a needle that has been guided into the suspicious material/mass.
- Needle biopsy: A procedure in which a core of tissue is obtained through a specially designed needle placed into the suspicious material/mass.
- Sentinal node (SLN) biopsy: A procedure in which the sentinel lymph node is removed and examined under a microscope to determine whether cancer cells are present. SLN biopsy is based on the idea that cancer cells spread in an orderly way from the primary tumor to the sentinel lymph node(s), then to other nearby lymph nodes.
- Incisional biopsy: A procedure in which a small portion or wedge of tissue is removed from a larger tumor mass.
- Excisional biopsy: A procedure in which the entire suspected tumor is removed with little or no margin of surrounding normal tissue for diagnostic purposes.
- Laparotomy: A surgical procedure involving an incision through the abdominal wall to gain access into the abdominal cavity.
- Laparoscopy: Also called minimally invasive surgery (MIS), band-aid surgery, or keyhole surgery, this is a modern surgical technique in which operations in the abdomen are performed through small incisions (usually 0.5–1.5 cm) as compared to larger incisions needed in traditional surgical procedures (Coleman, 2004; Szopa, 2005).
- Endoscopic surgery: A procedure that uses scopes going through small incisions or natural body openings in order to diagnose and treat disease. Another popular term is minimally invasive surgery (MIS), which emphasizes that diagnosis and treatments can be done with reduced body cavity invasion. Natural orifice transluminal endoscopic surgery (NOTES) is an surgical technique whereby "scarless" abdominal operations can be performed with an endoscope passed through a natural orifice such as the mouth, anus, or vagina and then through an internal incision in the stomach, colon, or vagina, thus avoiding any external incisions or scars (Halim & Tavakkolizadeh, 2008).

- Minor surgery is restricted to management of minor problems and injuries.

- Major surgery involves the more important, difficult, and hazardous operations.

- LASER therapy: The use of a laser, an intense beam of light, to precisely cut, burn, or destroy diseased tissues or treat bleeding blood vessels. Laser is an acronym for Light Amplification by Stimulated Emission of Radiation.

- Radiofrequency oblation (RFA): A type of electrical energy used to create heat in a specific location, at a specific temperature, for a specific period of time, and ultimately results in the death of unwanted tissue.

- Photodynamic therapy (PTD): Involves an intravenous injection of a light-sensitizing or photo-sensitizing agent that is absorbed by cancer cells, followed by exposure to laser light 24 to 48 hours later. This causes cancer cell death. The drugs only work after they have been activated by certain kinds of light (Coleman, 2004; Szopa, 2005).

- Portal vein injection to shrink tumor/liver lobe: Portal vein embolization (PVE) is a useful procedure in the preoperative treatment of patients selected for major hepatic resections. PVE is performed via either the percutaneous transhepatic or the transileo-colic route and is usually reserved for patients whose future liver remnants are too small to allow resection. The procedure causes atrophy or shrinking of a part of the liver and the hypertrophy or extra growth of the remaining liver and may reduce complications and shorten hospital stays after resection (Liu & Zhu, 2009).

6. Why is it important to know the previous history of the oncology patient undergoing surgery?

The surgical oncology patient requires nursing assessment and care similar to that required for any other surgical patient. The nurse must be aware of unique problems and complications related to treatment modalities for cancer and the disease process. The effect of cancer and previous cancer therapies may increase the risk for postsurgical complications. Special considerations include:

- Previous cancer therapy and the length of time since therapy completed;

- Current medications;

- Current and previous chemotherapy, biologic, and vaccine therapy;

- Radiation therapy;

- Side effects of any previous therapy;

- Allergies;

- Pain assessment (Surgical oncology patients may have greater needs for postoperative analgesia, particularly if the surgical procedure is for advanced disease or if the patients were previously receiving analgesics. Many oncology patients are not narcotic naïve and may have sources of chronic pain in addition to acute surgical pain);

- Nutritional interventions (Assessment of current nutritional status as well as the patient's baseline nutritional status); and

- Awareness of the effects of combined modality therapies or recent antineoplastic treatments (The interactive and compounding effects of chemotherapy, radiation therapy, and immunotherapy may produce problems and side effects for the postoperative patient. Postoperative wound healing may be compromised by effects of radiation therapy. Immunosuppression places the patient at a higher risk for wound infections and may have an adverse affect on wound healing. Antineoplastic agents have specific organ toxicities that place the surgical oncology patient at increased risk for pulmonary, renal, respiratory, hematologic, and cardiac complications) (Coleman, 2004; Gillespie, 2005).

7. What is the difference between neoadjuvant and adjuvant therapy?

- Neoadjuvant therapy is treatment given as a first step to shrink a tumor before the main treatment, which is usually surgery, is given. Examples of neoadjuvant therapy include chemotherapy, radiation therapy, vaccines, and hormone therapy. The use of effective neoadjuvant treatment modalities has led to a decrease in the extent of surgery in some instances.

- Adjuvant therapy is additional cancer treatment given after the primary treatment to lower the risk that the cancer will come back. Adjuvant therapy may include chemotherapy, radiation therapy, hormone therapy, targeted therapy, biologic therapy, and vaccines. Integrating surgery with other treatment modalities requires careful consideration of all effective treatment options (American Cancer Society [ACS], 2009).

8. What are important factors to be considered in the preoperative assessment of the patient having surgery for cancer?

- Complete pain assessment including the following: location; intensity; quality (nociceptive: aching, throbbing; neuropathic: burning, tingling, electrical, painfully numb); intensity; temporal patterns; aggravating and alleviating factors; meaning of pain; presence of suffering or distress; cultural factors; current medications (Miaskowski et al., 2005); pain score (e.g., numerical scale, visual analog scale, or verbal pain scale); psychosocial, which addresses patient's fears related to surgery and postoperative pain; answer questions or concerns at a level the patient can understand; explain proposed surgery and pain management strategies such as patient controlled analgesia to reduce patient anxiety; offer emotional support to the patient to help the patient through the surgical procedure and anticipated outcomes; supportive nurse–patient relationship promotes an atmosphere that allows the patient to voice fears and anxieties (Coleman, 2004).

- Evaluation of family support and/or other support systems: This is important to know in order to facilitate discharge planning, including any care of wounds, tubes, drains, ostomy, rehabilitation needs, etc.

- Thorough assessment of the patient's skin integrity: This is necessary for baseline temperature, color, turgor, and elasticity. Evaluate patient's skin for any injuries or breaks in the skin, bruising, pressure ulcers, rash, or impaired vascular circulation that may contribute to delayed wound healing or predispose the patient to other postoperative complications such as infection. Patients who have had preoperative radiation and chemotherapy are at increased risk for postoperative skin and wound complications (Coleman, 2004).

- Nutritional status: Includes baseline nutrition assessment to help guide postoperative care, especially if the patient had preoperative chemotherapy and/or radiation therapy and may be nutritionally depleted. Nutritional depletion places the patient at risk for poor wound healing, dehiscence or evisceration, infection, pneumonia, and increased morbidity (Coleman, 2004).

- Diabetes management: Necessary for anticipating glucose control postoperatively for adequate wound healing and minimizing vascular risk. Patients that undergo a total pancreatectomy will have surgically induced diabetes, if they were not a diabetic preoperatively. These patients, ideally, should have preoperative diabetes education with postoperative endocrine/diabetes education follow-up. Patients with more than 50% of their pancreas removed will need close monitoring for signs of diabetes after surgery and may need further evaluation for diabetes when discharged from the hospital (Coleman, 2004).

- Stage of cancer helps to determine treatment options. Most cancer treatment options are delineated in the National Comprehensive Cancer Network (NCCN) Clinical Practice Guidelines in Oncology (NCCN, 2010).

- A history of previous pulmonary embolism or deep vein thrombosis (DVT) is a concern for potential recurrence of vascular thromboembolism (VTE) after surgery. All preventive VTE measures and increased vigilance is necessary for these patients as coagulopathies and bleeding tendencies are not uncommon in the oncology patient. Hypercoagulability and thrombosis are associated with abnormal clotting factors found in some patients with cancer, placing them at increased risk for the development of VTE. Abdominal and pelvic surgery also predispose the patient to DVT (Coleman, 2004).

- Preoperative hemoglobin is essential as most patients with cancer have anemia of chronic disease. Patients who have had previous chemotherapy and/or radiation therapy will also have depleted blood cell stores. Meticulous care to control excessive bleeding and prevent administration of blood products are of benefit to the postoperative surgical oncology patient (Dionigi et al., 2009).

- Knowledge of comorbid conditions is necessary as many patients have other medical conditions that need concurrent treatment in the perioperative period.

- Rehabilitation potential of the patient needs to be evaluated, particularly if the intended surgery will significantly alter normal physiologic function.

- Quality of life issues need to be discussed with the patient as a surgical procedure may be technically feasible, but it may not be the best option in terms of quality of life.

9. What information regarding previous cancer therapy is important when obtaining a preoperative assessment?

Previous surgical history is important, including type of surgery, experience with anesthetic agents, blood transfusions, and surgical complications. Others information includes placement and current use of a vascular access device (VAD); impact of previous antineoplastic agents on proposed surgical procedure; bleeding; wound healing; potential bowel perforation; and metabolic alterations.

10. What is stereotactic surgery?

Stereotactic surgery is a form of radiation therapy, also called stereotactic radiotherapy. It is a highly precise form of radiation therapy initially used to treat tumors and other abnormalities of the brain. It delivers precisely targeted radiation at much higher doses than traditional radiation therapy while sparing nearby healthy tissues and organs. Stereotactic radiosurgery is also being used to treat cancer in other parts of the body in a procedure called stereotactic body radiotherapy (SBRT).

Three-dimensional imaging, such as computerized tomography (CT), magnetic resonance imaging (MRI), and positron-emission tomography (PET)/CT is used to locate the tumor or abnormality within the body and define its exact size and shape. These images—in which beams of radiation are designed to converge on the target area from different angles and planes— guide the treatment planning as well as the careful positioning of the patient for therapy sessions. Stereotactic radiosurgery works in the same way as other forms of radiation treatment. It does not actually remove the tumor; rather, it damages the DNA of tumor cells. As a result, these cells lose their ability to reproduce. Following treatment, malignant and metastatic tumors may shrink rapidly, even within a couple of months.

Stereotactic radiosurgery and SBRT are important alternatives to invasive surgery, especially for patients who are unable to undergo surgery and for tumors and abnormalities that are hard to reach, located close to vital organs, and subject to movement within the body. SBRT is currently used and/or being investigated for use in treating malignant or benign small-to-medium size tumors in parts of the body, including the lung, liver, abdomen, spine, prostate, and head or neck (Lo et al., 2010).

11. What is transarterial chemoembolization (TACE)?

It is an arterial chemotherapy infusion of the liver and chemoembolization of the liver (transarterial chemoembolization [TACE]) are similar procedures that are used for the treatment of liver cancers. In both procedures, chemotherapy is injected into the hepatic artery that supplies the liver tumor. The difference between the two procedures is that in chemoembolization, additional material is injected to block or embolize the small branches of the hepatic artery (Liapi, Georgiades, Hong, & Geschwind, 2007).

12. What are preoperative medications, including antineoplastic agents, that may place the patient at an increased risk for postoperative complications?

The medications include chemotherapeutic agents, targeted therapies, anticoagulants, immunotherapy, and antineoplastic agents (standard and experimental) being administered in a clinical trial.

Any of these agents may have specific side effects that may impact the patient in the perioperative period. Certain antineoplastics need to be stopped for a specific amount of time before the patient undergoes surgery. An example of an antineoplastic agent that needs to be stopped for 6 to 8 weeks prior to surgery is bevacizumab (Avastin) as this may put the patient at increase risk for bleeding and delay wound healing (Coleman, 2004).

13. What are the preoperative teaching needs of the patient having surgery for cancer?

- Emotional support is necessary as patients often only hear the words "cancer" and "surgery" and forget all of the preoperative instructions.

- Address the patient's fears, concerns, and perceptions about their situation.

- Promote an atmosphere in which the patient is encouraged to voice fears and anxieties (Rosén, Svensson, & Nilsson, 2008; Pritchard, 2009).

- Teach the patient about the planned procedure by explaining the operation, what to anticipate after surgery, potential complications, and expected outcomes.

- Use both written and verbal reinforcement to aid retention.

- Prepare the patient by explaining any particular preparation such as a bowel preparation, positioning during surgery, location of incision, placement of any tubes and/or wound drains, intravenous lines, or any other special attachments.

- Explain what will be expected of the patient postoperatively regarding deep breathing exercises, activity, diet advancements, and self-care to optimize recovery.

- Assess current pain management in terms of both needs and deficits. Ascertain if the patient is currently on any pain medications and, if so, which ones and at what dose because this will have an impact on postoperative doses. Address any patient fears of postoperative pain and explain pain management strategies, such as patient-controlled analgesia, epidural anesthesia, and the potential for intraoperative pain block.

- Facilitate discharge planning by assessing needs and available resources preoperatively: evaluate function in terms of abilities and deficits and evaluate support systems and any special needs (Coleman, 2004; Walker, 2007). Provide discharge instructions and incorporate multiple educational strategies such as verbal and written instructions or any media, such as CDs, with instructions for the patient to take home.

14. What are the roles of the family or significant others?

The family and/or the significant other have important roles. They are another set of ears to hear all information as well as to ask questions. They can be present for any patient teaching to also learn discharge instructions, wound care, nutrition needs, etc. The family and/or significant other can reinforce patient teaching and provide physical, emotional, and psychologic support.

15. What are some specialty services that need to be addressed prior to surgery?

Markings by ostomy nurse for potential ostomy sites prior to surgery help to optimize intraoperative stoma placement for esthetics and proper function (Vujnovich, 2008). Nutritional assessment with possible intervention may be important. Optimization of nutrition is necessary for postoperative wound healing and overall improved patient outcomes. Measures to improve nutrition, such as enteral or parental nutrition, may be instituted prior to surgery (Garth, Newsome, Simmance & Crowe, 2010).

Speech pathology for patients who undergo head and neck surgery, especially laryngectomy, will have speech disruption and should be counseled by speech pathologists prior to surgery. Education for vocal retraining is provided along with recommendations and instructions for speech assist devices and safe nutritional intake. Image recovery for appearance enhancement programs is designed to help patients understand and prepare for appearance changes that result from chemotherapy,

radiation therapy, and surgery. These programs educate patients about what to expect and how to prevent potential problems and help normalize physical appearance.

Social work provides psychosocial counseling for the patient and family, clarification of insurance concerns, as well as assistance with potential issues related to postoperative disposition and procurement of durable medical equipment. They can assist in referrals to community resources such as Reach to Recovery, Voicemasters, United Ostomy Association, and others (Coleman, 2004; Szopa, 2005).

16. What are important preparations for the patient prior to surgery for cancer?

Bowel preparation is widely used for bowel, major abdominal, and pelvic surgery for cancer to prevent anastomotic leakage and wound complications. This preoperative procedure is being reconsidered in many elective surgeries (Guenaga, Matos, & Wille-Jørgensen, 2009). Skin preparation may be performed to reduce hospital-acquired (nosocomial) surgical site infections that may occur after surgical procedures. Preoperative bathing or showering with an antiseptic skin wash product is the usual procedure for reducing skin bacteria. Currently, there is not clear evidence whether reducing skin microflora leads to a lower incidence of surgical site infection (Webster & Osbourne, 2007).

17. What are the most common postoperative complications?

The most common complications are infection, bleeding, and death. These complications may be seen in any postoperative patient but the patient with recent surgery for cancer is at increased risk. Vigilance by nurses caring for the postoperative surgical oncology patient can help prevent or stop life-threatening infection, hemorrhage, and multiple-organ failure (Friese & Aiken, 2008). Other considerations for common postoperative complications include respiratory problems including atelectasis and pneumonia; urinary tract infection from prolonged indwelling catheter; wound infection; DVT; and reaction to medications (Plauntz, 2007).

18. What are the potential postoperative long-term complications?

Consideration of the particular cancer surgery is necessary to determine any long-term complications. Some common complications are radical retropubic prostatectomy for incontinence and impotence; mastectomy may cause lymphedema, hematoma, and seroma; colorectal surgery can result in diarrhea and incontinence of stool; a pancreaticoduodenectomy (Whipple procedure) may result in pancreatic fistula and delayed gastric emptying in the immediate postoperative period and malabsorption, dumping, and diabetes as long-term complications; and headache and seizures may be a complication of brain surgery.

19. Are all oncology patients susceptible to immunosuppression?

All surgical patients are subject to immunosuppression, and cancer patients are generally already susceptible to immunosuppression as related to their disease. Nursing care in the perioperative period should be directed at assessing for causes of further depression of the immune system. Potential factors that may affect immune function include surgery, anesthesia, pain, opioid medications, temperature changes, blood transfusion, and physiologic and psychologic stress (Neil, 2007).

20. What is the risk of perioperative blood transfusion among cancer patients?

The need for allogeneic (taken from different individuals of the same species) blood transfusion is a known risk associated with surgical procedures. The risk of requiring transfusion of red blood cells, platelets, or other blood products varies with the diagnosis, stage of disease, extent, and type of surgical procedure planned. Transfusion rates may be very low in some cases involving solid tumors or may be extremely high in other procedures and tumor sites.

Immunosuppression associated with allogeneic transfusion, in addition to the presumed immunosuppression due to the cancer itself, is thought to be the underlying etiology for poorer outcomes reported among patients who received blood transfusion along with surgery for their cancer diagnosis. Allogeneic blood transfusion given perioperatively for multiple tumor types has been implicated as a factor leading to important outcomes such as increased rates of postoperative infection, increased risk of cancer recurrence, and overall survival (Weber, Jabbour, & Martin, 2008).

Nurses play an important role in assessing risk factors prior to surgery, including anemia. Low preoperative hematocrit and low postoperative hematocrit, as well as increased blood transfusion rates, have been associated with increased mortality, increased rates of postoperative pneumonia, and increased hospital length of stay (Neil, 2007).

21. What are the postoperative patient teaching needs?

- Schedule procedures for routine postoperative follow-up care.
- Teach changes in condition that should be reported to the healthcare team such as signs and symptoms of infection; persistent nausea, vomiting, or decrease in appetite; poor wound healing; changes in bowel or bladder patterns; changes in location, and persistent or increased severity of pain; and inability to resume functional ability within anticipated time frame.
- Identify potential community resources to meet unique demands of therapy and rehabilitation (Coleman, 2004).

22. What are the community resources needed postoperatively?

Assess the patient for need of community resources and make referrals for home care and/or support programs (e.g., Reach to Recovery, Voicemasters, Make Today Count, International Association of Laryngectomies, United Ostomy Association chapters, American Cancer Society) (Szopa, 2005). The postoperative needs of a patient having surgery for cancer will be dictated by the specific surgery.

23. Is there an increase risk for VTE, DVT, and pulmonary embolism among surgical oncology patients?

Patients with cancer undergoing abdominal surgery are at substantially higher risk for VTE than patients without cancer. The appropriate use of thromboprophylactic agents has significant implications for the clinical care and quality of life of surgical patients with cancer (Osbourne, Wakefield, & Henke, 2008).

24. What is the importance of quality of life from the patient's point of view?

Whatever the overall enjoyment of life is to the individual is that person's definition of quality of life. This may include aspects of an individual's sense of well-being and ability to carry out various activities. A surgical intervention may impact the aspects of a patient's quality of life and must be considered before undergoing any operation.

25. When should palliative care be introduced to the patient?

Palliative care is care given to improve the quality of life of patients who have a serious or life-threatening disease. The goal of palliative care is to prevent or treat as early as possible the symptoms of a disease, side effects caused by treatment, and psychologic, social, and spiritual problems related to a disease or its treatment. Palliative care may also be called comfort care, supportive care, and symptom management. Ideally, a patient with a diagnosis of cancer should be introduced to the concept of palliative care when the initial diagnosis is made (Ferrell, 2004).

26. What are important considerations for older adult patients?

More than half of all cancers and cancer deaths occur in older individual (over 65 years of age). No published data support the use of age alone as the primary means to determine contraindications for optimal cancer care. Currently, no evidence exists to withhold chemotherapy or standard treatment based solely on age. Effective therapy can be given to the older adult patient, and the outcomes and toxicities are the same as for younger patients for multiple tumor types. The most important considerations include functional or performance status, presence of significant comorbidities, medical and surgical history, prior therapies, and demographics. These are important indicators of the ability of a patient to tolerate surgery and anesthesia rather than chronologic age alone (Pasetto, Lise, & Monfardini, 2007; Audisio et al., 2004). Consideration of the patient's desire to have surgery after learning all the risks and benefits is also important.

27. What specialized care may impact perioperative outcomes in the patient having surgery for cancer?

Each of the following may have an effect on perioperative outcomes, from immediate postsurgical morbidity and mortality, to long-term rehabilitation and recovery of function.

- Tumor characteristics: biology and natural history of the specific malignancy is critical in surgery for cancer
- Patient characteristics: medical and surgical history, prior therapies, demographics, performance status, presence of significant comorbidities
- Pathology of tumor (if known)
- Staging of disease
- Consultation by medical and/or radiation oncology as indicated
- Discussion of the need for neoadjuvant therapy
- Documentation and communication of the goals of therapy
- Plans for immediate or delayed reconstruction, with consultation by plastic or reconstructive surgery, as needed
- Consultation with any other specialists who may need to be involved in surgery depending on the extent of the resection (e.g., urology in extensive colorectal or gynecologic surgeries; plastic surgery for reconstruction; vascular surgery for vessel reconstruction or replacement)
- Plans for rehabilitation, if needed
- Coordination of care; multidisciplinary or interdisciplinary care
- Environmental factors: specialized physician and nursing expertise; technology and surgical techniques; volume of cases preformed by the institution and by the attending surgeon with the patient's specific tumor type/stage; supportive care available; antibiotics, transfusions, nutritional supplementation, and related interventions
- Availability of specialized nursing care or specialty units, such as critical care; nutritional support services, social work, physical therapy, occupational therapy, speech therapy, etc. (Gillespie, 2005)

REFERENCES

American Cancer Society. (2009). Cancer Reference Information: Chemotherapy. Retrieved from http://www.cancer.org/docroot/CRI/content/CRI_2_4_4X_Chemotherapy_5.asp.

American Joint Committee on Cancer. (2010). What is cancer staging? Retrieved from http://www.cancerstaging.org/mission/whatis.html.

Coleman, J. (2004). Surgical therapy. In B. K. Shelton, C. R. Ziegfeld, & M. M. Olsen (Eds.), *Manual of cancer nursing* (pp. 107–119). Philadelphia: Lippincott Williams & Wilkins.

Dionigi, G., Boni, L., Rovera, F., Rausei, S., Cuffani, S., Cantone, G., et al. (2009). Effect of perioperative blood transfusion on clinical outcomes in hepatic surgery for cancer. *World Journal of Gastroenterology, 15*(32), 3976–3983.

Ferrell, B. R. (2004). Palliative care: An essential aspect of quality cancer care. *Surgical Oncology Clinics of North America, 13*(3), 401–411.

Friese, C. R., & Aiken, L. H. (2008). Failure to rescue in the surgical oncology population: Implications for nursing and quality improvement. *Oncology Nursing Forum, 35*(5), 779–785.

Garth, A. K., Newsome, C. M., Simmance, N., & Crowe, T. C. (2010). Nutritional status, nutrition practices and post-operative complications in patients with gastrointestinal cancer. *Journal of Human Nutrition and Dietetics, 23*(4), 393–401.

Gillespie, T. W. (2005). Surgical therapy. In C. H. Yarbro, M. H. Frogge, & M. Goodman (Eds.), *Cancer nursing principles and practice* (6th ed., pp. 212–228). Boston: Jones and Bartlett Publishers.

Guenaga, K. K. F. G., Matos, D., & Wille-Jørgensen, P. (2009). Mechanical bowel preparation for elective colorectal surgery. *Cochrane Database of Systematic Reviews*, (1), CD001544.

Halim. I., & Tavakkolizadeh, A. (2008). NOTES: The next surgical revolution? *International Journal of Surgery*, 6(4), 273–276.

Liapi, E., Georgiades, C. C., Hong, K., & Geschwind, J. F. (2007). Transcather arterial chemoembolization: current technique and future promise. *Techniques in Vascular Interventional Radiology*, 10(1), 2–11.

Liu, H., & Zhu, S. (2009). Present status and future perspectives of preoperative portal vein tembolization. *American Journal of Surgery*, 197(5), 686–690.

Lo, S. S., Fakiris, A. J., Chang, E. L., Mayr, N. A., Wang, J. Z., Papiez, L., et al. (2010). Stereotactic body radiation therapy: A novel treatment modality. *Nature Reviews. Clinical Oncology*, 7(1), 44–54.

Miaskowski, C., Cleary, J., Burney, R., Coyne, P., Finley, R., Foster. R., et al. (2005). *Guide for the management of cancer pain in adults and children* (No. 3). Glenview, IL: American Pain Society.

National Cancer Institute. (2004). *National Cancer Institute fact sheet. Staging: Questions and answers*. Retrieved from http://www.cancer.gov/cancertopics/factsheet/Detection/staging.

National Comprehensive Cancer Network. (2010). *National comprehensive Cancer Network clinical practice guidelines in oncology*. Retrieved from http://www.nccn.org/professionals/physician_gls/f_guidelines.asp.

Neil, J. A. (2007). Perioperative care of the immunocompromised patient. *AORN Journal*, 85(3), 544–560.

Osbourne, N. H., Wakefield, T. W., & Henke, P. K. (2008). Venous thromboembolism in cancer patients undergoing major surgery. *Annals of Surgical Oncology*, 15(12), 3567–3578.

Pasetto, L. M., Lise, M., & Monfardini, S. (2007). Preoperative assessment of elderly cancer patients. *Critical Reviews in Oncology Hematology*, 64(1), 10–18.

Plauntz, L. M. (2007). Preoperative assessment of the surgical patient. *Nursing Clinics of North America*, 42(3), 361–377.

Pritchard, M. J. (2009). Managing anxiety in the elective surgical patient. *British Journal of Nursing*, 18(7), 416–419.

Rosén, S., Svensson, M., & Nilsson, U. (2008). Calm or not calm. The question of anxiety in the perianesthesia patient. *Journal of Perianesthesia Nursing*, 23(4), 237–246.

Szopa, T. J. (2005). Nursing implications of surgical treatment. In J. K. Itano & K. N. Taoka (Eds.), *Core curriculum for oncology nursing* (4th ed., pp. 736–747). St. Louis, MO: Elsevier Saunders.

Vujnovich, A. (2008). Pre and post-operative assessment of patients with a stoma. *Nursing Standard*, 22(19), 50–56.

Walker, J. A. (2007). What is the effect of preoperative information on patient satisfaction? *British Journal of Nursing*, 16(1), 27–32.

Weber, R. S., Jabbour, N., & Martin, R. C. (2008). Anemia and transfusions in patients undergoing surgery for cancer. *Annals of Surgical Oncology*, 15(1), 34–45.

Webster, J., & Osbourne, S. (2007). Preoperative bathing or showering with skin antiseptics to prevent surgical site infection. *Cochrane Database of Systematic Reviews*, (2), CD004985.

CHAPTER 31

Ophthalmic Surgery

Susan J. Wolf, MPAS, MMS, PA-C

Most ophthalmic surgical procedures are elective and can be performed under local/monitored anesthesia care (MAC) anesthesia. The surgeon is responsible for making sure the patient understands when surgical intervention is appropriate and indicated, the risks and benefits to a procedure, as well as alternatives to surgery. The patient is responsible for making sure the surgeon understands his or her expectations as to the surgical outcome. It is also the patient's responsibility to ask appropriate questions to make an informed decision whether to proceed with surgery. Patients should never feel coerced but should always feel in control of the decision-making process. Working together, the surgeon and the patient can effectively manage the patient's as well as the surgeon's expectations.

1. How does the eye work?

Light enters the eye by passing through the cornea. It then passes through the pupil, which regulates the amount of light entering the eye by changing its size. The dilator muscle makes the pupil larger, whereas the constrictor muscle makes the pupil smaller. The light then passes through the lens and vitreous to the retina. Sensory receptors called rods and cones are then stimulated. The rods function in dim light whereas the cones function in bright light and detect color. Images that fall on the retina are transmitted to the optic nerve, which relays these sensory impulses to the visual area of the brain located in the occipital lobe. Once in the occipital lobe, these sensory impulses register as visual sensations.

2. What is ophthalmic surgery?

Ophthalmic surgery is any surgical procedure performed on the eye or the surrounding tissue. There are many reasons that ophthalmic surgery is performed; for example, to remove a cataract, replace a damaged cornea, straighten crossed eyes, reduce intraocular pressure, remove an eyelid or eye socket (orbital) cancer or some other mass, repair an orbital fracture, or repair a retinal tear or detachment. The most common purposes of ophthalmic surgery are to restore or improve vision or to enhance a patient's physical appearance.

3. What does a routine eye exam entail?

Visual acuity (VA) measures the resolving power of the eye. Each eye is tested by having the patient read letters of various sizes at a standard distance from a test chart (i.e., Snellen chart). The result is expressed as a fraction. For example, 20/20 is normal vision. This means that a person has the ability to see from a distance of 20 feet what a normal eye would see at that distance. A vision of 20/40 means a person sees at 20 feet what the normal eye would see at 40 feet. Patients with very poor VA may be recorded as having vision of counting fingers (CF), hand movements (HM), light perception (LP), or no light perception (NLP). Near vision can also be recorded in a similar manner by having the patient read a hand-held chart.

The visual field is the area within which objects can be seen with the eye in a fixed position (i.e., staring straight ahead). The extent of the visual field can be assessed in many different ways, including wiggling fingers in various areas, asking the patient to count the number of fingers held up in different areas, and more "formal" testing using a computerized instrument. Amsler grids are hand-held charts used to rapidly detect small central field abnormalities, particularly those due to macular disease. The patient can draw directly on the chart to indicate what he or she sees.

Pupils are examined for size and reactions to both light and near stimuli. The light reaction is produced by having the patient look at a distance, aiming a very bright, focused light toward the eye and noting the speed and extent of constriction of the pupil. The near reaction is induced by having the patient look first at a distant object and then at a letter or number held about 14 inches from the patient's eye. This should also result in constriction of the pupils.

The examination of extraocular movements usually begins with assessment of whether the eyes are correctly aligned. There are many reasons why misalignment of the eyes occurs. The most common patterns of ocular misalignment are esotropia, in which one or both eyes turn inward (i.e., crossed eyes), and exotropia, in which one or both eyes turn outward (i.e., wall eyes). Misalignment of the eyes usually results in double vision (diplopia), a condition in which the patient sees two images of what he or she is seeing. Diplopia may be horizontal, vertical, or oblique.

Examination of the anterior segment is done through a slit-lamp or with a flashlight and magnifying loupes and is used to evaluate the conjunctiva, cornea, sclera, iris, and lens.

Intraocular pressure is measured with a tonometer or Tono-Pen. This test is used to detect glaucoma. Ophthalmoscopy may be performed with or without pupil dilation. This is done to examine the retina (including the macula), retinal vessels, and optic disk (the part of the optic nerve within the eye).

4. What factors does the surgeon need to consider before recommending surgery?

The surgeon must review the clinical history, perform a complete evaluation, perform any ancillary testing, and determine if the surgical procedure will give the patient the desired outcome. In making this determination, the surgeon must consider coexisting eye pathology and concomitant medical conditions; assess and understand the patient's expectations; assess the risk–benefit ratio; discuss alternatives to surgery; and ascertain that the patient understands all of these issues.

5. What is the next step after it is determined that surgery is a viable option?

Once the patient and the surgeon decide that surgery is appropriate, the surgeon must obtain informed consent. Informed consent should include what the procedure involves, available nonsurgical options, an explanation of risks and benefits, a discussion of any alternatives to surgery, and a discussion of the consequences of not undergoing surgery. The surgeon should assess the patient's ability to understand all of this information and must inform the patient of the resident or fellow who will perform all or part of the procedure under his or her supervision.

6. What are the most common potential complications of ophthalmic surgery?

Potential complications include infection, bleeding, pain, scarring, failure to achieve the desired result, decreased vision or complete blindness, double vision, and complications related to the use of local or general anesthesia.

7. Where is ophthalmic surgery performed?

Most eye surgeries are outpatient procedures and can be performed in a surgicenter; however, some major procedures or procedures on infants require hospitalization.

8. What is required preoperatively?

Patients should inform their primary care physician that they are having eye surgery. Each medical facility has its own specific guidelines and requirements, such as a history and physical examination done within 30 days of the surgery; examination by patient's primary care practitioner or facility provider; consent; information (e.g., type of procedure, type of anesthesia, patient age, and concomitant medical problems); and laboratory tests, electrocardiogram, a chest x-ray, and a pregnancy test.

9. Do patients need to stop taking anticoagulants and blood-thinning medications prior to surgery?

The decision to stop anticoagulants or blood-thinners is at the surgeon's discretion. It is often dependant on the medical reason the patient is taking the medication as well as the type of surgery, length of the procedure, and type of anesthesia to be used. The surgeon and patient must weigh the risks and benefits of stopping these medications. Patients should be specifically asked about over-the-counter vitamins, minerals, pain medications, and herbal supplements as many of these substances are associated with an increased risk of bleeding or have an effect on anesthesia.

10. What are general care and instructions for patients who have undergone ophthalmic surgery?

If the patient requires postanesthesia care monitoring, the patient care includes hand-offs from anesthesia provider; vital signs, clinical assessment; and review of record; implement postoperative orders, evaluate patient; and assess readiness for inpatient transfer. Upon transfer or discharge, patients: are instructed to keep the eye patch in place until the surgeon removes it the day after surgery or to use it at night; may resume some of their normal activities the day after surgery; and are given restrictions provided in writing, which may include avoidance of heavy lifting (>10 lbs), bending over from the waist, strenuous activity, and lying on the operative side. Patients may be told to use stool softeners to avoid straining and to wear an eye shield at night. The patient should be made aware that when the patch is removed, the eye may look red or pink.

After surgery, patients may be prescribed eye drops that may include antibiotics, steroids, or nonsteroidal anti-inflammatory medications. Such patients are instructed on the proper method of instilling eye drops in the eye and should show that they understand how to do so. Patients are also told to call the surgeon's office immediately if they experience any problems like flashing lights, new floaters or a shower of floaters, decreased vision, increased pain, increased redness, eye pressure, or any unusual or unexplained symptoms.

11. What is local anesthesia, and how does it work?

Local anesthetic agents depress peripheral nerves and block pain. In ophthalmic surgery, these agents can be delivered topically or intraocularly. Topical anesthetic agents are instilled directly on the surface of the eye and can be administered during the procedure as needed. They have a very quick onset of action, typically 15 to 20 seconds. Once instilled into the eye, the effects usually last 15 to 20 minutes. Indications include adults who are undergoing short procedures involving the conjunctiva, cornea, or lens. It is inappropriate for children and adults with a strong blink reflex, who have difficulty fixating or focusing, and who have a difficult time following commands.

Intraocular anesthesia is usually used in combination with topical anesthesia for patients undergoing intraocular procedures such as cataract surgery. A major advantage of intraocular anesthesia in combination with topical anesthetic agents is that the patient is less aware of pain during intraocular manipulations.

12. How is regional anesthesia used in ophthalmic surgery?

Regional anesthesia for ophthalmic procedures involves injecting anesthetic medication directly into the orbit. This is delivered, most commonly, by injecting medicine into the space behind the eyeball (retrobulbar injection). Regional anesthesia can also be given by peribulbar injection, an injection around but not behind the eye.

Regional anesthesia numbs the cornea, conjunctiva, sclera, and intraocular structures as well as the extraocular muscles. Patients receiving regional anesthesia do not lose consciousness but experience loss of sensation and decreased mobility in the anesthetized area.

13. When and why is general anesthesia used in eye surgery?

In ophthalmology, general or total anesthesia is usually used in pediatric patients, as well as in adults undergoing strabismus (muscle) surgery; long procedures like vitreoretinal and orbital surgery; and complicated oculoplastic procedures such as orbital fracture repairs, tear duct procedures, or enucleation of the eye. General anesthesia can be used in patients who have trouble lying still, are mentally challenged, or who have had prior complications with local or regional anesthesia.

Major ocular complications of general anesthesia are usually related to postoperative nausea and vomiting, because nausea and vomiting increase intraocular pressure that can lead to wound dehiscence or intraocular hemorrhage, leading to loss of vision. Postoperative nausea and vomiting is preventable by certain drugs given during the perioperative phase.

14. What is a cataract, and how is it diagnosed?

A cataract is an opacity of the eye's natural lens, resulting in blurred or decreased vision. Cataracts may be congenital, traumatic, age-related, or due to systemic conditions. Certain medications, such as steroid drops, can also cause cataracts. Cataracts can usually be diagnosed when the eye is examined with a slit-lamp or an ophthalmoscope.

15. What is the goal of cataract surgery, and how is it performed?

The goal of cataract surgery is to remove the lens and replace it with an artificial lens that enables the patient to see normally. The most common procedure to achieve this goal is phacoemulsification surgery, in which a high frequency ultrasonic probe is used to break up the nucleus of the lens while simultaneously aspirating the nuclear fragments. The cortical material is removed by irrigation and aspiration. The posterior lining (capsule) of the lens is left in place. An intraocular lens (IOL) is then inserted into the eye. The use of a foldable, injectable intraocular lens implant allows a small incision that may not require any sutures to close it. After the procedure, a topical antibiotic is instilled in the eye and a patch (and sometimes an eye shield) is placed over the eye to protect it.

16. What are some of the possible complications of cataract surgery?

In approximately 20% to 50% of patients, the posterior capsule of the lens that is left in the eye during removal of the cataract becomes cloudy. This leads to hazy vision and can happen 6 months to several years after surgery. Patients in whom this occurs report their vision is not as sharp or clear as it was initially after the procedure. If this occurs, the surgeon can use a laser to make a hole in the capsule. This is often done the same day that the problem is noted and can usually be done in the surgeon's office.

Other potential complications of cataract surgery, while extremely rare, include infection, wound leak, retained lens fragments, loss of vitreous, retinal tear or detachment, displacement of the IOL, irregularly shaped pupil, corneal swelling, elevated intraocular pressure, and chronic inflammation.

17. What is glaucoma, and how is it diagnosed?

Glaucoma is a disorder in which fluid (aqueous humor) inside the eye builds up and causes an elevation of intraocular pressure (IOP) that damages the optic nerve. This, in turn, causes progressive, painless loss of peripheral vision and, eventually, complete blindness if the IOP is not lowered to normal. Glaucoma is diagnosed by measuring IOP, examining the optic discs, and performing a visual field test.

18. How is glaucoma treated?

Glaucoma may be treated with medications to lower the eye pressure or with various types of surgery. The three types of drugs most commonly prescribed for treatment of glaucoma are alpha agonists, beta-blockers, and carbonic anhydrase inhibitors. In most cases, the drugs are delivered topically; however, when they are given orally, electrolytes must be monitored.

19. What is the goal of glaucoma surgery, and how is it performed?

The goal of glaucoma surgery is to reduce the IOP so that further damage to the optic nerve does not occur and the patient does not go blind. Surgery usually is performed if medical treatment is not tolerated by the patient or is not lowering IOP to an appropriate level. The type of surgery that is performed depends on many factors but, in general, provides an outflow pathway for the fluid that has built up inside the eye. A laser can be used in some cases; in others, a surgical opening is made. In still others, a plastic tube is used to assist in fluid drainage. Most glaucoma surgery is performed under local/MAC anesthesia. Postoperatively, patients rest comfortably for about 1 hour, VA are taken, and, when ready, discharge instructions are provided.

20. What are potential complications of glaucoma surgery?

As with all surgical procedures, infection and bleeding may occur. In addition, the procedures may fail to lower the IOP or may lower it too much (hypotony).

21. What is the function of the cornea?

The cornea is a clear, protective tissue through which light enters the eye. Because it is free of blood vessels, it can be replaced with a transplant if it becomes diseased, swollen, or cloudy, which causes the patient to lose vision.

22. What are the diseases, problems, and symptoms that may indicate that a corneal transplant (also called a penetrating keratoplasty) is needed?

The cornea may be damaged by congenital as well as acquired disorders. Congenital cloudiness of the cornea may be due to trauma or may be a hereditary disorder that is present at birth. This condition needs to be corrected as soon as possible so that the child's vision can develop normally.

Corneal dystrophies are also inherited conditions that affect vision. These are most often bilateral and can involve the different layers of the cornea. Fuchs' dystrophy is the most common corneal dystrophy. It affects the endothelium of the cornea, resulting in corneal edema that causes a distortion or cloudiness in vision. If the visual loss is sufficiently severe, a corneal transplant may be indicated.

Corneal infections or injuries produce pain, tearing, redness, and blurred vision. If the infection is treated promptly, the cornea usually heals and normal vision is regained; however, in some cases, scarring or ulceration lead to permanent distortion or loss of vision, necessitating a corneal transplant.

Blunt trauma, severe nonhealing abrasions, lacerations, and chemical burns can also damage the cornea, leading to permanent loss of vision unless a corneal transplant is performed.

Keratoconus, a disease that causes the cornea to become cone-like or pointed, can also be an indication for corneal transplant. If the keratoconus becomes so severe that the cornea is stretched too much, it may cause tearing, pain, and erythema. In such cases, a corneal transplant may be performed.

The diagnosis of corneal disease can be made using a slit-lamp.

23. What is the goal of corneal transplant surgery, and how is it performed?

The goal of corneal transplant surgery is to replace the damaged cornea with a clear cornea so that the patient can see normally. Donor tissue is received from a tissue bank, and the surgeon examines it to determine if it is healthy enough to be transplanted.

The transplant itself requires removal of the center portion of the patient's damaged cornea. The donor graft is then sutured into place and the eye is patched.

24. What are possible complications of corneal transplant surgeries?

Unlike most surgical procedures, there is little or no risk of bleeding because the cornea has no blood vessels in it; however, infection, wound leak, increased IOP, and graft rejection may all occur.

25. What are the symptoms of a retinal tear or retinal detachment, and how are these diagnosed?

The symptoms of a retinal tear or detachment are the sudden occurrence of floaters, flashes of light, loss of a portion of the visual field, or a combination of these symptoms. Floaters are little black dots that cross through the field of vision. They float in the fluid of the eye (vitreous humor). Floaters are not uncommon and may occur spontaneously or from trauma, coughing or sneezing, straining to have a bowel movement, vomiting, or lifting heavy objects. Some floaters look like worms or amoebae. They tend to move when the eye moves. Flashes of light are usually visualized in a dark room but may also be seen in lit rooms or in daylight. These flashes are often described as resembling lightening, sudden star bursts of light, squiggles of light, or crescent-shaped lines of light. Even though floaters and flashes of light are common and often harmless, these symptoms should

be investigated if they are persistent, become larger, increase in number, or if the patient sees a sudden "shower" of floaters. Patients should also see an ophthalmologist immediately if they see a veil or curtain descending over the eye.

Retinal detachments are diagnosed with a slit-lamp and a hand-held, or contact lens, or a special type of ophthalmoscope that allows a three-dimensional view of the entire retina. In most cases, it is necessary to dilate the pupil in order to see enough of the retina to diagnose a retinal tear or detachment.

26. What is the goal of retinal reattachment surgery, and how is it performed?

The goal of retinal reattachment surgery is to restore the normal anatomy and function of the retina so that the patient's vision is stabilized or improved. Most retinal detachments occur because a tear or hole develops and vitreous fluid accumulates underneath the retina. A retinal detachment can be treated in many different ways, depending on its location, extent, and whether or not the patient has had previous ocular surgery (particularly cataract surgery). If diagnosed early, a small tear can often be treated by photocoagulation with a laser or cryotherapy (freezing). This causes an inflammatory reaction that helps the retina reattach. For large detachments, vitreous can be removed and gas can be injected, forming a bubble that holds the retina in the correct position while healing occurs. Silicone oil can also be injected into the eye to hold a detached retina in place. It is heavy and viscous and stays in place. Unlike gas that gradually resorbs, silicone oil is a foreign substance that does not dissipate over time and eventually needs to be surgically removed.

A scleral buckle can be used to treat certain types of retinal detachments. Once the hole or detachment is localized, the buckle is placed around the eye like a belt. This helps raise the tissue beneath the hole, which then allows fluid to drain away from under the retina. The retina then falls back into place. In some cases, a laser is used to help seal or tack the retina into place; in other cases, a hole is made in the eye underneath the detached retina so that the fluid can drain out. As this occurs, the retina flattens. A laser or cryoprobe is then used to produce an inflammatory reaction around the retinal tear or hole and a buckle may be placed.

If the vitreous is filled with blood or the vitreous, which is normally attached to the retina, is causing the detachment (traction detachment), a vitrectomy (removal of the vitreous) may be needed before the detachment is treated.

27. What are the potential complications of retinal reattachment surgery?

Potential complications of retinal reattachment surgery are failure to reattach the retina, bleeding, infection, increased intraocular pressure, production of new retinal tears, double vision, and loss of vision.

28. What specific instruction should the patient know before discharge?

If a gas bubble has been injected into the eye, patients are instructed to hold the head parallel to the ground as much as possible for an extended period of time (16 or more hours per day) determined by the surgeon. Holding the head parallel to the ground keeps the gas bubble centered over the area of the previous retinal detachment, thus holding the retina in place. The patient must even sleep with the head facing down.

If silicone oil is used, patients will have to have it surgically removed months after surgery. The length of time the oil stays in the eye is determined by the surgeon. Patients are given topical antibiotics and steroids postoperatively. If a scleral buckle has been used, pain medicine may also be prescribed. Patient must call the surgeon immediately for flashes of light, increased pain, persistent redness, or increased floaters.

29. What are the causes of eye muscle problems, and when is surgery needed to correct ocular misalignment?

The brain controls the six muscles around each eye, and it requires a great deal of work to have the eyes move in unison. Misalignment of the eyes due to an imbalance in the muscles is called strabismus.

The causes of misalignment of the eyes are numerous and include congenital and acquired muscle damage, nerve damage, and damage to the connections between the muscles and the motor nerves that control them. Patients with acquired strabismus usually complain of double vision (diplopia). Children with congenital strabismus usually develop amblyopia (lazy eye) and do not have diplopia.

Surgery is performed to restore binocular vision, improve cosmesis, or both.

30. What options are available prior to surgery to correct ocular misalignment, and, when needed, how is eye muscle surgery performed?

In some cases, successful treatment of the underlying condition (e.g., brain tumor, myasthenia gravis, hyperthyroidism) results in realignment of the eyes. In other cases, however, including congenital and infantile strabismus, surgery is required to straighten the eyes. Unlike cataract, glaucoma, and cornea surgeries, which are all intraocular procedures, eye muscle surgeries are extraocular procedures. Therefore, the risk of vision-threatening complications is much less.

Surgical correction of eye muscles can involve one or both eyes and can be performed on infants, children, and adults. Depending on the eye problems, muscles may be weakened (recessed or set back) or strengthened (resected or tightened). In many cases, a weakening procedure is performed on one muscle and a strengthening procedure on another. The weakening procedure is performed by attaching a suture to the muscle, taking the muscle off the eye, and putting the muscle back on the eye but further back than previously. The strengthening procedure is performed by attaching a suture to the muscle, removing the muscle from the eye, cutting a piece of the muscle away, and then reattaching the muscle to the eye. The principle is to weaken an overactive muscle and/or to strengthen an underactive muscle. Patients should be aware that correction often requires more than one surgery.

Eye muscle surgery can be quite uncomfortable due to manipulation of the eye during surgery and, therefore, is often done under general anesthesia. Manipulation of the muscles during surgery can produce significant bradycardia. The surgeon usually alerts the anesthesiologist before manipulating the muscles.

Children or adults may have adjustable suture muscle surgery to decrease the need for subsequent procedures. In this procedure, the muscle is put where the surgeon wants it, but the final knot is not tied and the muscle is held in place with a slip-knot. After the patient has recovered or awakened from general anesthesia, the surgeon evaluates the patient. The patient needs to be awake enough to follow instructions from the surgeon, including looking straight ahead and following an object by moving only the eyes. The surgeon can then decide if any further adjustment to the muscle is needed. Using anesthetic eye drops, the surgeon can adjust the eye muscle by loosening the slip-knot and either pulling the muscle forward or putting it back further. Once satisfied, the surgeon ties the suture permanently. The suture stays attached to the muscle for months, allowing the muscle to heal in the correct position. This adjustment is usually done within several hours postoperatively.

31. What are potential complications of eye muscle surgery, and what should a patient know prior to discharge?

Potential complications of eye muscle surgery include overcorrection or undercorrection resulting in persistent ocular misalignment and diplopia, torn muscles, scleral perforation, bleeding, and infection.

As a rule, the eyes are not bandaged postoperatively. The patient should be made aware that the eyes may look pink or red. The eyes may have blood around them and the patient may have bloody tears. The most common complaint after eye muscle surgery is headache.

32. What is ptosis and what are the common causes?

Ptosis is drooping of the eyelid. It may be unilateral or bilateral. Causes include a weakness in either the levator muscle or Müller's muscle, the two muscles responsible for raising the eyelid, dysfunction of the nerves that innervate these muscles, and problems with the connection between the nerves and the muscles (neuromuscular disease). Ptosis can also be caused by excess skin.

Ptosis may be congenital or acquired. Acquired causes include aging, causing stretching of the levator muscle tendon (levator dehiscence); third nerve palsy from stroke, tumor, or trauma; Horner syndrome; and myasthenia gravis.

Patients with ptosis may complain that their eyelids droop, making them look drowsy, that their eyebrows ache, or that they cannot see normally.

33. What are the goals of ptosis surgery, and how is it performed?

The goals of ptosis surgery are to raise the eyelids to improve vision, improve the patient's appearance, or both; however, before surgery is performed, it is first necessary to determine the cause of the ptosis. Special tests may be needed to evaluate suspected causes like myasthenia gravis or a third nerve palsy.

In patients with levator dehiscence, an incision is made along the natural crease of the upper eyelid. The incision is carried down through the orbicularis oculi muscle until the levator tendon is exposed. The tendon is then tightened. When weakness of Müller's muscle is the cause of ptosis, the eyelid is everted, and a portion of the muscle is removed, thus shortening the muscle and elevating the eyelid. In severe cases, particularly those in which the eyelid does not elevate at all, the upper lid may be attached to the brows so that forehead muscles actually do the lifting. This may be done using tissue or synthetic suture material. This is known as a frontalis sling or suspension procedure.

34. What are potential complications of ptosis surgery and specific care?

Potential complications of ptosis surgery are failure to achieve the desired elevation of the lid, infection, bleeding, and reduced vision. The patient may have a temporary inability to fully close the eye, in which case, a lubricating eye drop or ointment may be used to protect the cornea from becoming too dry. Specific care includes the use of an ice pack; prescribed antibiotic ointment; and no makeup, sunbathing, or direct exposure.

BIBLIOGRAPHY

Abel, R. Jr. (2004). The eye care revolution. New York: Kensington Publishing Company.

Albert, D. M., & Lucarelli, M. J. (2004). *Clinical atlas of procedures in ophthalmic surgery*. Atlanta: American Medical Association Press.

Albert, D. M., & Miller, J. W. (2008). *Albert and Jakobiec's principles and practice of ophthalmology*. Philadelphia: Saunders/Elsevier, Inc.

American Society of Ophthalmic Registered Nurses. (2003). *Ophthalmic procedures in the operating room and ambulatory surgery center*. Dubuque, IA: Kendall Hunt Publishing.

Ansons, A. M., & Davis, H. (2002). Diagnosis and management of ocular motility disorders. Malden, MA: Blackwell Science Ltd.

Arnold, A. (Ed.). (2006). Basic principles of ophthalmic surgery. San Francisco: American Academy of Ophthalmology.

Buckley, E. G., Plager, D. A., Repka, M. X., & Wilson, M. E. (2004). Strabismus surgery basic and advanced strategies. Oxford: Butterworth Heinemann Elsevier.

Foster, C. S., Azar, D. T., & Dohlman, C. H. (Eds.). (2004). *Smolin and Thoft's The cornea: Scientific foundations and clinical practice*. Baltimore: Lippincott Williams and Wilkins.

Garg, A., Fry, L. L., Tabia, G., Gutierrez-Carmona, F. J., & Pandey, S. K. (Eds.). (2004). *Phaco manual clinical practice in small incision cataract surgery*. New York: Taylor & Francis Group.

Garg, A. & Rosen, E. (2009). *Instant clinical diagnosis in ophthalmology: Oculoplasty and reconstructive surgery*. New York: McGraw Hill Medical.

Garrity, J. A., Henderson, J. W., & Cameron, J. D. (2007). *Henderson's orbital tumors* (4th ed.). Philadelphia: Lippincott Williams and Wilkins.

Higginbotham, E. J., & Lee, D. A. (2002). *Clinical guide to glaucoma management*. Woburn, MA: Butterworth Heinemann.

Kidd, D. P., Newman, N. J., & Biousse, V. (Eds.). (2008). *Neuro-ophthalmology: Blue books of neurology*. Philadelphia: Butterworth Heinemann Elsevier.

Kitchen, C. K. (2007). *Fact and fiction of healthy vision: Eye care for adults and children*. Westport, CT: Praeger Publishers.

Levine, M. R. (2003). *Manual of oculoplastic surgery*. Philadelphia: Butterworth Heinemann Elsevier.

MacEwen, C., & Gregson, R. (2003). *Manual of strabismus surgery*. Oxford: Butterworth Heinemann.

Miller, N. R., Newman, N. J., Biousse, V., & Kerrison, J. B. (2008). *Walsh & Hoyt's clinical neuro-ophthalmology: The essentials* (2nd ed.). Baltimore: Lippincott-Williams & Wilkins.

Palay, D. A., & Krachmer, J. H. (2006). *Primary care ophthalmology*. Philadelphia: Elsevier Mosby.

Riordan-Eva, P., & Whitcher, J. P. (2004). *Vaughn and Asbury's general ophthalmology*. New York: Lange Medical Books/McGraw Hill Medical Publishing Division.

Roy, F. H., & Arzabe, C. W. (Eds.). (2004). *Master techniques in cataract and refractive surgery*. Thorofare, NJ: Slack Incorporated.

Schachat, A. P. (2001). Retina. (pp.). In S. J. Ryan, D. R. Hinton, A. P. Schachat, & C. P. Wilkinson (Eds.), *Medical retina* (Volume 2, 3rd ed. pp. 875–1847). Philadelphia: Mosby.

Spaeth, G. (Ed). (2002). *Ophthalmic surgery: Principles and practice* (3rd ed.). Philadelphia: WB Saunders.

Spoor, T. C. (2009). *Atlas of neuro-ophthalmology*. New York: Taylor & Francis Group.

Stamper, R. L., Lieberman, M. F., & Drake, M. V. (2009). *Becker-Shaffer's diagnosis and therapy of the glaucomas*. Philadelphia: Mosby Elsevier.

Timby, B. K., & Smith, N. E. (2007). *Introductory medical-surgical nursing*. Philadelphia: Lippincott Williams and Wilkins.

Tsai, L. M., & Kamenetzky, S. A. (2006). The eye & ocular adnexa (pp. 976–992). In G. M. Doherty & L. W. Way (Eds.), *Current surgical diagnosis and treatment*. New York: Lange Medical Books/McGraw Hill.

Wilkinson, C. P. (2001). Retina (pp.). In S. J. Ryan, D. R. Hinton, A. P. Schachat, & C. P. Wilkinson (Eds.), *Surgical retina* (Volume 3, 3rd ed. pp. 1849–2601). Philadelphia: Mosby.

CHAPTER 32

Orthopedic Surgery

Susan Kulik, MSN, MBA, RN, ONC

INTRODUCTION

Orthopedic nursing is both an art and a science and therefore requires the nurse to have a comprehensive skill base as well as compassion for nursing practice. Orthopedic nursing practice involves both the prevention and care of musculoskeletal disorders. This chapter will help you provide care to orthopedic patients with varying diagnoses and help you to identify orthopedic emergencies.

1. What are the primary risk factors for complications associated with orthopedic injuries and procedures?

- Increased age
- Comorbidity (e.g., respiratory conditions, diabetes, immunosuppression, obesity, malnourishment)
- Drugs (e.g., warfarin, corticosteroids, NSAIDs, opioids, estrogen therapy)

2. What are the precipitating factors for acute confusion in the orthopedic patient?

Precipitating factors include low body temperature, acute metabolic imbalance, fluid and electrolyte imbalance, pain, hypoxia, infection, overmedication, and malnutrition.

3. What are the risk factors for pressure ulcer development?

Risk factors include impaired mobility/prolonged mobility, increased age, moisture/incontinence, depression, dehydration, altered tissue perfusion, hypotension, edema, altered level of consciousness, altered sensory perception, and length of surgical procedure.

4. Why is the orthopedic patient at a higher risk for pressure ulcer?

The orthopedic patient is at a higher risk for a pressure ulcer due to imposed mobility restrictions.

5. What are the complications of pressure ulcer?

Complications include osteomyelitis, septicemia, significant tissue necrosis requiring surgical intervention, development of scar tissue, need for amputation, body image disturbance, and increased length of stay.

6. Why is the orthopedic patient at risk for constipation?

Immobility decreases colonic activity and may lead to atrophy of the primary muscles of defecation.

7. What is the potential complication for the scenario below?

Mrs. Smith is a 58-year-old postoperative day 3 total knee replacement. She complains that she is bloated, has no appetite, and has a headache. You observe that she is passing flatus. Which of the following complications is most likely?

Bowel obstruction	Paralytic ileus
Constipation	Gastrointestinal (GI) bleed

8. What orthopedic procedures place the patient at a higher risk of hemorrhage?

Orthopedic procedures that place the patient at a higher risk of hemorrhage include revision arthroplasty, multilevel anterior/posterior spine procedures, and multitrauma.

9. Identify orthopedic procedures that place patients at a higher risk for developing pulmonary embolism.

Procedures involving the pelvis, hip, spine, or lower extremity place patients at a higher risk for developing pulmonary embolism.

10. What are the characteristic symptoms of pulmonary edema?

Characteristic symptoms include dyspnea, pleuritic chest pain, and hemoptysis.

11. What are risk factors for fat embolism?

- Fracture of a long bone
- Intramedullary nailing
- Multiple trauma
- Delayed open reduction internal fixation

12. What is fat embolism syndrome (FES) and what are its causes?

FES is the mobilization of fat and free fatty acids that lead to acute pulmonary insufficiency. This can be caused by fat from the marrow of broken bones embolized to the lung, which then occlude small pulmonary vessels. It can also be caused by stress response, which can lead to the release of catecholamines free fatty acids and mobilize in the lung and increase capillary permeability within the alveoli.

13. What are signs and symptoms of FES?

Signs and symptoms may occur in 12 to 48 hours after the event and may rapidly progress. They include confusion, agitation, anxiety, tachypnea, dyspnea, hypoxemia, tachycardia, hypotension, pyrexia, and petechiae.

14. What are the fat embolism prevention strategies in long bone fractures?

Prevention strategies include early splinting and immobilization.

15. What are the early symptoms of a tight cast, splint, or dressing?

Early symptoms include increased pain, increased swelling, numbness, and paresthesia.

16. What is the hallmark symptom of compartment syndrome?

The hallmark symptom includes severe pain that does not go away when you take pain medicine or raise the affected area.

17. What are the five "Ps" associated with compartment syndrome?

- Pain out of proportion to what is expected
- Paresthesia
- Pallor
- Paralysis
- Pulselessness

18. What is the first thing you want to do when you suspect acute compartment syndrome?

Relieve the sources of pressure such as with a bivalve cast, removing splint, removing or loosening a constrictive bandage, or releasing or decreasing traction.

19. What are the potential complications associated with clavicular fractures?

Potential complications include subclavian or carotid artery injury, pneumothorax injury, subclavian vein injury, nonunion, and malunion.

20. What is the most frequently dislocated joint in the human body?

The most frequently dislocated joint in the human body is the shoulder joint.

21. How does the dislocation of the shoulder joint occur?

Dislocation occurs either by a direct or indirectly blow due to force from a fall on the outstretched arm.

22. What are the complications of a severe thoracic scoliosis?

Pulmonary and cardiac function may be affected due to thoracic hypokyphosis decreasing the space between the vertebral bodies and the sternum.

23. What are the common conservative and surgical treatment options for scoliosis?

Curves less than 15°–20° are observed for progression. Curves between 20° and 40° in the growing child may require a brace. Bracing is ineffective in the mature patient. Surgery is recommended for curves greater than 40°.

24. Following spinal surgery, what will the nurse monitor that indicates signs and symptoms of a neurologic deficit?

- Muscle strength in both lower and upper extremities

- Sensation in upper and lower extremities and torso
- Complaints of numbness and tingling and increased radiating pain
- Urinary incontinence, inability to void, loss of rectal tone

25. What is a complication of spinal stenosis that is considered a medical emergency?

Cauda equina syndrome occurs when the nerve roots are compressed and paralyzed, cutting off sensation and movement. Nerve roots that control the function of the bladder and bowel are especially vulnerable to damage.

26. What are the key components of treatment after a pelvic fracture?

Key components include management of hemorrhage and hemodynamic instability.

27. What are the common causes of pelvic fractures?

Common causes include motor vehicle accidents, motorcycle accidents, falls from great heights, and crush injuries.

28. What diagnosis would you suspect of adolescents or young adults who present with anterior groin pain and pain with hip rotation?

The diagnosis would likely be femoroacetabular impingement (FAI). Recognition of FAI with early intervention before the degenerative process has begun may possibly delay the onset of osteoarthritis.

29. What is the current treatment of FAI?

The current treatment includes open surgical dislocation and hip arthroscopy to improve the clearance of hip motion and alleviate the FAI.

30. What are total joint precautions for anterior total hips?

Total joint precautions include no active abduction, no outward extension of the affected extremity, and no backward extension of the surgical leg (no crossing of the leg).

31. What are total joint precautions for posterior total hips?

Precautions include no bending of the affected hip beyond a 90° angle, no crossing of the legs, and no inward rotation of the toes on the affected extremity.

32. What are the indications for shoulder arthroplasty?

Indications include when pain and dysfunction result from structural damage to the glenohumeral articulating surface and the patient has failed conservative treatments.

33. What is the postoperative nursing care requirement of a shoulder patient with a sling?

A postoperative shoulder arthroplasty patient will arrive in the recovery area with a sling. The nursing care of a shoulder patient with a sling is to ensure that the sling holds the arm close to the body with no strain on the surgical site and provides adequate support for the arm.

34. What are postoperative nursing care requirements of the patient with traction?

- Maintain traction apparatus to ensure proper alignment of the body
- Assess skin integrity
- Assess for neurovascular compromise
- Assess for complications related to skeletal pain

35. What are postoperative discharge instructions would you give for patients with assistive device?

- With crutches, use the unaffected leg to go up the step first and use the affected leg to go down the step.
- In walking, lead with the strong, unaffected leg.
- Avoid rugs, electric cords, wet floors, or any obstruction on the way.
- Use sturdy and nonskid shoes.
- Take small steps and stand erect.

BIBLIOGRAPHY

Bidden, J. (2009). Treatment options in the hemodynamically unstable patient with a pelvic fracture. *Orthopaedic Nursing, 29*(3), 109–114.

Brown, F. (2008). Nursing care after a shoulder arthroplasty. *Orthopaedic Nursing, 27*(1), 3–9.

DeFazio Quinn, D., & Schick, L. (2004). *Perianesthesia nursing core curriculum.* St. Louis, MO: American Society of PeriAnesthesia Nurses.

Hart, E., Metkar, U., Rebello, G., & Grottkau, B. (2009). Femoroacetabular impingement in adolescents and young adults. *Orthopaedic Nursing, 28*(3), 117–124.

Maher, A., Salmond, S., & Pellino, T. (2002). *Orthopaedic nursing.* St. Louis, MO: Mosby.

Schoen, D. (2001). *Core curriculum for orthopaedic nursing* (4th ed.). Pitman, NJ: National Association of Orthopaedic Nurses.

CHAPTER 33

Thoracic Surgery

Peggy Lang, RN, MSN, ACNP and Stephen C. Yang, MD

INTRODUCTION

Thoracic surgery can be generalized to include any surgical procedures within the chest. Surgeons completing a cardiothoracic surgical fellowship often specialize in either adult cardiac or general thoracic surgery, but there can be overlap. This chapter will not discuss cardiac procedures but will limit itself to procedures of the lung, esophagus, chest wall, pleura, and mediastinum.

THE LUNG

1. Why are lung resections performed?

Most lung resections are performed because there is a concern, proven or not, for cancer. If a nodule or mass (nodule > 3cm) is biopsy-proven cancer, and the only site of disease, it should be resected to provide the best possibility of cure. Many times a lung nodule has not been biopsied or a biopsy is nondiagnostic, but the possibility for cancer is still high enough to warrant surgery. Many tests ordered before surgery are done to evaluate if the cancer is localized to just the lung or if it has it spread to lymph nodes or other organs. The goal of surgery is to remove everything known or thought to be cancer. If cancer has spread outside the lung, surgery will not provide the patient with a benefit, except in certain circumstances.

2. What is wedge resection?

Wedge resection is the removal of a small portion of the lung while leaving the hilar lymphatics and blood vessels intact. If a cancer originated from another organ and metastasized to the lung, it spread there through the bloodstream. Removing the nodule alone, without lymphatic and blood vessel resection, may provide an oncologic benefit. If the etiology of the nodule is unknown and the location of the nodule will permit, a video-assisted thoracic surgery (VATS) resection of the nodule will be performed followed by a frozen biopsy in the operating room (OR). If cancer is not found in the frozen specimen, no further resection is required. This surgery may also be performed in a patient with poor pulmonary function that could not tolerate a larger resection.

3. What is lobectomy?

Lobectomy is the removal of one lobe of the lung along with its arteries, veins, and lymphatics. If a biopsy proves primary lung cancer, meaning the cancer originates from lung tissue, or a nodule is suspicious for lung cancer based on appearance and risk factors, then the proper cancer operation providing the highest possibility of cure is to perform an anatomic lobectomy. This means removing the entire section of lung parenchyma separated from other lung parenchyma by anatomic borders, thus including the lymphatic and vascular drainage systems, which may have microscopic spread.

4. What is segmentectomy?

Segmentectomy is the removal of a segment or smaller section within a lobe of the lung along with its arteries, veins, and lymphatics. A segmentectomy is typically reserved for patients with marginal or poor pulmonary function who cannot tolerate a full lobectomy.

5. What is bilobectomy?

Bilobectomy is the removal of two lobes of the lung. If a mass crosses the fissure extending into another lobe, the second lobe is often removed (a bilobectomy). If a portion of the other lobe involving direct extension can be removed, such as a segment alone, that is preferable. If the nodule or mass is located at or near the carina of two lobes (i.e., the "Y" branching of the airways), it may be necessary to remove both lobes to attain negative margins. Typically, this is in the right upper lobe and right middle lobe or the right middle lobe and right lower lobe.

6. What is sleeve resection?

Sleeve resection is the removal of a circumferential portion of the trachea or mainstem bronchus. When a nodule, typically benign, is located only within the airway, removing parenchyma is not necessary. Resection of the airway alone can be performed.

7. What is sleeve lobectomy resection?

Sleeve lobectomy resection is the removal of one lobe of the lung (most commonly the right upper lobe or left upper lobe) and a sleeve portion of the main bronchus, and then reconnecting the remaining bronchus. There are times that the nodule or mass involves the lobar bronchus and a simple lobectomy cannot be done. A sleeve of the main bronchus needs to be resected. The lower lobe bronchus is reconnected to the main stem bronchus, thus preserving the lower lobe and saving lung parenchyma and lung function.

8. What is pneumonectomy?

Pneumonectomy is the removal of the entire lung. If a nodule or mass is located near the hilum, removing the entire lung may be necessary in order to attain negative margins. However, there must be sufficient cardiopulmonary reserve due to associated high surgical morbidity and mortality.

9. What is lung biopsy?

Lung biopsy is the surgical removal of a small portion of the lung parenchyma while leaving the lymph and blood vessels intact (similar to a wedge resection but typically smaller and multiple areas). Lung biopsies are performed at the request of a patient's pulmonologist. Specific respiratory diseases respond differently to medical management based on their pathologic characteristics. Taking a sample of lung tissue for diagnostic purposes can be performed by VATS or an open small thoracotomy. An open biopsy can be performed more quickly and is typically chosen when a patient's respiratory status is more tenuous, but exposure and sampling ability is limited compared to VATS.

10. What is a bronchoscopy, and why is it performed?

It is the insertion of a lighted scope into the bronchial tree for visualization and procedures; therefore, indications are both diagnostic and therapeutic. Flexible bronchoscopy can be performed in the operating room or at the bedside, whereas rigid bronchoscopy is only performed in the operating room under general anesthesia.

Bronchoscopy is often used by our pulmonary colleagues in the assessment and diagnosis of pulmonary nodules and respiratory disorders, and it is also a critical tool for thoracic surgeons. A flexible bronchoscopy should be performed by the operating surgeon before any lung resection to visualize the airways to verify operative intent, suction secretions, and rule out anatomic anomalies. Postoperatively, it should be used liberally for patients with difficulty clearing secretions or radiographic evidence of atelectasis. Rigid bronchoscopy is used for patients with aspirated foreign bodies, proximal airway obstruction, compression, or life-threatening hemoptysis. A combination of both types of bronchoscopies can be used to perform direct debridement, laser ablation, photodynamic therapy, brachytherapy, and stent placement (Sonnett, 2004).

THE ESOPHAGUS

11. What is an esophagectomy?

It is the removal of the thoracic esophagus and a portion of the stomach, along with local and regional lymph nodes while providing gastric continuity with either the stomach or colon.

The most common indication for removing the esophagus is for cancer. Other reasons for esophagectomy include achalasia, strictures, and perforation. Midesophageal tumors are more likely to be squamous cell carcinomas while lower esophageal and gastroesophageal junction tumors are most likely adenocarcinomas. Removing the esophagus and ensuring wide surgical margins (5–10 cms) provides for the best chance of cure. The stomach is modified and brought into the chest to function as a conduit, thus the nickname "gastric pull-up."

12. What are the different types of esophagectomy, and why is one chosen over the other?

The surgical approach varies but the most frequent include Ivor-Lewis (abdominal–right thoracotomy), three-incision or McKeown procedure (right thoracotomy-abdominal-cervical), or transhiatal (abdominal–cervical).

The approach depends on the tumor location, patient characteristics, and the surgeon's preference. The transhiatal approach avoids a thoracotomy, minimizes respiratory complications, and allows easy management of anastomotic complications. However, it does not allow visualization of the upper esophagus and does limit nodal dissection. The transthoracic approaches, on the other hand, allow for better visualization of the entire esophagus but includes the increased morbidity of anastomotic leak when an intrathoracic occurs, and the cardiopulmonary insult of a thoracotomy. Studies have not shown an advantage in morbidity, mortality, or long-term survival outcomes from one approach over another. When the use of the stomach is not an option, a section of colon or jejunum can be used to achieve gastric continuity but the risks with either of these surgeries are much higher (Reed, 2004).

13. What is an esophagoscopy?

It is the insertion of a lighted scope into the esophagus for visualization and performing procedures. Although performed most frequently by the gastroenterologist, this diagnostic and therapeutic modality is often utilized by thoracic surgeons. Esophagoscopy can be used to evaluate esophageal symptoms, pathology, and radiographic abnormalities. A flexible endoscope should also be used prior to any esophageal surgical procedure to verify pathologic findings and to evaluate response to preoperative therapy. It is often useful to leave the endoscope in the esophagus during the procedure to help locate lesions and to avoid penetration of the mucosal layer.

Therapeutic indications include the dilation of strictures, treatment of esophageal varices, removal of foreign bodies, and palliation of malignant obstruction using stents or laser therapy.

14. What is involved in the repair of an esophageal perforation?

Management of esophageal perforation (Boerhaave's syndrome) is a daunting challenge because the diagnosis carries a 25% chance of mortality. The consequences of perforation are related to extravasation of oral and gastric secretions into the mediastinum, which leads to septic shock. The infection can result in mediastinitis, empyema, or peritonitis depending on the location of the perforation. The symptoms at presentation depend on the location, extent, and duration of the injury. A small, contained perforation noted shortly after endoscopy is very different than a patient with Boerhaave's syndrome presenting to the emergency department as unresponsive. A barium swallow study and/or computerized tomography (CT) scan will help to diagnosis. A contained leak may be treated conservatively with "watchful waiting" while the patient is n.p.o. (nothing by mouth), given broad-spectrum antibiotics, and parenteral nutrition.

Primary esophageal repair should be considered if diagnosed within 24 to 48 hours of injury except in the setting of cancer or achalasia where resection would be preferred.

In cases of delayed diagnosis (over 48 hours), significant tissue necrosis and septic shock makes failure of the repair more likely. Operative drainage and irrigation of any contaminated spaces and creating a diverting esophagostomy to prevent further soilage should be utilized (Murthy & Rice, 2004).

15. What is an esophagostomy?

The cervical esophagus, above the perforation, is pulled out to the skin surface and opened into an ostomy to drain saliva. These are sometimes called a "spit fistula." Another operation is required to reverse the esophagostomy at a later date, but this can be performed after the leak has healed and the patient is stable.

THE MEDIASTINUM

16. What is a mediastinoscopy?

It is the insertion of a scope into the mediastinum. A 1 to 2 cm incision is made above the suprasternal notch and manual dissection is carried down to the pretracheal space. A mediastinoscope is advanced into this created tunnel for inspection and for taking biopsies.

Mediastinoscopy is used most commonly for lung cancer staging, and it is also useful for diagnosing granulomatous, infectious, and miscellaneous causes of lymphadenopathy. Lymph nodes accessed via mediastinoscopy (station 2, 4, and 7) positive for carcinoma will stage a patient with N2 disease, which is considered too advanced for positive outcomes from surgery. Often, a mediastinoscopy will be scheduled as the first part of a larger pulmonary resection, and, if nodes are found positive for cancer, the pulmonary resection will be aborted.

17. What is an anterior mediastinotomy (Chamberlain procedure)?

It is a parasternal incision that allows direct visualization of the mediastinum for lymph node or mediastinal mass biopsy. Mediastinotomy allows access to para-aortic and anterior mediastinal nodes on the left (station 5 and 6) and to anterior mediastinal masses for the purpose of biopsy. Some of these procedures are now performed by VATS.

18. What is a median sternotomy?

It is an incision from the suprasternal notch to below the xiphoid process. The sternum is divided with a saw and with the use of a sternal retractor, which allows access to the mediastinum. Closure of the sternum requires stainless steel wires.

Median sternotomy is used for a variety of procedures such as anterior mediastinal mass tumor resection (thymomas, lymphomas, teratomas, germ cell tumors, thymic carcinomas, and substernal goiters), bilateral lung volume reduction, and lower tracheal or carinal resections. Some mediastinal tumors, such as lymphoma, respond very well to chemotherapy so resection is not indicated.

CHEST WALL

19. What is a chest wall tumor resection?

It is the removal of tumor and surrounding structures, thus providing wide surgical margins while maintaining as much functional ability as possible, often requiring reconstruction. Chest wall tumors may be benign (lipoma, desmoid, or if arising from ribs osteochondroma, chondroma, and fibrous dysplasia), primary malignant (liposarcoma, malignant fibrous histiocytoma, chondrosarcoma, fibrosarcoma, Ewing's sarcoma, and osteosarcoma), or metastatic tumors that usually implant themselves through hematogenous route to the parietal pleura and, by extension, involve the other layers of the chest wall (Ruff, 2001).

Benign or primary malignant tumors can be resected to provide a survival benefit if an extensive work-up does not reveal metastatic disease. Metastatic tumors typically have other sites of disease requiring systemic therapy. Painful tumors can be palliated with radiation therapy.

20. What is a chest wall reconstruction?

It is the surgical repair of the chest wall following trauma, tumor resection, infection, radiation damage, or congenital anomalies.

Successful reconstruction requires the complete removal of the tumor, or radiated or infected tissues. Priorities include obliteration of intrathoracic dead space, stabilization of the rib cage, adequate soft tissue coverage, and return to function and form (Ruff, 2001). These cases use biologic (AlloDerm or bovine pericardium) and occasionally synthetic (Marlex mesh, Gortex, or methylmethacrylate) materials for reconstruction and are often performed in conjunction with plastic surgeons.

21. What is an Eloesser flap?

It is an open drainage procedure for an empyema created by removing two or three ribs and the attached intercoastal muscles. A flap of skin and subcutaneous tissue is brought internally into the drained empyema cavity and sutured to the pleura, creating an epithelium-lined sinus.

The Eloesser flap can be chosen in patients when the operative morbidity and mortality of an open decortication is prohibitive. It is most effective when an empyema is unilocular and located inferiorly or laterally or in patients with a chronic bronchopleural fistula.

THE PLEURA

22. What is a pneumothorax?

It is the presence of air in the pleural space.

23. What are the different types of pneumothoraces? What are their causes? What is the best treatment option for each type?

- Primary spontaneous pneumothorax: occurs without antecedent trauma to the thorax and the patient has no underlying lung disease. It is usually due to a rupture of an apical pleural bleb. If it is small and the patient has minimal symptoms, it can be observed and usually resolves spontaneously. If it is greater than 25%, the patient has significant persisting symptoms, if the disease presents in the contralateral lung, or if there is progression on serial radiographs, then a chest tube should be placed.

- Secondary spontaneous pneumothorax: occurs in the presence of underlying lung disease, most commonly chronic obstructive pulmonary disease (COPD). It is more life-threatening because these patients lack pulmonary reserve. Nearly all of these patients are symptomatic and need chest tube placement. If a persistent air leak exists after 5 to 7 days, the patient should undergo bleb resection and pleurodesis.

- Traumatic pneumothorax: results from a penetrating or nonpenetrating chest injury. The patient should be treated with a chest tube unless very small. If a hemopneumothorax is present, one chest tube should be placed in the superior aspect of the chest to evacuate air, while a second tube is placed inferiorly to remove blood. An iatrogenic pneumothorax occurs most commonly from a transthoracic needle biopsy, thoracentesis, or the insertion of central intravenous catheters. Treatment differs according to the degree of distress.

- Tension pneumothorax: a pneumothorax in which the pressure in the pleural space is positive throughout the respiratory cycle. It usually occurs during mechanical ventilation or resuscitative efforts. It is life-threatening because both ventilation is severely compromised and positive pressure in the mediastinum will decrease venous return to the heart and reduce cardiac output. Diagnosis is made clinically! (Do not wait to prove by x-ray.) The patient will have (1) unilateral decreased breath sounds with tympany to percussion, (2) hypotension and other signs of shock, (3) jugular venous distention, and (4) tracheal deviation away from the involved side (however, this is a late sign.) A large-bore needle should be inserted into the pleural space through the second anterior intercostal space. If a large amount of air escapes and vital signs normalize, the diagnosis is confirmed. The needle should remain in place until chest tube placement is complete (Light, 2005).

24. What is a pleural effusion?

The contained space that exists between the visceral and parietal pleurae is filled with a thin layer of fluid that acts as a lubricant. An effusion occurs when an imbalance in fluid production and absorption leads to a net accumulation. Progressive extrinsic compression of lung parenchyma leads to the hallmark symptom of dyspnea.

25. What is an empyema?

It is a pleural effusion that is infected.

26. What are the different types of effusions and how are they distinguished?

Pleural effusions are characterized as either transudative or exudative depending on the underlying etiology and the characteristics of the fluid composition. Transudative effusions are caused by altered osmotic or hydrostatic forces that produce excess fluid that is protein-poor (a systemic problem).

Exudative effusions develop from alterations in the pleura or its lymphatic drainage allowing accumulation of protein-rich plasma infiltrate (a local problem). It is critical to analyze a fluid sample because treatment will be dictated based on the results.

Fluid is analyzed using Light's criteria (Broder, 2001):

	Transudate *	*Exudate* **
Ratio of pleural fluid protein to serum protein	< 0.5	> 0.5
Ratio of pleural fluid LDH to serum LDH	< 0.6	> 0.6
Absolute pleural fluid LDH level	< 2/3 upper limit of normal for serum	> 2/3 upper limit of normal for serum

* All of the criteria need to be met to be called a transudate.
** Only one of the criteria must be met to be called an exudate.

Once fluid is identified as an exudate, additional evaluation is needed to help determine the cause. Amylase elevation is indicative of esophageal perforation, pancreatitis, or cancer. A low glucose levels is a sign of bacterial infections, cancer, or rheumatoid pleuritis. A pH level less than 7.2 indicates an empyema. It may also be helpful to send for cell counts, gram stains, and cultures (bacterial, fungal, and mycobacterial) (Broder, 2001).

27. What is the best treatment option for each type of effusion?

Transudative effusions occur most commonly from congestive heart failure. Other causes include cirrhosis, pulmonary embolism, and uremia. Their treatment should be focused on the underlying cause. Thoracentesis may be helpful for diagnosis and symptomatic relief but chest tube placement should be reserved for recurring effusion.

Exudative effusions result from pleural pathology such as malignancy (metastatic more common than primary mesothelioma). Other causes include, but are not exclusive to, pneumonia, collagen vascular disorders, drugs, intraabdominal abscess, esophageal perforation, pancreatitis, and chylous. Therapy should be guided toward treatment of the underlying problem; however, chest tube placement or surgical intervention is often re-quired. Surgery may include a pleural biopsy, decortication, pleurodesis, or placement of a Pleurx catheter (Broder, 2001).

28. What is a Pleurx catheter, and when is it appropriate to use?

A Pleurx catheter is a long-term, indwelling, removable catheter with a felt cuff and a one-way valved access port that is tunneled into the pleural space. The catheter can be connected to a vacuum collection bottle allowing patients to drain pleural fluid at home. Initially, drainage may take place daily, then with decreasing frequency over time. Over half of patients will exhibit spontaneous pleurodesis. It is solely used as a palliative measure for malignant pleural effusions. Other types of effusions should not undergo frequent thoracente-sis but require other treatment options.

29. What is a pleurodesis? Why is it performed?

It is the purposeful irritation of the pleural surfaces to produce an inflammatory pleuritis that promotes adherence of the visceral and parietal pleurae to obliterate the pleural space.

This procedure can be performed by chemical or mechanical means. Mechanical pleurodesis is performed in the operating room when the parietal pleura is physically abraded with a surgi-cal pad to cause the inflammation. This is often done in combination with other procedures. Pleurodesis can also be caused chemically by using bleomycin or talc. The chosen chemical is instilled through a chest tube and the patient is reposi-tioned on a timed schedule for more complete distribution.

A pleurodesis is performed for two major rea-sons: presence of a malignant pleural effusion or a persistent or recurrent spontaneous pneumothorax.

30. What is a decortication? Why is it performed?

It is the removal of an infected fibrous rind from around the lung. When an effusion, particularly a parapneumonic effusion, has persisted for a long period of time, it may become loculated or develop a rind or peel around its edge. Draining via thora-centesis or tube thoracostomy (chest tube place-ment) may not be sufficient. The goal with draining the fluid is to allow the lung to reexpand into its normal position with visceral and parietal pleura apposition. A decortication is the surgical removal of the fibrinous tissue from pleural surfaces and the surface of the lung to gain as much lung reexpan-sion as possible. It can be performed thoracoscopically or as an open procedure.

GENERAL CARE

31. What is a chest tube?

A drainage tube placed within the pleural space to allow unidirectional evacuation of air and liquid connected to a closed drainage system.

It is imperative to understand the physiology of breathing to understand chest tubes and drainage systems. The pressure in the pleural space is lower than atmospheric pressure and is referred to as negative. The pressure goes even lower before inspiration, which allows air to enter the lungs. When the pleura is entered surgically or by trauma, atmospheric (positive) pressure enters the pleural space, and the lung on that side collapses. A chest tube connected to a negative pressure closed drainage system allows air and fluid to drain from the pleural space and prevents air or fluid from entering back in. This accomplishes two basic purposes: (1) to aid in the expansion of the remaining portion of the lung as air (positive pressure) and fluid escape through the drainage tube, and (2) to reestablish negative pressure in the pleural space.

32. Why do surgery patient often have two chest tubes?

Two chest tubes are usually placed after pulmo-nary resections, although some surgeons only use one. The first is typically placed in the anterior pleural space and primarily removes the air from the pleural space. The second tube will be placed posteriorly and lower for drainage of fluid.

33. What is an air leak?

When the chest tube continues to drain air, a "leak" from the lung is suspected. This is a com-mon finding after surgery and should resolve within 1 to 2 days as the lung seals along the line of dissection. Persistent air leaks may indicate a secondary condition such as a rupture of a bleb, which is not uncommon in emphysema patients with friable lung tissue. These, too, will heal with time in most cases.

A new large continuous air leak may indicate a break in the system. Check that all connections are tightly sealed, that the drainage system is intact and free of damage, that the chest tube itself has not become partially removed, and that the chest tube holes are not outside the chest.

34. What does it mean when a chest tube is placed to water seal?

When a chest tube is connected to the drainage collection system, it will maintain a negative pressure. The water seal prevents air from reentering the tube and the pleural space and prevents fluid from siphoning back. Patency and function are assessed by tidal movement of fluid within the tube during the respiratory cycle and motion of the water seal level.

35. What does it mean when a chest tube is to suction? When should suction be used?

Applying suction to a chest tube promotes the closure of dead space, thus allowing better approximation of tissue surfaces. However, suction does not necessarily shorten the duration of an air leak. Therefore, it is used in select situations and not with every surgery. Suction should be used following a pleurodesis or decortication, following a new onset or worsening of a pneumothorax, or immediately following an operation when a large volume of space was created by surgery such as a bilobectomy. Suction should never be used in a pneumonectomy space (if a chest tube is used). (See question 20.)

36. What is a Heimlich valve, and when is it used?

A Heimlich valve is a one-way flutter valve that can be attached to the end of a chest tube to maintain negative pressure. Patients with persistent air leaks at 1 week after surgery and are stable on water seal can have a Heimlich valve attached to their chest tubes and can go home. They are monitored closely with frequent clinic visits and the tube removed typically in 7 to 10 days when it is clear that the air leak is closed.

37. When should a chest tube be clamped?

The two most common scenarios when chest tube clamping is appropriate for patients are postpneumonectomy and prepull trial.

Pneumonectomy patients will have a chest tube placed on the operative side, and it will be clamped leaving the OR. The surgical team will unclamp the chest tube for a few minutes each day to allow the mediastinum to slowly shift toward the operative side. The operative cavity will gradually fill with fluid. Patients may say they feel fluid "sloshing around" inside when they move until the entire cavity is filled, which takes a few weeks. The chest tube can also used to evaluate for a hemothorax or pneumothorax if the patient becomes hemodynamically unstable.

Nonpneumonectomy patients that have had a persistent air leak may undergo a clamping trial. The chest tube is clamped to simulate its removal. Serial x-rays are taken to evaluate for a pneumothorax. Clamping trials can last anywhere from 4 to 48 hours.

38. What should be done if a chest tube becomes disconnected from the drainage system?

The chest tube should be immediately clamped. Obstruct the end of the chest tube with your thumb or bend it 180° until a clamp can be applied. The ends of the tube and the drainage system should be wiped clean of obvious debris with an alcohol wipe then reconnected and taped securely. Remove the clamp and instruct the patient to cough forcefully several times. Sit the patient upright in the bed. Reassess breath sounds and vital signs. Notify the surgical team so a chest x-ray can be ordered immediately. If the patient is symptomatic, they will likely order suction to the chest tube.

39. What should be done if a chest tube is inadvertently removed?

This may or may not create a problem for the patient. The insertion site should be covered with Xeroform and gauze, then an airtight occlusive dressing. Notify the surgical team so a chest x-ray can be ordered. Sit the patient in an upright position in bed. Reassess breath sounds and vital signs. If the patient is asymptomatic, serial x-rays may be the only course of action. Gather the appropriate equipment to replace the chest tube immediately if the patient is symptomatic.

40. What is subcutaneous emphysema? How is it treated in a postsurgical patient?

The presence of subcutaneous emphysema typically indicates a kinked or blocked chest tube or a worsening air leak from the lung. It feels like "rice crispies" under the skin. Air that leaks from the lung but cannot exit via the chest tube will find the path of least resistance and exit through the chest tube insertion site. If it cannot escape through the skin, it dissects into the subcutaneous plane and can extend into the neck and face. Treatment is aimed toward relieving the obstruction to the chest tube or by placing a new one. Reassure the family that although the appearance is rather dramatic, it is a benign process and will resolve on its own (Von Fricken, 2001).

41. What is the importance of a nasogastric (NG) tube in esophagectomy patients?

An NG tube is used to prevent excessive distention of the gastric or bowel pull-up segment. Gastric atony will result in retention so gastric contents under pressure must have an egress. Vomiting would exert excessive force against the suture line and must be avoided. Anastomotic rupture has a high morbidity and mortality. Every effort should be used to maintain the NG tube so that it functions properly.

42. Why might an esophagectomy patient have a jejunal feeding tube?

An esophagectomy patient will be kept n.p.o. for several days after surgery to allow the anastomosis to heal. A swallow test will be performed around postop day 5 to 7. If the anastomosis has a leak, the patient will be kept n.p.o. for a longer period of time. The jejunal tube (J-tube) will be used to provide enteral nutrition during the immediate postoperative period and perhaps longer to provide supplemental feedings after discharge. Many patients have a J-tube placed preoperatively to sustain them during induction of chemoradiation therapy. J-tube feedings should be initiated slowly but early, typically postoperative day 3. There is no need to wait for bowel sound presence before initiation, but close monitoring for toleration should be done instead. Do not overinflate the balloon, if present.

43. What should be included in a routine assessment of a new J-tube?

The insertion site may have small amounts of bilious drainage, which will irritate the skin, causing redness, but drainage should not be purulent. The insertion site should be cleaned daily then covered with dry gauze and secured with tape, anchoring the tube to alleviate strain on the sutures. The skin around the sutures can become irritated and friable from drainage, and often, the sutures will eventually break through the skin if not kept dry. The tube should also flush easily when irrigated at least three times a day even when not used for feedings.

44. What are common problems with J-tubes?

- Site care: J-tubes may leak large amounts of bilious drainage when a patient is constipated, which is a frequent postoperative occurrence with narcotic use. The skin around the tube will become excoriated from this enzymatic drainage. Frequent site care is required. Diaper rash cream (zinc oxide) is an ideal choice for healing the skin and will function as a barrier toward future drainage. It is also economical and readily available for most patients.
- Clogging: J-tubes become easily clogged because they are typically smaller in diameter

than gastric tubes. Medications need to be carefully crushed or converted to liquid form when possible. Tubes should be consistently flushed every 8 hours, especially following medications. If resistance begins with flushes, using a carbonated fluid such as ginger ale may help improve patency. If complete obstruction occurs, a trial of pancreatic enzymes and sodium bicarbonate can be tried.

- Diarrhea: Remember, do not give bolus feedings! Jejunal feedings should always be given continuously on a pump. They are best tolerated if started at a slow rate for 24 hours then cycled faster to allow a patient an extended period of time disconnected from their tube. Work closely with a nutritional service if the patient is not tolerating the formula. Many options are available and fiber supplements can be added as well.
- Falling out: The tube needs to be reinserted as soon as possible. The tunneled track will begin to close within hours so reinsertion should not wait. Contact the surgical team to have it replaced.

45. What is pulmonary toilet (PT), and why is it important?

Keeping airways open and free of secretions is the best prevention for atelectasis and pneumonia. Coughing, deep breathing, use of incentive spirometry and/or flutter valve, and early and frequent ambulation all aid in preventing pulmonary complications following thoracic surgery. Nebulizations and/or chest PT are indicated in patients with rhonchi or other signs of retained secretions. Adequate pain control is essential for chest PT to be tolerated and beneficial. Bedside bronchoscopy may be deemed necessary in some cases.

46. How is postoperative pain managed?

Thoracic epidurals eliminate pain by blocking T6–T8 dermatomes and help ensure good analgesia for thoracotomy pain without having the sedating effects like opioids. Intercostal and paravertebral blocks are performed preoperatively to achieve 6 to 12 hours of good postoperative pain relief. Intrapleural catheters are placed along the chest tube during surgery. Bupivacaine 0.25% at 5 to 7 mL/hr is run at a continuous rate to help block the intercostal nerves, thoracic sympathetic nerves, and the nerve endings within the pleura. Patient-controlled analgesia pumps with opioids provide consistent pain relief readily available to the patient and lower toxicity rates if used appropriately. NSAIDs help reduce pain without having the sedating effect like opioids and often used in conjunction with opioids.

REFERENCES

Broder, K. (2001). Pleural effusions. In H. L. Karamanoukian, P. R. Soltoski, & T. A. Salerno (Eds.), *Thoracic surgery secrets* (pp. 152–155). Philadelphia: Hanley & Belfus.

Light, R. W. (2005). Disorders of the pleura, mediastinum, diaphragm, and chest wall. In D. L. Kasper, E. Braunwald, A. S. Fauci, S. L. Hauser, D. L. Longo, & J. L. Jameson (Eds.), *Harrison's principles of internal medicine* (16th ed., pp. 1565–1569). New York: McGraw-Hill.

Murthy, S. C., & Rice, T. W. (2004). Esophageal perforation. In S. C. Yang & D. E. Cameron (Eds.), *Current therapy in thoracic and cardiovascular surgery* (pp. 81–86). Philadelphia: Mosby.

Reed, C. E. (2004). Upper thoracic esophageal cancer. In S. C. Yang & D. E. Cameron (Eds.), *Current therapy in thoracic and cardiovascular surgery* (pp. 344–348). Philadelphia: Mosby.

Ruff, P. G. (2001). Chest wall reconstruction. In H. L. Karamanoukian, P. R. Soltoski, & T. A. Salerno (Eds.), *Thoracic surgery secrets* (pp. 174–176). Philadelphia: Hanley & Belfus.

Sonnett, J. R. (2004). Bronchoscopy: Diagnostic and therapeutic applications. In S. C. Yang & D. E. Cameron (Eds.), *Current therapy in thoracic and cardiovascular surgery* (pp. 36–39). Philadelphia: Mosby.

Von Fricken, K. (2001). Pneumothorax. In H. L. Karamanoukian, P. R. Soltoski, & T. A. Salerno (Eds.), *Thoracic surgery secrets* (pp. 149–151). Philadelphia: Hanley & Belfus.

CHAPTER 34

Liver and Kidney Transplantations

**Christine Mudge, RN, MS, PNPc, CNN, FAAN
and Susan Stritzel Diaz, RN, MSN, CPNP**

The hope of extending and improving quality of life through organ transplantation has intrigued and challenged us for many centuries. Organ transplantation became technically possible in the early 20th century and now is considered a life-saving reality for thousands of people with organ failure. The major challenge facing the future of organ transplantation continues to be the shortage of donor organs in addition to graft rejection and cost. Today, there are over 100,000 individuals in the United States waiting for organ transplantation (United Network of Organ Sharing [UNOS], 2010). The following section briefly reviews the major nursing considerations for the perianesthesia care of the liver and kidney transplant recipient.

1. What are the indications for liver transplantation?

The most common indication for liver transplantation is end stage liver disease (ESLD) that has been refractory to medical management. The causes of ESLD that can result in liver transplantation include cholestatic disorders (e.g., Alagille syndrome, biliary atresia, familial cholestasis, primary biliary cirrhosis, primary or secondary sclerosing cholangitis); parenchymal cirrhosis (e.g., autoimmune hepatitis, alcoholic cirrhosis [only when specific abstinence criteria are met], chronic hepatitis B or C, congenital hepatic fibrosis, cryptogenic cirrhosis, nonalcoholic steatohepatitis); acute liver failure (e.g., drug induced [e.g., acetaminophen overdose], fulminant hepatitis/necrosis, hypersensitivity, toxins [e.g., amanita]); metabolic liver diseases (e.g., alpha 1 antitrypsin deficiency, hemochromatosis, protoporphyria, tyrosinemia,

Wilson's disease); metabolic defects that involve extrahepatic organs or systems (e.g., Crigler–Najjar syndrome type 1, familial hypercholesterolemia type 2, glycogen storage disease, primary hyperoxaluria type 1, urea cycle defects [e.g., ornithine transcarbamylase deficiency]); generalized metabolic disorders (e.g., cystic fibrosis, familial amyloidosis, Niemann–Pick disease; vascular disease (e.g., Budd–Chiari syndrome, giant hepatic hemangioma, portal vein thrombosis; and malignancies (e.g., hepatoblastoma [objective response to chemotherapy], hepatocellular carcinoma, hemangioendothelioma, noncarcinoid neuroendocrine tumors [typically patients are considered candidates for transplant if there is no extrahepatic disease]).

2. What are the typical contraindications for liver transplant?

Contraindications to liver transplant typically include coma (with objective evidence of irreversible brain injury), active substance abuse, extrahepatic malignancy (unless the patient meets the standard of practice oncologic criteria for cure), sepsis unresponsive to treatment, insufficient social support (program specific), and noncompliance.

3. What is the liver allocation system and what is the Model for End-Stage Liver Disease/Pediatric End-Stage Liver Disease (MELD/PELD)?

Child-Turcotte-Pugh (CTP) Score was the scoring system used in the past to rank patients on the national transplant wait list. It was replaced by MELD/PELD in February 2002. MELD/PELD is the system that prioritizes liver allocation by the United Network of Organ Sharing (UNOS). It is an objective scoring system that determines medical need for liver transplantation. Factors used to calculate a MELD score are the most recent total bilirubin, international normalized ratio (INR), and creatinine. MELD scores can range from 6 to 40. A score of 40 indicates the most severe disease. A modification of this system is used for pediatrics (PELD). The designation of status 1 (predicated death within 7 days) is used for the most critically ill patients who are waiting liver transplantation, or the patient who is less than 18 years old with chronic liver failure that meets the pediatric UNOS status criteria. In some situations, there are exceptions or special cases. These are usually referred to the UNOS regional board for further review. See Table 34-1.

4. What are the clinical findings and causes of chronic end-stage liver disease?

The clinical manifestations of liver disease are often dependent on the primary diagnosis. In general, patients with end-stage liver disease present with fatigue, malaise, anorexia, and weight loss. Fibrotic scaring of the liver contributes to portal hypertension, resulting in ascites, varices, splenomegaly, thrombocytopenia, and an augmented risk for bleeding. There are also alterations in hemodynamic status and electrolyte balance. As the ability to detoxify estrogens, excrete bilirubin, and regulate serum cholesterol is reduced, patients begin to demonstrate spider angiomas (stigmas of cirrhosis), palmar erythema, jaundice, xanthomas, and progressive pruritus. Compromise in synthetic function leads to an increasing coagulopathy and further risk for easy bruising, petechiae, and bleeding. Impaired protein synthesis, manifested by a

decreased albumin level contributes to third spacing, ascites, peripheral edema, and poor nutritional status, a particular concern in children. Alteration in glucose metabolism can cause hypo/hyperglycemia. Other endocrine problems include gynecomastia, testicular atrophy, and decreased libido. Progressive hepatic encephalopathy is clinically manifested by behavioral changes, reversed sleep/wake cycle, asterixis, and confusion progressing to coma. Dyspnea is not uncommon due to an elevated diaphragm secondary to ascites. Alteration in renal function can be due to intrinsic renal dysfunction or hepatorenal syndrome. Compromise in kidney function often presents with alteration in fluids and electrolytes and elevated blood urea nitrogen (BUN) and creatinine.

5. What are the types of surgical procedures for liver transplant?

Organs for liver transplantation are either from living or deceased donors. The surgical approaches for liver transplant include whole organ, reduced sized graft, split graft, living-related left or right lobe, auxiliary transplant, and combined organ transplant (e.g., liver-kidney transplant). Reduced-sized grafts evolved to expand the donor pool. In reduced-sized grafts, the right posterior and anterior segments are resected, and the whole left liver with the vena cava are used. Split-liver transplantation is a surgical technique whereby the deceased donor liver is split between to recipients. In general, outcomes of split-liver transplantation have been shown to be equivalent to whole organ transplants. Living-liver transplantation (LLTx) is typically the donation of either the left lateral segment (segments 2 and 3), or the right lobe. With increasing experience, LLTx has become a well-accepted approach to liver transplantation. Auxiliary liver transplantation

TABLE 34-1. Outline Child-Turcotte Pugh (CTP) scoring system to assess severity of liver disease

Points	1	2	3
Encephalopathy	None	1–2	3–4
Ascites	Absent	Slight or controlled by diuretics	Moderate despite diuretics
Bilirubin	< 2	2–3	> 3
Albumin	> 3.5	2.8–3.5	< 2.8
Prothrombin time (seconds prolonged)	< 4	4.6	> 6
INR	< 1.7	1.7–2.3	> 2.3

is a surgical procedure in which the liver graft is implanted without removing the native liver. Although this approach is rarely used, it may have a place in the future. Combined liver-kidney transplantation (LKTx) has been performed in patients with end stage hepatorenal disease and hepatorenal syndrome. Patient and graft outcomes are influenced by the primary disease, severity of illness at the time of transplant, and location of the center performing the transplant. The surgical procedure is the same for single organ transplantation.

6. What is the process for donor liver surgical procedure?

Donor livers are matched to potential recipients based on blood type and body size. Typically, the donor and recipient are the same blood type. However, in cases of urgent need, donors with an incompatible blood type have been used. If the donor liver is too large, it can result in pulmonary compromise and, if it is too small, there may be hepatic insufficiency or a mismatch in vessel size, leading to stenosis or thrombosis. Donor and recipient weights within 20% of one another are generally considered a likely match. With the advancement in surgical techniques and the advent of the paired or reduced size graft surgical accommodations can be made for variation in donor size. Procurement of the donor liver is performed through a midline incision. The major vessels around the liver are dissected including the celiac truck and branches, portal vein, and the inferior vena cava. The common bile duct is transected with attempts to maintain maximum length of the duct for the recipient transplant operation. Cool saline is flushed into the biliary tree via the gallbladder to remove stagnate bile and protect the biliary mucosa. The liver is then flushed in situ with cool heparinized lactated Ringer's to remove old blood, and then with University of Wisconsin (UW) solution for preservation. The suprahepatic cava is transected at the right atrium and the infrahepatic cava just above the renal veins. This approach allows for preservation of the kidneys for possible transplant. The portal vein is divided at the confluence of the splenic vein and superior mesenteric vein; the abdominal aorta and hepatic artery are excised preserving the hepatic arterial supply. The liver is packed in UW solution, stored on ice, and transported.

7. How is the recipient surgical procedure approached?

The recipient surgery is generally done through a Chevron incision in adults and a transverse incision in infants and children. The recipient hepatectomy involves clamping the infrahepatic and suprahepatic inferior vena cava and dividing the portal vein. Venous return from the inferior vena cava is momentarily interrupted and the outflow from the infrahepatic inferior vena cava and portal vein is occluded. Decreased venous blood flow can led to engorgement of all subdiaphragmatic vessels causing an increase in portal hypertension and bowel congestion. Therefore, it is important to limit the time frame of the anhepatic phase to 30 to 45 minutes. The transplanted liver is placed orthotopically. There are five major anastomoses completed in the following order: suprahepatic inferior vena cava, infrahepatic inferior vena cava, portal vein, hepatic artery, and the biliary anastomosis. After the portal vein is anastomosed, the liver is reperfused with a warm hyperkalemic preservation solution that is vented through the anterior infrahepatic caval anastomosis. The reperfusion phase has been associated with electrolyte imbalances and coagulopathies.

8. What are the two approaches to biliary reconstruction?

A choledochocholedochostomy is an end-to-end anastomosis of the recipient and donor common bile ducts. In the presence of biliary disease or a biliary duct-to-duct mismatch, a choledochojejunostomy is performed. This is an anastomosis of the donor bile duct to the recipient's jejunum, also referred to as a Roux-en-Y.

9. What are the types of transplants?

See Table 34-2.

10. What are the potential complications following liver transplantation?

Liver transplant recipients are at risk for the same complications related to major abdominal surgery. In addition, they are also at risk for the multiple side effects of immunosuppressive therapy, rejection, and infection. Specific postoperative liver transplant complications are as follows:

- Primary nonfunction (PNF) is graft failure and should be differentiated from graft dysfunction or preservation injury, which is considered a spectrum ranging from mild graft dysfunction to severe dysfunction. Mild graft dysfunction is clinically manifested by elevated liver enzymes and mild alteration in synthetic function (e.g., elevated PT, INR). Whereas severe graft dysfunction is demonstrated by significant elevation in coagulation factors, hemodynamic instability and

TABLE 34-2. Types of transplants

Type of Graft	Description of the Type of Transplant
Allograft (homograft)	From a genetically nonidentical member of the same species (e.g., heart)
Autograft	From one part of a person's body to another location in the same person (e.g., skin)
Heterograft (xenograft)	Between species (e.g., pig to human)
Isograft (syngraft)	Between genetically identical people (e.g., monozygotic twins)
Orthotopic graft	An organ that is place in the normal anatomic position (e.g., liver)
Heterotopic graft	An organ that is place in a position other than the normal anatomic location (e.g., kidney)

associated multiorgan dysfunction. PNF is clinically manifested by hepatic cytolysis, coagulopathy, altered synthetic function (e.g., decreased albumin, and total protein, increasing PT and INR), lack of bile flow, high lactate levels, hyperkalemia, hypoglycemia, need for ventilatory support, hemodynamic instability and, often, acute renal failure. In the presence of PNF, there will be an initial elevation in serum transaminases followed by a dramatic decrease with coinciding prolonged coagulation studies. These findings suggest hepatocyte death requiring urgent retransplantation.

- Bleeding may develop during the first few days postoperatively. The primary causes of early post-liver transplant bleeding include fibrinolysis, heparin-like effect, persistent coagulopathy, preexisting splenomegaly and thrombocytopenia, portal hypertension with varices, compromised hepatic function, or graft failure, collapse of one of the vascular anastomosis, or stress ulcers. Coagulopathies may be managed with a continuous infusion of fresh frozen plasma, platelet administration, and/or cryoprecipitated plasma. However, it is not uncommon that patients return to the operating room for further evaluation and possible revision of one of the vascular anastomosis. Patients undergoing a split liver transplant are at increased risk of bleeding from the cut edge of the donor liver and should be monitored closely.

- Vascular complications following liver transplantation include hepatic artery thrombosis or stenosis and portal vein thrombosis or stenosis. To minimize the risk of vascular

complications, an abdominal ultrasound with Doppler is usually performed intraoperatively, immediately postoperatively, and the first postoperative day. Hepatic artery thrombosis (HAT) is the most severe vascular complication. Predisposition to HAT include anatomic problems (e.g., vessel size mismatch), hypercoagulable state, rejection, prolonged ischemic time, and transplant for sclerosing cholangitis. Early posttransplant HAT often presents with a severe coagulopathy, hemodynamic instability, encephalopathy, hypoglycemia, hyperkalemia, renal impairment, and subsequent liver failure. HAT may also contribute to severe biliary complications because the hepatic artery feeds the biliary system in the liver. Treatment of HAT is surgical revascularization if possible and more often urgent retransplantation. Hepatic artery stenosis is less common and usually presents at the anastomotic site. It can result in hepatic ischemia and/or infarction. Proposed treatment involves surgical reanastomosis or percutaneous balloon dilatation. Portal vein thrombosis (PVT) usually can be reversed if diagnosed early. Prompt surgical evacuation of the clot and reanastomosis with postoperative anticoagulation therapy may be successful. Clinical presentation can be insidious and may include increasing ascites or portal hypertension with variceal bleeding. Diagnosis is based on hepatic ultrasonography or angiography. Additional treatment options for PVT have included a combination of chemical thrombolysis and stent placement, and decompression of the splanchnic system through a splenorenal shunt or retransplantation. Portal vein stenosis usually results from either a mismatch in the size of the donor recipient portal vein or a problem with the surgical technique. Balloon venoplasty with stent placement has been successfully used to manage portal vein stenosis.

- Pulmonary complications during the early postoperative period include primarily atelectasis and right pleural effusion. These problems typically result in poor ventilation and oxygenation increasing the risk of pneumonia. Pulmonary complications are related to prolonged anesthesia; paralysis of the right diaphragm secondary to the retractors held during surgery, ascites, and graft larger than the native liver pressing against the diaphragm; and pain. It is important to correct contributing problems such as metabolic alkalosis and ascites, which can also interfere with proper ventilation. Vigorous pulmonary toilet, pain management, and early mobilization minimize the effects of a pleural effusion and atelectasis, thus, reducing the risk of pneumonia.

- Renal insufficiency can be observed in patients both pre- and post-liver transplant. Pretransplant disorders involving both the liver and kidney are extensive and can impact posttransplant patient and graft survival. Posttransplant renal insufficiency in the presence of normal renal function pretransplant, may be due to massive hemorrhage and hypotension, hypovolemia, infection, calcineurin inhibitors, antibiotic therapy, or graft failure. Efforts to preserve and/or resuscitate renal function posttransplant are imperative and include fluid, calculating appropriate antibiotic and immunosuppressive drug doses, reducing intra-abdominal pressure through paracentesis and close monitoring of renal function (e.g., urine output, creatinine, BUN).

- Biliary complications include bile leaks, strictures, and obstruction secondary to stones or biliary slugging caused by the shedding of the epithelial lining of the donor bile duct. Anastomotic biliary leaks that occur in the early postoperative period often result in either localized or generalized peritonitis and are often accompanied by peritoneal signs, acute abdominal pain, and fever. An elevation in total bilirubin is an indication for further investigation. Since the hepatic artery delivers blood to the biliary system, it is important that hepatic artery thrombosis be ruled out as a potential cause with all biliary leaks. Doppler ultrasound of the hepatic artery or hepatic angiography can be used to determine hepatic artery patency. Early management of biliary leaks typically involves surgical reexploration and revision of the biliary anastomosis to a Roux-en-Y choledochojejunostomy. Biliary strictures can involve both the intrahepatic and extrahepatic biliary tree. Strictures are usually successfully treated with balloon dilatation and stenting by ERCP or percutaneous transhepatic cholangiogram (PTC).

- Hepatic allograft rejection has been classified by histologic features, timing, response to therapy, and reversibility. A liver biopsy and histology remain the gold standard for diagnosing alteration in hepatic graft function. Hepatic histology allows rejection to be easily differentiated from viral hepatitis, bile duct obstruction, and other causes of hepatic dysfunction. The major targets of hepatic allograft rejection are the epithelial cells of the bile ducts and the endothelium of the hepatic arteries and veins; hepatocytes appear to be less vulnerable.

- Acute rejection post-liver transplant is usually a cell-mediated process developing within 3 weeks to 3 months posttransplant. Clinical manifestations may include fever, malaise, and/or fatigue. Laboratory manifestations often include an elevation in hepatic transaminases (AST, ALT, GGT), alkaline phosphatase, and, in some situations, bilirubin. Histologic findings are portal or periportal inflammation, bile duct damage, and venous endotheliitis. Rejection is treated based on histologic findings, patient response to therapy, transplant center, and provider.

- Chronic rejection is primarily a cell-mediated response often diagnosed 6 weeks or more post-liver transplant. It is defined as obliterate endarteritis with ischemic damage that may be accompanied by fibrosis, cirrhosis, and paucity of bile ducts (vanishing bile duct syndrome [VBDS]) with cholestasis. VBDS is characterized by loss of bile ducts in the absence of vascular rejection. Chronic rejection may improve with time augmentation of immunosuppressive therapy; however, retransplantation is not uncommon in this patient population.

- Recurrent disease can be a major problem for patients with viral hepatitis or hepatic malignancies, autoimmune hepatitis, nonalcoholic steatohepatitis, primary biliary cirrhosis, and primary sclerosing cholangitis. Diagnosis of recurrent disease is usually based on a liver biopsy and imaging studies. In the case of hepatitis, serum markers are also utilized. In general, the management of recurrent disease is treated much the same as in the native liver.

11. What are the signs of a functioning graft post-liver transplant?

The clinical indicators of a functioning liver graft are hemodynamic stability, normalization of coagulation factors, normalization of acid base balance, stabilization of vital signs and temperature, stable glucose metabolism, optimum bile production, optimum renal function and urine output, and stable/improving mental status.

12. What are the monitoring considerations immediately post-liver transplant?

In many centers, patients are admitted directly to the intensive care unit (ICU). They are often intubated and have multiple invasive lines and tubes. These may include a central line, arterial line, peripheral intravenous catheter, pulmonary artery catheter, Foley catheter, Jackson Pratt, and, less commonly, a T-tube (for biliary drainage). All lines and complications related to major abdominal surgery and liver transplantation should be monitored for closely and proper infection control protocols instituted.

Typical lab work to evaluate the status of the liver includes aspartate aminotransferase (ALT/SGPT), alanine aminotransferase (ALT/SGPT), gamma glutamyl transpeptidase (GGT), bilirubin, albumin, glucose coagulation factors (PT, INR, factor V, fibrinogen), which are an indication of synthetic function and serum lactate an indicator of metabolic function.

Specifically, metabolic alkalosis is often considered an optimum sign of graft function. It is often the result of diuretic therapy, or the administration of blood products. Citrate is the anticoagulant used in stored blood products. Following a blood transfusion, citrate is metabolized to bicarbonate in a functioning liver. If the graft is functioning properly LFTs, coagulation factors and serum lactate levels should normalize. Improving mental status or resolving encephalopathy are encouraging signs of graft function. An abdominal ultrasound with Doppler is usually performed postoperatively and, within 24 hours, to evaluate the liver and patency of the hepatic vessels, particularly the hepatic artery.

Patients often present hyperdynamic with a high cardiac output and low systemic vascular resistance that typically persists during the early postoperative period. Close monitoring for hypervolemia versus hypovolemia, cardiac stability, and possible arrhythmias are imperative. Hypertension may be the result of medications (e.g., steroids, calcineurin inhibitors), alteration in rennin-angiotensin system, or fluid administration intraoperatively. It is managed by optimizing medication dosing, diuretics, and antihypertensive therapy, which tends to be based on center protocol and provider. Hypotension may be related to bleeding or third spacing. Potential bleeding problems are assessed by monitoring coagulation factors, serial hematocrits, abdominal girth and drain output, incision site, hemodynamic status, and urine output. Treatment usually includes fluid resuscitation, blood transfusion, correction of the coagulopathy, and vasopressor support. It is not uncommon that patients undergo surgical reexploration to evacuate hematoma and for identification of ongoing bleeding. Third spacing may be the result of poor clinical and nutritional status pretransplant and patients may benefit from an infusion of albumin followed by diuretic therapy, in addition to hemodynamic support.

Pulmonary complications are common during the postoperative period. Contributing factors include a debilitated state pretransplant, nature of the incision, elevated right hemidiaphragm during surgery, possible phrenic nerve damage, and intraoperative fluids and massive fluid shifts. Management consists of appropriate ventilatory support and early extubation, careful attention to incentive spirometry, chest therapy, and early mobilization.

Careful monitoring of fluids, electrolytes, and renal function are imperative. It is not uncommon for patients to have alterations in electrolytes that need to be corrected. Magnesium levels are often low secondary to calcineurin inhibitors, and supplemental therapy is often required. Alteration in potassium levels are not uncommon and should be monitored frequently. Potassium levels may be elevated secondary to the calcineurin inhibitor, cell break down, and the graft preservation fluid. Hyperkalemia is usually managed by obtaining serial electrolyte levels, EKG monitoring, and diuretic therapy. Ionized calcium is checked frequently and should normalize. Replacement therapy may be necessary in patients who have received large volumes of blood products due to the citrate preservative in blood, which can decrease ionized calcium levels. BUN and creatinine are also monitored frequently to evaluate renal function.

Mental status can also be an indicator of graft function. Neurologic status may be compromised initially secondary to degree of encephalopathy pretransplant and the grafts ability to detoxify posttransplant. Regular neurologic checks are an important component of postoperative care. Pain management is essential, but periodically can be challenging regarding the need for prompt extubation or with changes in neurologic status.

13. What are the indications and listing criteria for kidney transplantation?

Kidney transplant is considered the optimum therapy for individuals in renal failure. The leading causes of renal failure in the United States are hypertension, glomerulonephritis, diabetic nephropathy, and polycystic kidney disease. Listing criteria for kidney transplant is end-stage kidney disease as manifested by a creatinine clearance of less than or equal to 20 ml/min or the initiation of dialysis. Organ allocation is based on a point system that incorporates blood type, time waiting, quality of the match, panel of reactive antibodies (PRA), and medical urgency with special dispensation given to pediatric patients. Further discussion of organ allocation can be found on the UNOS website. Organs for kidney transplant are from living or deceased donors. When compared to deceased organ transplants, living kidney transplants are often associated with improved graft survival, optimum general health of the recipient, shorter waiting times, and reduced cost. In an effort to expand the potential donor pool, the expanded criteria donor (ECD) has been established. ECD are older donors (over 55 years of age) or those who present with additional clinical features (e.g., diabetic, hypertensive or hypotensive, infected, abnormal organ function, history of malignancy). The ECDs are used in specific recipient situations. Regardless of the source or quality of the donor, the surgical procedure for the recipient is the same.

14. What are the disease indications for kidney transplantation?

Disease indicators for kidney transplant include congenital disorders, congenital nephritic syndrome (steroid resistant), hereditary nephropathies, polycystic kidney disease, Alport's syndrome, medullary cystic disease, familial nephritis, metabolic disorders, (e. g., primary hyperoxaluria [combined kidney-liver transplant], nephrocalcinosis,

amyloidosis, Fabry's disease), cystinosis, obstructive uropathy (e. g., congenital or acquired, reflux nephropathy), toxic nephropathies (e.g., lead nephropathy, analgesic nephropathy), trauma resulting in bilateral nephrectomy, renal vascular disease (e. g., renal artery occlusion, renal vein thrombosis, renal infarct), potential irreversible causes of acute renal failure, cortical necrosis, acute glomerulonephritis, hemolytic uremic syndrome, Henoch-Schönlein syndrome, acute tubular necrosis, inflammatory disorders, chronic pyelonephritis, membranoproliferative glomerulonephritis, focal segmental glomerulosclerosis, hypocomplementemic nephritis, Goodpasture's disease, systemic lupus erythematous, scleroderma, polyarteritis nodosum, Wegener's disease, tumors (e. g., renal carcinoma, Wilms' tumor, tuberous sclerosis), hypertensive nephrosclerosis, multiple myeloma, and macroglobulinemia.

15. How are the two approaches to kidney donation, open nephrectomy, and laparoscopic nephrectomy done?

The open donor nephrectomy involves a large abdominal muscle incision using the standard extraperitoneal flank approach, and occasionally, the removal of a rib. The kidney is removed, examined, and flushed with an iced preservation solution (e.g., Euro-Collins) to remove blood and decrease the core temperature of the kidney. Manipulation of the kidney is minimal to prevent nerve stimulation and vasospasm, which can result in thrombosis, stenosis, necrosis of the ureter, urinary leakage, and loss of graft. The donor incision is closed. The procedure takes approximately 4 to 6 hours. This approach to kidney donation requires an extended hospital stay and a prolonged recovery period, both of which have been considered disincentives to living kidney donation.

Laparoscopic live donor nephrectomy is less invasive and has become the standard for living kidney donation. The patient is placed in a modified lateral decubitus position at 45° and three laparoscopic ports are made. The first is lateral to the rectus muscle between the umbilicus and iliac crest, second at the umbilicus, and third in the midline midway between the xiphoid and the umbilicus. The camera is positioned at the umbilical port. The surgery is performed through the other ports. Carbon dioxide is introduced into the abdominal cavity. This allows for mobilization of the abdominal wall away from the organs to provide more operating space. The kidney, ureter, and vessels are separated and excised, and the kidney is removed through an incision just above the symphysis pubis. The procedure takes approximately 4 hours. Laparoscopic donor nephrectomy has been shown to decrease postoperative morbidity, cause less pain, provide a better cosmetic result, shorter hospital stay, and earlier return to work.

16. How is the recipient kidney transplant approached?

Transplanted kidneys are typically placed extraperitoneally in the iliac fossa in adults. This placement of the kidney provides close location of the graft to the vessels and bladder, and the ability to assess the graft posttransplant in the event a biopsy or surgical intervention are necessary. An oblique incision is made from the midline symphysis pubis, curving laterally and superiorly to the iliac crest. The anastomosis between donor and recipient are made in the following order: renal artery, renal vein, external iliac vein, and ureter. Circumstances that alter this procedure might include previous transplants, size mismatch between donor and recipient, pediatric recipients requiring intraperitoneal placement of the kidney, and/or multiple donor renal arteries. In some cases, the recipient is required to undergo a bilateral native nephrectomy prior to transplant. These cases might include, severe polyuria or electrolyte wasting, uncontrollable hypertension, severe proteinuria, recurrent pyelonephritis, and large cysts secondary to polycystic kidney disease to minimize the risk of infection.

17. What are the common complications post-kidney transplant?

Complications can be classified as the adverse side effects of immunosuppressive therapy, acute tubular necrosis, rejection, infection, and technical problems related to the surgery. Surgical complications are further categorized as vascular, urologic, lymphatic, and wound issues.

- Acute tubular necrosis (ATN) is a reversible condition lasting a few days to weeks. It is caused by alterations in the donor kidney due to oxygen interruption during renal procurement, prolonged cold or warm ischemic, preservation time, or handling. Cold ischemia time is the length of time the kidney is preserved on ice, if greater than 24 hours there is an increased risk of ATN. Warm ischemic time is defined as the length of time between cessation of renal circulation to adequate hypothermia in the donor organ. There are two types of ATN, oliguric and

nonoliguria. Oliguric ATN is characterized by prolonged oliguria or anuria lasting several days to 2 months. Nonoliguric or high-output ATN is characterized by a normal or greater than normal urine output with inadequate excretion of nitrogenous waste products. Both types present with an elevation in BUN and serum creatinine and electrolyte disorders. A renal scan may be performed to evaluate the presence of ATN; if present, there will be decreased uptake and excretion of the isotope. Renal biopsy histologically reveals tubular epithelial cell necrosis, mild edema, congestion, and inflammatory cell infiltration. Management strategies include judicious monitoring of fluids and electrolytes. Supportive dialysis may be temporarily needed during the early postoperative period.

- Rejection is one of major problems post-kidney transplantation. Although there have been major advancements in histocompatibility testing, immune modulating techniques, and immunosuppressive therapy, rejection continues to be problematic. The basic types of rejection are hyperacute, acute humoral antibody mediated, acute cellular, and chronic. A brief explanation of each is outlined.

- Hyperacute rejection occurs minutes to 24 hours after transplantation. Clinical manifestations are an immediate decrease in renal function, with a cessation of urine output. Intraoperatively, the kidney appears swollen, mottled, and cyanotic. Hyperacute rejection is caused by the presensitization of the recipient to the donor's class I human leukocyte antigens (HLA). The pathogenesis is an allograft specific coagulopathy initiated by preformed anti-donor HLA antigens on the vascular endothelium and platelets. Diagnosis is made by evaluation of the clinical manifestations, a renal scan that demonstrates lack of uptake or excretion by the allograft and/or surgical exploration. Histologic examination shows a diffuse intravascular coagulation in the glomerular capillaries and renal arterioles. Nonexistence of preformed HLA antibodies significantly reduces the risk of hyperacute rejection and humoral rejection episodes. Management and prognosis of hyperacute rejection is very poor and transplant nephrectomy is almost always required.

- Humoral antibody-mediated acute rejection usually develops 1 to 3 months posttransplant. Clinical manifestations include a brisk rise in serum creatinine and BUN, possible decline in urine output and hypertension. In some cases, patients may also present with fever, malaise, weight gain, and mild graft swelling and tenderness. The pathogenesis is based on the recipient's development of donor-reactive anti-HLA antibodies and maybe non-HLA antibodies. Diagnosis of humoral-antibody mediated rejection is usually based on laboratory data, radiologic findings, and renal biopsy (gold standard). Management of acute rejection involves close monitoring of renal function, aggressive treatment with immunosuppressive therapy based on center protocol and provider, degree of renal involvement, and the patient's response to therapy.

- Acute cellular rejection generally develops within the first 6 to12 months post-kidney transplant. Clinical manifestations include, a gradual increase in serum creatinine and BUN, and increasing hypertension, without a noticeable decline in urine output. The pathogenesis of acute cellular rejection involves a delayed type hypersensitivity reaction and activation of cytotoxic CD8+ T lymphocytes and a number of soluble mediators such as cytokines, lymphokines, chemokines, vasoactive substances, and growth factors. Diagnosis is made based on laboratory findings and renal biopsy. Treatment typically involves augmentation of immunosuppressive therapy.

- Chronic rejection usually occurs months to years after kidney transplant. Chronic rejection has an insidious onset with a slow rise in serum creatinine, increasing proteinuria, and hypertension. It is typically unresponsive to an increase in immunosuppressive therapy and often presents as a relentless downward trajectory in renal function. Clinical manifestations are highly variable depending on the degree of renal function. Patients often experience proteinuria secondary to increasing glomerular permeability, increasing BUN and creatinine, decline in urine output, fluid retention, alteration in electrolytes, and an increase in renin production resulting in hypertension. The pathogenesis of chronic rejection includes both immunologic (HLA mismatch, early rejection episodes, and late rejection episode) and nonimmunologic factors (ischemia injury, nephrotoxic drugs, viruses, hypertension, and hyperlipidemia). Renal biopsy is the most definitive method of diagnosing chronic rejection. Treatment of chronic rejection focuses on graft preservation and delaying retransplantation or dialysis. Management of chronic rejection is similar to progressive end-stage renal disease involving changes in medication and diet, fluid restriction, monitoring of electrolytes, blood pressure control, help in maintaining activity level, education, and support. In some cases, a transplant nephrectomy may be indicated for chronic symptoms, infection, or severe reflux nephropathy.

- Infection is a common complication posttransplant. Factors that predispose patients to infection include administration of immunosuppressive medications, preexisting uremia, systemic disease (e. g., diabetes, systemic lupus erythematosus [SLE], or malnutrition), alterations in the host's defense, the surgical procedure (break in the skin, the first line of defense), invasive lines, catheters, and intubation. Wound and urinary tract infections (UTIs) are the most common bacterial infections postrenal transplant. The clinical presentation of a UTI often includes one or more of the following: fever, tachycardia, tachypnea, chills, suprapubic or lower back pain, burning on urination, bladder spasms, frequency, urgency, hesitancy, incontinence, nocturia, hematuria, pyuria, cloudy, foul smelling urine, nausea, and diarrhea (more common in infants). Diagnosis is typically based on a complete blood count with differential, urinalysis, and urine for culture and sensitivity, although other tests may be ordered. The results of the urinalysis demonstrates bacteria, pus, red blood cells (RBCs), white blood cells (WBCs), casts, and an increased urinary pH. A complete blood count reveals an elevated WBC with a shift to the left. Blood cultures should be performed if there is a suspected bacteremia. Treatment includes systemic antibiotics, augmentation of fluids, antipyretics, analgesics, and, in some situations, antibiotic bladder irrigations if the catheter remains in place for 14 to 21 days.

- Renal artery thrombosis (RAT) is complete blockage of arterial flow to the kidney. RAT is a serious early complication that results in graft infarction and failure. The initial clinical finding is usually abrupt anuria suggesting a lack of blood supply to the graft. There is also accompanying elevation in BUN and creatinine, tenderness over the graft, and increasing edema of the thigh and leg on transplant side. Diagnosis of renal artery thrombosis is suspected with a sudden decrease in urine output particularly during the early postoperative period. A missed diagnosis of renal artery thrombosis usually results in graft loss and transplant nephrectomy. Diagnosis is made by emergent Doppler ultrasound. Findings demonstrate lack of flow to the transplanted graft. Management includes emergent surgical exploration and revision of the vascular anastomosis. In circumstances where the thrombosis cannot be corrected, a transplant nephrectomy is usually indicated.

- Renal artery stenosis (RAS) usually occurs at the site of the anastomosis secondary to vessel size mismatch, torsion of the renal artery, or intimal damage during procurement, preservation, or transplantation. RAS is manifested by uncontrolled hypertension, increased serum BUN and creatinine, and an arterial bruit over the renal allograft or femoral artery close to the inguinal ligament. Hypertension is the result of hypoperfusion to the graft stimulating renin production and augmenting the renin-angiotensinogen mechanism. Diagnosis is based on Doppler examination and renal angiography. Depending on the degree of the stenosis, treatment may be based on medical managed, percutaneous transluminal renal angioplasty, or surgical revascularization.

- Renal vein thrombosis (RVT) is caused by an irregular intimal surface of the vessel, intimal damage during procurement, preservation or transplantation, or a mechanical occlusion of the donor vein. It results in an embolus, usually in the renal vein and occasionally in the iliac vein. Clinical findings include declining renal function, proteinuria, hematuria, and graft enlargement. In some situations, iliac flow will be altered, causing engorgement ipsilaterally on the affected side. Diagnosis is made by venography showing no outflow of the radioisotope from the graft. Management concentrates on systemic anticoagulation and early surgical intervention with anastomotic revision. In severe cases, nephrectomy may be indicated if damage is extensive.

- Graft rupture (GR) is rare. It typically occurs within 2 weeks of surgery. The etiology of graft rupture includes acute rejection with accompanying extensive swelling, renal biopsy, ischemic damage during procurement, urinary obstruction, emboli, lymphatic occlusion, or trauma. Clinical findings consist of pain and edema over the graft, abdominal swelling and tenderness, bleeding at incisional site, oliguria, increased BUN and creatinine, hypotension, tachycardia, cool and clammy skin, and mental status changes. Close monitoring is imperative to prevent the risk of vascular collapse secondary to blood loss and shock. Diagnosis is based on clinical features and confirmed by ultrasonography, computerized tomography (CT) scan, or surgical exploration. Management mandates emergent surgical intervention. Attempts are made to repair the kidney; however, in most circumstances, a transplant nephrectomy is necessary.

- Urologic complications primarily encompass urinary leaks, fistulas, and obstruction. Damage to the donor ureter during the donor nephrectomy procedure is the most common cause of urinary extravasation or fistula post-transplant. It results in injury to the donor ureteral blood supply causing ischemic necrosis of the donor ureter. Other contributing factors include insufficient closure of the cystotomy and preexisting bladder abnormalities. Patients at higher risk for urologic complications are those with small contracted dysfunctional bladders who have a history of multiple urologic procedures, some with urinary diversion and insulin-dependent diabetics. Clinical findings typically develop within 5 weeks of transplant. Clinical manifestations of a ureteral extravasation or fistula are decreased urine output, pain and swelling over the graft, fever, elevation in serum BUN and creatinine, and cutaneous and urinary drainage over the surgical incision site. Diagnosis is made primarily by clinical features and ultrasonography revealing a peri-ureteral fluid collection or hydronephrosis. Management strategies to minimize the risk of bladder extravasation are meticulous attention to the bladder anastomosis during the transplant procedure, decompression of the bladder with a Foley catheter (monitor for kinks), and the avoidance of bladder overdistention. Placement of a ureteral stent is often indicated in patients undergoing surgical reanastomosis. Surgical reconstruction depends on the status of the ureter. Extensive necrosis of the ureter usually requires an alternate surgical approach.

- Ureteral obstruction is an uncommon early complication that is often caused by a tight submucosal tunnel of the ureter into the bladder or torsion or the ureter. If it occurs later, it is usually the result of ureteral ischemic secondary to inadequate blood supply to the distal ureter. Lymphocele is the most common cause of extrinsic ureteral obstruction. Clinical findings present with a decreased in urine output, rise in serum BUN and creatinine, local pain, with impending signs of sepsis. Accompanying symptoms might include abdominal tenderness or pain and urinary leakage along the suture line. Diagnosis is made by radioisotope renal scan or ultrasonography, which reveals marked narrowing at the stenotic or obstructed area and dilation of the ureter above the stenosis, with varying degrees of hydronephrosis. Management strategies often involve external drainage or a percutaneous stent placed anterograde or cystoscopically. In some cases, surgical reconstruction is required for ureteral obstruction.

- A lymphocele is the collection of extraperitoneal fluid in the transplant fossa secondary to a leak of lymphatic fluid. It is the consequence of insufficient ligation of the lymphatics during surgery. Clinical findings vary depending on their location. Small lymphoceles can be completely asymptomatic. However, large lymphoceles can cause compression on the ureter, resulting in a deterioration in renal function and hydronephrosis. In general, clinical manifestations include increased BUN and creatinine, decreasing urine output, mild lower abdominal pain, and genital and/or ipsilateral edema of the extremity on the effected side. In severe cases, the lymphocele may compress the transplanted ureter or iliac vein resulting in bladder extravasation or extreme ipsilateral edema of the extremity on the affected side. Diagnosis is confirmed by the observance of a lymphatic fluid collection easily detected on ultrasound or computerized tomography. Management strategies vary depending on the size of the lympocele. Small nonobstructive asymptomatic lymphocele may involve serial observation with ultrasonography and monitoring renal function. Larger symptomatic lymphoceles are often treated with external puncture and percutaneous drainage or surgical intervention with fluid evacuation and internal marsupialization of the lymphocele cavity into the peritoneal

cavity to allow for subsequent drainage of the fluid.

18. What are the important monitoring considerations post-kidney transplant?

The immediate postoperative considerations include airway management and successful extubation, optimizing hemodynamic parameters, pain management, and monitoring fluid status to ensure graft perfusion and graft function. A complete blood count, chemistry profile, coagulation studies, electrocardiogram, and chest x-ray are also regularly obtained. Ongoing assessment of volume status is vital to avoid volume overload or depletion. Initially, posttransplant there is large diuresis usually resulting from a high osmotic load secondary to pretransplant uremic, elevated glucose levels often caused by steroids, intravenous fluids, diabetes, and intraoperative fluids administration. Fluid replacement is given to match urine output and diuretics are administered to secure continued diuresis. In patients who do not respond to therapy, ATN should be suspected. Overhydration can lead to congestive heart failure, pulmonary edema, promote electrolyte disturbances, or contribute to hypertension. In an effort to enhance gas exchange, management strategies for overhydration often include oxygen, nitroglycerin as precardiac load reducer, and morphine sulfate to relieve pain. If treatment is unsuccessful, emergent hemodialysis is necessary. Inadequate fluid replacement can progress to oliguria and impaired renal function. Dehydration can cause a reduction in renal perfusion and subsequent graft damage.

Renal function requires diligent monitoring and is confirmed by the immediate and continued flow of urine, decline in serum BUN and creatinine, and the stabilization of electrolytes. Abrupt cessation of urine output must be immediately evaluated. Urinary obstruction can result in allograft failure; therefore, it is imperative that the bladder remain decompressed and the urinary catheter remains free of clots. Obstructive ureteral problems are related to a variety of causes and may be as simple as a kink in the catheter. Blood clots are the most common cause of catheter occlusion and diminishing urine output in the early postoperative period. If aseptic irrigation is unsuccessful in removing the clots, the catheter should be replaced after consulting with the surgeon. If urine flow is not reestablished, bladder distention and pressure on the ureteral anastomosis may result in a leak. Decreased urine flow may also suggest ATN, rejection, technical complications (e. g., anastomotic collapse), decrease in circulating volume, or obstruction (e. g., vascular thrombus, ureteral stenosis). If other clinical manifestations of hypovolemia are present, such as hypotension, a fluid bolus is often administered to improve renal perfusion and urine output. Depending on the type of anastomosis, the urinary catheter is typically left in place for 2 to 5 days. This allows close monitoring of urinary flow, urine characteristics, and bladder decompression. Bladder spasms may develop, causing pain. Treatment varies between centers and providers but may include belladonna and opium suppositories (B & O), oxybutynin chloride (Ditropan), and propantheline bromide (Pro-Banthine). To allow for complete bladder emptying, treatment of bladder spasms should be stopped 24 hours before the catheter is removed.

Electrolytes are monitored closely. Patients with potential electrolyte disturbances typically undergo EKG monitoring. Hypocalcemia and hypomagnesemia are not uncommon in the presence of a brisk diuresis. Hyperkalemia is anticipated when urine output is low, and may be observed in the presence of ATN or acute rejection. Other factors that can cause hyperkalemia include administration of potassium, blood transfusions, and surgery, resulting in cell damage, causing the release of intracellular potassium ions to the extracellular space, administration of calcineurin inhibitors, and the presence of acidosis or hyperglycemia, contributing to ionic shifts. Hyperkalemia is initially treated with diuretics. However, if potassium levels are greater than 6.5 mEq/L, other forms of therapy should be implemented, such as hemodialysis. Hypokalemia is usually the result of massive diuresis, excessive use of diuretics, large gastrointestinal losses, or lack of appropriate potassium replacement. Hypokalemia is treated promptly with intravenous potassium replacement, EKG monitoring, and accurate measurement of gastrointestinal losses, which are high in potassium. Hyperglycemia is often associated with the initial high doses of corticosteroids on glucose metabolism, use of tacrolimus, exacerbation of preexisting diabetes mellitus, familial tendency toward diabetes, or the administration of large volumes of dextrose-containing intravenous fluids. Clinical manifestation of hyperglycemia include polydipsia, polyuria, glycosuria, weakness, fatigue, headache, blurred vision, nausea, vomiting, and abdominal cramps. Polyuria is the result of an osmotic diuresis caused by hyperglycemia, which can lead to dehydration. Dehydration causes decrease perfusion to the newly transplanted kidney and can result in damage. Thus, glucose monitoring is imperative to minimize the secondary risks of dehydration.

There are a number of cardiovascular disorders associated with end-stage renal disease, hypertension, atherosclerosis, left ventricular hypertrophy and dysfunction, and/or a history of pericarditis or pericardial effusion. Blood pressure monitoring is performed hourly or more frequently to ensure optimum cardiovascular function. Postoperative hypertension is often related to preexisting disease, volume overload, medications, or renal artery stenosis and is routinely treated with diuretics and antihypertensive agents. Hypertension caused by renal arterial stenosis usually requires surgical intervention and reanastomosis of the affected vessels. Hypotension is usually the result of volume depletion or occurs in response to one of the medications. It subsequently leads to decreased renal perfusion and exacerbation of ATN if present. A single hypotensive episode can also result in collapse of the patient's arteriovenous (AV) hemodialysis vascular access. Aspects of preserving the patient's dialysis vascular access include frequent monitoring for a bruit and thrill, and protection of the involved extremity by eliminating cuff pressures, blood draws, and intravenous line placements. During the surgical procedure, the kidney is anastomosed to the iliac vessels. A vascular thrombosis of these vessels can occur, causing decrease perfusion to the effected extremity. Frequent assessment of femoral, popliteal, and pedal pulses will allow for early detection and prompt intervention of this problem.

Respiratory problems posttransplant often develop secondary to preexisting disease, history of smoking, pulmonary edema secondary to volume overload, atelectasis, and pulmonary infiltrates secondary to infection. Methods of ensuring adequate oxygenation and maintenance of pulmonary function include pain management, deep breathing, use of respiratory devices, early mobilization, oxygen therapy if indicated, and regular assessment of breath sounds, respiratory rate and effort, sputum, oxygen saturation, and patient color. If there is a change in pulmonary function, arterial blood gases and chest radiography are ordered to evaluate respiratory status. If pulmonary edema or infiltrates are observed on chest radiography, diuretic therapy is typically the first line of therapy.

19. What are the typical immunosuppressive medications used posttransplant?

The goals of immunosuppressive therapy are to optimize patient and graft survival, decrease the risk for rejection, minimize the risk for infection, reduce drug toxicities and side effects, minimize the risk malignancy, reduce cost, and enhance compliance. How these medications are prescribed is dependent on the type of transplant, patient response, center, and provider. Typically, one medication from each class of drug is given to minimize the risk of side effects. Medications used posttransplant typically include corticosteroids, a calcineurin inhibitor, and an antiproliferative agent. Additional medications, such as antilymphocyte antibodies and interleukin (IL) 2-receptor antagonists, may also be used. The action of these drugs is briefly outlined. Corticosteroids (methylprednisolone [Solu-Medrol], prednisone, and prednisolone) cause a rapid decrease in circulating T lymphocytes, inhibit production of IL-1, decrease the production of IL-2 and interferon-gamma, and inhibit the production of inflammatory mediators. Calcineurin inhibitors include cyclosporine (CSA) and tacrolimus (Prograf). In general, these drugs inhibit T-cell activation and proliferation, prevent the release of gamma interferon, and B-cell activating factors. Antiproliferative agents include azathioprine, cyclophosphamide, mycophenolate mofetil (Cell-Cept) and sirolimus (Rapamune). These drugs work through different pathways to prevent mitosis and proliferation of cells—specifically, T and B lymphocytes. Antilymphocyte preparations include both polyclonal and monoclonal antibodies. Polyclonal preparations include antithymocyte globulin, equine (Atgam [ATG]) and antithymocyte globulin, rabbit (Thymoglobulin [rATG]). Antithymocyte globulin is a polyclonal IgG antibody preparation derived from the hyperimmune serum of horses or rabbits who have been immunized with human thymus lymphocytes. It is used as a lymphocyte selective immunosuppressant to reduce the number of circulating thymus-dependent lymphocytes. The antilymphocyte effect is thought to reflect an alteration in the function of T lymphocytes, which are responsible for cell-mediated immunity and humoral immunity. Muromonab-CD3, Orthoclone (OKT3) is a monoclonal antibody to the CD3 antigen of human T lymphocytes. It blocks the function of the CD3 molecule on the T-cell membrane, rendering it ineffective. This action inhibits antigen recognition by T cells. The inhibited lymphocytes are eliminated from the circulation by the reticuloendothelial system. Patients receiving antibody preparations are typically premedicated with acetaminophen, diphenhydramine, and Solu-Medrol and are closely monitored for serious adverse events. IL-2 receptor antagonists include basiliximab (Simulect) and daclizumab (Zenapax), which are monoclonal antibodies that act as IL-2 receptor agonists. They block IL-2 receptors sites on

activated T cells and subsequently prevent proliferation of T-cell activity. Daclizumab is humanized (90% human and 10% murine) and basiliximab is chimeric (70% human and 30% murine).

20. What medications are used to minimize the potential side effects of the immunosuppressive medications typically administered posttransplant?

Prevention and treatment of opportunistic infections related to immunosuppressive therapy include antibiotic, antiviral, and antifungal prophylaxis. Most patients receive antibiotics intraoperatively and early postoperatively to minimize the risk of a bacterial infection. Antiviral treatment is usually comprised of either valganciclovir (Valcyte), ganciclovir, or acyclovir and is focused on the prevention of cytomegalovirus (CMV) and herpetic viruses. Antifungal therapy focuses on the prevention of pneumocystic carinii pneumonia (PCP) and oral/perianal candidiasis. PCP prophylaxis typically includes treatment with biweekly trimethoprim/sulfamethoxazole (Septra/Bactrim), daily Dapsone, or monthly inhaled pentamidine. Mucocutaneous candida prevention includes one of the following: Fluconazole once a week or oral Nystatin, which is swished and swallowed four times a day (often used in infants and children). It is not uncommon for patients to receive a protein pump inhibitor (PPI) such as omeprazole (Prilosec) for gastric protection, baby aspirin to minimize platelet aggregation in an effort to ensure vascular flow, antihypertensive therapy, and electrolyte supplementation. As immunosuppressive therapy is tapered, these medications will also be tapered and or discontinued depending on the center, provider, organ transplanted, and the patient's clinical status and response to treatment.

BIBLIOGRAPHY

Bennett, J., & Bromley, P. (2006). Perioperative issues in pediatric liver transplant. *International Anesthesiology Clinics*, 44(3), 125–127.

Berrocal, T., Parron, M., Alvarez-Lupque, A., Prieto, C., & Santamaria, M. L. (2006). Pediatric liver transplant a pictoral essay of early and late complications. *Radiographics*, 26(4), 1187–1209.

Bucuvalas, J. C., & Alonso, E. (2008). Long-term outcomes after liver transplant in children. *Current opinions in Organ Transplant*, 13(3), 247–251.

Cheung, C. Y., Chan, H. W., Liu, Y. L., Chau, K. F., & Li, C. S. (2009). Long-term graft failure with tacrolimus and cyclosporine in renal transplant paired kidney analysis. *Nephrology*, 14(8), 758–763.

Collins, A. J., Foley, R. N., Herzog, C., Chavers, B. M., Gilbertson, D., Ishani, A., et al. (2010). Excerpts from the US renal data system 2009 annual data report. *American Journal of Kidney Disease*, 55(Suppl 1), S1–420.

Danovitch, G. M. (2010). *Handbook of kidney transplantation* (5th ed.). Philadelphia: Wolters Kluwer, Lippincott, Williams & Wilkins.

Feng, S. (2008). Long-term management of immunosuppressive therapy in pediatric liver transplant; is minimization or withdrawal desirable or possible or both? *Current Opinions in Organ Transplant, 13*(5), 506–512.

Fisher, R. A., Cotterell, A. H., Maluf, D. G., Stravitz, R. T., Ashworth, A., Nakatsuka, M., et al. (2009). Adult liver donor versus deceased donor liver transplant: A 10 year prospective single center experience. *Annals of Hepatology, 8*(4), 298–307.

Fraser, S. M, Rajasundaram, R., Aldouri, A., Farid, S., Morris-Stiff, G., Baker, R., et al. (2010). Acceptable outcome after kidney transplant using "expanded criteria donor" grafts. *Transplantation, 89*(1), 88–96.

Hedegard, W., Saad, W. E., & Davies, M. G. (2009). Management of vascular and nonvascular complications after renal transplant. *Techniques in Vascular and Interventional Radiology, 12*(4), 240–262.

Jaskowski-Phillips, S., McGhee, B., & Reyes, J. (2003). *Pediatric liver, intestine and multivisceral transplantation: A manual of management and patient care.* Hudson, OH: LexiComp.

Kim, J. Y., Akalin, E., Dikman, S., Gagliararid, R., Schiano, T., Bromber, J., et al. (2010). The variable pathology of kidney disease post liver transplant. *Transplantation, 89*(2), 215–221.

Knight, E. R., & Morris, P. J. (2010). Steroid avoidance or withdrawal after renal transplant increases the risk of acute rejection but decreases cardiovascular risk; a meta analysis. *Transplantation, 89*(1), 1–14.

Lankarani, M. M., Assari S., & Nourbala, M. H. (2009). Improvement of renal transplant outcomes through matching donor and recipients. *Annals of Transplantation, 14*(4), 47–51.

Lida, T., Ogura, Y., Oike, F., Hatano, E., Kaido, T., Egawa, H., et al. (2010). Surgery-related morbidity in living donors for liver transplant. *Transplantation, 89*(10), 1276–1282.

Lock, J. F., Schwabauer, E., Martus, P., Videv, N., Pratschke, J., Malinowski, M., et al. (2010). *Liver Transplant, 16*(2), 172–180.

Lopez-Benitez, R., Barragan-Campos, H. M., Richter, G. M., Sauer, P., Mehrabi, A., Fonouni, H., et al. (2009). Interventional radiologic procedures in the treatment of complications after liver transplant. *Clinical Transplant, 23*(21), 92–101.

Mendez National Institute of Transplantation. About. Retrieved from www.transplantation.com/

Mudge, C. L., Carlson, L., & Brennen, T. (2006) Transplantation. In A. Molzahn & E. Butera (Ed.), *Contemporary nephrology nursing.* Pitman, NJ: American Nephrology Nurses' Association.

Rastogi, A., & Nissenson, A. R. (2009). Technological advances in renal replacement therapy: five years and beyond. *Clinical Journal of the American Society of Nephrology, 4,* S132–S136.

Segev, D. L., Muzaale, A. D., Caffo, B. S., Mehat, S. H., Singer, A. L., Taranto, S. E., et al. (2010). Perioperative mortality and long term survival following live kidney donation. *Journal of the American Medical Association, 10*(303), 959–966.

Taylor, C. J., Kosmoliaptsis, V., Sharpler, L. D., Prezzi, D., Morgan, C. H., Key, T., et al. (2010). Ten-year experience of selection omission of pre-transplant cross match test in deceased donor kidney transplant. *Transplantation, 89*(2), 185–193.

Transplant Living. (2010). Information and resources just for you. Retrieved from www.transplantliving.org

United Network for Organ Sharing. (2010). Learn. Retrieved from http://www.unos.org

United States Renal Data System. (2010). USRDS. Retrieved from www.usrds.org

University of California San Francisco, Department of Surgery (2009). Kidney Transplant Housestaff Manual.

University of California San Francisco, Department of Surgery (2010). Liver Transplant Housestaff Manual.

U.S. Department of Health and Human Services. (2010). Organ procurement and transplant network. Retrieved from http://optn.transplant.hrsa.gov/

Yudkowitz, F. S., & Chietero, M. (2005). Anesthetic issues in pediatric transplant. *Pediatric Transplant, 9*(5), 666–672.

CHAPTER 35

Vascular Surgery

Deborah Tabulov, RN, CRNP

Vascular surgery is the specialty that treats problems in the extracranial carotid arteries, thoracoabdominal aorta, abdominal aorta, visceral arteries, renal arteries, and peripheral extremity arteries, typically treating occlusive, aneurysmal, stenotic, or thromboembolic disease in these vessels. Vascular surgery also treats venous disease. The discussion of all of the problems noted is beyond the scope of this chapter. Therefore, this will deal with some of the important basic concepts in dealing with postoperative vascular patients with common, life threatening, and less frequently seen vascular problems.

1. What are the essential components of a vascular examination?

The essential components of a vascular examination include taking a thorough history and performing a thorough physical examination. The examination includes auscultation of the heart noting rate rhythm and murmurs, auscultation of the lungs noting the appearance of the thorax and pectus deformities (carinatum, excavatum) that may indicate underlying vascular problems such as Marfan's syndrome. Blood pressure is taken in both arms unless there is an absolute contraindication such as the presence of a dialysis access. If blood pressure is unequal, it may signal a blockage in the subclavian artery or an aortic dissection. The presence or absence of the peripheral pulses is checked starting with the temporal pulses. A strong temporal pulse, palpated anterior to the ear, usually indicates a patent common and external carotid

artery. Next, note the quality of the carotid pulses by palpating at the lower part of the neck between the midline trachea and the anterior border of the sternocleidomastoid. There may be a palpable pulse if the internal carotid artery is occluded as long as the external carotid artery is patent. Look for pulsatile masses. A pulsation seen in the base of the right neck in persons with longstanding hypertension is often mistaken for an aneurysm. Next, auscultate over the carotid arteries for bruits and then listen over the infraclavicular and supraclavicular areas for bruits. Bruits are caused by turbulent flow and may indicate stenosis in the artery. Moving downward with the patient in a supine position, observe the abdominal wall for aortic pulsation then palpate the aorta (normally, the aorta is the width of the persons thumb), noting any tenderness. Auscultate for bruits over the aorta that may indicate mesenteric or renal artery stenosis. At the umbilicus, the aorta bifurcates; listen over the aorta, visceral renal, and iliac arteries for bruits; listen over the femoral arteries for bruits; assesses the lower extremities for quality of the femoral, popliteal, dorsalis pedis, and posterior tibial pulses; check the extremities for skin color, temperature, hair distribution, edema, sensation, movement, ulcerations, gangrene, or microembolic phenomenon. If the pulses are questionable, check for a Doppler signal.

2. What is carotid artery stenosis?

Carotid artery stenosis is atherosclerosis that occurs at the carotid bifurcation, bulb, or origin of the internal carotid artery. This accounts for 50–75% of embolic strokes in the carotid territory per year.

3. How is carotid artery stenosis found?

Most commonly, a bruit is assessed during examination by the healthcare professional. Bruits suggest turbulent flow through a stenotic or tortuous vessel. Carotid bruits are best heard with the bell of the stethoscope over the anterior border of the scalene muscle midway between the clavicle and mastoid process. The intensity of the bruit is not an accurate predictor of the degree of stenosis. Bruits occur in 2–5% of the elderly population and are known to increase stroke risk. Approximately 25% of those with a carotid bruit will have a significant stenosis.

4. What is a Hollenhorst plaque?

A Hollenhorst plaque, seen by an ophthalmologist, is a cholesterol embolus from atherosclerotic disease in the carotid or innominate arteries that occludes a retinal or branch artery. It may be asymptomatic or cause transient monocular blindness called amaurosis fugax, which is often described as a shade dropping over the eye that lasts seconds to minutes. It is considered a stroke equivalent and occurs on the same side as the stenosis.

5. What other symptoms may be observed?

If carotid stenosis is symptomatic transient ischemic attacks (TIAs) or cerebrovascular accident (CVA) with any combination of symptoms of hemiparesis, paralysis dysarthria, dysphagia, aphasia, and facial droop may be seen.

6. What testing is done for both asymptomatic and symptomatic carotid artery stenosis?

Carotid duplex, a low risk, noninvasive, accurate, safe, and cost-efficient test, is most often ordered. It images the extracranial carotid arteries and measures blood flow velocity across a stenotic area. The blood flows more rapidly through a stenotic area, and degree of stenosis is then quantified. Plaque characteristics are seen with carotid imaging.

7. What other tests can be done?

Magnetic resonance angiography (MRA) is often ordered. It gives information about the aortic arch and arch anatomy but often overestimates the degree of stenosis. This test requires administration of gadolinium. People with metallic implants, implantable cardioverter defibrillators (ICD) and pacemakers are not candidates. It is difficult for people with claustrophobia, respiratory, cardiac, and back problems due to length of time required to be immobile in a supine position. This procedure is moderately expensive compared to ultrasound and computerized axial tomography (CAT) scan.

Angiography is still considered as the gold standard. However, it is infrequently done as it carries an estimated 1–3% risk of stroke, requires dye, which is nephrotoxic, and is expensive.

8. What is the treatment?

Treatment depends on the degree of stenosis and symptomatology. If the stenosis is less than 69% and asymptomatic, it can be managed with best medical therapy, which includes antiplatelet therapy, antilipid therapy, beta-blockade, and smoking cessation.

If the stenosis is significant, more than 70%, and the patient is a good candidate or there are symptoms of cerebrovascular insufficiency, then, operation such as carotid endarterectomy (CEA) or carotid angioplasty and stenting (CAS) may be considered.

If a carotid artery is occluded, there is no surgical corrective treatment. These patients are given best medical therapy and monitored closely for contralateral carotid disease.

The decision to operate is based on patient symptomatology, operative risk, comorbidities, and benefit, which is stroke-free survival. The results of several clinical trials are considered.

North American Carotid Endarterectomy Trial (NASCET) and the Asymptomatic Carotid Atherosclerosis Study (ACAS) are the two major studies that demonstrated the efficacy of CEA in patients with symptomatic and asymptomatic high-grade carotid stenosis in stroke prevention over best medical therapy.

9. What are the surgical treatments?

CEA is an open operation done since the 1950s and is still considered the gold standard in treating carotid stenosis. It carries a 1–2% risk of stroke and/or death. Most commonly, it is done under general anesthesia, but may be done under local or regional anesthesia. Some surgeons will order intraoperative EEG monitoring. Use of an intraoperative shunt to supply blood flow during the clamping of the internal carotid artery is used to decrease ischemia. Patch angioplasty using a Dacron patch to close the endarterectomy site can be used to decrease the incidence of restenosis.

Anesthesia is reversed in the operating room (OR), where the patient is checked for any indication of neurologic deficit (e.g., difficulty waking from anesthesia, aphasia, clumsiness of movement, or paralysis of the contralateral side). If any of these exist, a Doppler exam followed by immediate reoperation is performed, as it is assumed that thromboembolism from the endarterectomy site or residual plaque may be the culprit. Delay beyond even 1 hour decreases the chance of successful reoperation.

A diffuse neurologic deficit is caused by intraoperative hypotension, causing a watershed infarct. Postoperative stroke occurring within the first 24 hours is presumed to be embolic. CT scan is not helpful and delays the reoperation treatment. If symptoms develop after the first 24 hours, a CT scan is done to rule out intracranial bleeding. Postoperatively, patients are admitted to a critical care unit for overnight monitoring. Most patients are discharged on the first or second postoperative day.

10. What are the unique postoperative nursing care needs after CEA?

Neurologic checks done frequently according to policy should include arousability, orientation, strength of hand grasp, shoulder shrug, fluency of speech, position of the tongue (which should be midline), and facial symmetry at rest and with movement is critical. Cranial nerves may be injured during surgery causing hoarseness and voice fatigue; these deficits are usually transient.

Monitor the drain output. A Jackson Pratt or other drain may be inserted postoperatively, and any increase in output should be reported promptly, as it indicates bleeding in the operative area requiring return to the OR.

Monitor the operative site for neck swelling and hematoma. Approximately, 2–5% of patients undergoing CEA will develop a hematoma. A large hematoma requires evacuation and control of bleeding sites. Dysphagia, change in voice, tracheal deviation, and stridor are late signs of bleeding at the operative site.

Low-molecular weight Dextran (LMD) is a glucose polymer that may be infused for the first 24 hours postoperatively to decrease platelet aggregation.

Control of hypertension is essential. If untreated, it can lead to postoperative stroke and/or myocardial infarction (MI). The systolic blood pressure is kept between 120 and 160 mm Hg. In a patient who has uncontrolled hypertension preoperatively, the upper limit is used to prevent hypoperfusion, leading to watershed infarction. Nipride and beta-blockers are commonly used. Apresoline (hydralazine) IV should be used with caution as it can produce sudden hypotension that could lead to a cerebral infarction.

Control tachycardia. If untreated, tachycardia can lead to myocardial ischemia and infarction. Use of perioperative beta blockade is commonly used. Causes of tachycardia include hypoxia, pain, and hypovolemia. This should be considered and treated appropriately.

The head of the bed should be elevated 30°–45°, which should decrease edema, improve venous return, and facilitate deep breathing.

Carotid angioplasty and stenting (CAS) is a newer treatment for carotid stenosis. It is a catheter-based procedure and requires use of a cerebral protection device to prevent embolization. Dye is used for visualization as CO_2 cannot be utilized in intracranial imaging. The catheter is usually inserted in the groin, then advanced through the aorta. If the aorta is atherosclerotic chances of embolization to the extremities, renal arteries, and viscera are increased. Clinical trials have been done, none of which demonstrate that carotid stenting is superior to CEA. In select patients (i.e., those with recurrent stenosis after CEA or in patients who have radiation to the neck), this may be a good option. The postoperative care is basically the same as for CEA. Additionally, the site used for vascular access needs to be monitored for swelling and bleeding. The extremity needs to be monitored for color, sensation, and movement.

11. What is an aneurysm?

An aneurysm is a localized dilatation of a vessel to 1.5 times or greater than the normal diameter of that particular vessel. It may occur in any vessel but is most common in the infrarenal abdominal aorta.

12. What is the incidence of aneurysms?

Aneurysms occur in approximately 5% of the population. Risk factors include being over the age of 65 years, male gender, hypertension, hyperlipidemia, PAD, atherosclerosis, smoking, chronic obstructive pulmonary disease (COPD), and a family history of aortic aneurysm. Of aneurysms, 90% are located in the infrarenal aorta (AAA) and 10% involve the descending and thoracoabdominal aorta (TAA). Many aneurysms are an incidental finding on the physical exam or diagnostic testing done for another problem because they are usually asymptomatic.

13. What are the etiologies of aneurysms?

The etiology of aneurysms is multifactorial and includes changes in the elastin and collagen makeup of the arterial walls causing degeneration, atherosclerosis, trauma, infection (rarely, syphilis) inflammatory processes (e.g., Takayasu's arteritis), and genetic and connective tissue disorders (e.g., Ehlers–Danlos syndrome type IV, Marfan's syndrome, Loewi's–Dietz syndrome).

14. How are aneurysms classified?

They are classified by appearance, saccular or fusiform; by location, ascending aorta, arch, descending thoracic (TAA), thoracoabdominal (TAAA), abdominal (AAA) (infrarenal, suprarenal, juxtarenal or by cause); inflammatory; degenerative (atherosclerotic); traumatic; and infectious (mycotic).

15. What are the treatment considerations?

- Risk of rupture is dependent on size. For example, if smaller than 4 cm, risk is 0%; at 4 to 5 cm, 3 5% per year; 6 to 7 cm, 10–20%; and 8 cm, 30–50% per year. In general, the threshold for repair of a TAA is 6 cm and 5.5 cm for an AAA. It is not common for an AAA smaller than 5 cm to rupture, but if the patient is female, has Marfan's syndrome, a chronic dissection, or the aneurysm is growing rapidly; and is greater than 5 mm per year, the repair may be done at a smaller size.

- Proximal extent of the aneurysm is an important prognostic and treatment feature. Operative morbidity and mortality increase the more proximal the aorta has to be clamped, as more organs are ischemic, the higher the clamp.

- Presence of comorbidities such as cardiac disease, pulmonary disease, or renal insufficiency make postoperative management challenging.

- There is a limited life expectancy due to advanced cancer or dementia.

16. What are factors that increase the risk of aneurysm rupture?

Factors include being a smoker, having COPD, rapid expansion of the aneurysm over 1 cm/yr, poorly controlled hypertension, and eccentric shape of an aneurysm.

17. How are aneurysms repaired?

Aneurysms can be repaired using a traditional open approach. The aneurysm sac is opened and a prosthetic graft is sewn to the normal aorta proximally and distally. The aneurysm sac is then closed over the prosthetic graft to protect it from infection and erosion into the bowel.

Endovascular approach utilizes a stent graft consisting of fabric covering metal supports, which then attaches to aorta by fixation devices. The stent graft directs blood flow through it, thereby taking pressure off the aortic wall. The aneurysm is still there, but is said to be excluded. Many companies now produce these stent grafts. Which graft is used often depends on the operator's preference and/or the patient's anatomy.

18. What are the advantages and disadvantages of open repair?

Advantages include good exposure, the aneurysm is destroyed, it is a durable procedure, use of a left retroperitoneal approach may decrease pulmonary problems, and ileus and mobility problems. Disadvantages include increased early mortality, longer hospital stay, and prolonged recovery time when compared to stent graft.

19. What are the complications of open repair?

Complications of open repair include death, myocardial infarction (MI), cerebrovascular accident (CVA), infection, bleeding, distal embolization, deep vein thrombosis (DVT), kidney failure, ischemic colitis, paraparesis/paralysis for TAA and TAAA repair, abdominal compartment syndrome, graft infection, aortoenteric fistula, anastomotic aneurysm, and sexual dysfunction (e.g., retrograde ejaculation).

20. What are the advantages and disadvantages of endovascular aortic aneurysm repair (EVAR) and thoracic aortic aneurysm repair (TEVAR)?

Advantages include shorter hospital stays, decreased early mortality, and is minimally invasive (when compared to open repair). Disadvantages include the cost of the stent grafts; costs associated with follow-up; the aneurysm is excluded but not gone, so the patient will require lifetime monitoring with MRA, CT scan, or ultrasound to check stent graft placement and monitor for aneurysm sac growth. A contraindication includes anatomy being unfavorable for stent repair either because of access, the site of the aneurysm, or its configuration.

21. What are the complications of endovascular repair?

Complications include but are not limited to access artery injury, such as dissection or rupture; microembolization to distal arteries, including the renals, which may lead to renal infarction and/or renal failure; the mesenteric arteries, causing ischemia or gangrene of the bowel and to the extremities; plaque embolization, causing blue toe syndrome, a painful condition affecting the toes causing color changes, blisters, skin loss, and gangrene. Other complications include groin hematoma, seroma, or lymphocele; groin incision infection; and or dehiscence.

Postimplant syndrome may occur in up to 50% of patients undergoing EVAR and is characterized by a fever up to 40°C, leukocytosis, general malaise, depression, and back pain due to thrombosis in the aneurysm sac.

Endoleak is a failure to exclude the aneurysm sac fully from the arterial circulation. If the sac remains pressurized, it may require additional interventions such as embolization or open repair. Endoleaks are classified as type I, at the attachment site; type II, retrograde into the sac via a lumbar artery or the IMA; type III, fabric tear; type IV, ooze through the fabric; and type V, endotension where the sac continues to be pressurized and grow but the endoleak cannot be found.

22. What are the unique nursing care needs in the postoperative period after aneurysm repair?

Maintain normothermia. Hypothermia during TAAA repair is thought to be protective for the spinal cord and for prevention of tissue ischemia. If the core temperature is below 36°C (96.8°F) postoperatively, it can result in coagulopathy due to increased blood viscosity and platelet dysfunction. Hypothermia can also cause myocardial ischemia, can affect drug distribution, and is a major risk factor for surgical site infection (SSI).

Ventilatory support is needed in most patients for at least for the first 24 to 48 hours after an open repair. Monitor O$_2$ saturation and peak inspiratory pressures. Wean the patient as soon as possible to prevent complications such as ventilator-acquired pneumonia (VAP) and barotrauma. Reintubation is associated with a higher incidence of morbidity and mortality.

Avoid hypotension. Identify the cause of the hypotension and treat it as quickly as possible to avoid complications such as MI and end organ damage due to malperfusion. There may be bleeding in the retroperitoneum or chest cavity, both require emergency reoperation. In the immediate postoperative period, these patients require large amounts of fluids, often vasopressors, as well as blood administration. Maintain mean arterial pressure (MAP) as ordered. After a TAA repair, MAP is monitored closely and is often kept at greater than 80 mm Hg. Hypotension can cause decreased spinal cord perfusion and may lead to temporary or permanent paralysis from spinal cord ischemia (SCI). Perioperative hypotension (MAP <70 mm Hg) was found to be a significant predictor of SCI. Therefore, careful monitoring and prompt correction of arterial pressure is essential in preventing the development of paraplegia.

Paralysis after a TAA repair decreases the 1 year survival rate to less than 50%. Preoperatively, a spinal drain is placed in patients undergoing both stent graft and open repair TAA to both avoid and treat this complication.

Frequent assessment of neurologic function, for at least every 2 hours, allows for early detection and prompt intervention. Check for any asymmetry in spontaneous movement of the upper and lower or between the right and left lower extremities. There is only a 2-hour window before irreversible damage occurs. Check spinal drain tubing for kinks and monitor drain function. If these changes occur, reduction of the CSF pressure by drainage fluid is useful.

Abdominal compartment syndrome should be considered in the presence of oliguria and hypotension that is not responsive to fluids or pressors, increased abdominal girth, and increased ventilatory requirements. Easily overlooked or mistaken for other events, such as hypovolemia, the clinician must consider and be alert to this possibility. In this set of patients, the increased intraabdominal pressure is the result of a prolonged operation and fluid resuscitation, resulting in edema of the abdominal organs, which then compress the inferior vena cava. This compression results in decreased preload and cardiac output, raised intrapleural pressure and decreased lung compliance resulting in hypoventilation, hypoxemia, hypercapnia, and acute onset of renal insufficiency. Decrease in cardiac output results in more injury/ischemia to the intraabdominal organs causing metabolic acidosis and rising lactate levels. A bladder pressure of over 20 to 30 mm Hg is diagnostic. Treatment is emergency decompression laparotomy. Once the abdomen is decompressed, the intraabdominal pressure returns to normal, and there is resolution of the previously mentioned signs. The abdomen is packed and closed secondarily in a staged manner.

23. What is an aortic dissection?

A dissection is a defect in the aortic wall, initiated by an intimal tear, which allows blood to flow in a channel called a false lumen, created between the intimal and medial layers of the vessel wall. It is most common in the 40- to 60-year-old age group and are more common in males (3:1) compared to females. Most of these patients have a history of severe hypertension, often not well controlled. There are also genetic defects that are associated with dissection. Dissection is distinct from aneurysm.

24. What factors predispose to aortic dissection?

The predisposing factors include hypertension, trauma, atherosclerosis, perforation of an aortic plaque or ulcer, aortic coarctation, Marfan's syndrome, and pregnancy, especially in the third trimester.

25. How are aortic dissections classified?

There are two widely used classification systems: DeBakey and Sanford. Both systems provide an anatomic description of the aortic dissection. De-Bakey categorizes the dissection based on where the original intimal tear is located and the extent of the dissection (localized to either the ascending aorta or descending aorta), or involves both the ascending and descending aorta. In the DeBakey system, a type I originates in the ascending aorta, propagates at least to the aortic arch, and often beyond it distally. Type II originates in and is confined to the ascending aorta. Type III originates in the descending aorta and rarely extends proximally, but will extend distally.

In the Stanford system, type A dissection involves the ascending aorta usually originating just above the aortic valve. Type B dissection only involves the descending aorta, usually originating just distal to the left subclavian artery.

26. What are the signs and symptoms of aortic dissection?

Usually, there is an abrupt onset of severe pain commonly described by the patient as tearing that is not controlled by narcotics. The patients are often hypertensive, but if there is an associated rupture, hypotension may be seen. Blood pressure and pulses in the extremities may be asymmetrical. Cardiac tamponade can occur with rupture, producing the classic triad of jugular venous distension (JVD), muffled heart sounds, and pulsus paradoxus. The pain often occurs in the chest, neck, and jaw for an ascending and in the back for a descending dissection. Acute congestive heart failure (CHF) may occur in ascending dissection because of aortic valve insufficiency, acute MI may occur if the dissection involves the coronary artery ostia, or stroke if it involves the arch vessels or if it extends to the carotid artery. Other signs and symptoms caused by the compression of adjacent structures from an expanding intramural hematoma may include Horner's syndrome (unilateral miosis, ptosis, anhydrosis) from compression of the brachial plexus; SVC syndrome (dilatation of the chest veins, edema of the face, neck and upper torso, orthopnea, change level of consciousness or syncope); compression of the left laryngeal nerve that causes hoarseness. If the trachea or bronchus is compressed, stridor and dyspnea may occur. Compression of the esophagus produces dysphagia.

Abdominal pain occurs because of the dissection itself or if the mesenteric vessels are involved and there is visceral ischemia. Signs include hypoactive bowel sounds, bloody stools, and an increasing lactate level. Renal involvement will cause increased serum creatinine.

Malperfusion of the extremities may produce the 5 Ps: pain, pallor, pulselessness, paresthesias, and, if not treated, paralysis.

Paralysis of the lower extremities without ischemic changes suggests spinal cord ischemia.

27. How is an aortic dissection diagnosed?

Chest x-rays may demonstrate widening of the mediastinum, leading to more definitive studies such as a CT scan and MRA. Angiography is used to determine the extent of the dissection and to determine and possibly correct visceral and peripheral compromise.

28. What is the treatment of a type B aortic dissection?

In an uncomplicated dissection (i.e., absence of organ or extremity malperfusion), medical management is preferred. Aggressive control of blood pressure (SBP 100–120 mm Hg) is the mainstay of treatment. Nipride is used in conjunction with beta-blockers reduces the heart rate, blood pressure, and, consequently, stress on the aortic wall. Avoid the use of diazoxide—a direct acting vasodilator that may cause hypotension, tachycardia, and CHF—and hydralazine, which increases wall stress.

If there is organ malperfusion, open surgery, percutaneous intervention (e.g., fenestration, stenting), or a combination of the therapies can be used to reestablish flow.

29. What is the treatment of type Stanford A/DeBakey I and II?

Emergent surgery is done to prevent death from cardiac tamponade or aortic regurgitation with heart failure and is done under circulatory arrest. The mortality is 1% to 3% per hour.

30. What are the types of mesenteric ischemia, its causes and treatments?

Acute mesenteric ischemia:

- Classically, the patient has severe generalized abdominal pain out of proportion to the abdominal exam (i.e., peritoneal signs are usually absent), nausea, vomiting, and diarrhea may occur, so bowel sounds may be present. There may be leukocytosis. If not recognized early as bowel ischemia worsens, fever, metabolic acidosis, bloody diarrhea, peritoneal signs, hypovolemia, and septic shock may occur at a later phase. The clinician needs to have a high suspicion for this diagnosis.

- Causes are embolism secondary to dysrhythmias (especially in elderly with atrial fibrillation), thrombosis, low-flow states (CHF or hypovolemia), and by penetrating or blunt traumas (e.g., seatbelt trauma).

- Diagnostic modalities include CT angiography to assess the vasculature and bowel for evidence of ischemia, perforation, or free air, and early angiography if indicated.

- Treatment includes emergency laparotomy, visceral bypass, resection of the ischemic bowel, fluid resuscitation, and anticoagulation.

Chronic mesenteric ischemia:

- Classically, the patient will present with complaints postprandial abdominal pain typically dull or crampy epigastric discomfort that occurs 30 minutes to 1 hour after eating and lasts about 4 hours (abdominal angina) and presents with early satiety. This leads to food fear and weight loss. An abdominal bruit may be heard on exam.

- Causes include atherosclerosis, extrinsic compression (pancreatic neoplasm), and median arcuate ligament compression syndrome (MALS) caused by compression of the celiac axis by the median arcuate ligament of the diaphragm during expiration.

- If chronic, a gastrointestinal (GI) workup, including endoscopy, barium studies, abdominal ultrasound, and CT scan, may be done to rule out other causes such as ulcers, gastritis, and cholelithiasis, among others. A mesenteric duplex will demonstrate abnormal flows in the celiac axis and superior mesenteric artery. Angiography is the most reliable diagnostic tool.

- Treatment options include angioplasty and stent, median arcuate ligament release, visceral bypass, and endarterectomy of the affected vessel(s).

- Postoperatively, these patients should be monitored for return of bowel function and ability to tolerate a diet without symptoms.

31. What is May-Thurner syndrome?

May-Thurner syndrome is not a disease, but an anatomic variant where there is compression of the left iliac vein by the right common iliac artery. Patients usually present with a swollen, painful left leg. An iliac vein DVT is found on workup for left leg swelling.

The mainstay of treatment in the past was anticoagulation with heparin and Coumadin. This treated the clot but did not prevent valvular damage, which produced chronic leg edema. More recently, catheter-directed thrombolysis followed by angioplasty and stenting of the iliac vein has been used with some success.

32. What is phlegmasia?

Phlegmasia is a condition that occurs when there is an extensive iliofemoral DVT. Venous and lymphatic outflow are obstructed, and the leg becomes markedly edematous. If untreated, arterial circulation to the lower leg and foot is compromised. Hypovolemia from the third spacing of fluid may cause a decrease in cardiac output, thereby increasing the risk of thrombus extension and pulmonary embolism. About 50% of the cases are associated with a malignancy. Other causes include hypercoagulable states, trauma, and surgery. It can occur at any age, but is more common during the fifth and sixth decades of life. The incidence is higher in females than in males.

33. What is phlegmasia alba dolens?

Phlegmasia alba dolens is the less severe form of phlegmasia. The extremity is painful, edematous, and pale but there is no neurovascular compromise or ischemia. In the past, it was called "milk leg," and was associated with the third trimester of pregnancy caused by pressure of the gravid uterus on the iliac vein.

34. What is phlegmasia cerulea dolens?

Phlegmasia cerulea dolens is the most severe form of phlegmasia. The extremity is grossly edematous, cold, and blue; there are often bullae and petechiae. At this point, the patient is at risk for neurovascular compromise and arterial insufficiency; if not treated, it can progress to venous gangrene involving the skin subcutaneous tissue and muscle. When venous gangrene occurs, it has a similar distribution with the cyanosis. Arterial pulses may be present when the venous gangrene is superficial. If the gangrene involves the muscular compartment, it may result in increased compartment pressures and a loss of palpable pulses. The arterial pulses are difficult to appreciate because of the significant edema, and use of a Doppler to detect arterial signals is appropriate.

Treatment is initiated with heparin. Thrombolytic therapy is initiated (if there are no absolute contraindications) to decrease the clot burden if there is impending or existing gangrene. After the acute phase, the patient is anticoagulated with low-molecular weight heparin (LMWH) such as Lovenox and/or Coumadin.

During the infusion of thrombolytics, the patient is in the ICU and monitored closely for bleeding. The patient's neurologic status should be monitored

SECTION I

SECTION II

SECTION III

for change in mental status or headache, as there is a potential for intracranial bleeding. The extremity is monitored closely for changes in color, edema, sensation, and movement. Pain must be adequately controlled. Any puncture site is monitored for bleeding. The patient should be on bedrest, with limited mobility and skin integrity must be maintained. Surgical thrombectomy is done infrequently. Waist-high compression garments are used to control the edema. Improvement in the edema usually occurs 6–12 months after surgery, as the body develops collateral pathways.

BIBLIOGRAPHY

Becquemin, J. (2001). Endovascular treatment of carotid disease. In J. Hallett Jr., J. Mills, J. Earnshaw, & J. Reekers (Eds.), *Comprehensive vascular and endovascular surgery* (pp. 533–546). New York: Mosby.

Bethel, S. (1999). Use of lumbar cerebrospinal fluid drainage in thoracoabdominal aortic aneurysm repairs. *Journal of Vascular Nursing, 17*(3), 53–58.

Black, J. (2009). Technique for repair of suprarenal and thoracoabdominal aortic aneurysms. *Journal of Vascular Surgery, 50*(4), 936–941.

Bower, T. (2001). Acute and chronic mesenteric ischemia. In J. Hallett Jr., J. Mills, J. Earnshaw, & J. Reekers (Eds.), *Comprehensive vascular and endovascular surgery* (pp. 285–293). New York: Mosby.

Chutter, T., & Schneider, D. (2010). Abdominal aortic aneurysms: Endovascular treatment. In J. Cronenwett & K. Johnston (Eds.), *Rutherford's vascular surgery* (7th ed., pp. 1972–1993). Philadelphia: Saunders.

Clouse, W., & Cambria, R. (2010). Complex aortic aneurysm: Pararenal, suprarenal, and thoracoabdominal. In J. Hallett Jr., J. Mills, J. Earnshaw, & J. Reekers (Eds.), *Comprehensive vascular and endovascular surgery* (pp. 445–478). New York: Mosby.

Conrad, M., & Cambria, R. (2010). Aortic dissection. In J. Cronenwett & K. Johnston (Eds.), *Rutherford's Vascular Surgery* (7th ed., pp. 2090–2109). Philadelphia: Saunders.

Cuthbertson, S. (2000). Nursing care for raised intra-abdominal pressure and abdominal decompression in the critically ill. *Intensive and Critical Care Nursing, 16*(3), 175–180.

Executive Committee for the Asymptomatic Carotid Atherosclerosis Study. (1995). Endarterectomy for asymptomatic carotid artery stenosis. *JAMA, 273*(18), 1421–1428.

Greelish, J. P., Mohler, E. R., III, & Fairman, R. M. (2010). Carotid endarterectomy: Preoperative evaluation; surgical technique; and complications. Retrieved from http://www.uptodate.com/patients/content/topic.do?topicKey=~QQggvHGWdl88SWsQ

Hallett, J., Brewster, D., & Rasmussen, T. (2001). *Handbook of patient care in vascular diseases* (4th ed.). Philadelphia: Lippincott Williams & Wilkins.

Hoel, A., & Thompson, R. (2004). Pathophysiology and natural history of abdominal aortic aneurysms. In J. Hallett, Jr., J. Mills, J. Earnshaw, & J. Reekers (Eds.), *Comprehensive vascular and endovascular surgery* (pp. 391–407). New York: Mosby.

Mackey, W., & Naylor, R. (2001). Carotid artery disease: Natural history and diagnosis. In J. Hallett, Jr., J. Mills, J. Earnshaw, & J. Reekers (Eds.), *Comprehensive vascular and endovascular surgery* (pp. 521–531). New York: Mosby.

Mohler E. R., III, & Fairman, R. M. (2010). Natural history and management of abdominal aortic aneurysm. Retrieved from http://www.uptodate.com/patients/content/topic.do?topicKey=~jCGxCpeU4JIYU7x&selectedTitle=1~99&source=search_result

Naylor, A., & Mackey, W. (2001). The surgical treatment of carotid disease. In J. Hallett, Jr., J. Mills, J. Earnshaw, & J. Reekers (Eds.), *Comprehensive vascular and endovascular surgery* (pp. 547–569). New York: Mosby.

North American Symptomatic Carotid Endarterectomy Trial Collaborators. (1991). Beneficial effect of carotid endarterectomy in symptomatic patients with high grade carotid stenosis. *New England Journal of Medicine, 325*(7), 445–453.

O'Hara, P. (2001). Abdominal aneurysm—Open repair. In J. Hallett, Jr., J. Mills, J. Earnshaw, & J. Reekers (Eds.), *Comprehensive vascular and endovascular surgery* (pp. 425–443). New York: Mosby.

Papia, G., & Cina, C. (2010). Postoperative management. In J. Cronenwett & K. Johnston (Eds.), *Rutherford's vascular surgery* (7th ed., pp. 501–516). Philadelphia: Saunders.

Tan, K., Oudkerk, M., & van Beek, E.(2001). Deep vein thrombosis and pulmonary embolism. In J. Hallett, Jr., J. Mills, J. Earnshaw, & J. Reekers (Eds.), *Comprehensive vascular and endovascular surgery* (pp. 625–663). New York: Mosby.

Upchurch, G., & Patel, H. (2010). Thoracic and thoracoabdominal aortic aneurysms: Evaluation and decision making. In J. Cronenwett & K. Johnston (Eds.), *Rutherford's vascular surgery* (7th ed., pp. 2014–2030). Philadelphia: Saunders

van Sambeek, M., van Dijk, L., & Hendriks, J. (2001). Abdominal aortic aneurysms—EVAR. In J. Hallett, Jr., J. Mills, J. Earnshaw, & J. Reekers (Eds.), *Comprehensive vascular and endovascular surgery* (pp. 409–423). New York: Mosby.

Wilterdink, J. L., Furie, K. L., & Kistler, J. P. (2010). Evaluation of carotid artery stenosis. Retrieved from http://www.uptodate.com/patients/content/topic.do?topicKey-=~ssYcTCKU5bl4on&selectedTitle=1~150&source=search_result

Woo, Y. J., & Mohler, E. R. III, (2010). Management and outcome of thoracic aortic aneurysm. Retrieved from http://www.uptodate.com/patients/content/topic.do?topicKey=~ak1Fp.Msh4ZEsLk&selectedTitle=1~30&source=search_result

CHAPTER 36

Cardiovascular Interventional Procedure

Laurel Stocks, RN, MSN, ACNP/BC, CCRN, CCNS

The cardiac catheterization laboratory is a combination of cardiac telemetry, critical care, and outpatient care. Most patients come from home to have a routine diagnostic catheterization or are admitted for the emergency or cardiac departments for emergent percutaneous intervention (PCI). Patients without coronary artery disease (CAD) are discharged home the same day. The range of stability runs from no additional medications or sedation to a level I transfer to cardiac surgery. The postprocedure care is primarily focused on the patient's recovery from moderate sedation and the vascular assessment of the femoral arterial sheath site if the patient had a diagnostic procedure. For the PCI patient monitoring for dysrhythmias, new onset ischemia, or infarct and initiation of postprocedure, fibrinolytics are as important as the mechanic removal of the arterial and/or venous sheaths is usually done in the postprocedure period or later if the patient is transferred to an inpatient unit after the activated clotting time (ACT) or partial thromboplastin time (PTT) has returned to baseline. A nursing background in cardiac surgery, telemetry, or intensive care nursing is recommended, but is not a prerequisite. Most units have an orientation program and require each nurse to be current in basic life support (BLS) and advance cardiac life support (ACLS). Key skills are recognition of dysrhythmias, prompt correction of vasovagal reactions or allergic reactions, clinical assessment of the heart and lungs, and coordination with the cardiology attending on local procedures based on American Heart Association (AHA) protocols.

1. What is coronary artery disease?

Coronary artery disease (CAD) is atherosclerosis of the coronary arteries, which produces blockages in the vessels that provide blood flow to the myocardium. Atherosclerosis is a disease of the endothelium, which causes the smooth walls to become jagged and allows plaque to accumulate both in the wall and along the lining, producing arterial narrowing. A sudden clot formation may occlude the lumen entirely, spasms may causes occlusion, or a restricted blood flow may not be able to provide adequate oxygen when increased demand arises from exercise or stress. Myocardial ischemia, injury, and death produce electrocardiogram (ECG) changes, blood markers, and symptoms ranging from mild discomfort to severe pain and sudden death. Over 99% of plaque rupture is clinically silent.

2. What are the major types of myocardial infarction (MI)?

One major type is non-ST segment elevation myocardial infarction (NSTEMI) or non-Q-wave MI. The heart attack, or MI, does not cause typical changes on a 12-lead ECG. Chemical markers in the blood may indicate that damage has occurred to the heart muscle. Chemical markers serum CPK-MB and troponin I are the most commonly measured. Troponin T and C reactive proteins are also markers of cardiac disease.

Another type is ST segment elevation myocardial infarction (STEMI) or Q-wave MI. This MI is caused by a prolonged period of blocked blood supply. It usually affects a large area of the heart muscle and may lead to acute failure and pulmonary edema. Commonly, there are changes on the ECG, but some MIs, such as a right ventricular infarct, are not seen on the traditional 12 lead except in V4 as ischemia and may need a 15 lead or right-sided chest lead ECG in order to diagnose. Unstable angina (UA) may produce similar ST segment depression that resolves with rest or nitrates.

3. What is angioplasty or percutaneous coronary intervention (PCI)?

Angioplasty or PCI was previously called percutaneous coronary transluminal angioplasty or PTCA. In this procedure, a catheter is placed in the femoral artery or brachial artery to allow access to the left heart. The provider can then use a catheter-delivered balloon, rotoblades, or a laser to open blocked or narrowed coronary arteries. Once in place, the balloon is inflated to push the plaque outward against the wall of the artery. This widens the artery and restores the flow of blood. Noncritical coronary lesions are less than 50% of the diameter of the vessel lumen.

Angioplasty can improve blood flow to myocardial tissue, relieve chest pain/ischemia, and reduce heart tissue damage. Sometimes, a small mesh tube called a stent is placed in the artery to keep it open after the procedure. A chemotactic drug coating or drug eluting stent may reduce the incidence of restenosis.

4. What can be assessed by a cardiac catheterization?

- The size of the vessel and number of coronary arteries involved the location and the percentage of blockage that can be reached by angioplasty (TIMI flow)

- Left atrial, left ventricular pressures, direct cardiac output/stroke volume, or left ventricular gram (ejection fraction measurement)

- Each patient should be evaluated and the procedure planned that will best treat their disease, but some rural area units may need to perform an evaluation and then transfer the patient to a referral center for an intervention.

5. Which patients should have a cardiac catheterization instead of coronary-artery bypass graft (CABG) or mini coronary-artery bypass (CAB)?

Diabetics, patients with tortuous arteries, and patients with more than two diseased arteries may have better results from a CABG. If a patient has a very low ejection fraction (EF) or severe congestive heart failure (CHF) and cannot tolerate the time

lying flat, he or she may need to be intubated and stabilized in a coronary care unit until the procedure can be tolerated.

6. The AHA provides algorithms for the care of acute coronary syndromes (ACS). What is the standard for detection of coronary thrombosis (critical lesions)?

The left heart catheterization with IV radioactive dye is the gold standard for the detection of coronary atherosclerosis and left ventricular (LV) ejection fraction during the LV gram. Other noninvasive tests include a positron-emission tomography (PET) scan or computerized axial tomography (CAT) scan of the chest and two-dimensional echocardiogram can determine cardiac EF, but only during the time of the test.

7. What interventions (PCI) are performed to reduce the ischemia and injury of a coronary occlusion by the interventional cardiologist?

Most catheterization labs can perform diagnostic procedures, but if intervention is required, the unit or hospital must have a contingency plan for a perforated coronary artery or ventricular puncture during PCI. Either an on-site CT surgical capability or emergency transfer agreement should be in place. As the patient advocate, you should ensure the patient's safety is paramount prior to beginning a PCI.

8. What types of interventional procedures might be done during angioplasty?

- Balloon angioplasty: During this procedure, a specially designed catheter with a small balloon tip is guided to the point of narrowing in the artery. The balloon is inflated to compress the blockage or plaque into the artery wall and stretch the artery open to increase blood flow to the myocardium.

- Cutting balloon or laser: The cutting balloon catheter has a special balloon tip with small blades or laser tip to reduce the plaque or occlusive clot form the arterial lumen.

- Stent: A stent is a small metal mesh tube that acts as a scaffold to provide support inside your coronary artery. A balloon catheter is placed over a guide wire and then inserted into the narrowed coronary artery. Once in place, the balloon tip is inflated and the stent expands to the size of the artery. The elasticity of the intima and the stretched wire then mesh and hold the arterial wall open. The balloon is deflated and removed, while the stent stays in place permanently. Some stents contain medicine, such as drug-eluting stents, and are designed to reduce the risk of reblockage or restenosis.

- Atherectomy: The catheter used in this procedure has a hollow cylinder on the tip with an open window on one side and a balloon on the other. When the balloon is inflated it pushes against the fatty matter. A blade (cutter) within the cylinder rotates and shaves off any fat that protruded into the window. The shavings are caught in a chamber within the catheter and removed. This process is repeated as needed to allow for better blood flow. Like rotoblation, this procedure is rarely used today.

9. Which drugs can be given through the catheter directly into the coronary arteries by the interventional cardiologist?

Medications are not approved by the Food and Drug Administration (FDA) for administration via the intracoronary route but the same medications that are given for coronary vasospasm via the venous route may be directly injected into the coronary arteries during the PCI for severe vasospasms and to facilitate stenting. Nitroglycerine, adenosine, and nicardipine are three such medications that maybe given through the lumens in a dilute microgram per milliliter concentration. Continuous monitoring and patient response should be documented.

10. What sedation do most patients receive for a cardiac catheterization or PCI?

Most patients receive a preprocedure anxiolytic such as oral Valium or intravenous (IV) versed and local anesthetic at the cannulation site. The most common site is the femoral vein, as these are large and relatively easy to compress after the procedure. The ambulatory patient will most likely come from a referral and be hemodynamically stable. A local anesthetic only at the femoral sheath would not require continuous airway monitoring, but the cath lab staff must be prepared to treat arrhythmias and allergic reactions to the radio opaque dye used in any procedure.

A patient with active chest or arm pain may be given small doses of morphine and then a fentanyl IV for severe pain. This becomes moderate sedation and the RN should be credentialed in airway maintenance and the use of sedative hypnotics. ACLS is a prerequisite in most institutions prior to administering IV sedation.

Many elderly are very sensitive to narcotics and/or have an adverse reaction to midazolam (Versed).

[P]atients over 60 years of age and debilitated or chronically ill patients should have only 1–1.5 mg IV titrated slowly (max infusion rate 0.75 mg/min); wait two or more minutes to evaluate the sedative effect; continue to titrate, if necessary, using small increments to the appropriate level of sedation (Micromedex, 2009).

Elderly patients will require approximately half the amount of midazolam than healthy, young patients if narcotic premedication or other central nervous system (CNS) depressants are used.

10. What should preprocedural assessment include?

- Baseline history and physical (H&P), 12-lead, complete blood count (CBC), blood chemistry (chem) or basic metabolic panel, chest x-ray (CXR), vital signs (VS; blood pressure, pulse, temperature, and respirations) and neurologic assessment
- Allergies, especially iodine, shellfish, x-ray dye, latex, or rubber products (e.g., rubber gloves or balloons); or penicillin-type medications

11. How often should the cardiac patient be assessed?

Reassessment of sedation level and pain should be at least every 15 minutes, and continuous pulse oximetry is required during moderate sedation. ECG should be monitored continuously and the ST segment evaluated. Noninvasive blood pressure (NIBP) should be every 3–5 minutes during the procedure: A constant arterial waveform from the femoral or brachial pressure should be compared to the cuff pressure for determination of need for volume or vasoactive medications. Most cardiologists will set a systolic or mean arterial blood pressure (MAP) goal and desire that the patient be pain free after the stenosis has been opened.

12. What happens when the patient is actively having chest pain?

An emergent or emergency department patient with active symptoms or signs of acute injury on 12-lead ECG will be monitored by the RN, but may not be given any sedation until the catheter is placed and the neurologic assessment is completed.

PCI is the treatment of choice if the door to balloon time can be achieved in less than 90 minutes, fibrinolytics are contraindicated, or for restenosis of previously placed stents. Your location and provider preference are also factors. Most community locations do not have cardiothoracic surgical back-up in case of a vessel perforation.

Expect to repeat the 12-lead ECG after the procedure in the recovering area. Cardiac enzymes (creatine kinase-MB, troponin I, troponin T) and CBC should be repeated every 4–6 hours.

13. What are the potential complications of femoral artery cannulation?

Injury to the vessel, bleeding, hematoma, pseudoaneurysm, and clot or occlusion of the vessel causing a loss of the distal pulse should be monitored frequently while the catheter or sheath is in place and postprocedure until the coagulation times are within normal ranges. The pulse can still be assessed just above the insertion site and the distal pulses should be assessed prior to the cannulation and at routine intervals postprocedure. Most suggest assessing every 15 minutes for the first 1–2 hours after removal, then every hour until the patient is discharged or is ambulatory. The American Association of Critical-Care Nurses (AACN) procedure manual is an excellent reference on the removal and monitoring of the arterial catheter.

14. Can a nurse remove the femoral sheath?

Yes, a nurse can remove the femoral sheath if he or she is trained and credentialed by your institution. Be sure the patient has a patent IV; another nurse or provider must be available to monitor and treat potential vasovagal syndrome or dysrhythmias while the sheath is removed and the arterial pressure is applied. The ACT or PTT should be measured prior to the removal and no signs of hemodynamic instability should be noted. Your lab will provide the normal values, but most institutions would like the ACT below 180 and the PTT/internalized international unit (INR) normalized.

15. What devices can be used to seal the artery after removal?

- angio-Seal
- safeguard
- femoStop
- star close
- perclose

See the manufacturer's guidelines and your hospital's policies for care of each type of device. The goal is to reduce the bedrest time and allow discharge or early ambulation to avoid pressure sores, back pain, DVT, and other risks of immobility.

16. After the procedure, how long should the patient be monitored?

Angio-Seal patients should be on bedrest for 4 hours post-Angio-Seal placement if there is no GPIIb–IIIa infusion, such as eptifibatide, initiated during the procedure. On GPIIb–IIIa, the patient should be supine for 6 hours with head elevated gradually to less than 30°. Discontinue sheaths when ACT is less than 180–200 sec.

If no closure device was used, bedrest should be for 4–6 hours postsheath removal with gradual head elevation and ambulation prior to discharge. Difficult or multiple femoral cannulations should receive individualized care with additional observation time.

17. Is a sand bag or IV bag appropriate to provide pressure on the groin site after a sheath removal?

There is no evidence that supports the use of a sandbag. The weight is neither sufficient (less than 10 lb), nor applied directly to the artery and, thus, only hides the site from the staff. A clear dressing or very small occlusive dressing without antimicrobial ointment should be applied to the site and direct observation and palpation for hematoma should be performed to assess the site.

18. Many patients have a vasovagal response to the sheath removal. How should the bradycardia be treated if the patient is symptomatic?

For an adult, follow AHA guidelines: Give 0.5–1 mg of Atropine IV every 5 minutes. For asystole: 1 mg IV should be given every 5 minutes, with a maximum total dose of 3 mg or 0.04 mg/kg.

19. What injuries should I assess for?

Remember the pneumonic "NAVAL" (for nerve, artery, vein, and lymph, and includes the deep inguinal lymph nodes located medial to the femoral vein) when assessing or removing the arterial sheath. Assess from the lateral hip to the medial groin: nerve, artery, vein, and ligament.

Numbness, tingling, or severe pain should all be followed up and the provider notified. Repositioning of the hip and/or knee with a roll or pillow will reduce pressure on the femoral nerve and/or sciatic nerve on the patient's dorsal side. Offload the heel with a device or pillow to avoid a pressure ulcer. Reduction of shear stress and offloading reduces pressure points. Retroperitoneal bleeding may occur gradually.

20. What conditions should be reported to the provider?

- bradycardia or tachycardia
- temperature greater than 38°C
- bleeding at site or a developing hematoma
- hypotension/hypertension above a 20% change for the patient

- chest pain or change in ST segments
- shortness of breath/unrelieved nausea

21. What medications should I have ready to give in the postprocedure catheterization lab?

Most patients can take oral medications and clear liquids while they are on bed rest. Elevation of the head to 15° or reverse Trendelenburg helps reduce chance of aspiration and improves comfort. Narcotics, Tylenol, antihistamine, antiemetics, aspirin, clopidogrel, beta-blockers, angiotensin-converting inhibitors, or calcium channel blockers for preexisting hypertension are often prescribed. Unfractionated heparin is turned off prior to sheath removal. Hydration with normal saline and oral fluids are encouraged to reduce potential acute tubular necrosis and subsequent renal insufficiency from contrast administration.

Other renal protective strategies include premedication with acetylcysteine and bicarbonate drips are used with varying results. Rarely, vasopressors such as nitroglycerin or norepinephrine maybe needed. Coronary vasospasm, reocclusion of a vessel, or severe bleeding necessitate emergent recatheterization, or transfer to the operating room (OR) or intensive care unit.

22. What complications of an acute myocardial infarction (AMI) might occur in the first 24 hours?

- Decreased cardiac output leading to fulminant CHF.
- Ventricular and A-V block dysrhythmias.
- Ventricular rupture or aneurysm usually followed by cardiogenic shock.
- Papillary muscle rupture associated with the inferior wall MI and mitral regurgitation.
- Acute ventral septal defect requiring surgical repair.
- Puncture of a coronary artery during catheterization may induce cardiac tamponade: cardinal signs include pulsus paradoxus (widening pulse pressure), muffled heart sounds leading to cardiovascular collapse.
- Global hypoperfusion, leading to myocardial stunning and cardiogenic shock.
- Late: pericarditis as evidenced by global ST segment elevations, new onset friction rub, and aching chest pain not relieved by nitrates.

23. What discharge instructions should the nurse emphasize?

- Avoid eating or drinking, except clear liquids until the groin sheath is removed because

nausea and/or hypotension can occur during this time.

- Once the patient is allowed to eat, he or she will be advised to follow a low-cholesterol and low-salt diet. Patient should be admitted to the hospital overnight after a PCI or for complications postprocedure to a monitored unit.

24. What are the indications for placement of a permanent pacer?

A pacemaker sends electrical impulses to the heart muscle to maintain a suitable heart rate and rhythm. Leads may be placed on the atria and ventricles. A pacemaker may be inserted for fainting spells (syncope), congestive heart failure, tachybradyarrhythmias, and hypertrophic cardiomyopathy (such as the SA node, AV node, or HIS-Purkinje system).

The pacemaker has two parts: the leads and a pulse generator. The pulse generator houses the battery and a tiny computer, and resides just under the skin of the chest. The leads are wires that are threaded through the veins into the heart and implanted into the heart muscle. They send impulses from the pulse generator to the heart muscle, as well as sense the heart's electrical activity. Biventricular pacers use three leads: one placed in the right atrium, one placed in the right ventricle, and one placed in the left ventricle (via the coronary sinus vein). The provider programs the minimum heart rate. When the patient's heart rate drops below that set rate, the pacemaker generates (fires) an electrical impulse that passes through the lead to the heart muscle. Overdrive pacing may be set as well to control the ventricular rate of tachyarrhythmias.

25. What is cardiac resynchronization therapy (CRT)?

CRT is a biventricular pacer used to treat heart failure such as hypertrophic cardiomyopathy and as a bridge to transplant.

26. How is the pacemaker assessed just after insertion?

Assess the patient's pulse; arterial waveform; and perfusion including capillary refill, mentation, MAP, and urine output. If the electrical stimulus does not produce ventricular ejection, no cardiac output will be present and, thus, no blood pressure. Increasing the MA until capture is advisable. The newly placed lead may have become dislodged or moved adjacent to damaged myocardial tissue, which no longer conducts. If this occurs, a pacer-dependent

TABLE 36-1. The NASPE/BPEG Generic (NBG) Pacemaker Code

Position	I	II	III	IV	V
Category	Chamber(s) Paced	Chamber(s) Sensed	Response to Pacing	Programmable Functions: Rate Modulating	P = Multisite Pacing; S = Shock
	O - None	O - None	O - None	O - None	O - None
	A - Atrium	A - Atrium	T - Triggered	R - Rate modulated	A - Atrium
	V - Ventricle	V - Ventricle	I - Inhibited		V - Ventricle
	D - Dual (A + V)	D - Dual (A + V)	D - Dual (A + V)		D - Dual (A + V)
Manufacturer's designation only	S - Single (A or V)	S - Single (A or V)			

Note: North American Society for Pacing and Electrophysiology (NASPE); British Pacing and Electrophysiology Group (BPEG). NGB Code is universally used to code pacemaker operation (2002). Adapted from VITHaS (n.d.).

patient should be transcutaneously paced until the lead can be replaced.

27. What instructions should be given to a patient who has a pacemaker and/or internal cardiodefibrillator (ICD) or cardiac internal electronic device (CIED)?

All patients should carry their identification card and wear a bracelet that identifies them as having a pacemaker. The ICD/pacing functions should be noted on their card and bracelet. Precautions are highly variable, but all pacemaker patients should not have an MRI and need to stay away from highly magnetized areas.

28. What is the common pacemaker code?

See Table 36-1.

29. What is arrhythmia ablation?

Nonsurgical ablation is used for many types of arrhythmias in a special area called the electrophysiology (EP) laboratory. During this nonsurgical procedure, a catheter is inserted into a specific area of the heart. A defibrillator is used to direct joules through the catheter to small areas of the heart muscle, identified through mapping, that are causing the dsyrhythmia. This energy disconnects the pathway of the abnormal rhythm. It can also be used to disconnect the abnormal electrical pathways between the upper chambers (atria) and the lower chambers (ventricles) of the heart.

30. What is a modified maze procedure?

In a modified maze procedure, a special catheter is used to deliver energy that creates controlled lesions on the heart and, ultimately, (AV) node. The scar tissue formed by the procedure blocks the abnormal electrical impulses from being conducted through the myocardium and promotes the normal conduction of pathway. One of four energy sources may be used to create the scars: radiofrequency, microwave, laser, or cryotherapy (cold temperatures).

31. What type of arrhythmias require ablation therapy?

- Symptomatic atrial fibrillation and flutter (which is refractory to other treatments including multiple medication trials) refractory to medical management (i.e., treatment with medication).
- Ventricular or supraventricular rhythms with accessory pathways

32. What are the advantages of ablation therapy?

In addition to reestablishing a normal heart rhythm in patients with certain arrhythmias, ablation therapy can help control the heart rate in those with rapid arrhythmias and can reduce the risk of blood clots and strokes.

33. A patient received pulmonary artery (PA) catheters under fluoroscopy for both diagnosis and treatment of cardiac conditions. What are the normal pressures you should observe for pulmonary artery or right heart catheter?

The normal values for pressures obtained with a PA catheter include the following:

- Right atrium mean (CVP): 0–8 mm Hg
- Right ventricle systolic/diastolic: 15–25/0–8 mm Hg
- Pulmonary artery systolic/diastolic: 15–25/8–12 mm Hg
- Pulmonary artery (occlusive) wedge: 6–12 mm Hg

34. Why would the femoral vein be cannulated during a cardiac catheter or pacemaker insertion?

The central vein is often cannulated to provide additional IV assess and to provide the team with the ability to inject dye into both the arterial and venous systems. The venogram may provide important information about retrograde flow and other vascular abnormalities requiring intervention. An intraaortic balloon pump (IABP) maybe inserted for cardiogenic shock or for transport to surgery.

35. What is the indication for a ventricular assist device (VAD), and how would the patient be monitored?

A VAD, a single-chamber or double-chamber cardiac assist device, may be inserted in the cath lab emergently by a cardiologist or vascular surgeon. The new term is a mechanical circulatory support device. The patient may not have a pulse pressure due to the linear nature of this pump, thus a Doppler may be needed to obtain a noninvasive BP. The arterial waveform will reflect the augmented blood pressure.

36. What is the TIMI Risk Score?

See Table 36-2.

37. What is the thrombolysis in myocardial infarction (TIMI) flow grading system postcardiac catheterization?

See Table 36-3.

38. What additional skills are recommended for post-cardiac catheterization recovery nurses that may not be included in perianesthesia competencies?

- ECG interpretation should include recognition of ischemia, injury, and infarct, and the use of the cardioactive medications per the ACLS protocols.
- Pacing with the transvenous and transcutaneous pacer, defibrillation, cardioversion, and

TABLE 36-2. TIMI Risk Score for UA/NSTEMI

From the Thrombosis in Myocardial Infarction trial (AMA, 2000), based upon data from 15,000 patients with an STEMI eligible for fibrinolytic therapy, is an arithmetic sum of eight independent predictors of mortality. • Age ≥ 75 years — 3 points • Age 65–74 years — 2 points • History of diabetes, hypertension, or angina — 1 point • Systolic blood pressure <100 mmHg — 3 points • Heart rate >100/min — 2 points • Killip class II to IV — 2 points • Weight <76 kg — 1 point • Anterior ST elevation or left bundle branch block — 1 point • Time to reperfusion therapy > 4 hours — 1 point

Note. There is a continuous relationship between mortality and score; a score of 0 to > 8 was associated with a 30-day mortality of 0.8–36% (UpToDate.com, 2010).

set-up; and monitoring a patient with a femoral, brachial, or radial arterial line.

- 12-lead ECG; drawing blood from central and arterial lines
- Management of heparin, IIb/IIIa fibrinolytics, Argatroban or lepirudin infusions; IV vasopressors like nitroglycerine, dopamine, milrinone
- IV moderate sedation credentials and assisting with sterile procedures

TABLE 36-3. TIMI Flow Grading System

Grade 0	Complete occlusion of the infarct related artery
Grade 1	Some penetration of contrast material beyond the point of obstruction, but without perfusion of the distal coronary bed
Grade 2	Perfusion of the entire infarct vessel into the distal bed but with delayed flow compared with a normal artery
Grade 3	Full perfusion of the infarct vessel with normal flow

Source: Chesebro et al., 1987.

REFERENCES

Antman, E. M., Cohen, M., Bernink, P. J. L. M., McCabe, C. H., Horacek, T., Papuchis, G., . . . Braunwald, E. (2000). The TIMI risk score for unstable angina/non-ST elevation MI. *JAMA, 284*(7), 835-842.

Chesebro, J. H., Knatterud, G., Roberts, R., Borer, J., Cohen, L. S., Dalen, J., et al. (1987). Thrombolysis in myocardial infarction (TIMI) trial, phase I: A comparison between intravenous tissue plasminogen activator and intravenous streptokinase. Clinical findings through hospital discharge. *Circulation, 76*(1), 142–154.

Thompson Reuters. (2010). MICROMEDEX gateway. Retrieved from http://www.thomsonhc.com/hcs/librarian

UpToDate.com. (2010). Left upper pulmonary vein on transesophageal echocardiogram. Retrieved from http://www.utdol.com/online/content/image.do;jsessionid=B05E17F18B1F52CCE77DA749DB5B678A.1002?imageKey=CARD%2F3138

VITHaS. (n.d.) The NBG code. Retrieved November 29, 2010, from http://www.pacemaker.vuurwerk.nl/info/nbg_code_naspe.htm

BIBLIOGRAPHY

American Society of PeriAnesthesia Nurses. (2008). Standards of perianesthesia nursing practice 2008–2010. Cherry Hill, NJ: Author.

American Association of Critical-Care Nurses. (2001). *The AACN Procedure Manual for Critical Care* (4th ed.). Philadelphia, PA: Saunders.

American Heart Association. (2006). ACC/AHA/SCAI practice guidelines. *Circulation, 113*(7), e166–e286.

American Heart Association. (n.d.). SCM order set: PCI post procedure orders. Retrieved from http://www.americanheart.org/downloadable/heart/1226007298138BMC%20Post%20PCI%20Order%20Set.pdf

Chair, S. Y., Thompson, D. R., & Li, S. K. (2007). The effects of ambulation after cardiac catheterization on patient outcomes. *Journal of Clinical Nursing, 16*(1), 212–214.

Kalra, S., Duggal, S., Valdez, G., & Smalligan, R. D. (2008). Review of acute coronary syndrome diagnosis and management. *Postgraduate Medicine, 120*(1), 18–27.

Kumar, A., & Cannon, C. (2009). Acute coronary syndromes: Diagnosis and management: Part I. *Mayo Clinic Proceedings, 84*(10), 917–938.

National Heart Lung and Blood Institute. Disease and conditions index. What is angina? Retrieved from http://www.nhlbi.nih.gov/health/dci/Diseases/Angina/Angina_WhatIs.html

Society of Critical Care Medicine. (2007). Fundamentals of critical care support (4th ed.). Mount Prospect, IL: Author.

Wound, Ostomy and Continence Nurses Society. (n.d.). Clinical fact sheet: Quick assessment of leg ulcers. Retrieved from http://www.wocn.org/pdfs/WOCN_Library/Fact_Sheets/C_QUICK1.pdf

CHAPTER 37

Endoscopic/Laparoscopic/ Minimally Invasive Procedures

Donna Beitler, MS, RN, CGRN

Endoscopy can be traced back to 1807 when Phillip Bozzini used a candle as a light guide for various tubes to be introduced into orifices. Since that time, the endoscope has developed into a high-definition technology allowing the viewer to see clearer images showing minute details. The first laparoscopic cholecystectomy was performed in 1987 by French physician Mouret, opening a whole new arena for minimally invasive surgery (MIS). Using small incisions, this technique has grown to include not only the gastrointestinal (GI) tract, but almost all anatomic areas in an attempt to leave the body as naturally intact as it was prior to surgery. Using the body's natural orifices, endoscopic and laparoscopic surgery has advanced as the future of surgical procedures.

ENDOSCOPIC/LAPAROSCOPIC PROCEDURE

1. What is an endoscopy or endoscopic procedure?

An endoscopy is a procedure that involves inspection of body organs or cavities by the use of an endoscope. The endoscope may have a rigid or flexible tube and provides an image via a light and camera lens.

2. What are the most common upper endoscopic procedures (UEP)?

- Esophagogastroduodenoscopy (EGD) is an endoscopic procedure that allows direct examination of the esophagus, stomach, and duodenum. The examination takes approximately 30 to 60 minutes and is usually well

tolerated with minimal discomfort. EGD may be used to evaluate abdominal pain, heartburn, persistent nausea and vomiting, dysphagia, upper GI bleeding or bloody stools, and chest pain in the absence of cardiac disease. It may also be used for periodic surveillance to control bleeding or to remove foreign bodies. It can detect ulcers, inflammation, hiatal hernias, abnormal growths, or other precancerous conditions.

- Endoscopic ultrasound (EUS) utilizes high frequency ultrasound during endoscopy to provide detailed images within and beyond the walls of the digestive tract. It is used to stage GI cancers by determining the depth of tumor penetration. It can also detect tumors in the pancreas and stones in biliary ducts. A fine needle aspiration (FNA) may be performed during ultrasound to obtain a biopsy or fluid to determine pathology or presence of metastasis. The procedure takes approximately 1 to 2 hours.

- Endoscopic retrograde cholangiopancreatography (ERCP) allows for examination of the biliary tree, including the liver, gallbladder, bile, and pancreatic ducts. Using fluoroscopy and endoscopy, the physician injects dye into the ducts in the biliary tree and pancreas so they can be seen on x-rays. ERCP is used primarily to diagnose and treat conditions that block the bile ducts, including gallstones, inflammatory strictures (scars), leaks (from trauma and surgery), and carcinoma. It may also be performed on patients with unexplained recurrent pancreatitis, jaundice, and abnormalities of liver chemistries. If x-rays show a blockage of the papilla or the duct systems, interventions may be performed. Common treatments include sphincterotomy, balloon dilatation (stretching), stenting, and placement of drainage tubes. Biopsies of suspicious lesions can also be done. It is also required in patients being considered for liver transplantation.

3. What are the most common complications of UEPs?

Complications from EGDs are rare; patients may experience a mild sore throat and some abdominal distention. Bleeding from biopsy sites or perforation may occur more often in EUS and/or ERCP. Pancreatitis is the most common complication of ERCP; it occurs in 3% to 5% of patients. Infection can occur in the bile ducts or pancreas after ERCP, especially when there is duct obstruction, which cannot be treated by the ERCP procedure. Antibiotics would then be required and possibly a surgical intervention.

4. What are the most common lower endoscopic procedures?

Colonoscopy is an endoscopic procedure that examines the interior of the large intestine from the rectum to the terminal ileum. It can be used to detect abnormal growths, inflammation, and to assist in diagnosing changes in bowel habits, blood in stool, and unexplained anemia and weight loss. It is also recommended as screening to detect early signs of colorectal carcinoma, and biopsies may be taken or polypectomy may be performed.

Flexible sigmoidoscopy is an endoscopic procedure that examines the rectum and lower portion of the colon.

5. What are the most common complications of lower endoscopic procedures?

While complications are rare, cramping and bloating may occur. If biopsies or polypectomy are performed, bleeding may be seen and perforation may also occur.

6. What is an endoscopic polypectomy?

An endoscopic polypectomy involves removal of a polyp via the endoscope. This can be done either in the upper or the lower GI tract. Polyps can be smaller (less than 5 mm) and removed more easily with the use of biopsy forceps, which reduce the risk of colonic perforation. Polyps may also be removed by fulguration using argon plasma

coagulation to destroy the polyp. The disadvantage of this technique is that no tissue is obtained for histologic analysis. Larger polyps are classified into two categories: sessile and pedunculated. Pedunculated polyps are growths that typically have stalks connecting them to the colon. If the stalk of the polyp is smaller, the removal is typically easier with hfewer complications. Patients with thicker stalks are at increased risk for bleeding postremoval secondary to blood vessels that are often located in the stalk.

Sessile polyps are typically flat colonic lesions that can present challenges for removal. A technique called endoscopic mucosal resection (EMR) is often used for removal of these growths. EMR involves the injection of saline or other liquid to elevate the growth and make it less difficult to resect. Cautery is also used in this technique. This method has an increased risk for perforation and bleeding postprocedure.

7. What are special considerations if my patient is at risk for upper GI bleeding?

Upper GI bleeding can present many challenges. The most common causes of upper GI bleeding include peptic ulcer disease, gastric erosions or ulcers, and esophageal varices. The first priority in management of the patient with active GI bleeding is to stabilize the patient. It may require volume replacement, hemodynamic stabilization, and correction of existing coagulopathy. Patients with the potential for upper GI bleeding should always have two large bore intravenous (IV) lines for rapid fluid boluses or blood transfusions. Protection of the airway is always a priority with upper GI bleeding. Intubation should be considered with any active bleeding and prior to endoscopic procedures where bleeding is suspected.

8. What are special considerations if my patient has lower GI bleeding?

The most common causes of lower GI bleeding are diverticulosis, inflammatory bowel disease (IBD), and malignant neoplasms of the small and large intestine. Again, the first priority in the management of these patients is resuscitation. These patients should receive two large bore intravenous catheters and isotonic crystalloid infusions with transfusions of blood products as needed. The patient may need to return to the operating room (OR) if the bleeding is unable to be controlled for further treatment. Surgical treatment is indicated if the patient continues to bleed and if nonoperative management is unsuccessful or unavailable.

9. What if a perforation occurs during the endoscopic procedure?

GI perforations are a rare but potentially dangerous complication that can occur anywhere in the GI tract. There are three main causes of GI perforations during an endoscopic procedure. Mechanical perforations occur when the scope tears the wall of the GI tract, either from too much force being used or at a diseased segment. Pneumatic perforations are caused by overdistension with air, and therapeutic perforations occur after removing a polyp, lesion, or while attempting to control bleeding. Patients with colonic perforation will typically develop severe abdominal pain soon after the procedure with persistent abdominal distention. Other symptoms include fever, tachycardia, and elevated WBCs. Smaller perforations may be capable of closing on their own with antibiotics and conservative treatment. However, larger perforations will require surgery to fix them. Diagnosis is obtained through x-ray, CT scan, and fluoroscopic procedures.

10. What type of anesthesia is commonly used for endoscopic procedures?

Upper and lower endoscopic procedures are commonly done under moderate sedation. With this type of sedation, a combination of a benzodiazepine and narcotic may be used. This allows the patient to maintain and move into certain positions, which may be required for the procedures. Moderate sedation may be administered by the registered nurse or an anesthesia provider. For more interventional type procedures, such as ERCP or EUS/FNA, a deeper sedation may be required. In some instances, propofol may be administered by the nurse during the procedure. This varies from state to state and is governed by the Nurse Practice Act for each state.

MINIMALLY INVASIVE OR LAPAROSCOPIC SURGERY

11. What is laparoscopic or MIS?

Laparoscopic surgery, also called MIS, is a surgical technique in which operations are performed through small incisions, usually 0.5 to 1.5 cm. It is any procedure, surgical or otherwise, that is less invasive than open surgery used for the same purpose. These procedures typically involve the use of laparoscopic devices and remote controlled instruments. This technique uses specialized techniques, miniature cameras, tiny fiber-optic flashlights, and high-definition monitors. Carbon dioxide (CO_2) is introduced into the abdominal cavity for increased visualizations. Initially used in abdominal surgeries, the technique has grown to include many specialties.

12. What are the most common surgeries performed using the laparoscopic or minimally invasive method?

- Laparoscopic cholecystectomy is the removal of the gallbladder and is accomplished through four small incisions, one around the umbilicus and three underneath the ribs on the right side. Both the artery and bile duct to the gallbladder are divided between metal clips. The gallbladder is then detached from the liver and removed through the umbilical incision site.

- Gastric bypass involves the creation of a small 15 to 30 ml pouch from the upper stomach, accompanied by bypass of the remaining stomach. This reconstruction of the GI tract can be either proximal or distal. This restricts the volume of food, which can be eaten. It is indicated in morbid obesity and is the most common bariatric surgery performed in the United States.

- Hernia repair involves two small incisions in the lower abdomen. The hernia defect is reinforced with a mesh (synthetic material made from the same material as sutures) and secured in position with stitches, staples, titanium tacks, or tissue glue, depending on the preference of the surgeon.

- Nissan fundoplication is used to treat refractory gastroesophageal reflux disease (GERD). In a fundoplication, the gastric fundus (upper part) of the stomach is wrapped or plicated around the lower end of the esophagus and stitched in place, reinforcing the closing function of the lower esophageal sphincter.

13. What are the most common complications following laparoscopic and minimally invasive surgeries?

The most common complication occurs from residual CO_2 in the abdominal cavity. When a pocket of CO_2 rises in the abdomen, it pushes against the diaphragm and can exert pressure on the phrenic nerve. This produces pain in the shoulder region and may also cause pain while breathing. This pain is transient and will be eliminated through respiration. Instruct the patients to lie flat with their buttocks elevated to facilitate relief. The most significant risks are bleeding from injury to blood vessels or organs, which usually result from trochar injury. Infection can occur, resulting from peritonitis in abdominal laparoscopic surgeries.

14. What is robotic surgery?

Robotic surgery is the use of a robot in performing surgery. Three major advances aided by surgical robots have been remote surgery, MIS, and un-manned surgery. Some major advantages of robotic surgery include precision, miniaturization, smaller incisions, decreased blood loss, less pain, and quicker healing time. Further advantages are articulation beyond normal manipulation and three-dimensional magnification. The most com-mon robotics system is the da Vinci Surgical Sys-tem, which is composed of a console with four arms to assist the surgeon. Three of these arms hold objects such as scalpels while the fourth is an endoscopic camera, which gives the surgeon full view from the console. This method of MIS allows the surgeon more range of motion and decreased trembling while maintaining full control.

15. What are the general preoperative instructions for endoscopic and minimally invasive procedures?

Because most of these procedures require a general anesthetic, patients are instructed not to eat or drink anything after midnight the night before the surgery. Anticoagulants and nonsteroidal inflam-matory drugs (NSAIDS) are usually discontinued 3 to 7 days before the operation and may vary depending on the procedure and the preference of the surgeon. The American Society for Gastrointes-tinal Endoscopy (ASGE) and the Society of Ameri-can Gastrointestinal and Endoscopic Surgeons (SAGES) have guidelines published for discontinu-ation of these medications. If a colonoscopy or colon surgery such as resection is performed, the patient will need to have the bowel prepped prior to the procedure to ensure maximum visualization. Preparations may include a combination of dietary restrictions, including clear liquids for 24 to 48 hours before the procedure, saline solutions, cathartics, and enemas. For all procedures requiring anesthesia or sedation, the outpatient must have a person to accompany them home.

16. What are general discharge instructions for endoscopic and minimally Invasive procedures?

Patients are instructed to expect some soreness in their shoulder area or chest. This is caused from residual CO_2. This can be relieved by walking or moving. They may also lie flat and elevate their buttocks to help facilitate elimination. Patients

may also experience a sore throat from intubation, which can be relieved with warm saline rinses. Strenuous activity should be avoided for 3 to 5 days postsurgery and heavy lifting should be avoided for 1 to 2 weeks depending upon the procedure. Patients may also experience tenderness, swelling, and bruising around any wound or puncture sites, especially the umbilicus. Because of the anesthetic agents administered, patients should avoid alcohol for 24 hours and be instructed not to sign anything legal or make important decisions for the same time period. They should call their doctor immediately for fever, bleeding, drainage from any wounds or puncture sites, continued nausea and vomiting, or excessive pain not relieved by pain medications.

17. What are the most common anesthesia techniques for this procedure?

The choice of anesthesia techniques for upper abdom-inal laparoscopic surgery is mostly limited to general anesthesia with muscle paralysis and tracheal intuba-tion. It is important to avoid stomach inflation during mechanical ventilation as this increases the risk of gastric injury during insertion of laparoscopic equip-ment. Intermittent positive pressure ventilation (IPPV) is used to ensure airway protection and control of pulmonary ventilation to maintain normocarbia.

18. Why do abdominal laparoscopic patients require intubation for these surgical procedures?

These patients need to be intubated because a neuromuscular blocking agent or paralytic is usually administered to minimize movement and decrease the probability of puncturing adjoining organs. Respirations are then con-trolled by mechanical ventilation. For laparo-scopic abdominal surgeries, a large amount of CO_2 may be introduced, which could block the diaphragm from functioning properly and de-crease respiratory effort.

19. What are the benefits of minimally invasive procedures?

MIS is any technique involved in surgery that does not require a large incision. There are a number of advantages to the patient with laparoscopic surgery versus an open procedure. These include smaller incisions, which result in minimal scarring and a superior cosmetic outcome, faster recovery time with less pain, and a decreased need for postsurgi-cal pain medication. There is also a shortened length of hospital stay associated with reduced recovery time and increased overall patient produc-tivity allowing earlier return to work. The smaller incision means reduced tissue trauma, which results in a reduced risk of incision-related complications such as wound infections, hernias, and development of adhesions.

20. What are the disadvantages of minimally invasive procedures?

Not all surgical procedures or patients are candidates for the minimally invasive approach. This technique requires difficult hand-eye coordination and handling of instruments. MIS is considered more technically demanding than traditional open surgical methods. The surgeon's vision is often restricted, and there is no tactile perception. The operating time may be longer that the traditional open technique. Additionally, as previously discussed, general anesthesia is required, whereas some of the open alternate operations can be performed under epidural or local anesthesia. The risk for trauma to other organs may also be increased due to limited visibility. More experience is needed to mature and refine surgical procedures, techniques, equipment, and surgeon skills.

21. What are future trends for laparoscopic or MIS?

Once considered a surgical trend, almost all surgical specialties now are performing MIS procedures on almost all anatomic areas. What began in the GI tract has advanced to include orthopedics, genitourinary, gynecologic, ear nose and throat, bariatric, and even cardiac surgery. MIS has now grown to include natural orifice translumenal endoscopic surgery (NOTES). Surgeons must be given the opportunity to acquire the knowledge and skills necessary to safely and efficiently perform MIS. Therefore, residency programs have incorporated extensive programs into their curriculum, which include the use of MIS simulation.

22. What is NOTES?

NOTES is an acronym for natural orifice transluminal endoscopic surgery. This technique involves the use of the patient's natural orifices (e.g., mouth, anus, vagina) to pass instruments into the peritoneal cavity as access for surgical procedures. First described by Dr. Anthony Kalloo at Johns Hopkins in 1998, the first human procedure was a transgastric appendectomy performed in India in 2005. In 2007, the first transvaginal removal of the gallbladder was performed in the United States. In 2009, the first human kidney was removed transvaginally by Dr. Robert Montgomery at Johns Hopkins Hospital. As of this writing, more than 100 cases have been performed worldwide using transgastric (through the stomach) and transvaginal (through the vagina) techniques. NOTES could be the next major paradigm shift in surgery, just as laparoscopy was the major paradigm shift during the 1980s and 1990s.

BIBLIOGRAPHY

American Society for Gastrointestinal Endoscopy. (2003). Preparation of patients for GI endoscopy. *Gastrointestinal Endoscopy, 57*(4), 446–450.

Berci, G., & Forde, K. A. (2000). History of endoscopy: What lessons have we learned from the past? *Surgical Endoscopy, 14*(1), 5–15.

Bragg, K., VanBalen, N., & Cook, N. (2005). Future trends in minimally invasive surgery. *AORN Journal, 82*(6), 1016–1019. Retrieved from http://www.ncbi.nlm.nih.gov/pubmed/16478082

Fletcher, R., & Jonson, B. (1984). Deadspace and the single breath test for carbon dioxide during anaesthesia and artificial ventilation. Effects of tidal volume and frequency of respiration. *British Journal of Anaesthesia, 56*(2), 109–119.

Gharaibeh, H. (1998). Anesthetic management of laparoscopic surgery. *Eastern Mediterranean Health Journal, 4*(1), 185–188.

Giday, S. A., Kantsevoy, S. V., & Kalloo, A. N. (2006). Principle and history of natural orifice transluminal endoscopic surgery (NOTES). *Minimally invasive therapy and allied technologies, 15*(6), 373–377.

Harrell, A. G., & Heniford, B. T. (2005). Minimally invasive abdominal surgery: Lux et veritas past, present, and future. *American Journal of Surgery, 190*(2), 239–243.

Johns Hopkins Medicine Gastroenterology and Hepatology. (2010). Diseases and conditions. Retrieved from https://www.hopkins-gi.org/GDL_DiseaseLibrary.aspx?SS=&CurrentUDV=31

Kalloo, A. N., Singh, V. K., Jagannath, S. B., Niiyama, H., Hill, S. L., Vaughn, C. A., et al. (2004). Flexible transgastric peritoneoscopy: A novel approach to diagnostic and therapeutic interventions in the peritoneal cavity. *Gastrointestinal Endoscopy, 60*(10), 114–117.

Kantsevoy, S. V., Hu, B., Jagannath, S. B., Vaughn, C. A., Beitler, D. M., Chung, S. S., et al. (2006). Transgastric endoscopic splenectomy: Is it possible? *Surgical Endoscopy, 20*(3), 522–525.

Kantsevoy, S. V., Jagannath, S. B, Niiyama, H., Chung, S. S., Cotton, P. B., Gostout, C. J., et al. (2005). Endoscopic gastrojejunostomy with survival in a porcine model. *Gastrointestinal Endoscopy, 62*(2), 287–292.

Marco, A. P., Yeo, C. J., & Rock, P. (1990). Anesthesia for a patient undergoing laparoscopic cholecystectomy. *Anesthesiology, 73*(6), 1268–1270.

National Digestive Diseases Information Clearinghouse. (2010). Upper GI endoscopy. Retrieved from http://digestive.niddk.nih.gov/ddiseases/pubs/upperendoscopy/index.htm

Natural Orifice Surgery Consortium for Assessment and Research. (2010). FAQ. Retrieved from http://www.noscar.org/faq.php

Saunders, B. (2007). Removing large or sessile colonic polyps. *World Organization of Digestive Endoscopy*. Retrieved from www.omed.org/downloads/pdf/publications/how_i_doit/2007/omed_hid_removing_large_or_sessile_colonic_polyps.pdf

Selzer, D. J., & Lillemoe, K. D. (2005). Laparoscopic cholecystectomy. In T. M. Bayless & A. M. Diehl (Eds.), *Advanced therapy in gastroenterology and liver disease* (5th ed., pp. 748–753). Hamilton, Ontario: BC Decker.

Weeks, J. C., Nelson, H., Gelber, S., Sargent, D., & Schroeder, G. (2002). Short-term quality-of-life outcomes following laparoscopic-assisted colectomy vs open colectomy for colon cancer: A randomized trial. *JAMA, 287*(3), 321–328.

Wexner, S. D., Beck, D. E., Baron, T. H., Fanelli, R. D., Hyman, N., Shen, B., et al. (2006). *ASGE/ASCRS/SAGES guidelines for bowel preparation prior to colonoscopy.* Retrieved from http://www.sages.org/publication/id/BOWEL

Zuckerman, M. J., Hirota, W. K., Adler, D. G., Davila, R. E., Jacobson, B. C., Leighton, J. A., et al. (2005). ASGE guideline: The management of low-molecular-weight heparin and nonaspirin antiplatelet agents for endoscopic procedures. *Gastrointestinal Endoscopy, 61*(2), 189–194.

CHAPTER 38

Interventional Radiology Procedure

Kathleen A. Gross, MSN, RN-BC, CRN

Interventional radiology (IR) is a newer, emerging specialty in medicine that offers patients less invasive alternatives for both diagnostic and therapeutic purposes. These alternatives are often preferred by hospitals, insurers, and patients alike due to faster throughput and decreased medical costs, risk, and recovery time. Whether the patient is an inpatient or outpatient, nursing care is essential for preprocedure, intraprocedure, and postprocedure care of IR patients. Screening, assessment, sedation/analgesia, monitoring, and teaching are vital components of nursing care for patients having interventional procedures not only in the interventional department but also in the computed tomography (CT), ultrasound (US), or magnetic resonance imaging (MRI) areas. Nurses in specialties other than radiology nursing need to have some basic understanding of the care of IR patients who may be admitted to their units pre- or post-IR procedure.

PREPROCEDURE

1. Why is it important to have current coagulation studies available prior to a biopsy procedure?

Coagulopathy or abnormal clotting studies may increase the risk of bleeding after a biopsy. A partial thrombin time (aPTT), prothrombin time (PT), international normalized ratio (INR), and platelet count are usually requested. In the event the values are outside the normally accepted values, the physician performing the biopsy procedure should determine acceptable coagulation study

values in view of the organ or site to be biopsied. Prior to the procedure, a medication reconciliation should be performed to assess for any medications (prescription, over-the-counter, or herbal) that affect coagulation. For outpatients, this should be done in advance so that scheduled procedures are not unnecessarily canceled. For inpatients, the floor nurse should be notified in advance if any heparin infusion is to be discontinued. Coagulation studies also should be performed prior to interventional procedures where there would be a risk of bleeding (e.g., an angiogram with vascular puncture, tube placement, spinal procedure). A baseline hemoglobin (Hgb) and hematocrit (HCT) should be available for comparison status postprocedure in the event of hemorrhage and per any sedation and analgesia protocols.

2. Why is it important to include questions about any past contrast media reaction in the preoperative nursing assessment?

Patients who have experienced a reaction to contrast media in the past may be more prone to another reaction. It is important to ask the patient if he or she knows the type of contrast that was used, when this reaction occurred, what happened (including severity of reaction), and what, if known, was done to treat the problem. The physician should be notified of this situation. Premedication with a steroid and antihistamine may be necessary. Ideally, premedication is given (p.o.) in advance but may be given (intravenous [IV], intramuscular [IM] just prior to a procedure in an urgent situation. Two protocols are recommended by the American College of Radiology: for example, prednisone 50 mg p.o. given at 13 hours, 7 hours, and 1 hour; and diphenhydramine (Benadryl) 50mg IV, IM, or p.o. 1 hour before contrast media injection. Methylprednisolone (Medrol) 32 mg p.o. 12 hours and 2 hours before injection with an antihistamine is another choice for premedication. Alternatives to performing a contrast study may include performing the procedure without contrast or choosing an alternative study (e.g., ultrasound or magnetic resonance imaging [MRI]). Medical grade carbon dioxide (CO_2) may be used in a limited number of angiographic procedures for the patient with a contrast allergy.

3. What is the rationale for assessing renal function prior to a contrast media study?

Contrast media is excreted via glomerular filtration. Contrast-induced nephrotoxicity (CIN) can occur after the administration of contrast media. Although the exact etiology of CIN is not known, hemodynamic changes in the kidney and tubular toxicity from the contrast are believed to be factors. Patients are at risk for CIN if they have preexisting renal insufficiency. Dehydration, cardiovascular disease, use of diuretics or other nephrotoxic drugs are believed to be additional risk factors. The osmolality and volume of contrast used may be contributing factors that can be controlled. Serum creatinine (Scr) has been used as a convenient, readily available test for renal function. The Scr may not, however, be the most reliable test. A creatinine based eGFR (from either of two commonly used formulas, the Cockroft-Gault formula or the Modification of Diet in Renal Disease formula) may be ordered. The limitations of these two formulas should be known.

4. What specific discharge instruction should be given to the noninsulin dependent diabetic patient who is taking metformin or a metformin combination drug for glucose control?

The biguanide oral antihyperglycemic medication metformin may not be excreted if decreased renal function occurs after the administration of contrast media. This may lead to lactic acidosis. Lactic acidosis is stated to be rare, occurring in 0 to 0.084 of cases per 1,000 patient years, but the mortality associated with lactic acidosis is 50% (American College of Radiology [ACR], 2010). Current recommendations for patients with multiple co-morbidities and normal renal function include discontinuing metformin when intravascular contrast is given and having the patient

withhold the medication for 48 hours. Renal function should be evaluated before the medication is resumed although it may not be necessary to repeat a serum creatinine if the practitioner does not believe it is warranted (ACR, 2010). In patients with reanal dysfunction taking metformin, discontinue metformin at the time of injection and determine time to reinstitute metformin medication by renal function assessment.

5. What does ALARA mean?

ALARA is an acronym for as low as reasonably achievable. It is used to describe efforts to reduce the amount of radiation exposure to a patient during an examination. The effects of radiation are considered to be deterministic or stochastic in nature. Deterministic effects are related to a threshold dose of radiation received. Skin erythema and hair loss are examples of deterministic effects. Stochastic effects are related to the probability of the occurrence of a change (e.g., a cancer developing from radiation exposure or genetic changes).

6. Why is glucagon requested for use during placement of a percutaneous gastrostomy tube?

Glucagon slows gastric peristalsis. The usual dose is 0.5 to 1 mg given intravenously. (Caution: Glucagon is packaged in 1 mg and 10 mg vials. It is prepared with the manufacturer's diluent just prior to use.) The radiologist should notify the nurse as to when to administer the glucagon.

7. What is the indication for fallopian tube recanalization?

This procedure is performed when the patient has documented fallopian tube blockage and comes for treatment of infertility. The procedure should be scheduled to coincide with the patient's follicular phase of the menstrual cycle. A pregnancy test should be done on the day of the procedure to document absence of pregnancy per institutional policy. The patient is usually given doxycycline 100 mg p.o. to take for prophylaxis prior to coming for the procedure. The nurse should document compliance with the antibiotic prophylaxis. Pelvic infection is a contraindication to this procedure.

8. Why is it important to know the patient's weight prior to interventional radiology or computed tomography (CT) procedures?

Interventional radiology procedure tables have table weight limits. It would not be safe to place a patient on the procedure table if their weight exceeds the specified limit. The same applies to the

CT table. In CT, there are also limitations related to the bore/gantry diameter. This factor may preclude the patient being able to be scanned. Always check with the radiologist or the radiologic technologist when in doubt.

9. Why is an inferior vena cava (IVC) filter sometimes placed in the absence of a known pulmonary embolism or deep vein thrombosis (DVT)?

IVC filters are sometimes placed in a patient with a known malignancy due to a hypercoagulable state that may result in a thromboembolic event. A prophylactic IVC filter may be used in the treatment of the multiple trauma patient or placed preoperatively in a patient at risk. A contraindication to anticoagulation or known problems from anticoagulation is an indication for IVC filter use. Retrievable filters (sometimes referred to as optional filters) are now available for use when the need is for a specific time frame.

10. Why is n-acetylcysteine (Mucomyst) sometimes ordered before an interventional arterial study?

CIN is a major concern for the at-risk patient and prevention is important. Various medications have been used in the past as preventive agents. N-acetylcysteine (NAC) is sometimes given on the day before and the day of the procedure as a preventive measure. Whether this is effective has not been proven, but it is believed to be helpful. The taste and smell of N-acetylcysteine is not pleasant and is difficult for patients to take by mouth. This effect can be diminished by mixing it in juice or other desired liquid. (Caution: Check NPO guidelines on the day of the procedure.) Intravenous sodium bicarbonate ($NaHCO_3$) has been given with N-acetylcysteine as a renal protective measure. The ACR recommends sufficient hydration as a significant preventive measure against CIN (ACR, 2010).

11. How will the patient be positioned for a vertebroplasty or kyphoplasty procedure?

The patient will be placed prone on the procedure table for these procedures. It is important to assess whether the patient will be able to lie in this position prior to the procedure to avoid canceling the procedure at the last minute. In addition to local anesthesia, patients will be given intravenous sedation and analgesia for the procedure. Any issues that may interfere with the patient's breathing in the prone position should also be assessed. The patient's airway status may be compromised due to comorbid conditions. An anesthesia consult is needed for patients where airway problems are present, when the inability to lie prone exists, or when the amount of medication needed is anticipated to be above the safe limits of that given by a nonanesthesia provider.

12. Why is it important to assess distal pulses prior to an arteriography?

It is important to note baseline pulses (e.g., dorsalis pedal and posterior tibial for a femoral access site and radial and ulnar pulses for a brachial or axillary access) due to the potential complication of arterial thrombosis or distal embolization with loss of pulses. During the initial assessment, the quality of the pulse should be noted along with presence or absence. If the pulse is not present on light palpation, it should be checked by a Doppler device. The site where the pulse was felt or heard should be marked for comparison to the postprocedure pulses. Any significant neurologic or sensory deviations should also be noted with the initial evaluation. It is important to note any extremity hair loss, existing wounds, or skin ulcerations on the initial assessment as these can be signs of poor circulation.

13. Where can parents find information on radiation exposure in children?

Radiation exposure is a concern that is gaining more interest in the medical and nonmedical communities. Parents should be encouraged to ask the radiologist about radiation exposure questions prior to the child's procedure. Questions can be addressed at the time consent is obtained. Parents can also be directed to the website for The Alliance for Radiation Safety in Pediatric Imaging (http://www.pedrad.org/associations/5364/ig/). This website offers educational information for different healthcare providers as well as for parents. Parents may use a downloadable brochure and card for recording a child's procedures involving radiation exposure, available at this site.

14. What is the measure used to designate the strength of the magnetic field in MRIs?

Tesla is the unit of measure of the strength. Strengths can be referred to as low- or high-field strength. Common magnet strengths are 1.0 and 1.5 Tesla with 3.0 Tesla magnets being used in some clinical settings. (Magnets used for research can be much higher in strength.) All patients undergoing an interventional magnetic resonance imaging (iMRI) procedure should be thoroughly screened for any contraindications, including but not limited to cardiac devices, brain clips or coils, cochlear implants, and periorbital metal fragments. MRI safety also includes screening for pregnancy. Personnel should be thoroughly trained in recognized MRI zoning and the danger of ferromagnetic objects in the MRI field. All instruments used for a procedure should be iMRI compatible and appropriately labeled. The superconducting magnet of the MRI is always on so safety should be a priority. Detailed information about MRI safety can be found at the website for the American College of Radiology (www.acr.org).

15. What intravenous contrast agent is used for MRI studies?

A gadolinium-based contrast media is used. Although reactions to gadolinium are rare, patients should be screened for prior reaction and pregnancy.

16. What is radiofrequency (RF) thermal ablation?

Radiofrequency (RF) thermal ablation is a technique that involves placing a long electrode into a tumor. Alternating RF current is then passed through the electrode, which heats the area. This heat leads to coagulation, necrosis, and cell death. RF ablation has been utilized in the treatment of lung, liver, renal, bone, and other tumors. It is important that a grounding pad be properly placed on the patient prior to the procedure. Saline that has been cooled may be needed to cool the edges of the pad that is closest to the electrode. This will prevent a burn from occurring.

POSTPROCEDURE

17. What possible complications can occur following a drainage catheter placement into an infected fluid collection?

Bacteremia and shock may occur following catheter placement into an infected fluid collection in the kidney, biliary system, or liver. This may occur rapidly as noted by a change in the patient's heart rate and blood pressure. Fever, hypothermia, chills, or rigors may ensure. Prompt recognition of the condition is needed along with appropriate antibiotic therapy and fluid administration, if necessary. Transfer of the patient to a higher level of care should be considered.

18. What treatment is indicated in the case of contrast extravasation following peripheral contrast media extravasation?

The radiologist may order either warm or cold compresses to the site of a local contrast extravasation. The ACR recommends the site should be

evaluated by a radiologist prior to the discharge of an outpatient as the extent of the injury may not be apparent at the onset. The patient's discharge instructions should include information for follow-up in the event of any decline in neurologic, sensory, or circulatory symptoms or skin blistering. Severe extravasations may necessitate a surgical consultation. Compartment syndrome is a rare occurrence. The extravasation, symptoms, treatment, and patient education/discharge information should be documented in the medical record.

19. What medications are used to treat bronchospasm due to a contrast media reaction?

The patient should be given supplement oxygen for bronchospasm and a beta-agonist inhaler (metaproterenol, terbutaline, or albuterol) should be used. For severe bronchospasm unresponsive to inhaler therapy, epinephrine (1:1,000, 0.1 to 0.3 mg SC or IM) is given. (Caution: Epinephrine comes in two concentrations.) It may be necessary to activate a rapid response team or other teams for additional assistance.

20. What medication is given for urticaria after a contrast media injection?

Diphenhydramine is given for urticaria after contrast media injection. This medication may be given p.o., IM, or by IV depending on the clinical situation and per the physician. The patient should be observed for other signs and symptoms of a reaction and treatment given. Outpatients who receive diphenhydramine for a reaction should be informed of the sedative effect of diphenhydramine and have a responsible adult to drive them home.

21. What are some general principles and information to include when teaching the patient about flushing a drainage catheter?

Patient education should include the following information:

- The drainage bag should be kept at a lower level than the tube insertion site and drainage catheter to facilitate gravity drainage.

- The tube may be secured by a commercial catheter holding apparatus and secured to clothing by a pin or leg via the use of a leg bag with straps. There should be some slack in the tubing to allow for a change of position.

- Catheters usually require gentle flushing to maintain patency. The radiologist should provide guidelines for this. For example, 10 ml of normal saline may be used to forward flush the catheter twice a day. (Aspiration should not be performed unless specifically instructed.) Sterile technique should be used. If the catheter has a stopcock attached, the patient should be instructed about the different positions and when the catheter is open to drainage or in the closed position. Patients will need a prescription to obtain the necessary supplies for catheter care, such as syringes, sterile saline, and alcohol wipes. It is advisable for the patient (or caregiver) to return a demonstration prior to discharge.

- Dressing care and skin care at the tube insertion site should be given per the radiologist's instructions.
- Symptoms of a blocked drainage catheter, including decreased output, or symptoms of infection should be given. The patient should also be instructed to report any pain, especially increased pain. The patient should be instructed to report any fever or signs of infection, leaking around the catheter insertion site, skin breakdown, or signs of infection at the insertion site. Recording of the catheter output may be needed in some instances. In such a case, patients should be told to bring a record of the output to the next visit. Drainage bags should be emptied as needed with care not to allow overfilling of the bag. Nephrostomy tubes may be connected to a larger drainage bag for overnight use (leg bags hold smaller volumes). Patients should be informed that tube changes will be necessary if the tube is to remain for any length of time. These changes maybe done every 4 to 6 weeks on average. The patient should be told that if the catheter is accidentally dislodged, it should be reported immediately. The more time the catheter is out, the more difficult it may become to reinsert another catheter, as the tract (pathway) will close.
- Instructions should include information on activities of daily living (e.g. bathing, care not to dislodge drainage catheter, diet, medications, who to contact in an emergency, next appointment time). Verbal instructions should be reinforced in a written document that is signed by the patient.

22. What should be monitored in the patient who has had a percutaneous nephrostomy tube placement?

Bleeding and sepsis are two complications of percutaneous nephrostomy. Status postpercutaneous nephrostomy tube placement, the patient's urine may show gross hematuria (pink to dark pink or red in color). This is caused by bleeding from small intrarenal veins and small arteries. The urine should become clear (or return to baseline color). Any frank bleeding or clots should be reported to the radiologist. Continue to monitor the patient for bleeding or clots in the urine and signs of infection. Antibiotics may be ordered if the urine was believed to be infected. A sample of urine is usually sent for urinalysis, culture, and sensitivity at the time the nephrostomy tube is placed to determine appropriate antibiotic coverage. Also monitor the tube insertion site for any leakage of urine, volume of urine output, and any pain the patient would report. The patient may initially report some discomfort at the tube insertion site.

23. Why does the patient who has had an internal double-J ureteral stent placed report feeling a sense of frequency or urgency to void?

The internal double-J ureteral stent is used for treatment of ureteral obstruction. One end of the nephroureteral stent is situated in the renal pelvis and the other end sits in the bladder. This is perceived as a foreign body at first and acts as an irritant. Reassure the patient this feeling should diminish over time. The patient should talk with the physician if the feeling persists.

24. What medication maybe used in an arterial infusion to control gastrointestinal bleeding?

Vasopressin (Pitressin) has been used for control of gastrointestinal bleeding found during a visceral angiogram by causing constriction. The intra-arterial infusion should be given via an infusion pump with all lines clearly marked per institutional protocol. Vasopressin has an antidiuretic hormone (ADH) effect and may cause decreased urine output.

The patient should be monitored in an intensive care setting. The patient should also be observed for a reaction, cardiovascular changes, abdominal cramping, nausea, or vomiting. Embolization of the bleeding vessel maybe the preferred treatment for gastrointestinal bleeding.

25. What medication maybe needed in the event the postprocedure patient, who has had midazolam (Versed) for sedation, has a drop in the pulse oximetry reading with decreased respirations?

Flumazenil (Romazicon) maybe used for the patient who desaturates and fails to respond to manual airway opening, oxygen administration, and stimulation. This drug should be used with caution in the patient who has a history of long-term benzodiazepine use, as a seizure may occur. The patient should be monitored for resedation after administration of flumazenil. Follow all facility policies and procedures for use of reversal agents and transfer the patient to a higher level of care for observation per requirement.

26. What is postembolization syndrome (PES)?

PES follows the intentional disruption of the blood supply to an area. Procedures that may have this as a side effect include uterine fibroid embolization and hepatic arterial embolization. The patient may complain of nausea (with vomiting) and pain in the affected area. Fever and increase in the white blood cell count may occur. These symptoms usually diminish over 24 to 72 hours. Analgesics, antiemetics, and antipyretic medications are used to treat the symptoms.

27. What are some possible complications of a puncture site?

The method used for hemostasis following vascular puncture should be documented. Intraprocedural anticoagulation will influence when the catheter or sheath can be removed. Hemostasis is often obtained by direct manual pressure or use of a mechanical device (e.g., Compressar or FemoStop), vascular suture devices (e.g., Perclose), vascular plugs (e.g., VasoSeal, Angio-Seal), or topical pads (e.g., Syvek, Clo-Sur PAD) may be used. All manufacturer guidelines and institutional protocols should be followed. Time to ambulation will be partly determined by the method used for vascular closure and hemostasis. Closure devices may be used for a select group of patients given criteria are met. These may be used when outpatient procedures are performed and early ambulation is desired. Regardless of the method of hemostasis, the puncture site should be carefully observed for any complications. Possible vascular puncture site complications include bleeding (with possible hematoma formation at the puncture site), retroperitoneal hemorrhage, pseudoaneurysm formation (false aneurysm), nerve damage, thrombosis, arteriovenous fistula formation, or infection.

28. What is a TIPS procedure?

TIPS stands for transjugular intrahepatic portosystemic shunt. TIPS is useful in treating ascites in patients with portal hypertension, esophageal varices (prophylactic or during active bleeding), and Budd-Chiari syndrome. Under ultrasound guidance, the right internal jugular vein is used for access to the liver. A long sheath is placed into the inferior vena cava and the right hepatic vein is accessed. A tunnel is made through the liver parenchyma. A connection is made from the hepatic vein to the portal system via the right portal vein. Some variations may be necessary based on anatomy. A stent is placed to provide a diversion for blood flow. An ultrasound examination is typically performed within 24 hours and at specified intervals to assess velocities within the vessels and shunt. The patient should be assessed for signs of liver failure, hepatic encephalopathy, and cardiac failure after the procedure. If the shunt occludes, a revision using angioplasty of the stent maybe performed.

29. What complication of endovascular procedures is common?

Restenosis is a known postprocedure problem. Neointimal hyperplasia, thrombosis, and remodeling are three contributing factors. Pharmacologic prophylaxis may be ordered. It is important to stress the importance of patient compliance with any medications ordered (e.g., aspirin) when giving discharge instructions.

30. What complication maybe noted in a patient who is status post-lung biopsy or central venous access?

Pneumothorax may occur. The patient may complain of some shortness of breath or pain when taking a breath. They may appear apprehensive. The patient's respiratory rate, character, and pulse oximetry readings should be recorded and reported to the physician along with the patient's complaint. Pneumothorax is diagnosed by an upright chest x-ray. A small pneumothorax (minimal lung collapse) may not need treatment if the patient is not symptomatic. A follow-up chest x-ray may be ordered. For more symptomatic pneumothorax, a small catheter with a Heimlich valve may be placed as soon as possible. A chest tube placed by a chest surgeon may be needed for a large pneumothorax. A tension pneumothorax is an urgent situation, and immediate action is necessary. Patient monitoring is important.

31. How can postcatheterization pseudoaneurysms be treated?

Pseudoaneurysm development is a complication that occurs after a puncture site access for vascular interventions. Depending on the nature of the pseudoaneurysm, direct pseudoaneurysm compression may be done using an ultrasound transducer. Direct percutaneous thrombin injection is another pseudoaneurysm treatment option. A specified period of bedrest will be ordered after the repair of the pseudoaneurysm. A follow-up Doppler may be ordered shortly after the repair and at certain intervals thereafter.

32. How are contrast reactions categorized, and what are the symptoms of a contrast reaction?

Reactions to medication should be ruled out as a cause when there is any change in a patient's condition. A reaction to contrast media may not fall into a discrete category. It may start with one symptom and progress to others; therefore, observation of the patient is very important. The ACR separates reactions into three categories: mild, moderate, and severe. A few small scattered hives, nasal stuffiness, or nausea and vomiting may be considered a mild reaction. A moderate reaction might be noted by tachycardia or mild hypotension. Laryngeal edema, profound hypotension, or cardiovascular collapse are examples of severe reactions. A severe reaction can start with the appearance of a mild reaction, so observation and rapid recognition and treatment are needed (See ACR, 2010).

33. What are salient aspects of nursing care for the patient undergoing thrombolytic therapy for arterial occlusion?

The patient who is undergoing thrombolytic therapy will require close monitoring (e.g., in an intensive care setting or appropriate step down unit). The nurse should be knowledgeable about the patient's status, indications, and potential complications of the thrombolytic agent used (e.g., tissue plasminogen activator [t-PA], reteplase [r-PA], tenecteplase [TNK], or urokinase [UK]). A systemic lytic state can occur. Thrombolytic agents should be delivered via an infusion pump with all lines clearly marked with the flow rate and location of the catheter or delivery wire. Preprinted order sheets are often used. The patient should be monitored per order or at least every hour for vital signs, vascular access site stability (groin), and affected extremity progress, including pulse and neurovascular status. The patient's neurologic status should also be monitored. Changes in any of these parameters should be reported to the physician without delay. Fibrinogen level, complete blood count, and coagulation studies will be monitored in addition to other labs (e.g., electrolytes and creatinine). Patients may be given a clear liquid diet, but before lysis is reevaluated, the patient should be NPO. Lysis will be monitored by scheduled checks or emergent need. Lysis is clinically evaluated by an improved pulse, extremity warmth, and decreased complaints of pain. Patients

may, however, experience a period of worsening pain during thrombolysis. Handheld Doppler devices and cutaneous marking of pulses are helpful to nursing and medical staff. It is essential that no intramuscular injections are given during the process of thrombolysis. It is advisable for the patient to have more than one venous access device in place prior to the initiation of thrombolysis. One site can be used for phlebotomy and the other for intravenous fluid and medication administration. Bedrest is needed during this period. Positioning and patient comfort can present nursing challenges.

34. Can thrombolysis be used in the venous system?

Endovascular thrombolysis can be used for deep vein thrombosis (DVT).

35. How does the healthcare provider know if the patient's port can be used for power injections?

When ports are placed, patients are usually given a wallet card with information (e.g., type of port, manufacturer, lot, location of vessel, implantation date, and location) to carry with them. Patients, however, may not have this card available and the medical record may not be accessible. Some manufacturers help practitioners identify the ports with a certain shape or projections (bumps). Imaging over the area with fluoroscopy maybe helpful to determine the type of device. It is imperative that only a special needle is used to access the port intended for a power injection and that power injectable ports are in place.

36. How long will the interventional radiology patient need to stay in the postanesthesia care unit (PACU) status postprocedure?

The amount of time the patient will need to stay in the PACU will vary greatly according to the patient's status and specific procedure done. If the patient's procedure is intended as an outpatient procedure, the order sheet should include information when the patient can be discharged along with procedure-specific discharge instructions. The patient's condition should be at baseline (or within reasonable limits due to procedure), pain (and nausea/vomiting) should be managed, and prescriptions (for pain, nausea, antibiotics, other) given per physician. The patient should be released with a responsible adult and have appropriate arrangements for care at home. Some procedures will require an overnight (or longer stay) either due to the nature of the procedure or patient condition. All procedure-specific orders should be followed before transfer to another level of care. Many universal elements of care as for all postanesthesia care patients will be addressed. Good communication between caregivers during the transfer of care is needed.

37. What is the significance of a fibrin sheath?

A fibrin sheath can occur on the end of a catheter, preventing use of a venous catheter. A thrombolytic medication may be instilled and allowed to dwell in the catheter in an attempt to treat. Other treatment options include exchanging the catheter or placing another catheter at a new site. Balloon angioplasty and fibrin sheath stripping via transfemoral venous access may be used in some situations.

REFERENCE

American College of Radiology. (2010). Manual on contrast media version 7. Available at http://acr.org/SecondaryMainMenuCategories/quality_safety/contrast_manual.aspx

BIBLIOGRAPHY

American College of Radiology. (2010). MR safety. Available at http://www.acr.org/SecondaryMainMenuCategories/quality_safety/MRSafety.aspx

Cowper, S. E. (2010). The International Center for Nephrogenic Fibrosing Dermopathy Research (IC-NFDR). Available at http://www.icnfdr.org/ image gently. (n. d.). Alliance for radiation safety in pediatric imaging. Available at http://www.pedrad.org/associations/5364/ig/

RadiologyInfo.org. (2010). Transjugular intrahepatic portosystemic shunt (TIPS). Available at http://www.radiologyinfo.org/en/info.cfm?PG=tips

Sasso, C. (2008). *American Radiological Nurses Association core curriculum for radiologic and imaging nursing* (2nd ed.). Pensacola, FL: American Radiological Nurses' Association.

Society of Interventional Radiology. (2010). Available at www.sirweb.org

Note: Page numbers followed by *f* indicate figures and those followed by *t* indicate tables.

anesthetic agents
  benzodiazepines, 91, 92*t*
  categories, 91, 91*t*
  narcotics, 92–93
  nonnarcotic analgesics, 92
aneurysm, 309
  classification, 310
  etiologies of, 309–310
  EVAR, 310–311
  incidence, 309
  open repair, 310
  postoperative nursing care needs, 311
  TEVAR, 310
  treatment, 310
aneurysm repair surgery, 205
angioplasty, 316–317
angiotensin I, 63, 63*f*
angiotensin II, 63–64, 63*f*
angiotensin-converting enzyme (ACE), 63–64, 63*f*
angiotensinogen, 63, 63*f*
anterior mediastinoscopy, 287
anticonvulsants, 32, 34
antidiuretic hormone (ADH), 63, 223
antiseizure medications, postcraniotomy, 261
antithymocyte globulin, 305
anxiety
  pain and, 36–37
  pediatric patient and, 170–171
anxiety disorder, 145
  medications, 147*t*
  perianesthesia nursing strategies, 146–147
  therapeutic medical interventions, 146
aortic dissection, 311–312
Apfel Simplified Risk Assessment Tool, 50, 51*f*
APG. *See* ambulatory payment group
Apgar score, 254–255
appendectomy, 199
appendicitis, laparoscopy vs laparotomy, 202
aprepitant, 52, 53*t*
Apresoline (hydralazine), 309
APS. *See* American Pain Society
aPTT. *See* partial thrombin time
ARDS. *See* acute respiratory distress syndrome
ARF. *See* acute renal failure
arrhythmia ablation, 320
arrhythmias, cardiac surgery and, 208
arterial blood gas (ABG)
  analysis, 70–71
  cardiac surgery, 209
  compensation, 71
  geriatric patients and, 135
  normal range, 70
arterial oxygen (PaO$_2$), 23–24
arthritis, 109
ASA. *See* American Society of Anesthesiologists; American Stroke Association
ASAM. *See* American Society of Addiction Medicine
ASGE. *See* American Society for Gastrointestinal Endoscopy

Asperger syndrome, 153–154
aspiration, airway management, 27
aspiration biopsy, 265
aspirin
  adverse effects, 39
  arthritis, preoperative considerations, 109
  immunosuppressive medications and, 305
  rectal administration, 35
ASPMN. *See* American Society for Pain Management Nursing
ASPMN Position Statement: Pain Management in Patients with Addictive Disease, 39
Association of Critical-Care Nurses (AACN), 318
asthma, 107
  pediatric patient, 174
  postoperative implications, 108
  preoperative considerations, 107–108
Asymptomatic Carotid Atherosclerosis Study (ACAS), 308
atelectasis, airway management, 27
atherectomy, 317
Ativan. *See* lorazepam
ATN. *See* acute tubular necrosis
attention deficit hyperactivity disorder (ADHD), 152–153
AUB. *See* abnormal uterine bleeding
autism spectrum disorder (ASD), 153–154
azapirone, 147*t*
azathioprine, 305

B
balloon angioplasty, 316
bariatrics
  patients
    cardiovascular system and, 100
    critical care, 116
    healthcare professionals and, 104
    intraoperative concerns, 100
    OSA, 99–100
    other disorders, 100
    preoperative concerns, 100
    pressure-induced rhabdomyolysis, 116–117
    respiratory system and, 99–100
    special considerations, 100
    weight-loss surgery considerations, 100
  surgery
    anastomotic leak, 103
    benefits of, 102
    combination procedures, 101, 101–102
    DVT, 103
    fluid requirements, 103–104
    history of, 101
    malabsorptive procedures, 101–102
    postoperative cardiovascular interventions, 103
    postoperative intubation, interventions for, 103
    postoperative respiratory status, 102
    respiratory complications, interventions, 102
    restrictive procedures, 101
    skin integrity, 103
Bartholin cysts, 249

normothermia, pediatric patients, 176–177
North American Carotid Endarterectomy Trial
    (NASCET), 308
nose, 20
NOTES (natural orifice transluminal endoscopic
    surgery), 327
nothing by mouth (NPO), 12, 12*t*
NPUAP. *See* National Pressure Ulcer Advisory Panel
NRS. *See* numerical pain rating scale
NSAIDs. *See* nonsteroidal antiinflammatory drugs
NSQIP. *See* Veterans' Administration National Surgical
    Quality Improvement Program
NSTEMI. *See* non-ST segment elevation myocardial
    infarction
numerical pain rating scale (NRS), 30, 178
Nursing Delirium Screening Scale, 120
Nystatin, 305

O

OA. *See* osteoarthritis
obesity, morbid, 110
    postoperative implications, 111
    preoperative considerations, 111
observation care, 123
    admission criteria, 125
    discharge, 127
    documentation requirements, 126
    ICU patients and, 126
    level of care, 128
    monitoring requirements, 126
    nurse–patient ratio requirement, 125
    nursing personnel types, 125–126
    outpatient qualifications, 124–125
    PACU criteria for, 123–124
    patient management, responsibility, 126
    Phase II level and, 127
    short stay, 124
    staffing requirements, 125
    standard of care, 125
    time limitation, 124, 126
    transport policies, 127
    types of orders and, 128
    vital signs, frequency, 126
obsessive-compulsive disorder (OCD), 145
obstetrics surgeries
    abnormal bleeding, pregnancy and delivery, 255
    ACLS, pregnant patient, 255–257, 256*t*
    Apgar score, 254–255
    cerclage, incompetent cervix, 254
    cesarean section, 254
    eclampsia, 254
    ectopic pregnancy, 253
    fetal monitoring, 254
    labor anesthesia, 254
    labor, signs of, 254
    newborn examination, 255
    perioperative medications, 253
    postpartum bleeding, 256
    preeclampsia, 254

pregnancy, physiological changes, 253
    resuscitation, pregnant patient, 255
    trauma risks, pregnant patient, 255
    uterine massage, post delivery, 256
obstructive sleep apnea (OSA), 27, 108
    bariatric patients, 99–100
    pediatric patient, 174
    postoperative limitations, 108
    preoperative considerations, 108
occupational health, infection prevention, 86
OCD. *See* obsessive-compulsive disorder
oliguria, 243, 246
omentum, 252
omeprazole (Prilosec), 305
ondansetron, 52, 53, 53*t*
open donor nephrectomy, 299
open reduction internal fixation (ORIF), 222
ophthalmic surgery, 273
    anesthesia, 275
    anticoagulants, blood-thinning medications, 274–275
    cataracts, 275–276
    complications, 274
    corneal transplant, 276–277
    discharge instructions, 278
    eye exam, 273–274
    eye, function, 273
    eye muscle surgery, 278–279
    factors, for, 274
    general care instructions, 275
    glaucoma, 276
    ocular misalignment, 278
    preoperative requirements, 274
    ptosis, 279
    retinal reattachment, 277
opioid antagonists, 40–41
opioid-naïve patient, 34, 37
opioids, 32
    addiction, 37–38
    adverse effects, 40–41
    clinically significant opioid-induced respiratory
        depression, 42–44, 43*t*
    first-line, 33–34, 33*t*
    geriatric patients, 141
    IV titration, 33–34
    opioid-tolerant patient and, 38
    opioid-tolerant vs opioid-naïve patient, 37
    sedation assessment and, 41, 42*t*
OPPS. *See* outpatient prospective payment system
oral airway, 24
oral infections
    cause of, 220
    fatality, 220–221
    hospitalization, criteria, 220
    toothache, 220
    treatment for, 220
orchidectomy, 264
orchiectomy, 245
ORIF. *See* open reduction internal fixation
orif mandible, 221–222
orotracheal sedation, 201

palliative care, 270–271
patient previous history, 266
patient quality of life, 270
perioperative blood transfusion, risk, 270
postoperative community resources, 270
postoperative complications, 269–270
postoperative patient teaching needs, 270
preoperative assessment, 267
preoperative medications, postoperative complications and, 268
preoperative patient teaching needs, 268–269
presurgery services, preparations, 269
previous cancer therapy, 268
purpose of, 263–264
role of, 264
specialized care, perioperative outcomes and, 271
staging, 264–265
stereotactic surgery, 268
surgical interventions, types, 265–266
TACE, 268
VTE, DVT, pulmonary embolism risk, 270
surgical site infections (SSIs), 14
Surviving Sepsis Campaign, 114–115
syndrome of inappropriate ADH secretion (SIADH), 63, 226

T

TACE. *See* transarterial chemoembolization
tachycardia
 CAD, postoperative implications, 106–107
 CEA, postoperative, 309
tacrine, anesthetic drug interactions and, 154
tacrolimus (Prograf), 305
tattoos, hepatitis C and, 76
TBW. *See* total body water
TEE. *See* transesophageal echocardiogram
temazepam (Restoril), 92t
temperature measurement, 56
temporomandibular joint (TMJ) ankylosis, 221
TENS. *See* transcutaneous electrical nerve stimulation
tension pneumothorax, 288
tension-free vaginal taping (TVT), 250–251
TEP. *See* tracheoesophageal puncture
terbutaline (Brethine)
 bronchospasm, 332
 pregnant patient, 192
Tesla, magnet strengths, 331
TEVAR. *See* thoracic aortic aneurysm
thermoregulation
 febrile patient management, 57
 geriatric patient, 138–139
 MH, 57–60
 pediatric patients, 176–177
 perioperative thermoregulation, 55–56
 temperature measurement, 56
 UPH, 56–57
Third National Health and Nutrition Examination Survey (NHANES III), 110
thoracic aortic aneurysm repair (TEVAR), 310
thoracic incision, 197

thoracic surgery, 284
 chest tubes, 289–290
 chest wall, 287
 esophagus, 285–286
 jejunal feeding tube, 291
 lung, 284–285
 mediastinum, 286–287
 NG tube, 290–291
 pleura, 287–289
 postoperative pain, 291–292
 PT, 291
 subcutaneous emphysema, 291
thoracotomy, 205
thrombolysis, endovascular, 335
thrombolysis in myocardial infarction (TIMI), 321, 321t
thrombolytic therapy, 335
thyroid storm, 223
thyroidectomy, 223–224, 237
thyrotoxic crisis, 223–224
TIA. *See* transient ischemic attack
timeout/hands-free report, 13–14
TIMI flow grading system, 321, 321t
TIMI Risk Score, 321, 321t
TIPS procedure, 334
TIVA. *See* total intravenous anesthesia
TJC. *See* The Joint Commission
TMJ ankylosis. *See* temporomandibular joint ankylosis
TNM Staging System, 265
To Err is Human: Building a Safer Health System (IOM), 80
toddler. *See also* pediatric patients
 anatomy, physiology, 168
 definition, 167
 physical, cognitive, social stages of development, 179–180, 182t
tolerance, 37
tonometer, 274
Tono-Pen, 274
tonsillectomy, 230–231
total body water (TBW), 61
 antidiuretic hormone, 63
 RAA secretion, 63–64
total intravenous anesthesia (TIVA), 50
total joint precautions, 283
total laryngectomy, 234–235, 236t
total proctocolectomy, 199, 263
trachea, 20
tracheoesophageal fistulas, 197
tracheoesophageal puncture (TEP), 234
tracheomalacia, pediatric patient, 174
tracheostomy, 232–233, 236t
TRAM. *See* transverse rectus abdominus myocutaneous
transarterial chemoembolization (TACE), 268
transcutaneous electrical nerve stimulation (TENS), 197
transesophageal echocardiogram (TEE), 206
transient ischemic attack (TIA), 106
transperitoneal endoscopic technique, 251
transsphenoidal hypophysectomy, 225–226
transsphenoidal surgery, 259–260, 262
transurethral resection of bladder tumor or bladder neck (TURBT), 244
transurethral resection of the prostate (TURP), 65